AF673190

Role of Dietary Fibers and Nutraceuticals in Preventing Diseases

Role of Dietary Fibers and Nutraceuticals in Preventing Diseases

Dr. K. T. Augusti, M.Sc. Ph.D.

(Fellow of the Kerala Acad.Sci; Rted.Prof and Head,
Dept. Med. Biochem. School of Health Sciences, Kannur University,
Thalassery Campus, 670661 Kerala, India. and Former Prof. of Biochemistry of
Kerala and M.G. Universities and Common Wealth Academic Staff Fellow,
University of New Castle Upon Tyne, U.K.
E-mail: ktaugusti@yahoo.co.uk

Mr. P. Faizal M.Sc. and K. Suneesh MSc.

Lecturers in Med.Biochem. SHS, Kannur University, Thalassery Campus, Kerala.

Dr. Paul Augustine M.S, Fellow NCI (USA),

Surgical Oncologist, Regional Cancer Centre,
Thiruvananthapuram, 695011, Kerala.

Dr. Regi Jose MD, DPH, DNB

Assistant Professor of Community Medicine,
Dr. Somervell Memorial CSI Medical College, Karakonam,
Thiruvananthapuram, Kerala.

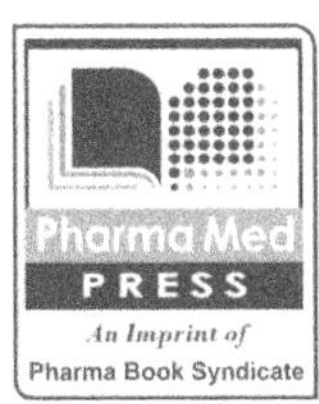

PharmaMed Press

An imprint of Pharma Book Syndicate

4-4-309/316, Giriraj Lane,
Sultan Bazar, Hyderabad - 500 095.

Published by

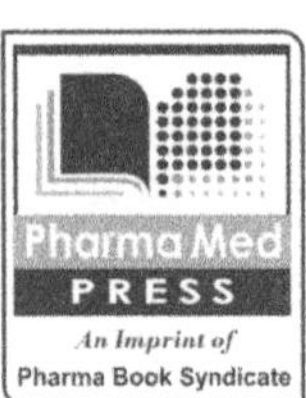

PharmaMed Press

An imprint of Pharma Book Syndicate

4-4-309/316, Giriraj Lane, Sultan Bazar, Hyderabad - 500 095.

Phone: 040-23445605, 23445688; Fax: 91+40-23445611

E-mail: info@pharmamedpress.com

ISBN : 978-93-52300-61-7 (HB)

DEPARTMENT OF MEDICAL MICROBIOLOGY AND MEDICAL BIOCHEMISTRY
SCHOOL OF HEALTH SCIENCES
KANNUR UNIVERSITY
Thalasscry Campus, Palayad P.O., Kcrala, India. Pin 670661

Dr. P.C. Ravindran
DIRECTOR

FOREWORD

I am extremely happy to introduce the Book entitled **"Role of Dietary Fiber and Nutraceuticals in Preventing Diseases"** being published by Professor K.T. Augusti, presently Ph.D Guide in Medical Biochemistry of this School as the Chief Editor. This is the outcome of the National Seminar on the **"Evaluation of Nutraceuticals that Prevent Diseases"** held under the auspices of the School of Health Sciences of Kannur University at Thalassery campus in 2006, when Dr. Augusti was Professor and HOD of Medical Biochemistry of this School and also the Organizing Secretary of the Seminar.

As the authors of various articles in this book include very Eminent Medical Doctors and Scientists from Kerala and outside viz; Drs. Arun Bordia, Rtd.Cardiologist of RNT Medical College, Udaipur; Banjamin Lau, Rtd.Immunolgist of Lorna Linda Medical School, California; K. Madhavan Kutty, Rtd. D.M.E. of Kerala; K. Bhaskaran, Principal, Pariyaram Medical College. Kannur; K.P. Paulose, Physician, SUT Hospital, Tvm.; M. Iqbal Ahammed, Director, Malabar Cancer Centre, Thalassery; Regi Jose, Asst. Prof. of Community Medicine at Dr. Somervell Memorial C.S.I Medical College, Karakkonam, Tvm.; Sathiagopal of Cholayil Sanjeevanum, Thalassery; R.Kuttan, Director of Amala Cancer Research Centre, Thrissur; K.Polasa, Deputy Director of NIN, Hyderabad, P.R.Sudhakaran, Prof. & Head, Dept of Biochemistry, Kerala University; B.Nagarajan, Scientist, Cancer Institute of Chennai; Venugopal Menon, Prof. and Head, Dept of Biochemistry & Dean, Faculty of Science, Annamala University; Dr. P.K. Jospeh. Rtd. Prof. of Biochemisry, St.John's Medical College, Bangalore; R.D.Gupta, Director of NHRDF, Nasik; U.P.Singh, Rtd.Prof. and Head, Dept of Mycology, B.H.U., Varanasi; Ruby John, Senior Scientist, R.G.C.B.T., Tvm.; Jasmin Maret, Prof. and Head, Dept of Computer Studies, St. Kevin College, Newzealand and many others, this book contains a good collection of informations to justify its title.

As the English say **"An apple a day keeps the doctor away"** many of the authors in this book praise the Medicinal values of Dietary Fiber and Functional Foods like barley, beans, ginger, turmeric, garlic, onions, pomegranate, broccoli, amla, tomatoes, carrots etc., because each of them contains fiber or sufficient number of Nutraceuticals that can lower cholesterol, boost up our immune system, drive away viral diseases, and keep our body healthy and free from many fatal diseases like cancer and C.H.D. I congratulate each of the authors and editors of this book in their unique endeavor to enlighten the readers.

Dr. P.C. Ravindran

EDITORIAL

This book is the outcome of a National Seminar on the **"Evaluation of Nutraceuticals that prevent diseases"** which was conducted by the School of Health Sciences of Kannur University at Thalassery as myself as its organizing secretary in November-December 2006.

It was supported with grants from Kannnur Uty (UGC fund), ICMR, CSIR and KSCSTE (Govt. of Kerala). On this context I am much obliged to Dr. P. Chandramohan, Vice Chancellor of Kannur University, Dr. P.C.Ravindran, our Director and also the staff of the University and students of our school for their unrelenting support in conducting the Seminar and also in compiling the articles required for this book. Apart from the Seminar topics dietary fibre is also included in this book. Further I thank particularly my two colleagues K. Suneesh and P. Faizal and my son Dr. Paul Augustine who spent months with me for putting in order the various articles. Again I thank Dr. P.C.Ravindran for writing a good foreword for this book and also all the authors and editors for their contributions in shaping this book on a scientific putting.

At this moment I remember with gratitude my PhD guide Late Dr. H.D. Brahmachari of BITS, Pilani, Post doctoral guides, Drs. S. Gurnani of RRL, Hyderabad, R. Aiman of Christian Medical College, Vellore and H.A. Diwar. Rtd. Cardiologist of Royal Victoria Infirmary in the University of Newcastle Upon Tyne, UK. and my benefactor and Senior Co-worker Dr. P.A. Kurup, Rtd Professor and Head Department of Biochemistry at Kerala University (Tvm) for building up the biochemist in me with specialization in functional foods. The quotations I have taken from the pioneers in this field and given under a section later justify the need of this book for the present generation.

Most of the nutraceuticals are antioxidants and they are present in our functional foods viz; onions, garlic, turmeric, ginger, limes, oranges, carrots, tea, amla, papaya, pomegranate, grapes, apples, mangoes, sweet potatoes, green leaves, mushrooms etc. Therefore regular addition of one or more of these dietary components in our food shall prevent various cancers, CHD, dementia, Alzheimer's disease and ageing. These are compiled from the panel discussion on Nutraceuticals at the National Seminar on the "Evaluation of Nutraceuticals that prevent diseases," held under Kannur University at Thalassery Campus during 28th Nov. to 2nd Dec. 2006.

Panel members:

Dr. Arun Bordia, Rtd. Cardiologist of RNT Medical College, Udaipur, Rajasthan.

Dr. K. Bhaskaran, Prof. of Pharmacology and Principal, Pariyaram Medical College, Kannur.

Dr. B. Nagarajan, Prof. of Oncology, Cancer Inst. Chennai-20.

Dr. P.R. Sudhakaran, Prof and Head of the Dept. of Biochemistry, Kerala Univerisity.

Dr. K.T. Augusti, Prof. and Head of the Dept. of Medical Biochemistry, School of Health Sciences, Kannur University Campus, at Thalassery and Organising Secretary of the Seminar.

This book is the outcome of their combined efforts.

Dr. K.T. AUGUSTI
Chief Editor

Contents

Chapter 3

Terpenes, Carotenoids and Phytosterols

Chapter 4

Phenolics of the Functional Foods

Chapter 5

Nutraceuticals of Alliums

Section 6

Nutraceuticals Vs Diseases

Section 7

Role of Allium Principles as Anticancer Agents

Section 8

Cancer and Ageing – Causation and Prevention

Section 9

Laboratory Experiment

Section 10

Certain Functional Foods in the Prevention of Diseases

Some Excerpts from the Articles of Great Scientists on the use of Herbal Products in Health and Diseases

Plants are the fountain head of medicine

Excerpts from the Presidential address of Dr. K. Madhawan kutty, Former Director of Medical Education, Govt. of Kerala at the National Seminar on Nutraceuticals.

Plants provide us nearly 35% of the medicines and drugs that we use, so much so, that many pharmaceutical companies have collecting centres specially for plants used as drugs in many forests of the 3rd world. The list of such drugs is endless.

Neem, Opium, Olive, Iris, Sarpagandhi, Vinca rosea, Thulasi, Turmeric, Ginger, Eucalyptus, Lemon Grass, Aarogyapacha (a green plant used for health by tribes), Ginseng, Sandal wood, Cinchona, Vep, Lime, Onion, Garlic, Cashew, Tomatoes, Coccinia Indica, Black pepper, Garcinia Cambogia (Kodampuli), Bitter gourd, Ash gourd, Amla (goose berry) Sugar cane , Moringa, Pomegranate, Papaya, Betel leave and various spices are on the list (More than 200 plants).

Many of these have been our household articles of food from times immemorial and perhaps have given way for more modern (fashionable) vegetables. *For as Mark Twain put it humorously "Training is every thing". For many, peach was once a bitter almond, a cauliflower is nothing but a cabbage with college education.*

In fact the WHO is now actively encouraging developing countries to use herbal medicines, which they have been traditionally using for centuries and have identified 3000 plants which come from the forest of India and other tropical countries. The active ingredients from these plants are worth nearly Rs.20000 millions for U.S. market alone and nearly 8 times that for the world market.

The papers being presented here have great relevance for solving the problems of the present world. Let us encourage the so called functional foods viz; items of food enriched with antioxidants/nutraceuticals etc.

Only when we gave up all these things and resorted to a cola, hamburger, pizza, fast food culture, did our country become the world capital for obesity/diabetes etc.

Editors comments: Many medical people slowly recognize now that functional food contains medicinally active compounds called nutraceuticals other than vitamins, minerals etc., and that they can function as antioxidants and prevent many fatal diseases like Cancer, CHD, DM, Dementia etc. Mushrooms are the latest addition to the list of functional foods. Ganoderma, a Chinese mushroom is a remarkable one with miraculous medicinal properties.

Make you feel good

Although there are reports to document the antifertility, antidiabetic and antibacterial effects of several plant extracts or compounds, a good majority of plant extracts have been employed to improve the general health. Thus there are preparations from plants which claim to improve one's memory, resistance to disease, body complexion, digestive power, general health etc. It is to be noted that these preparations essentially can be grouped under the category of **"make you feel good"** and have to be taken over a period and do not have dramatic effects if taken for shorter duration. This is due to the fact that many of them have profound antioxidant activity and it is well known that antioxidants are powerful scavengers of free radicals, which attack the biological macromolecules. During oxidative phosphorylation (ETC in mitochondria) which results in generation of energy in all eukaryotes, reactive oxygen species (free radicals) are generated and these attack proteins, lipids and nucleic acids in cells and cause cellular death. It leads to diseases such as arthritis and senescence inducing damages in eukaryotic cells. Fruits and vegetables are excellent sources of natural antioxidants such as ascorbic acid, tocopherol, carotenoids and polyphenols.[1].

1. **Dr. A. Jaganadha Rao,** CSIR Emeritus Scientist, Dept. of Biochem. Indian Institute of Science, Bangalore – 560012.

Oxygen radical absorbance capacity (ORAC)

Oxygen radical absorbance capacity (ORAC) of a phytochemical is an index of its antioxidant action. A plant with highest ORAC value is "Gojibery" which is found in Himalayas. It has a ORAC value of 23,300 units while pomegranate has 3,307 units. As the results of various studies on ginger, turmeric, garlic, onions, pomegranate and fenugreek are encouraging, more human studies should be undertaken, particularly with reference to cancer, coronary diseases and memory[2].

2. **Dr. Arun Bordia**, Rtd. Cardiologist, RNT Medical College, Udaipur, Rajasthan

   Note: N.B. Functional foods with high ORAC values are Red wine> Black tea> Green tea> Black currant juice> Orange juice> Apple> Onion.(According to a table by **Brook Bond Centre,** Bangalore in India, they somehow missed garlic which is better than onion)

Garlic is a panacea for all diseases

Antitumor, antimicrobial, antiplatelet, antithrombotic, antihyperlipidemic, antihypertensive and antiasthmatic effects as well as immune stimulatory properties are attributed to garlic and other Alliums[3]. Consumption of garlic and other Alliums is said to reduce cancer risk including prostate cancer[4]. Extracts and components of garlic effectively block experimentally induced tumors. Information on biological activity of genus Allium plants and Allium compounds can be easily obtained via a web search using PubMed(http://www.ncbi.nlm.nih.gov/entrez/query.fcgi), the free search and the retrieval system of the National Center for Biotechnology Information (NCBI) of the US, National Library of Medicine(NLM). Using the terms 'garlic', 'allium', 'allicin', 'ajoene', 'diallyl trisulfide' and 'vinyl dithiin' generates more than 3000 references.

3. **N.B.** Dr. Block is a pioneer scientist on Allium Research.
4. **Dr. Eric Block,** Dept. of Chemistry, State University of New York at Albany. Albany New York- 12222, U.S.A

Ginger should be a food supplement for everybody

Ginger contains up to 3% of an essential oil that causes the fragrance of the spice. The main constitutents are sesquiterpinoids with (-) Zingiberene as the main component. Lesser amounts of other sesquiterpenoids are beta sesquipellandrene, bisabolene and farnesene with a small amount of monoterpenoid fraction of beta phellandrene, cinol and citral. The pungency of ginger is due to non-volatile phenyl propanoids particularly gingerol and zingerone and diarylheptanoids viz; gingerols and shoagoles. Cooking ginger transforms gingerol into zingerone which is less pungent and has a spicy sweet aroma[5]. Ginger principles possess antioxidant, anti-inflammatory, antiulcer, antiemetic, antimotion sickness, antithermogenic, anticlotting of blood, anticarcinogenic, hypocholesterolemic properties. They are promoters of circulatory system also. Based on the above findings Paul Schulick states that literally hundreds of thousands of lives can be saved by ginger, it should be in every one's daily supplement routine.

5. **Dr. Schulick. P.** Author of Ginger, Common Spice or Wonder drug? Ginger, Herbal Free Press, Brattleboro 1994, Vermont.USA.

   N.B.: It is a pity that Kerala is the abode of ginger, but there very little research work has been done on it.

Diet, nutrition & Cancer – the Indian Scenario

The National Institute of Nutrition, Hyderabad has conducted studies on several aspects of diet – cancer inter-relationship. These include studies on metabolic susceptibility, case- control approach to determine the risk factors and intervention studies to determine the role of nutrients and non-nutrient components on preneoplastic events. Extensive work has been carried out demonstrating the antimutagenic/anticarcinogenic potentials of some commonly consumed spices and vegetables such as turmeric, mustard, green leaf/ and allium species of vegetables[6]. Dietary intervention for cancer prevention is needed to control the disease, besides avoiding risk factors such as smoking and alcoholism and exposure to genotoxicants.

6. **Drs. K. Krishnaswamy and K. Polasa**. Scientists from National Institute of Nutrition, Hyderabad.

Garlic extracts are truly Immune Boosters, antistress and anticancer effectors

Our body employs five major branches of protection against diseases.

B Lymphocytes, T Lymphocytes, Phagocytes/Macrophages, Killer Cells and Natural Killer Cells. The B Lymphocytes respond to various stimuli by producing antibodies, which help fight off many common infections. The other four types of immune cells directly attack foreign invaders, such as cancer cells, bacteria, viruses or fungi. Several studies have demonstrated that components of garlic are immune boosters. One study by us showed that lymphocytes and macrophages were attracted to the site where garlic principles were injected. Others also noticed that garlic extract attracted immune cells. A group of mice maintained on the regular diet plus 25mg/day/mouse of a special garlic powder (SGP), tolerated a stress including exercise far better than a group maintained only on the regular diet. The stress hormone corticoid level of blood was only $1/5^{th}$ in the garlic group as compared to the normal control group. Comparing garlic's effectiveness alongside standard anticancer agents, we discovered that garlic showed significantly more positive results than BCG, a live vaccine currently used to treat bladder cancer. In fact after five treatments of garlic injected directly into the tumors, no cancer cells were present, garlic actually cured the bladder cancer in the mice.

Diallyl sulfides, ajoene and a special protein are the various active components of garlic[7]. Regular consumption of Allium Plants (onions, garlic, leeks, scallions, shallots and chives) lowers the risks of developing heart diseases and cancer and improves immunity.

7. Dr. Benjamin Lau M.D. of Loma Linda University, California

Garlic, Ginger Combination is a super functional food

Garlic preparations have shown to lower the level of serum cholesterol, triglycerides and incidence of CHD through inhibition of biosynthesis of the former two as well as the inhibition of the oxidation of low density lipoprotein. The garlic and onion alliins (S-allyl and S-methyl cysteine sulfoxides), their various decomposition products, e.g; allyl and methyl sulfoxides and their polymers like ajoene are endowed with hypocholesterolemic and antidiabetic actions.

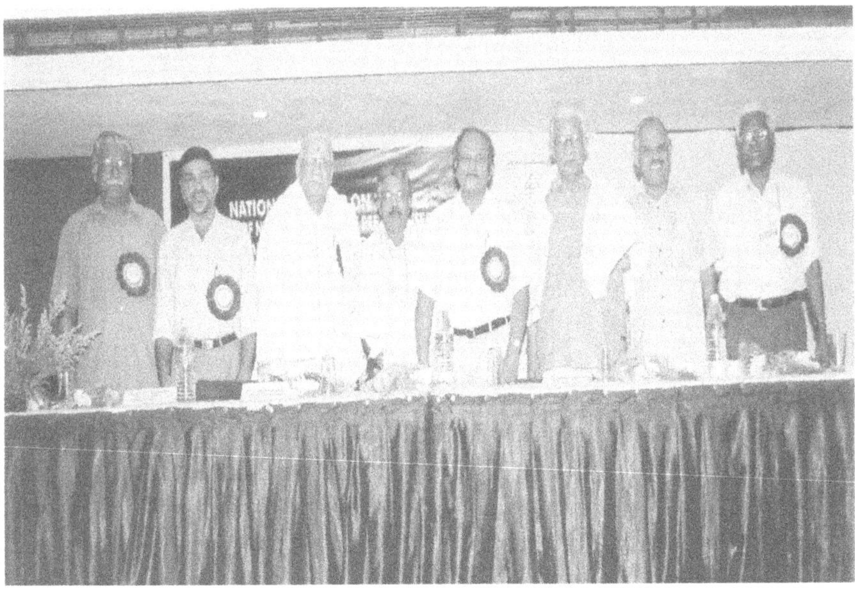

Top Group Photo: Speakers at the inauguration function of the National Seminar on Nutraceuticals at Thalassery on 29th November 2006.

L to R: Dr. P.C. Ravindran (Director SHS), Sri. A.P. Kuttikrishnan(Syndicate member), Dr. K. Madhavan kutty(Chairman of the Session), Dr. Anandha Bhanu(Speaker), Dr. P. Chandramohan(V.C. who conducted the inauguration), Dr. Arun Bordia(Speaker), Prof. K. Kunhikrishnan(P.V.C.), Dr. K.T. Augusti(Organising Secretary)

A combination of garlic and ginger has been claimed to be superior to garlic alone in reducing serum lipids as well as blood glucose in normal rats[8]. Studies with aged garlic showed that it stimulates the proliferation of mouse spleen cells, release of cytokines, increase in NK activities

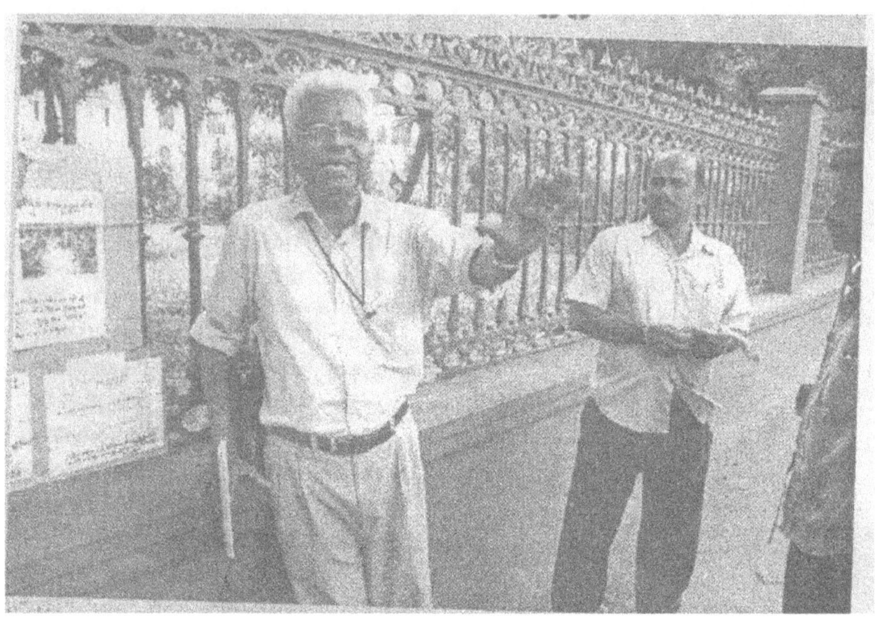

Bottom: Editor in action, in front of the Secretariate, TVM on 15th Sept.2007 to spread the news that Ginger-Allium-Black pepper food supplement is a good medicine to use against viral fevers both prophylactically and curatively.

and phagocytosis of peritoneal macrophages. Garlic powder supplementation to cholesterol rich diet is more advantageous than aspirin alone because it has the beneficial effects on both blood clotting and plasma cholesterol level. Some steroidal saponins isolated from fresh garlic bulbs also exhibited inhibitory effect on blood coagulability. Besides these properties, garlic extracts have very many actions against chicken and plant pathologens e.g. candida albicans and certain fungi.

Dr. U.P. Singh, Rtd. Prof of Mycology and Plant Pathology, Institutte of Agric. Sciences B.H.U. Varanasi & President: Assoc. Allium Workers in India.

An apple a day keeps the Doctor away (English Saying)

An Allium (garlic) a day keeps the virus away (Dr. Banjamin Lau US Immunologist)

Gandhiji and Nutraceutical Rich Goat's Milk

Goat's Milk was a Link Between Gandhiji and Nutraceuticals

Gandhiji used to drink only goat's milk. He and his goat were very much projected in News papers during 1940s, particularly whenever his health status was discussed after a prolonged fast. After breaking his fast; every time after achieving some thing for the right of the Nation, goat's milk always found a place in his menu as a means to boost his health.

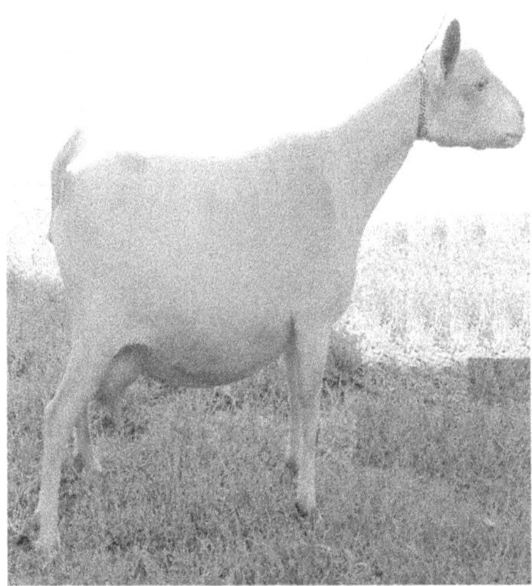

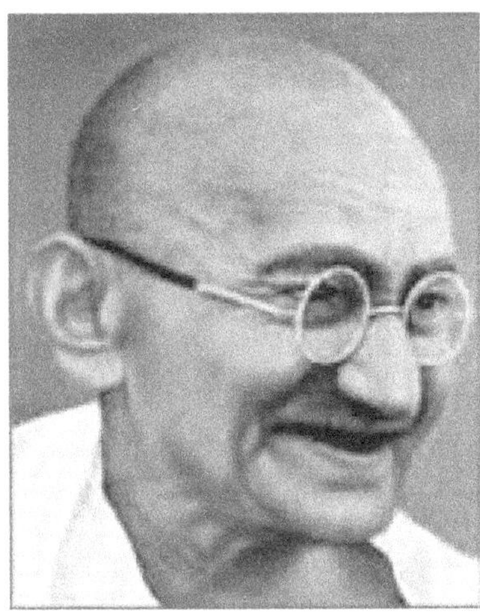

You may wonder why Gandhiji preferred goat's milk to cow's milk; this was because goat's milk is enriched with nutraceuticals while cow's milk is not so. Ayurvedic practitioners usually prescribe goat's milk for infants who cannot breast feed.

There are two reasons for this:

1. Goat grazes on all types of grasses and herbs which are endowed with nutraceuticals particularly terpenes, carotenoids, flavonoids etc. which in due course become a part of the milk.
2. The fat content of goat's milk is relatively low as compared to cow's milk and it helps the children and old people in digestion and the nutraceuticals in the milk build up immunoresistance of the body against diseases.

(Editors)

References

1. Jaganatha Rao, A; Use of herbal products in health and diseases in the Proceedings of the National symposium on current trends in the development of herbal drugs and 27th Annual Conference of IABS. Nov. 25-27 2006. Thiruvananthapuram.P.57.

2. Bordia, A; Recommendations made by Dr. Arun Bordia to ICMR and other sponsors of the seminar in: Proceedings of the National Seminar on the "Evaluation of Nutraceuticals that Prevent diseases" Nov. 28 – Dec 2nd 2006. Thalassery Campus of Kannur University p 9.

3. Eric Block. Biological activity of Allium Compounds: Recent results in: Proceedings of the 4th International symposium on Edible Alliacea. April 21-26 2004. Beijing P.41-57.

4. Hising, A.W; Chokkalingam, A.P. et al. Allium vegetables and risk of prostate cancer: a population study. J. Natl Cancer Inst.94 (2002) 1648-51.

5. Grant, W.B. A multicountry ecology study of risk and risk reduction factors for prostate cancer mortality. Eur. Uro l.45 (2004) 271-279.

6. McGee Harold on food and cooking. The science and Lore of the Kitchen (2nd Edn. 2004) New York. Scribner PP 425-426.

7. Kamala Krishnaswamy & Kalpagam Polasa,. Diet, nutrition & Cancer – the Indian Secenario Indian,. J. Med. Res. 102(1995) 200 – 209.

8. Lau, BHS. Garlic Research Update. Published by Odyssey Publishing Inc. 2135 West 45th Avenue. Vancouver, B.C. Canada. 1991. PP 13-23

9. Lau, BHS, Fred Lam and Rebekah Wang – Cheng – Effect of an odor modified garlic preparation on blood lipids. Nutrition Res. 7 (1987) 139-149.

10. Lau, BHS, Yamasaki, T and Daila S.G. Garlic compounds modulate macrophage and T-lymphocyte functions. Mol. Biother 3(1991) 103-107.

11. Ahmed, R.S. and Sharma, S.B. Biochemical studies on combined effects of garlic (Allium sativum Linn) and ginger. (Zingiber officinale Rosc) in albino rats. Indian J. Exp. Biol, 35 (1997) 841.

12. Kyo.E; Uda, N et al, Immunomodulation and antitumor activities of aged garlic extract. Phytomedicine, 5(1998) 259.

13. Keskin, E; Durgan, Z et al. Effect of garlic and aspirin on some coagulation parameters in hypercholesterolemic rabbits. Med. Sci: Res. 26(1998) 413.

14. Peng. J.P; Chen, H et al. Two new steroidal saponins from Allium sativum and their inhibitory effect on blood coagulability. Yao Hsueh Hsueh Pao, 31 (1996)607.

15. Singh U.P., Prithiviraj B et al. Role of garlic (Allium sativum L) in human and plant diseases. Indian Jour Exp. Biol. 39(2001) 310-312.

Chapter – 1

Dietary Fiber and Essential Macronutrient

1.1 Dietary Fiber: An Essential Macronutrient

Dr. M. Indira
Department of Biochemistry, University of Kerala
Kariavattom Thiruvananthapuram
E-Mail: indiramadambath@yahoo.co.uk

What is Dietary Fiber?

Even today this is an unanswered question. No consensus has been arrived at the definition of fiber. As early as 1929 it was defined as unavailable carbohydrate by Mcchance and Lawrence. But Hipsley who defined dietary fiber as unavailable carbohydrate from plant cell wall is attributed with first definition of dietary fiber. But these definitions have undergone a lot of changes. *Trowell in 1972 defined dietary fiber as that part of plant material in our diet, which is resistant to digestion by secretions of human digestive tract. As this definition did not include polysaccharides present in some food additives such as gums, algal polysaccharides, pectins, modified starches; Trowell et. al. (1972) extended this definition to include all polysaccharides and lignin that are undigested by endogenous secretions of human digestive tract. But then there is the question whether the source of fiber is solely from plant sources.*

The definitions based on analytic methods may include fiber from animal sources. Thus chitosan and glycosaminoglycans are often included in reported fiber values. The National Academy of Sciences, Institute of Medicine Food and Nutrition Board formed a committee to determine the definition of dietary fiber and a second panel to determine the physiologic effects of dietary fiber and its relation. The definitions determined by these panels are as follows.

Dietary fiber consists of nondigestible carbohydrates and lignin that are intrinsic and intact in plants. Functional fiber consists of isolated nondigestible carbohydrates that have physiological effects in humans. Total fiber is the sum of dietary fiber and functional fiber. In 1998 the president of American Association of Cereal Chemists (AACC) appointed a scientific review committee and assigned the committee the task of reviewing, and if necessary, updating the definition of dietary fiber.

According to this committee the definition of fiber is "dietary fiber is the edible parts of plants or analogous carbohydrates that are resistant to digestion and absorption in the human small intestine with complete or partial fermentation in the large intestine. Dietary fiber includes polysaccharides, oligosaccharides, lignin, and associated plant substances. Dietary fibers promote beneficial physiological effects including laxation, and/or blood cholesterol attenuation, and/or blood glucose attenuation."

Constituents of Dietary Fiber

Non-Starch Polysaccharides and Resistant Oligosaccharides

Cellulose, Hemicellulose, Arabinoxylans, Arabinogalactans, Polyfructoses, Inulin, Oligofructans, Galactooligosaccharides, Gums, Mucilages, Pectins.

Analogous Carbohydrates

Indigestible Dextrin, Resistant Maltodextrins (from corn and other sources)

Resistant Potato Dextrins, Synthesized Carbohydrate Compounds Polydextrose, Methyl cellulose, Hydroxypropylmethyl Cellulose, Indigestible ("resistant") Starches.

Lignin is made up of phenyl propane polymer units.

Substances Associated with the Non-Starch Polysaccharide and Lignin Complex in Plants

Waxes, Phytate, Cutin, Saponins, Suberin, Tannins.

The major components of dietary fiber are cellulose, hemicellulose, pectins, gums, mucilages, algal polysaccharides, modified cellulose and lignin. Most of these are carbohydrates, but classified as non-starch polysaccharides (NSP).

Based on the solubility, dietary fiber is classified as soluble and insoluble fiber. Soluble fiber comprises of pectins, gums, and mucilages, whereas insoluble fiber includes celluloses, hemicelluloses and lignin.

The backbone of plant cell wall is cellulose which is a polymer of linear $\beta(1 \rightarrow 4)$ linked glucose molecules, with several thousand molecules in length. The mammalian enzymes cannot break β linkages; these polysaccharides are not digested and absorbed. Cellulose fibers are aligned side by side in plant cell, linked by hydrogen bonds between hydroxyl groups forming a strong intermolecular bond. Cellulose is intimately associated with hemicellulose and lignin in the plant cell wall. Cellulose is having water holding capacity and is insoluble in water.

The hemicelluloses are a diverse group of fibers containing xylans, galactans, or mannans as their backbone and varying degrees of branching and contain 150-200 molecules of different sugars such as arabinose and galactose.

Pectins are biologically cementing substances which bring cells together through ionic bonds. They have galacturonic acid as their backbone that differ in their degree of esterification with methyl or acetyl groups, this in turn affects their solubility and viscosity. Principal cross linkages are provided by the helical $(1\rightarrow 4)$ α galactosyluronic groups from adjacent polysaccharide and condensation with calcium converts soluble pectin into rigid structures.

Lignin, the main noncarbohydrate portion of fiber is a unique aromatic polymer containing phenylpropane polymer units such as guaiacyl, syringyl, propane, and P. coumaryl. In the plant cell wall, lignin is laid down with cellulose and hemicelluloses to produce an essentially inert structural material.

Gum is a complex of acidic heteropolysaccharide made up of galactose, arabinose, rhamnose, glucuronic acid and uronic acid residues.

Mucilages are made up of main chain galactose-mannose, glucose mannose, arabinose xylose, galacturonic acid, p rhamnose and side chain containing only galactose. These are synthesized by plant secretory cells.

Cutin is a fatty substance and this insoluble biopolyster made up of hydroxyl and epoxy fatty acids of C_{16} and C_{18} families.

Silica, the mineral component of fiber probably provides major parts of silica in human nutrition.

Analysis of Fiber

Different methods have been employed to quantify the amount of fiber present and this led to a lot of confusion. The earlier method was crude extraction with hot dilute acid followed by dilute alkali. This crude fiber method is good for analyzing the fiber content of diet for cattle but not for humans. Hence newer methods were used. The acid detergent method, which involves boiling samples with sulfuric acid, was used to estimate fiber component of celluloses and lignin in feeds and forges. But this was not suited for the determination of soluble fiber. Alternatively the neutral detergent fiber method involved boiling the material with sodium lauryl sufate and EDTA-borate at a pH of 7. It adequately determined the plant cell wall components such as cellulose, lignin, hemicellulose, but again it was not good for the soluble fiber. This method was modified for the analysis of human foods. In this modification fat was extracted followed by treatment with amylase to break down the starch. Later Van Soest method was developed combining the acid detergent and neutral detergent methods. But this method was also inadequate to quantify soluble fibers.

The best method to be developed for the complete analysis of soluble and insoluble fibers is Southgate fractionation system. In this method nonfibrous material is removed first followed by removal of pectic substances with hot water and a chelator. Hemicelluose is extracted in several fractions by first adding sodium hydroxide under nitrogen to precipitate the material. This step is repeated with alcohol to get second component of hemicelluloses. Finally under the strong sodium hydroxide and nitrogen the final fraction of hemicellulose is obtained (hemicellulose A, B, & C). Cellulose is extracted by precipitation in 17.5% NaOH. Finally lignin is extracted by the addition of 72% sulfuric acid. Even though good results were obtained with these method it was laborious and time consuming and expensive.

The greatest breakthrough came with the development of enzymatic method or the Prosky method. Here enzymatic removal of protein and starch from fat extracted food occurs first. Then 95% alcohol is used to precipitate the soluble dietary fiber. Residual protein is then quantified and sample is corrected for ash and protein content. Finally fiber is determined gravimetrically. This method may sometime over estimate the fiber by not completely removing non fibrous materials.

Physical and Physiological Properties of Fiber

Fiber can be regarded as a physical agent passing along the gastrointestinal tract i.e. sponge. Such a sponge will have water holding and cation exchange capacities. It acts as an adsorbant and it provides a matrix and catalytic surfaces. However in the cecum fiber is profoundly affected by flora. Fiber may pass unchanged or modified in physical properties through the cecum to descending column. Alternatively the fiber can be partially or completely hydrolyzed. The end products of which may be reabsorbed from the cecum to the portal vein or the hydrolyzed products themselves may have biological effects within the lumen of colon. The chemical composition of dietary fiber may affect its metabolism in the colon.

Water holding capacity and fermentation products

The water holding capacity of fiber is one of the most important physical properties. Hydration of fiber occurs by adsorbtion of water to the surface of the macromolecules and by entrapment within the interstices of the fibrous gel. The given fiber's ability to hold water is enhanced by the presence of monomers that have free polar groups such as OH, COOH,

SO_4, and C=O groups. Hence pectic substances, mucilages, and hemicellulose have the greatest water holding capacity. In the small intestine hydration of fiber will contribute to the formation of a gel matrix. This can increase the viscosity of the contents within small intestine and slow the rate of absorption of food products.

Fiber is subject to bacterial degradation in the colon. Pectins, mucilages and gums appear to be almost completely fermented in the small intestine, while cellulose is only partly degraded. The extent of degradation depends upon the physical structure of the plant itself. The fibers derived from fruits and vegetables appear to be more fermentable than those from cereals. Acetic, butyric, and propionic acids are produced during bacterial fermentation. **These fatty acids can be used as an energy source for colon mucosal cells as well as be absorbed into the portal circulation. These fatty acids are hypothised to be protective against colon cancer.**

Fiber as a sequestrent of sterols and an agent to decrease transit time of feces.

Another important physical property of dietary fiber is that it may bind intestinal materials such as bile acids, cholesterol, and toxic compounds. Lignin seems to be very efficient in binding bile acids present in the intestinal tract. Pectin and other acidic polysaccharides also appear to bind bile acids. But cellulose has little ability to bind bile acids. It is this property that is responsible for the hypocholesterolemic effect of fiber to an extent. The cation exchange or metal binding capacity of fiber may have potential consequences in terms of nutrient absorption and requirements.

Dietary fiber is also known to interact with other components in the diet, particularly protein and carbohydrate. Cellulose and hemicellulose reduce the activities of pancreatic trypsin, amylase and lipase.

The most important physical activity of the fibers is their ability to alter the bulkness and composition of feces as well as their transit time. Noncellulose polysaccharides such as gums, mucilages and pectin are ineffective bulking agents due to almost complete degradation via bacterial fermentation. Cellulose, hemicellulose and lignin are more efficient bulking agents.

The amount of energy contributed by fiber is a matter of debate. According to some it is negligible because of some interference with absorption of energy containing macronutrients coupled with a very small contribution to metabolizable energy through production of absorbed fermentation products. In the United States dietary fiber is assigned an energy value for food labeling process of 0 kcal/g if it is insoluble and 4 kcal/kg if it is soluble.

Diets naturally high in fiber can be considered to bring about five main physiological consequences:

1. Improvements in gastrointestinal health
2. Improvements in glucose tolerance and the insulin response
3. Reduction of hyperlipidemia, hypertension and other coronary heart disease risk factors
4. Reduction in the risk of developing some cancers
5. Increased satiety and hence some degree of weight management

Contributions on fiber research by the Department of Biochemistry, University of Kerala

Department of biochemistry under the able leadership of Dr.P.A.Kurup was one of the pioneer institutions to do research on dietary fiber. Our interest in the development of strategies for the management of cardiovascular diseases revealed that consumption of black gram *(Phaseoles mungo)* led to reduction in the serum lipids (Devi and Kurup.1970, 1973) and analysis of fiber content of different cereals and purified starches showed that black gram polysaccharide had the highest content of fiber and maximum hypocholesterolemic effect (Vijayagopal, Devi and Kurup 1973). There was significant excretion of bile acids and bile salts. Studies revealed that fiber caused significant binding of bile acids when it was shaken with natural or pure bile acid solutions.

Findings with Neutral detergent Fiber

Further studies with neutral detergent fiber (NDF) isolated from blackgram fed at a level of 30% of the diet showed significantly lowered cholesterol both in the chicks and rats (Menon PV, Kurup PA.1976; Indira and Kurup1989; Jayakumari and Kurup1979). Its effect was much more than that of pure cellulose. This indicated that the action had a definite relationship with its composition. Detailed studies revealed that hemicellulose is the most active component of the isolated NDF. The lipid lowering effect was due to greater hepatic degradation of cholesterol to bile acids as the latter is removed speedily by fiber from the intestine. *In vitro* studies showed significant binding of bile acids by NDF. NDF from black gram could also reduce ethanol induced hyperlipidemia(Indira and Kurup 1982). NDF isolated from banana (M. paradisiaca) (Usha, Vijayammal, Kurup 1989) and coconut (Cocos nucifera L) (Sindhurani and Rajamohan 1998) also had similar effects. Dietary fiber isolated as neutral detergent residue from unripe banana altered the concentration of aortic glycosaminoglycans in rats fed cholesterol free and cholesterol diet (Usha, Vijayammal, Kurup 1991). Hemicellulose of coconut fiber was also found to be the active component involved in the reduction of lipids in the body.

In order to examine how chemically diverse fibers differ in their hypolipidaemic activity, mucilages of varying chemical composition isolated from three different sources were administered to experimental animals and the metabolism of lipids and lipoproteins was studied (Boban et. al. (2006)). The mucilages used were a galactomannan isolated from fenugreek (Trigonella foenum-graecum) seeds, a glucomannan from Dioscorea esculenta tubers and an arabinogalactan from Colocasia esculenta tubers. All these mucilages decreased lipid levels both in serum and tissues. Among these mucilages, glucomannan showed the most hypolipidaemic effect followed by galactomannan and arabinogalactan. Comparison of relative viscosity and water-holding capacity showed that mannan-rich mucilages like galactomannan and glucomannan, which showed greater hypolipidaemic effect, had greater relative viscosity and water-holding capacity.

Carbohydrate Metabolism

The effect of the administration of blackgram fiber on the metabolism of carbohydrates was studied in rats fed 30% NDF diet. Absorption of glucose and cholesterol was lower in rabbits fed blackgram NDF than in rabbits fed a fiber-free diet (Indira and Kurup 1989). Detailed *in vivo* studies revealed that the blackgram fiber exhibits significant hypoglycemic action in experimental animals (Boby and Leelamma 2003). The rats fed 30% blackgram NDF showed a significant increase in liver glycogen level and blood glucose. Significant increases in the activities of glycogen phosphorylase, hexokinase, fructose-1, 6-diphosphatase, glucose-6-phosphate dehydrogenase and isocitrate dehydrogenase were observed in the experimental group. The activities of phosphoglucomutase and glucose-6-phosphatase were significantly lower in rats fed the fiber diet.

Similar studies with dietary fiber from banana on the metabolism of carbohydrates in the liver showed that fiber fed rats had significantly lower levels of fasting blood glucose and higher concentration of liver glycogen. Activities of the enzymes involved in the glycolysis and glycogen metabolism were also affected (Usha, Vijayammal and Kurup 1989).

Fiber of Coconut Kernel

The effect of NDF from coconut kernel in rats fed 5%, 15% and 30% level on the concentration of blood glucose, serum insulin and excretion of minerals revealed that increase in the intake of fiber resulted in significant decrease in the level of blood glucose and serum insulin (Sindurani and Rajamohan 2000).

Editor's comment: *As our ancestors used coconut kernel more than coconut oil, they had no problem of hypercholesterolemia.*

Cancer

Chicks given NDF from blackgram at 30% level of the diet showed significantly lowered bacterial as well as tissue β glucuronidase activity indicating the lower activity of intestinal microflora (Indira et. al. 1982). This observation is relevant since the activity of microflora is positively correlated with the incidence of colon cancer. Later studies with fiber isolated from black gram and coconut kernel (Manoj et. al. 2001) on the metabolic activity of intestinal and fecal beta glucuronidase activity during 1,2-dimethylhydrazine induced colon carcinogenesis were conducted. The results indicated that the inclusion of fiber from black gram and coconut kernel generally supported lower specific activities and less fecal output of beta-glucuronidase than did the fiber free diet. This study suggests that the fibers isolated from coconut or black gram may potentially play a role in preventing the formation of colon tumors induced by the carcinogen 1,2-dimethylhydrazine by reducing the activity of the intestinal as well as fecal beta-glucuronidase. The influence of NDF from coconut kernel on the antioxidant status in rats treated with the colon specific carcinogen 1,2-dimethylhydrazine (DMH) in rats fed a high-fat diet for 15 weeks showed that coconut kernel fiber can protect cells from loss of oxidative capacity with the administration of the procarcinogen DMH (Pillai, Thampi, Menon, and Leelamma 1999). Experiments with dietary fibers from Musa paradisiaca and Artocarpus heterophyllus on intestinal mucosal and bacterial beta-glucuronidase activity in hexachlorocyclohexane-treated rats also showed similar results (Serji and Saraswathy, 1993).

Interaction with cations and bile acids

Blackgram NDF could also bind to inorganic cations, glucose bile acids and cholesterol. *in vitro* studies revealed significant binding of inorganic cations and bile acids by blackgram NDF. It showed different binding affinities for different bile acids, with maximum binding observed with chenodeoxycholic acid, and minimum binding with deoxycholic acid (Indira and Kurup1989).

Fecal excretion of Cu, Cr, Mn, Mg, Zn and Ca was found to increase in rats fed different levels of coconut fiber when compared to fiber free group (Sindhurani and Rajamohan 2000). Fecal excretion of inorganic cations (Mn++, Mg++, Cu++, Fe, Zn++, Na+ and K+) was greater in rats fed blackgram NDF than in rats fed a fiber-free diet (Indira and Kurup 1989). Fiber rich diet could also reduce the toxic effects of an insecticide malathion (Indira and Kurup 1980).

Soluble fiber

We have also conducted certain studies with pectin isolated from cucumber (Cucumis sativius L) on carbohydrate metabolism. Level of blood glucose was significantly lowered and the level of glycogen in the liver was significantly increased in pectin-administered rats. The regulatory role of protein kinase C (PKC) in glycogen metabolism in pectin fed rats was also investigated. Administration of pectin led to inhibitory effects on PKC activity in the liver of rats. In the brain and pancreas, PKC activity was significantly higher in pectin treated rats as compared to the control group. Glycogen synthase activity was enhanced, while glycogen phosphorylase enzyme showed inhibition in pectin-treated rats. Results indicated that pectin administration might have caused an increase in the secretion of insulin, which in turn, had a stimulatory effect on the PKC activity in the pancreas. The decreased PKC activity in the liver and increased PKC activity in the brain and pancreas on pectin administration indicated enhanced glycogenesis and reduced glycogenolysis. .

Conclusion

Dietary fiber is an essential nutrient. Inclusion of it in the diet offers some protection against hyperlipidemia (leading to atherosclerosis), glucose intolerance and cancer. Even though there is a slight increase in the excretion of minerals it is insignificant since the intake of minerals is usually high.

Editor's Comment: *Some workers reported that soluble fiber increases TAG level in the body while insoluble fiber has no such action and both of them are hypocholesterolemic in action. These differences in action may be due to the insulin production in soluble fiber fed animals.*

References

1. "Advanced human nutrition" edited by Robert E.C Wildman Denis M Medeiros 2000 CRC press LLC pp 89-97
2. "AACC Report Cereal foods world" The Definition of Dietary Fiber. March 2001, Vol. 46, No. 3 112-126
3. Boban PT, Nambisan B, Sudhakaran PR.Hypolipidemic effect of chemically different mucilages in rats: a comparative study. Br J Nutr.2006; 96(6):1021-9

4. Boby RG, Leelamma S. Blackgram fiber (Phaseolus mungo): mechanism of hypoglycemic action. Plant Foods Hum Nutr. 2003 58(1):7-13.

5. Devi KS, Kurup PA. Effects of certain Indian pulses on the serum, liver and aortic lipid levels in rats fed a hypercholesterolaemic diet. Atherosclerosis. 1970 11(3):479-84

6. Devi KS, Kurup PA. Hypolipidaemic activity of Phaseolus mungo (blackgram) in rats fed a high-fat--high-cholesterol diet. Isolation of a protein and polysaccharide fraction. Atherosclerosis. 1972 15(2):223-30.

7. Devi KS, Kurup PA. Hypolipidaemic activity of the protein and polysaccharide fraction from Phaseolus mungo (blackgram) in rats fed a high-fat-high-cholesterol diet. Atherosclerosis. 1973 18(3):389-97.

8. Hipsley, E.H. 1953. Dietary "fibre" and pregnancy toxaemia. British Medical Journal 2:420-422.

9. Indira M, Kurup PA. Effects of neutral detergent fiber from blackgram (Phaseolus mungo) in rats and rabbits. J Nutr. 1989 119(9): 1246-51

10. Indira M, Kurup PA. Effect of blackgram fiber on toxic effects of organophosphorus insecticides. Indian J Exp Biol. 1980 18(12): 1529-30

11. Indira M, Kurup PA. Effect of blackgram fibre on ethanol-induced hyperlipidemia in rats. Atherosclerosis. 1982 41(2-3):241-6.

12. Indira M, Vijayammal PL, Menon PV, Kurup PA. Effect of dietary fiber on intestinal bacterial beta-glucuronidase activity in chicks fed a cholesterol-containing diet. Cancer. 1980 1;46(11):2430-2

13. Jayakumari N, Kurup PA. Dietary fiber and cholesterol metabolism in rats fed a high cholesterol diet. Atherosclerosis. 1979 33(1):41-7.

14. Manoj G, Thampi BS, Leelamma S, Menon PV. Effect of dietary fiber on the activity of intestinal and fecal beta-glucuronidase activity during 1,2-dimethylhydrazine induced colon carcinogenesis. Plant Foods Hum Nutr. 2001; 56(1):13-21.

15. Menon PV, Kurup PA. Dietary fibre and cholesterol metabolism: effect of fibre rich polysaccharide from blackgram (Phaseolus mungo) on cholesterol metabolism in rats fed normal and atherogenic diet. Biomedicine. 1976; 24(4):248-53.

16. Pillai MG, Thampi BS, Menon VP, Leelamma S. Influence of dietary fiber from coconut kernel (Cocos nucifera) on the 1,2-dimethylhydrazine-induced lipid peroxidation in rats. J Nutr Biochem. 1999 10(9): 555-60.

17. Prosky L., Asp N-G., Furda I., DeBreis J. W., Schweizer T. F., Harland B. F. Determination of total dietary fiber in foods, food products and total diets: interlaboratory study. J. Assoc. Off. Anal. Chem. 1984; 67:1044-1052

18. Serji K, Devi KS. Dietary fiber from Musa paradisiaca and Artocarpus heterophyllus on intestinal mucosal and bacterial beta-glucuronidase activity in hexachlorocyclohexane-treated rats. Bull Environ Contam Toxicol. 1993 50(2):293-9

19. Sindurani JA, Rajamohan T. Effects of different levels of coconut fiber on blood glucose, serum insulin and minerals in rats. Indian J Physiol Pharmacol. 2000 44(1):97-100.

20. Southgate DAT. Determination of carbohydrates in foods II unavailable carbohydrates. J. Sci. Food Agri. 1969 20 331-335

21. Sudheesh S, Vijayalakshmi NR. Role of pectin from cucumber in modulation of protein kinase C activity and regulation of glycogen metabolism in rats. Indian J Biochem Biophys. 2007, 44(3):183-5.

22. Trowell, H., and Burkitt, D.R. Crude fiber, dietary fiber and atherosclerosis, Atherosclerosis .1972 16: 138-140

23. Usha V, Vijayammal PL, Kurup PA. Effect of dietary fiber from banana (Musa paradisiaca) on metabolism of carbohydrates in rats fed cholesterol free diet. Indian J Exp Biol. 1989 27(5):445-9

24. Usha V, Vijayammal PL, Kurup PA. Aortic/glycosaminoglycans alterations in antiatherogenic action of dietary fiber from unripe banana (Musa paradisiaca). Indian J Med Res. 1991 94:143-6

25. Vansoest, P.J. Use of detergent in the analysis of fibrous feeds. IV determination of plant cell wall constituents, J. Assoc. of Anal. Chem. 1967 50: 50-55

26. Vansoest, P.J. Use of detergent in the analysis of fibrous foods. A rapid method for the determination of fiber and lignin, J. Assoc. of Anal. Chem. 1967 46: 829-835

27. Vijayagopal P, Devi KS, Kurup PA. Fibre content of different dietary starches and their effect on lipid levels in high fat-high cholesterol diet fed rats. Atherosclerosis 1973; 17(1):156-60.

1.2 Dietary Fiber for Good Health

Dr. D.S. Sheriff,

Professor, Department of Biochemistry, Jubilee Mission Medical College, Thrissur, Kerala.

Dietary Fiber is only found in plants, and functions sort of like a skeleton for the plants to help maintain shape and structure. Humans cannot digest fiber so it passes through the small intestine into the colon and helps to keep the colon healthy[1]. Some disorders like diverticulitis, constipation and irregularity may be connected with not getting enough fiber in the diet.

Types of Dietary Fiber

Insoluble fiber is the type of dietary fiber found in high fiber foods like whole grains, nuts, wheat bran and vegetables. Insoluble fiber or neutral detergent fiber (NDF) does not dissolve in water so it helps to move material through the colon faster by increasing the bulk of the stool. This can be very helpful to people who suffer from constipation or irregularity[2-4]. Diets high in insoluble fiber may also decrease the risk of Diabetes.

Soluble fiber is also found in many high fiber foods like oats, citrus fruits, apples, barley, psyllium, flax seeds and beans. Soluble fiber absorbs water, which helps to soften stools making them easier to eliminate from the body. Some soluble fibers called beta glucan bind to bile acids which contain cholesterol. A high fiber diet with this type of soluble fiber has been shown to reduce cholesterol closer to healthy levels[5, 6].

High Fiber Foods

According to the Institute of Medicine: *The recommended intake for total fiber for adults 50 years and younger is set at 38 grams for men and 25 grams for women, while for men and women over 50 it is 30 and 21 grams per day, respectively, due to decreased food consumption.*

People who currently have low fiber diets may want to increase their daily intake of high fiber foods slowly because some fiber may increase gas and bloating. The body adjusts the increased amount of fiber over time and the gas and bloating will decrease. Fiber content of certain vegetables are given below. One half cup cooked or baked item is taken as one unit.

Fiber Content of Various Vegetables and Cereals

Cooked navy beans - 9.5 g	Frozen mixed vegetables, cooked – 4 g
Baked beans, canned – 9 g	Raw blackberries – 3.8 g
Cooked lentils – 7.8 g	Canned pumpkin – 3.5 g
Cooked black beans – 7.5 g	Cooked whole-wheat spaghetti – 3.4 g
Dates – 7.1 g	24 almonds – 3.3 g
Raisin bran cereal – 3.5 g	One apple with skin – 3.3 g
Cooked kidney beans – 6.5 g	Cooked barley 3 g
Cooked lima beans – 6.7 g	Broccoli – 1.2 g
Canned tomato paste – 5.9 g	One red sweet pepper – 2.4 g
Cooked garbanzo beans – 6.2 g	One nectarine – 2.3 g
Bean with ham soup – 5.6 g	28 peanuts – 2.3 g
Frozen red raspberries – 5.5 g	One slice whole grain bread – 2 g
Cooked artichoke – 4.5 g	15 walnut halves – 2 g
Frozen peas, cooked – 4.4 g	Medium bran muffin - 5 g
Oatmeal – 2 g	Half Asian pear – 5 g

Fiber Supplements

Fiber supplements are available and may be added to a low fiber diet, however fiber supplements shouldn't replace high fiber foods in your diet. High fiber foods are usually high in nutrition as well.

In general, a food that is high in fiber would have at least 5 g of fiber per serving or more. Those that are good sources of fiber have at least 2.5 g of fiber per serving. You can also look for these high fiber foods (they have 5 g of fiber or more per serving): Barley, Navy Beans, Baked Beans, Split Peas, Lentils, Wheat Flour, Oat Bran Dates, Refried Beans, Raspberries, Asian Pears, Green Peas, Kellogg's All-Bran Cereal, Couscous, dry Prunes, Kellogg's Raisin Bran Cereal, Spinach, Spaghetti and Meatballs, Artichokes, Brussels sprouts, Progresso Healthy Classics Lentil Soup, Shredded Wheat Cereal, Broccoli, Pears, Kellogg's Frosted Mini-Wheats Cereal, Raisins, General Mills Total Raisin Bran cereal, other high fiber foods include other bran cereals, bran muffins, etc.

Foods that are still pretty good sources of fiber (about 2 to 4.9 g of fiber per serving), at least as compared to other foods without fiber, but not as high as the high fiber foods listed above, include:

Mixed Vegetables, Strawberies, Carrots, Potatoes (with the skin on), Corn Rice, Figs, General Mills Cheerios cereal, Apples (with the skin on), Oranges, Air Popped Popcorn, Oatmeal, Applesauce, Tomato soup, Fruit Cocktail Graham Crackers, Whole Wheat Bread, General Mills Honey Nut Cheerios cereal, Pistachio Nuts, Peanuts, Celery.

Foods that have some fiber, but not as much as most persons think include grapes, melons, granola bars, non-bran cereals, oatmeal cookies, lettuce, and apples without the skin on them. High fiber diet shall fill up the stomach without much calories, but with a food to satisfy one's hunger and at the same time protect him from CVD[7]

Mark Twain said "part of the secret of success in life is to eat what you like most and let the food fight it out inside." Michael Pollan in his book *The Omnivore's Dilemma (Penguin 2006) q*uestions why one must forego the pleasures of food, while foregoing nutritionism, the quest for nutrients as medicine, a pursuit that may be, paradoxically, fail to enhance health.

Eat less means eat less calories, shun means avoid in between snacks, move more means balance your diet with your physical activity.

Let us remember the concept *"doctor diet, doctor quiet and doctor merry man" can keep you healthy.*

In a world of haste and hustle, stress and strain, fast food and burgers may satiate our hunger but in such busy world of modern man nutraceuticals may help the hungry as well as the ill.

References

1. Burkitt, DP. Epidemiology of large bowel diseases, the role of fiber. Proc. Nutr. Soc. 32(1973) 145-149
2. Anderson, JW; Major, AW. Pulses and lipemia, short and long term effect: Potential in the prevention of Cardiovascular diseases; Brit. J Nutr. 88(2002) suppl. 3S ; 263-271
3. Brown, L; Rosener, B et. al. Cholesterol lowering effects of dietary fiber: A meta analysis. Am. J Clin. Nutr. 69(1999) 30-42
4. Life Sciences Research Office. 1987. Physiological Effects and Health consequences of Dietary fiber. Pilch, SM ; Ed. Federation of American Societies for experimental Biology, Bethesda, M.D
5. Anderson, JW; Story, L et. al. Hypocholesterolemic effect of High fiber diet rich in water soluble plant fiber. Long term studies with oat bran and bean supplemented diet for hypercholesterolemic subjects. J Cancer Diet Assoc. 45(1984) 140-149
6. Mozaffaraian, D; Kumanyika, SK et. al. Fruit and vegetable fiber intake and the risk of cardiovascular disease in elderly individuals. JMA. 289(13) 2003. 1659-66
7. The relationship of dietary fiber and heart disease. In: Trends in Atherosclerosis Research 1987. Dept of Biochem. Univ. of Kerala. 117-124

1.3 Beneficial effects of Neutral Detergent Fiber of Barley in Cholesterol Diet Fed Rats as compared to that of Garlic Oil with respect to Serum and Heart Lipid Profile and Serum Enzymes.

B.S. Vinod* & Dr. K.T. Augusti**

**School of Health Sciences, Thalassery Campus, Kannur University, Palayad, 670661

*Rajiv Gandhi Centre for Biotechnology, Thiruvananthapuram

Abstract

Feeding a diet containing 2% cholesterol to rats for a period of two months significantly increased their lipid profile and altered their enzyme levels in serum and tissues. Incorporation of 20% neutral detergent fiber (NDF) isolated from barly in the above diet or simultaneous feeding of garlic oil (100ml/kg/day) significantly ameliorated the deleterious effects of cholesterol in diet. This work supports the necessity of fibers[1-2] and antioxidants in our diet. The effects of edible fibers present in cereals, pulses and many vegetables are beneficial to health. This work was done at the School of Medical Education of M.G. University, Kottayam as a part of M.Sc. Project of Mr. Vinod.

Introduction

Edible fibers are the endogenous components of plant materials in the diet which are resistant to digestion by enzymes produced by humans[1]. They have been classified into soluble and insoluble fibers[2]. The latter is also called a Neutral Detergent Fiber (NDF)[3]. The hemicellulose component of coconut kernel, NDF showed very good hypocholesterolemic effect[4].

Fibers with a high water holding capacity such as pectin, gums and psyllium have been referred to as soluble fiber. Fibers act as bile acid sequestrants. NDF may be binding glucose and cholesterol also.

The NDF contains all fiber components except pectin and other water soluble polysaccharides. Barley offers mainly insoluble fiber. Insoluble fibers are largely cell wall components of fruits and vegetables and consists of cellulose, hemi cellulose and lignin. See the list of fiber contents in various edible items.

Fiber contents of edible items			
Items	**NDF g/100g**		**NDF g/100g**
Rice bran	69.3	Beans	28.0
Coconut cake	53.6	Snakegourd	28.0
Amaranthus	40.5	Cucumber	21.5
Moringa leaves	37.8	Ladies Finger	21.0
Banana Stalk	36.9	Brinjal	20.5
Black gram	36.0	Tomatos	19.6
Peas	34.0	Barley	17.0
Banana	32.0	Raggi	14.9
Goose berry	28.1	Wheat	12.9
		Onion	12.8

Merits and demerits of different Fibers

Generally adequate quantities of insoluble fiber like cellulose decreases intestinal transit time and increases fecal bulk. On the other hand, soluble fibers such as pectin and guar may delay gastric emptying and increase small intestinal transit time because of their gel formation.

Solube fiber may enhance the chances of cholesterol and TAG absorption into blood than that with insoluble fiber.

Therefore in the present study we have selected barley as a source of NDF in order to assess its hypocholesterolemic effect as compared to that with garlic oil which has been proved to be a good serum cholesterol lowering agent[5].

Materials and Methods

- Garlic oil was prepared from methanolic extract of fresh garlic homogenate, from which the ether soluble fraction was separated and used.
- Neutral detergent fiber was prepared from powdered and defatted barley with neutral detergent solution as described by Goring and Vansoest [6](1970) yield 17g/100g
- Male Sprague Dawley strain ablbino rats 6-8 months old and weighing 180-230 g were divided into four groups of six each. They were maintained on diet with NDF or garlic oil supplements as described below for two months.

In normal diet 61.8% corn starch, 20% casein, 8% ground nut oil, 4% salt mixture, 5 yeast tablets, 1% shark liver oil and 0.2% choline chloride were used.

In cholesterol diet 2% cholesterol, 10% coconut oil and 57.8% corn starch with the other components as above were used for groups 2 and 4.

The same diet made with 20% NDF and 41.8% corn starch was used in group 3.

Garlic Oil (G.O) was orally administered to group 4 in normal saline at a dose of 100 mg/kg/day. Thus the various groups of rats are numbered below with the pattern of their diet.

1. Normal diet fed.
2. 2% cholesterol diet fed.
3. Do +20% NDF fed.
4. Do + G.O. fed (100 mg/kg/day).

Collection of Blood and Tissues for Estimations

After two months feeding as above, the rats were deprived of food overnight, stunned by a blow at the back of the neck and blood was collected in dry test tubes by cutting the jugular veins and allowed to clot to separate the serum.

After decapitation of the rats their heart tissues were collected in ice cold containers and various parameters of both serum and tissues were determined by standard methods (Augusti et. al. 2005).

Results on Cholesterol diet fed rats with NDF & G.O are shown in Table 1.

The results depict the beneficial effects of neutral detergent fiber (NDF) isolated from barley as compared to garlic oil on serum lipid profile and atherogenic index (AI), in cholesterol diet fed rats for two months.

Table 1

Results on cholesterol diet fed rats with NDF

Beneficial effects of neutral detergent fiber (NDF) isolated from barley as compared to garlic oil on serum lipid profile and atherogenic index (AI), in cholesterol diet fed rats for two months.

Values are mean of six rats ± S.D. for each group (mg/100ml)

	Groups and Diet	TAG	TC	LDLc	HDLc	AI	FFA
1.	Normal diet (8% ground nut oil)	76.3 ± 2.1	78.7 ± 2.6	46.6 ± 4.6	30.0 ± 2.6	1.9 ± 0.2	86.1 ± 2.1
2.	2% chol. diet (10% coconut oil)	120.3 ± 6.9	163.6 ± 4.3*	79.2 ± 8.6*	60.3 ± 2.2*	3.06 ± 0.2*	126.1 ± 6.9*
3.	Do + 20% NDF	90.9 ± 2.7*	113.9 ± 3.9*	44.3 ± 4.7*	61.3 ± 2.7*	1.86 ± 0.06*	96.8 ± 3.3*
4.	Do + G.O. (100 mg/kg)	88.2 ± 2.3*	107.2 ± 4.0*	36.1 ± 5.3*	64.5 ± 3.2*	1.7 ± 0.11*	87.6 ± 2.9*

Student ct-to ct. level of clg nl floance $p<0.001$

HEART LIPID PROFILE

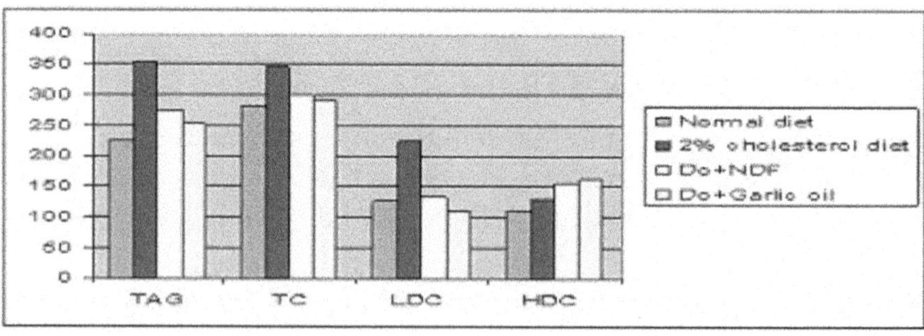

Fig. 1 Beneficial effects of NDF from Barley as compared to G.O on heart lipid profile in cholesterol diet fed rats for two months. Values are mean of six rats for each group (mg/100g)

In group 2 control, lipd values significantly increased over the normal and in groups 3 & 4 values other than HDLc significantly lowered from that of the control and HDLc significantly increased.

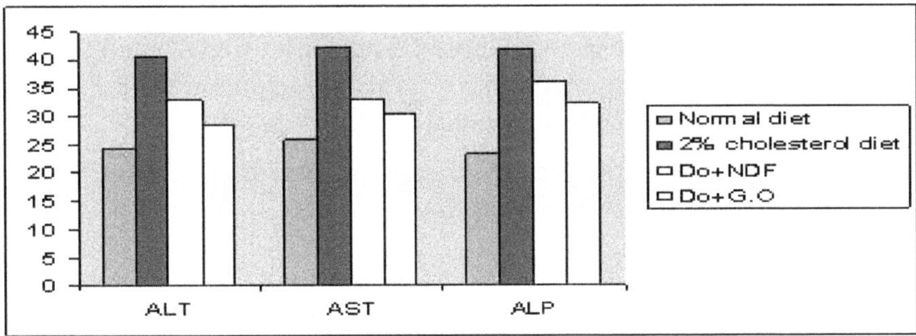

Fig. 2 Serum enzyme values of Alanine transaminase (ALT). Aspartate transminase (AST) and alkaline phosphatase (ALP) of groups shown in Table 1. Values are mean of six rats in each group (IU/L).

In group 2 control, enzyme values increased significantly over the normal and in groups 3 & 4 values decreased significantly from the control.

Results on cholesterol diet fed control

Cholesterol diet fed rats showed significant rise in their serum levels of TAG, TC, LDL chol. (P<0.001) and in HDL cholesterol (p<0.01) as compared to normal values. The atherogenic index in serum i.e. total cholesterol/HDL cholesterol ratio increased by 61% over the normal value.

A similar pattern of lipid profile was also obtained in the heart tissue with an atherogenic index of 31% over the normal value (P<0.01).

Results on NDF treated rats

On the contrary barley NDF feeding to a similar group showed significant decreases both in serum and heart TAG and total and LDL cholesterol and a significant rise in HDL cholesterol.

With respect to these parameters a better effect was shown by feeding of garlic oil to the cholesterol diet fed rats (P<0.01).

Similarly FFA levels also increased in the serum of cholesterol diet fed rats and the same decreased significantly on feeding fiber or garlic oil as compared to their control (P<0.001).

In the case of serum enzymes viz; ALT, AST and ALP all of them significantly increased in the serum of cholesterol diet fed rats (P<0.001). However each of them decreased significantly on feeding NDF or garlic oil in groups 3 and 4 respectively (P<0.001).

Conclusions

- The results clearly establish that barley NDF and G.O are significantly active and comparable to ameliorate the deleterious effects of a 2% cholesterol diet.
- NDF helps to remove cholesterol from our system and reduces Carbohydrate and fat absorption.
- Generally activity of them is in the order G.O.> NDF.
- Fiber/garlic oil and even garlic can be included in the diet as functional foods.

References

1. Usha V et. al. (1984). Effect of dietary fiber from banana (Musa paradisiaca) on cholesterol metabolism Indian Jour. Expt. Biol.22:550-554.
2. Gomathy R et. al. (1989). Hypolipidemic principle of the inflorescence stalk of plantain (Musa Sapientum) J Biosci. 14(3) 301-309.
3. Jayakumari N and Kurup P A. Black gram. Fiber Atherosclerosis, 33.41
4. (a) Sindhurani J A & Rajmohan T (1998). Effect of dietary fiber from coconut (cocos nucifera) on cholesterol metabolism J Clin. Biochem Nutr. 24.125-132.
   (b) Hypolipidemic effect of hemicellulose component of coconut fiber. Indian Jour. of Exp. Biol. (1998) 36: 786-89.
5. Farva.D Goji, I.A et. al. Effects of garlic oil on STZ diabetic rats maintained on normal and high fat diets. Indian Jour. Biochem. & Biophys. 23.(1986)24, 27
6. Georing, H.K. and Vansoest. P.J. Forage analysis. Agricultural analysis in Agric. Hand Book. No.379. 1970 ARS, USDA. Washington DC.

Chapter – 2

Sources of Nutraceuticals and the Chemistry of their Functions

2.1 Nutraceuticals or Nutritional Medicines

Dr. K. Bhaskaran
B.Sc.D.H.M.S.M.B.B.S.M.D.
HOD.Pharmacology & Principal
Pariyaram Medical College.Kannur, Kerala.

During the past few years an increasing number of dietary supplements are available the medical shops for purchase without a valid prescription. They are also available in the open market and health shops. The concept of nutritional medicine came into the mind of the researchers while thinking about deficiency diseases and their treatment. The health status of the population determines the economic development of the state. Nutraceutic is a new branch of Pharmaceutical science which deals with natural products used for the proper maintenance of normal health. Large number of varoius preperations are being poured out into the Pharmaceutical market claiming their magical effect on health. Many of these preparations are not well studied scientifically or their effects are not being experimentally proved. Because of their simplicity of manufacturing process and less toxicity and their wide publicity they are being accepted widely. Their authenticity is questionable.

Dr. Stephen De Felice first coined the term nutraceutical in 1989 while he was presenting a paper in a conference, and he defined the nutraceuticals as “food or parts of food that provide medical or health benefit including the prevention and treatment of diseases”. The term functional food is also used to refer nutraceuticals. In States of Canada and Great Britain, a functional food is essentially a food, but a nutraceutic is in an isolated form or concentrated form.

Many of these new products are being promoted to treat various diseased states which find their origin in the plant kingdom. This is an obvious choice, as many plants produce secondary compounds as alkaloids to protect themselves from infection and these constituents may be useful in the treatment of human infection. Many of the phytomedicines are typical examples. The fact that all the living plants have their own natural method of keeping healthy and strong and also keep aloof from the noxious infections is the basic principle of using them against human diseases. Even preparations very similar to natural human hormones are now synthesized from plant sources. Various phytochemicals are now available for replacement therapy in endocrine deficiencies.

To bring a medicine to the market will take about five to ten years and the effort will cause millions of rupees; where as to market a nutraceutical needs only a fraction of this. The government is not having any regulatory system over the manufacturing of these agents at present. So large number of such products are coming into the market. Various classification of nutraceuticals are now adopted depending upon their uses and their source. The difference between pharmaceutical and nutraceutical is sometimes difficult to define, depending only on regulatory issues.

The United States Congress in 1990 defined a medical food "as food which is formulated to be consumed or administered internally under the supervision of a physician and which is intended for specific dietary management of a disease or condition, for which distinctive nutritional requirements based on a recognized scientific principle and established by medical evaluation". Since the introduction of nutraceutical is very simple and risk free, many of the multinational pharmaceutical firms are switching over to nutraceutical manufacturing.

The old proverb; "an apple a day will keep the doctor away" is now replaced by "a nutraceutical a day will keep the doctor away". Consumers are turning increasingly to food supplements to improve the well being when pharmaceuticals fail. The phytochemicals are thought to be the active principle of causing the beneficial effects of nutraceuticals in various human ailments.

Active hexole correlated compounds {AHCC} increase the level of the natural killer cells, T cells, macrophages and interleukin 1 & 2. Genistein combined polysaccharide had shown anticancer, anti-inflammatory and antiangeogenesis activity in early bladder carcinoma and prostatic carcinoma.

As consumers in United States of America, Japan and Europe rely increasingly on nutraceuticals, to improve their health, regulators and lawmakers are reacting to develop appropriate regulations; given that most health claims accompanying these products are supported by little or no research.

Nutraceuticals now include a wide variety of products, such as Echinacea, St.John's wort; oil from fish and flaxseeds, glucosamine and chondroitin, calcium-fortified juices and plant sterols. Iceland's largest diary company recently introduced the world's first milk to lower high blood pressure. In United States alone six out of ten consumers take some type of food supplement and thirty to forty percent take herbal supplement. Even some physicians are recommending natural products before prescribing pharmaceuticals. The trend also reflects the growth of a new paradigm "self care". **A recent study in the United States reveals that 72% take food supplements to feel better, 67% to prevent illness, 50% to live longer, 37% to build muscle and strength, 12% for weight management, and 33% on the advice of their physician. 53% said nutraceutical offer better benefits not matched by conventional drugs and 56% said they offered benefits comparable to drugs but with few side effects. Remarkably 95% were satisfied with supplements.**

An epidemiological study by a Canadian research group indicated that vitamin E may have a protective effect against Parkinson's disease; moreover the interactions between drugs and nutraceutical are rarely documented. Recently the scenario has changed. Various reports of nutraceutical interaction with modern drugs and other drugs of Ayurveda, Siddha etc. had come into light.

The substances that have hormonal actions such as DHEA and androstenidiones are having clear drug like action, but they are regulated as nutraceuticals in USA. The nutraceuticals being studied are changing continuously; for example about one fifth of the Americans used natural products such as Echinacea, Ginseng, Ginkobiloba, St. John's wort, and fish oils in descending order. But today consumption of fish oil is high up and others are down.

The regulatory environment is ever changing worldwide. Europe has become stricter in nutritional supplements. **"Nutraceuticals are bioengineered foods"**. The recently proposed FDA regulation supports the emerging nutraceutical industry and a new regulatory process must be created to foster scientific researches.

Related References

1. Jack. D.B. Mole Med Today 1995:118-21
2. Brower. B. Nat Botecnol 1998: 16; 728-33.
3. Mannion. M. Am J Nat. Med 1998; 5; 30-33.
4. Mazza.G. Functional Foods. Technomic Publishing Company inc 1998.
5. Cockbill. C.A. British Food Journal 1994; 96;3-4.
6. Aarts. T.A J Nutr FunctionMedFoods 1998; 1; 45-47.
7. Senior. K. MolMedToday1996; 60-64.

8. Newall. C.A, Anderson.L.A, Phillipson.J.D., HerbalMedicines; Pharmaceutical Press 1996.

9. Herbal Medicines Controls moves to Europe Pharm.J.1999; 263;775.

10. The Medicines Act 1968 London.

11. Shaw. D, Leon C, Kolev S, Murray V, Traditional remedies and food suppliments. A five year Toxicological Study., Drug safety 1997;17: 342-56.

12. Bidlack WR, Omaye ST, Meskin MS, Jahner D. Phytochemicals: US Technomic Publishing Company Inc 1998.

2.2 Nutraceutical Foods

Mrs. Jiji Thomas Kunnethedam.
B'-Canti. Jawaharnagar. Trivandrum-3.

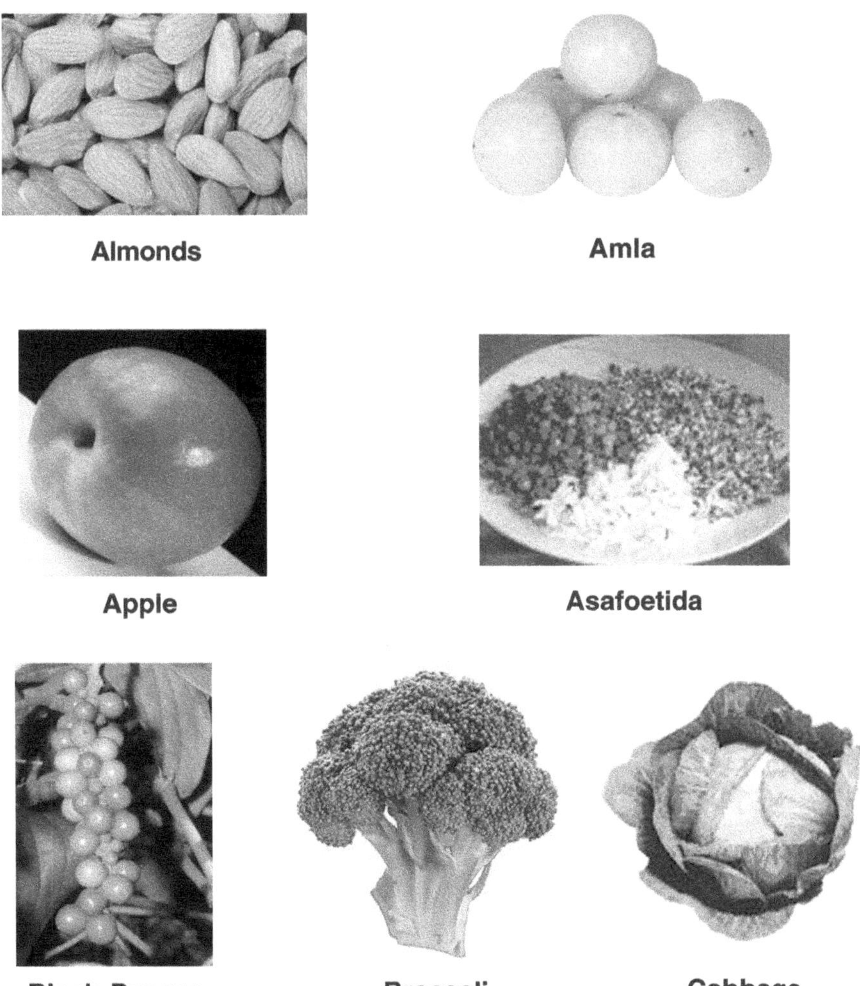

Almonds

Amla

Apple

Asafoetida

Black Pepper

Broccoli

Cabbage

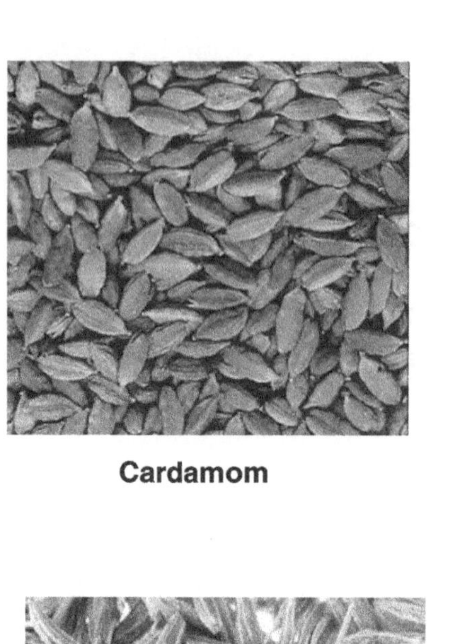

Cardamom

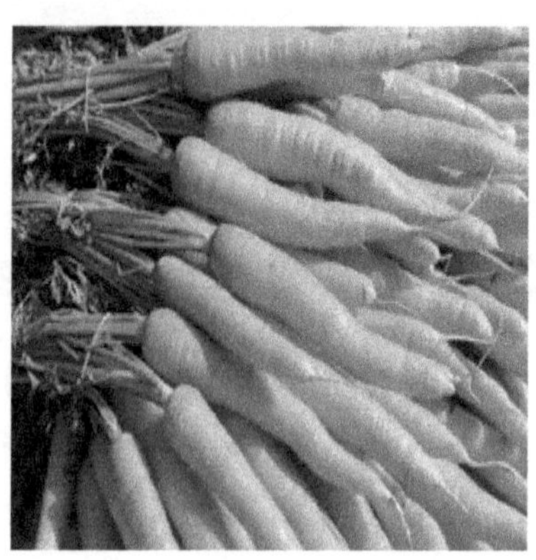

Carrot

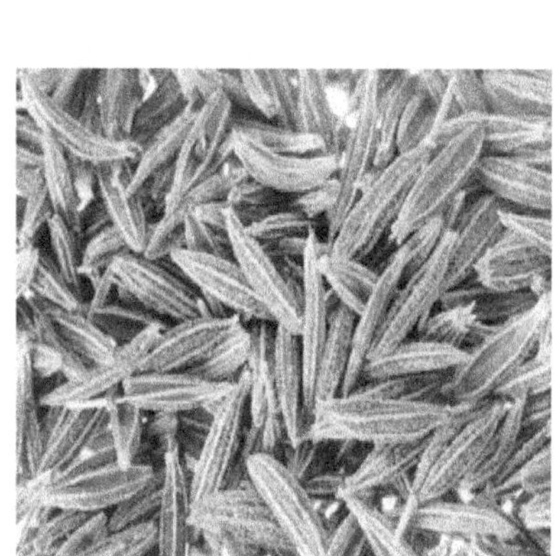

Cumins

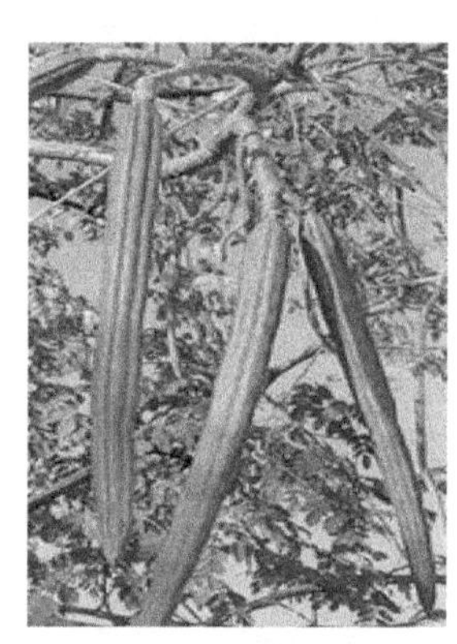

Drumstick

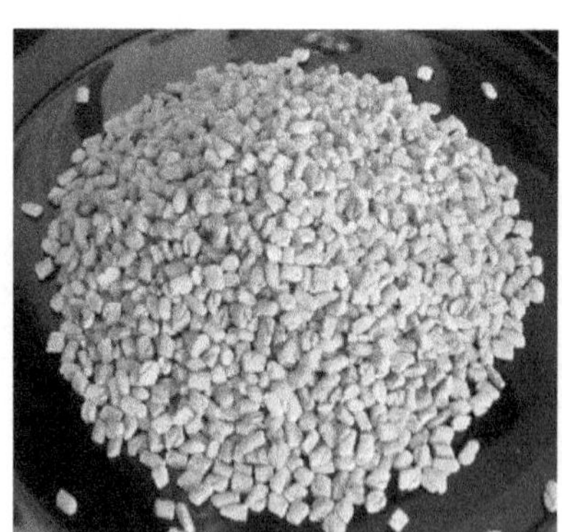

Fenugreek

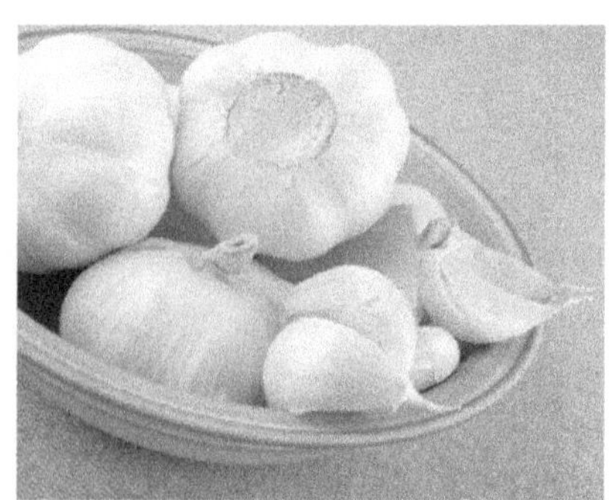

Garlic

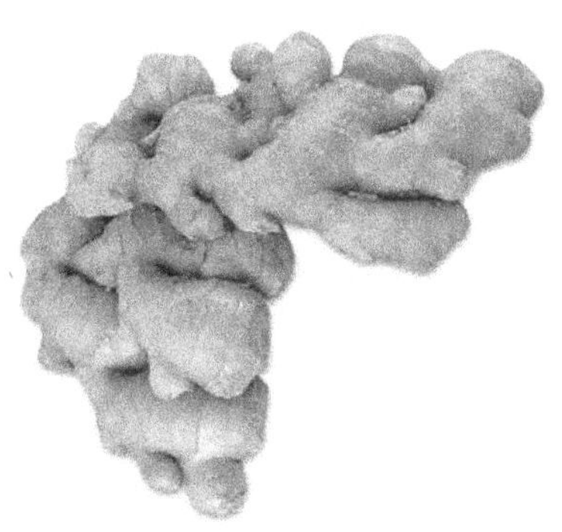

Ginger

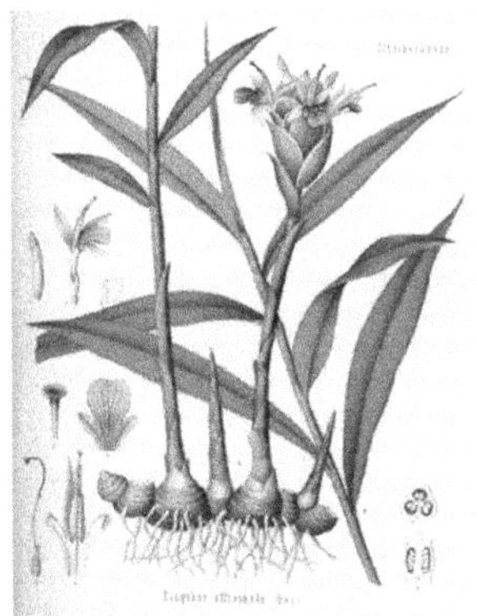

Ginger plant

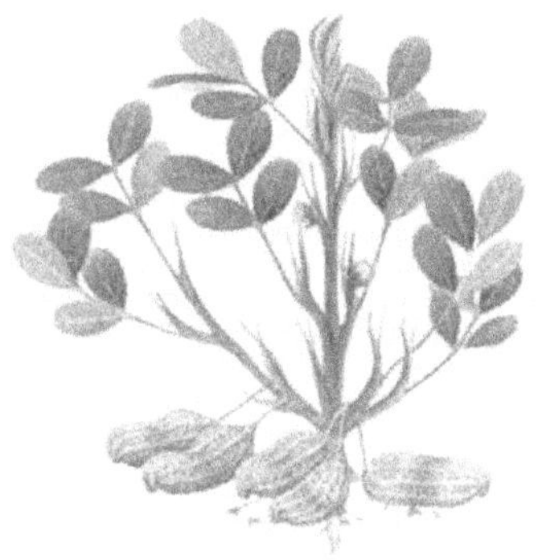

Groundnut

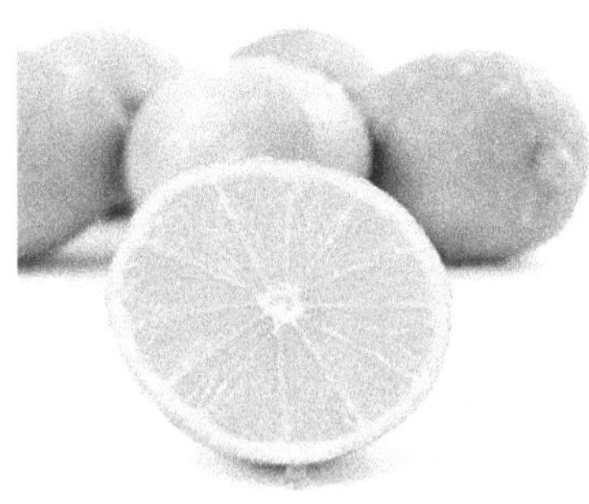

Lime

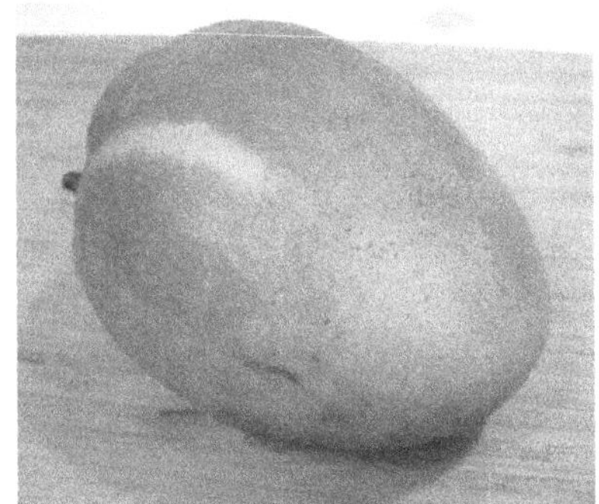

Mango

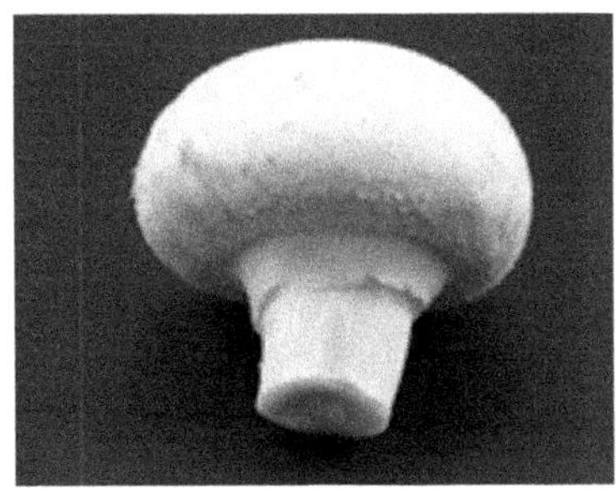

Mashroom

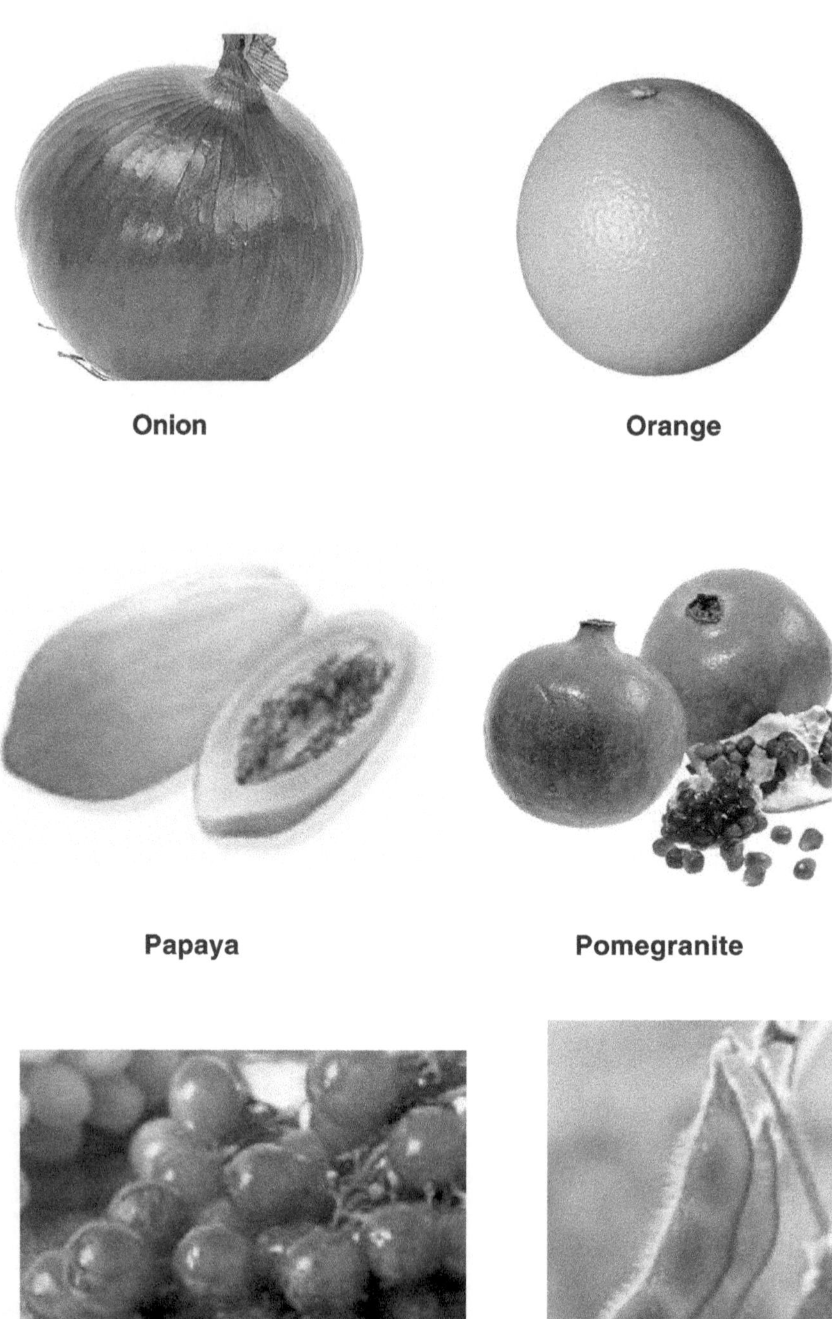

Onion

Orange

Papaya

Pomegranite

Red Grapes

Soybean

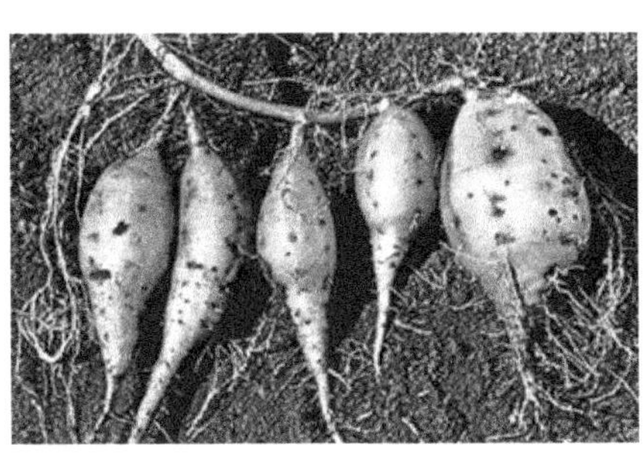

Sweet Potato

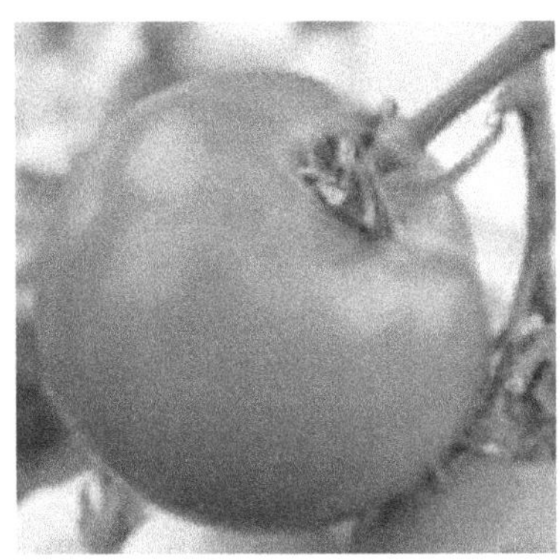

Tomato

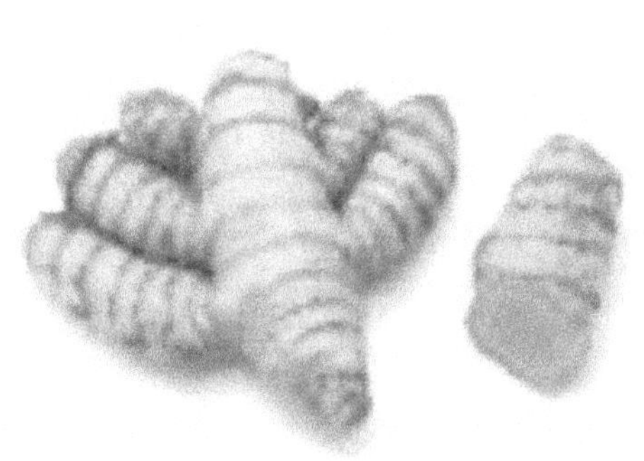

Turmeric

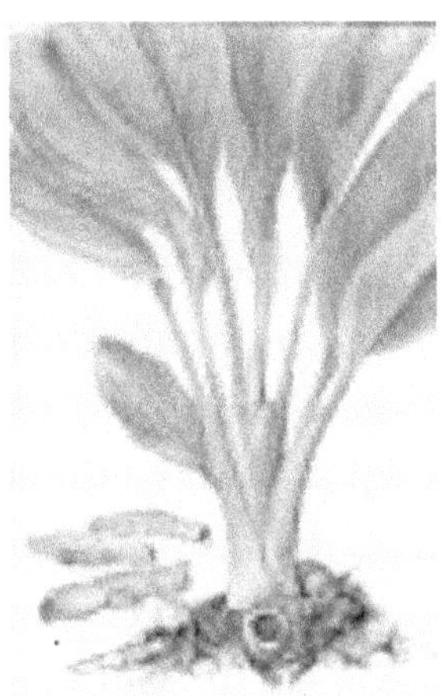

Turmeric plant

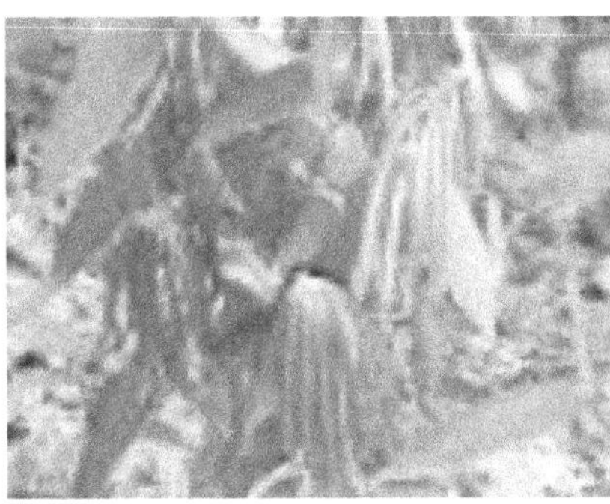

Vanila

2.3 Nutraceuticals, their Sources, classification and role A Review

Sastraratna Dr. K.T. Augusti,
Rtd Prof.& HOD, Medical Biochemistry, School of Health Sciences,
Thalassery Campus of Kannur University,
E-mail: ktaugusti@yahoo.co.uk

Nutraceuticals are variously called as functional foods, phytonutrients, antioxidants/free radical scavengers etc. Nutraceuticals are soon to revolutionise the global food industry. The word nutraceutical combines 'nutrition' and pharmaceuticals to mean that food extracts can be used as preventive drugs or food supplements. The entire concept is building on the research studies that link the importance of diet in combating diseases in man. What is new about this concept is the science's added knowledge about the disease preventing phytonutrients which are ever present in food stuffs. Minerals like ***selenium*** that function as cofactors for enzymes are also included in this class. Briefly any edible substance that helps to prevent a disease is a nutraceutical.

Sources: These functional foods according to Binoo P Bonny of Kerala Agricultural University, Trichur cover every thing from break fast cereal that has been pumped full of vitamins to benecol, a margarinesque spread that actually lowers cholesterol. Vegetables of all sorts particularly the colored ones among fruits, leaves, tubers such as carrots, ginger, curcuma-longa and beetroots, bulbs of alliums & cabbage, various grains, tomatoes, papaya, gooseberries (amla), pomegranate, citrus fruits, grapes, brinjal, bitter gourd, soyabeans, drum stick and guva are a few to be mentionad. Among the leaves amaranthus, broccoli, moringa and spinach are of special mention. Among the spices black pepper, green pepper, cloves, cardamom, cumin etc. top in the sources for nutraceuticals.

Calassification and Functions: The major phytonutrients identified to have nutraceutical properties include **terpenes, phytosterol, polyphenols, Flavanoids and Theols**. The identification is based on their protective functions, the physical and chemical characteristics of their molecules.

1. **Terpenes:** They represent the largest class of phytonutrients. Terpenes are found in green foods, ginger, soya products and grains. Carotenoids and limonoids are the two major terpene subclasses. Carrotes, tomatoes, parsley, orange and spinach are rich sources of carotenoids. They act as vitamin A precursor and have preventive action against many eye diseases.

   They can also prevent the oxidation of vitamin A, C and E. Thus they have a role to maintain a better blood levels of these vitamins too.

   A terpene isolated from Salacia oblonga Wall demonstrated hypoglycemic, hypocholesterolemic, hypolipidemic and antioxidant actions in diabetic rats. It stimulated the activities of antioxidant enzymes such as catalase and superoxide dismutase (SOD) and suppressed lipid peroxidation in liver and heart[1] and critrus peel can act as nutraceuticals supplying limonoids. They act as antioxidants and protect lung tissues from free oxygen. Limonene and nomilin are the two major terpenoids found in citrus fruits such as lemon, lime, orange and grape fruit. Both these compounds have been found to induce activities of the detoxifying enzyme glutathion-S transferase. The increased enzyme activity has been correlated with the ability of the compounds to inhibit chemically induced carcinogenesis, in laboratory animals. Limonin and nomilin inhibited the formation of tumors induced by benzo (a) pyrene (BP) in mice[2]. Addition of nomilin and limonin to the diet inhibited BP induced lung tumor formation in A/J mice. The inhibition of lung tumor was correlated with inhibition of the formation of BP-DNA adducts in lungs[3]. This shows that metabolic conversion of BP to its hydroxy derivatives that form adducts with DNA was blocked by the terpenoids. This preventive step protects DNA from mutation which is a prerequisite for tumor formation. In U.S.A. D-limonene has a safe status for use as an added flavoring agent. Carotenoids of various vegetables, β-Carotene of carrots and lycopene of tomatoes all belong to the class of terpenoids and they act as good antioxidants/free radical scavengers and thereby act as inhibitors of carcinogens. Isoprenoids are active against free radicals in the body. Thus they reduce oxidative damage (i.e. destruction of any component of cell by removal of hydrogen and addition of oxygen) of tissues, where as tocopherols (vitamin E) found in grains and palm oil inhibit breast cancer. Vitamins A and E have isoprenoid units in their side chains. In Kerala there is rarely any Ayurvedic decoction without dry ginger. Many wondered why it is so. Now we know that ginger contains a sesquiterpene, Zingiberene and the medicinal effects of ginger is partly due to this compound and related aldehydes, ketones and alcohols. The ginger compounds possess anti-inflammatory, antioxidant and immunostimulatory actions. This may be the reason why Chinees use a rasayana of ginger and garlic in the ratio of 1:4 in vinegar to fight against all viral diseases. The author advocated the use of this in Kerala to drive off viral fevers during 2006-07.

2. **Phytosterols:** They belong to the plant products which are water soluble and lather forming. The author and his guide Dr. Brahmachari[4] reported hypoglycemic activity of an aqueous extract of the bark of ***Ficus religiosa Linn***. Ambika and Rajaramarao[5] isolated β-sitosterol-D glucoside from the above bark and demonstrated its hypoglycemic action in fasting rabbits at 2 hrs to a tune of 34 % on i.v. adminstration of 7.5 mg/kg weight. In oral administration 25 mg dose was required to show a 20% reduction in FBS at 5 hrs. The bark contains both β-sitosterol and its glycoside according to the above workers. The bark of Terminalia Arjuna also contains β-sitosterol. These compounds come under a group of saponins that are present in various parts of the plants. viz; bark, leaves, rhizomes and fruits. They are endowed with very many biological actions. The beneficial effects of saponins on hypercholesterolemia have been reported by Venugopalan and Sreevastava[6]. Other rich sources of phytosterols include yellow vegetables, seeds of pumpkins and yamas. β-sitosterol competes with dietary cholesterol for uptake in the intestine thereby blocking cholesterol absorption into the body. It also facilitates the excretion of cholesterol from the body and prevents the development of tumor in breast and prostate glands. Kutkosterol and related compounds present in picrorhzia Kurroa gives protection to liver from several ailments. Its decoction is reported to produce reduction in serum cholesterol and coagulation[7].

   Saponins are also abundant in soyabeans. Related to other food stuffs, soyabean seeds contain high levels of four classes of compounds which demonstrated anticancer activity. They are glycosides, phytosterols, protease inhibitors and phytic acid. The saponins most extensively investigated for anticancer activity have been glycyrrhizin and its aglycone[8]. Dietary saponins were found to enhance natural killer cell activity[9], presumably with an initial effect on the mucosal immune system due to its poor absorption[10]. Saponins were also found to be cytotoxic to sarcoma 37 cells. ***In vivo and in vitro*** studies have shown saponins to reduce colonic cell proliferation rates and to decrease growth and rate of DNA synthesis of various tumor cells. The suggested anticarcinogenic mechanism of saponins involves their ability to bind bile acids and cholesterol. Vegetarians who frequently consume soyabean based meat substitute are at decreased risk of breast and colon cancer[11]. Soyabean saponin completely inhibited HIV-induced cyto pathic effects and virus specific antigen expression, 6 days after infection at concentration greater than 0.25 mg/ml.

3. **Polyphenoles/Flavonoids**: Phenols comprise of a large group of phytonutrients with profound importance in preventive medicine. Tea, berries, grapes and egg plants, are rich in phenolic content. Phenols are toxic only if it contains a single hydroxyl group as in carbolic acid (Phenol). When the number of phenolic groups increases they become polyphenols as in tannins, catechins and reserveratrol of red wine. Flavanoids also come under polyphenols with an oxide ring in particular and all of them develop antioxidant activity just like vitamin E which is also active because of its phenolic group. Terminalia arjuna W.et A contains[12] tannins including pyrocatechol tannins which are good antioxidants that protect tissues including that of heart and liver from lipid per oxidation and inflammation. Resveratrol a polyphenol present in red wine and red skins of graps is a good antioxidant. Broccoli contains 17 polyphenols with antioxidant activity and it is a good item for salad

   Flavonoids, anthocyanidines (flavanals), their precursors viz; leucocyanidines and isoflavones are the major subclasses coming under the phenolic group. Epicatechin is a polyphenol with hypoglycemic activity and it was isolated from the stem and bark of pterocarpus marsupium by Chakravarthy et. al.[13]. Flavonoids were once grouped as vitamin P but later deleted for want of specific deficiency disease symptoms. However it has been proved that those phytochemicals can enhance the effectiveness of vitamin C. They can also act against allergies, ulcers, tumors and platelet aggregation. It is effective in controlling high blood pressur and can reduce the risk of estrogen induced cancer. Anthocyanidines or flavonals have a significant role in collagen protein synthesis. They are important in sports medicine also. Athletes who exercise a lot produce free radicals that are tackled by anthocyanidins. Isoflavones largely present in soybeans can prevent tumor growth as in breast cancer. Beans and other legumes are rich sources with nutraceutical properties. Important isoflavones, genstein and daidzin found in soyabeans have nutraceutical properties against cancer.

4. **Flavonoids/Isoflavonoids/Polyphenols of Various Nature**

   People who consume traditional diets rich in soya food rarely experience breast, uterus and prostate Cancer. The herb ***pueraria lobata*** also contains isoflavones that can be used in treatment against alcoholism. Isoflavones alter the speed at which the enzyme alcohol dehydrogenase converts alcohol into aldehydes. This causes good tolerance for alcohol and reduces the pleasure response to drinking. The kik is due to the production of acetaldchyde by the above enzyme which is slowed down by isoflavones. When the aldehyde acts on the neurons the kick is generated and the drunkard is presuaded to do any dirty thing.

The author isolated three flavanols from the bark of ***Ficus bengalensis*** (pipal tree) and demonstrated their hypoglycemic, hypolipidemic and antioxidant activities. They are glycosides of leucocyanidine, leuco pelargonidine and leucodelphinidine[14-16]. The second one demonstrated protective action as good as garlic oil and vitaime E against damages induced in liver by carbon tetrachloride[15]. The antiperoxidative effects of the flavonoids from ***Punicagranatum Linn*** were demonstrated by Sudheesh and Vijayalakshmi[17]. According to the work of Francis et. al.[18] flavonoids such as kaempferol, morin, fisetin, biochanin A, and the glycoside rutin exhibit a dose dependent inhibition of mutagenic activity of AFB_1 in strain TA98 by 150%. Flavonoides are generally lipid soluble compounds. They act as potent antioxidants, metal chelators and free radical scavengers. Chalcone, a precousor of flavonoids, has recently been shown to inhibit chemically induced mammary tumor formation in rats and pulminory tumor formation in mice by acting as a suppressing agent. The flavonoids querectin and luteolin present in fruits and vegetables (e.g. the former is present on the skins of onions and apples) were found to be potent inhibitors of protein tyrosine kinase, products of oncogenes in cell membranes from cancer cells. A flavonoid epicatechin was found to be active in alloxan diabetic rats and regenerated pancreatic β cells and controlled hyperglycemia[13].

These compounds also inhibited epidermal growth factor stimulated protein tyrosine kinase and cellular proliferation. Naringenin a flavanone present in citrus fruit is effective in inhibiting the oxidation of nifedipine and the activation of aflatoxin B_1[19]. Naringenin has also been shown to inhibit the hydroxylation of B(a)P, aminopyrene N-demethylase and to a lesser extent bifenyl 4-hydroxylase activities[20]. B(a)P only in the hydroxylated form makes adduct with DNA and mutate it. Flavonoids appear to be promising anticarcinogenic agents that warrant further study. Picrorrhiza kurroa contains several flavonoid glycosides that produce 40% blood sugar reduction in diabetic rats[21].

Polyphenols present in fruits like amla (Emblica officinalis) are ellagic acid[22] and phyllemblic acid[23]. Other components present in amla include ascorboc acid, tannins, trigalloylglucose, flavonoids etc. Ascorbic acid present in plants is associated with poly phenols[24] and its reducing activity was shown to be heat stable. Jeena and Kuttan[25] ascribed the stronger antioxidant activity of amla to water soluble poly phenols. This extract was found to be a potent inhibitor of lipid per oxidation and scavenger of hydroxyl and super oxide radicals *in vitro*. Further the ellagic acid (condensed polyphenols) which is commonly found in grapes, strawberries, amla and certain nuts has been shown to inhibit B(a)P induced lung and fore stomach tumour in mice, N-Nitrosobenzyl methylamine induced oesophagal tumour in rats, and the mutagenicity of aflatoxin B_1[26]. Glutathione –S-transferase activity was increased significantly in the liver and fore stomach of mice by tannic and ellagic acids. This could result in an increased conjugation leading to faster excretion of the reactive carcinogen metabolites[27]. Caffeic acid and ferulic acid are hydroxy derivatives of cinnamic acid which are present in a wide variety of fruits and vegetables including garlic. They are shown to be potent blocking agents that prevent nitrosamine formation ***in vitro and in vivo***[28]. Nitrosamines are carcinogens. Therefore plant phenolics may block ***in vivo*** nitrosations that leads to cancer formation in stomatch when high levels of nitrates (preservatives) are consumed. Such a protection is possible by garlic as it contains many phenolics (See article by U.P.Singh) and allyl sulfides[29] Curcumin (Diferuloyl-methane) the principal phenolic compound present in turmeric is a potent inhibitor of tumor promotion by phorbol esters. The inhibitory effects of curcumin and its analogues on chemical carcinogenesis in culture and in mouse skin have been investigated[30]. Curcumin was reported to inhibit 98% of the TPA induced tumour promotion on mouse skin. Intensive studies on the action of curcumin in various biological systems have indicated that this compound has engaged in multiple antitumour promotion pathway and blocked tumour promotion[31].

Pomegranate Fruit (PF) is the richest source of flavonoids and many workers[32] studied its biological properties. The ethyl acetate extracts of the PF suppressed the damages induced by lead salts and alcohol in rats and the results are presented in this seminar by Andrews. [Proceedings of the National Seminar on Nutraceuticals held at Thalassery, Kerala pp.65-70, 28th Nov. to 2nd Dec. 2006]

5. Theols (Mainly Organosulfur Oxides/Polysulfides)

Theols are a class of sulfur containing phytonutrients with antioxidant activities. The food sources having theolic nutraceutical properties include garlic, onions, mustard and other cruciferous vegetables like cabbage and turnip. Important subclasses under theols are rich sources of glucosinates. They activate liver detoxification enzymes and can reduce tumour. Allylic and related sulfides (CH_2=CH-CH_2-S-) are mild hypoglycemics and potent hypocholesterolemic, hypolipidemic, hypotensive and anticarcinogenic agents[33]. They protect against damages induced by nicotine[34,35] Carbon-tetrachloride[15] and lead salts[35(b)] (Ref: Augusti's papers). They also give protection against cardiovascular diseases[36,37] and tumour growths[38]. They can block the activity of toxins produced by bacteria and virus thereby building up immunity against diseases[39.] Garlic, onions and cabbage[40] are the most potent members of this class. Allylic or related sulfides are also present in leeks, shallots and chives. Phytonutrients get released from plants only when it is cut or smashed due to the action of enzymes like alliinase. S-allyl cysteine sulfoxide (SACS), S-propenyl cysteine sulfoxide (SPCS) and S-methyl cysteine sulfoxide (SMCS) are the main precursors of garlic, onion and cabbage oils respectively. These precursors have lesser effect as compared to the oils (R-S-S-R and R-S(O)-S-R) produced by them. Here R=CH_3, C_3H_5, C_3H_7 etc. When alliinase acts on these precursors they decompose into alkyl polysulfides and their oxides like allicin. Allicin on storage get converted into ajoene which is a stronger product than allicin as a nutraceutical.

The sub class indoles are found in citrus and amla (gooseberry) fruits. They are also effective against cancer. ***In China to prevent all infectious diseases they make a 'rasayana' of ginger and garlic in the ratio 1:4 and keep it in vinegar. Regular use of this preparation give us immunity to viral and bacterial infections and keep our memory and eye sight properly.*** The hepatoprotective and immunostimulatory effects of garlic were found by various workers[15, 39, 41].

Dr. Stephen De Felice coined the word "Nutraceutical" from "Nutrition" and "Pharmaceutical", in 1989. Any substance that helps nutrition and at the same time prevents diseases come under this group and usually vitamins are not included in them. They are also the functional foods that aids in the prevention and or treatment of diseases or disorders other than anemia. Further nutraceuticals must not only supplement the diet but should also aid in the prevention of diseases and be represented for use as a conventional food or as the sole item of diet.

Conclusion: When a functional food aids in the prevention and treatment of disease(s) and or disorder(s) (except anemia), it is called a nutraceutical. The five classes of them are described above. More of them are yet to come. Most of our traditional food items are endowed with nutraceuticals, however refined food or fast foods are deficient of them.

In addition to the above listed sources of nutraceuticals, various spices and honey are also rich in them. List of spices are attached. **It is advisable to put two to three of them in our diet daily to drive away all types of diseases by stimulating the defense cell system.**

***NB*:** Goat's milk is endowed with many nutraceuticals as it grazes over all kinds of medicinal plants. Gandhiji used to drink only goat's milk. Honey is also enriched with many nutraceuticals as the bees collect them from different flowers.

Functional Foods:

Functional foods with high oxygen radical absorbance capacity (ORAC) are in the order – red wine > black tea > green tea > black currant juice > orange juice > apple > onion according to a table published by book bond centre Bangalore.

ORAC is an index of anti oxidant action. A plant with highest ORAC is Gojibery.

***Spices*:** Caraway, Ginger, Fenugreek, Cardamom, Mustard, Poppy seed, Black cumin, Hyssop, Curry leaf, Cinnamon, Pepperment, Asafoetida, Saffron, Camboge (Malabar tamarind), Pepper, Clove, Nutmeg, Mace, Cumin, Staranise, Long pepper, Basil, Tamarind, Mint, Anise, Turmeric, Coriander, Greater galanga, Red Chilly, Vanila, Garlic, Fennel, All spice, Thyme, Celery.

The order of edible foods with nutracuetical contents is approximately as follows.

Garlic>Ginger>Turmeric>Pomegranate>Citrus fruits > Onion >Apple> Carrot

Additional Information: September issue of the Am. Jour. Med.(2006) reports that the risk of **Alzheimer's** was reduced by 76% for those who drank fruit juices more than three times a week compared with others who drank them less than once a week. The antioxidants in juice are protecting brain from oxidative stress according to the scientists from U.S. and Japan.

Author: He is a Retired Professor of Biochemistry from Kerala and M.G. Universities who is presently Research Professor of Medical Biochemistry in the School of Health Sciences, Thalassery Campus, Palayad (PO) 670 661, India. Recipient of Sastraratna award (2005) from Indian Inst. Scientific Heritage, Trivandrum. The award was presented to him by Dr. K. Mohandas.V.C. of Commen Wealth Universities and Director of SCTIST –Thiruvananthapuram.

References

1. Krishnakumar.K; Augusti..K.T; Vijayammal.P.L., Pharmaceutical Biology 37 (1999)1-5; Ind Jour. Physiol & Pharm. 43 (4) (1999) 510-514
2. Lam-L.K.T., Hasegawa S.Nutrition and Cancer; 12 (1989) 43-45.

3. Luke. K.T.; Hasegawa S. Food phytochemical for cancer prevention II (1994). 209-219. American Chemical Soc.. Washington D.C.
4. Brahmachari.H.D. and Augusti.K.T; J.Pharm and Pharmacol 14(1962) 254
5. Ambika. SH and Rajaramanna Rao.M.R. The Indian Jour. Pharm. 29(1967) 91-94.
6. Venugapalan.C and Srivastava.K.N. J.Food Sci.Technol.33 (1996) 389.
7. Tiwari.N.S. and Jain.P.C. J.Res.Ayur.Siddha I(1) (1980) 121.
8. Nishino,.H. et. al. JPN. J. Cancer Res.77 (1986) 33-38.
9. Chavali.S.R. et. al. Clinical Exp. Immunol. 74 (1988) 675-683.
10. Chavali.S.R. et. al. Int. J. Immunopharmac. 9(1987) 675-683.
11. Nair P.V. et. al. J.Clin.Nutr.40 (1984) 927-930
12. Nakashina H et. al. AIDS 3 (1989) 655-658.
13. Chakravarthy.B.K. et. al. Life Sciences 29 (1980) 2043-2047.
14. Vinod Kumar.R. et. al. Indian Jour. Bichem & Biophys 26(1989) 400-404 and 29 (1992) 380-382.
15. Agusti.K.T. et. al. Indian.J. Exp.Biol 43 (2005) 437-444
16. Geetha.B.S. et. al. Ind.J. Physiol. Pharmacol. 38 (1994) 220-222
17. Sudheesh.S. and Vijayalakshmi.N.R. Fitoterapia 76 (2) (2005) 181-186.
18. Francis. A.R. et. al. Mutation Research 222 (1989) 393-401
19. Guengerich, F.P. and Kim, D.H. Carcinogenesis 11(1990) 2275-2279.
20. Beyeler.S and Bernal.T. Biochem.Pharm. 37 (1988) 1971-1979.
21. Joy.K.L. and Kuttan.R. Jour. Ethnopharmacology 167 (1999) 143-148
22. Damodaran. M and Nair.K.R. Biochem.J. 30 (1936) 1014-1020
23. Pillay.P.P. and Iyer.M.K. Current Sci. 27 (1988) 266-267.
24. Brahmachari.H.D. and Gupta.V.S; Indian J.Appl.Chem.21(1958) 173-174
25. Jeena.K.Jose and Kuttan.R; J.Clin Biochem. Nutr.19(1995) 63-70
26. Ather.M. et. al. Carcinogenesis 11 (1990) 55-61

27. Sayer.J.M. et. al. J.American Chem.Soc 104 (1982) 5562-5564
28. Kuenzing.W. et. al. Carcinogenesis 5 (1984) 309-313.
29. Mei.X et. al. Acta Nutr Sinica 4 (1982) 53.
30. Kuttan.R et. al. Cancer Letters 19. (1985) 197-202
31. Huang.M.T. and Conney.A.H. Cancer Res. 47 (1987) 3012-3032.
32. Sumner.M.D. et. al. AM. J. Cardiol 96(2005) 810
33. Augusti.K.T, Indian J.Exp. Biol 34 (1996) 634-640
34. Helen.A. et. al. Vet Human Toxicol 41(1999) 316-319
35. (a) Helen.A. et. al. Toxicology Letters 116 (2000) 61-68
    (b) Augusti.K.T.: Andrews A et. al. Proceedings of the 19th Kerala Sciences Congress pp.791-93. 29-31 Jan.2007. Kannur
36. Fulder.S. Cardiology in Practice 7(1989) 30-35
37. Bordia.A et. al. AM. J. Clin.Nutr 34 (1981) 2100
38. Lau.B.H.S et. al. J. Urol. 136 (1986) 701-705
39. Lau.B.H.S et. al. Jour Nutr. Res. 10(1990) 937
40. Tarfa.S.P. et. al. Current Sci. 57 (1988) 32-33
41. Haripriya.M. and Girija.K. Amala Res. Bulletin 19(1999) 82-89

2.4 Structures of various Nutraceuticals such as Sulfides, Terpenes, Flavonoids, Poly Phenols etc. present in Functional Foods

Composed by Mohind C. Mohan and Dr. K.T. Augusti,
School of Health Sciences, Kannur University

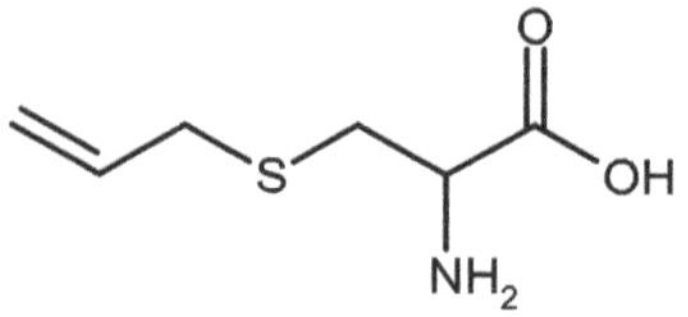

Alliin (Allyl-cysteine)

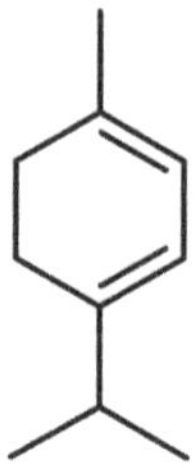

Alpha-terpinene

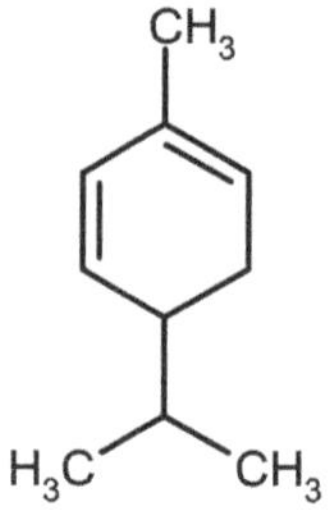

Alpha-phellandren

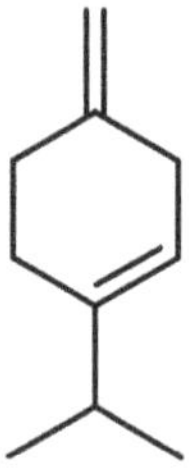

Beta-terpinene

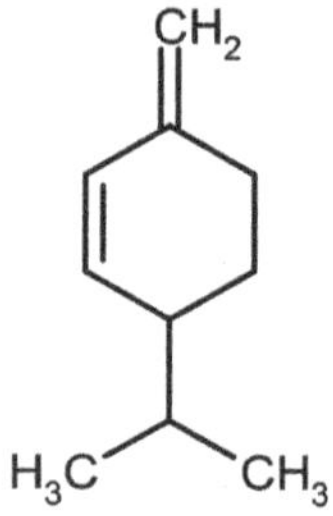

Beta-phellandren

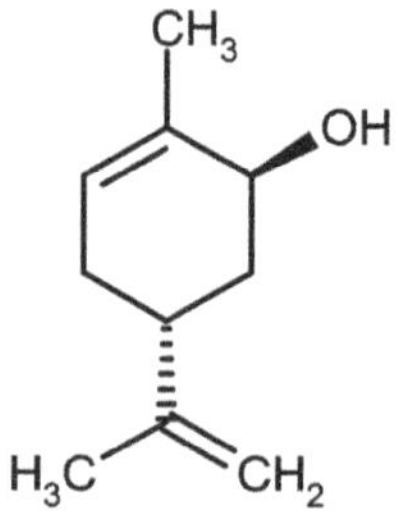

Carveol

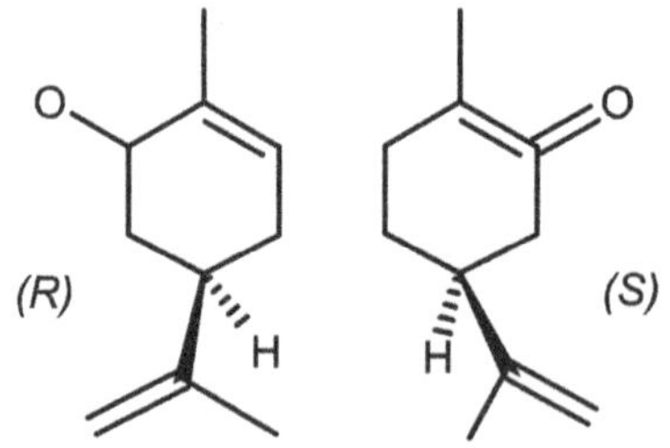

Carvone (Isomers)

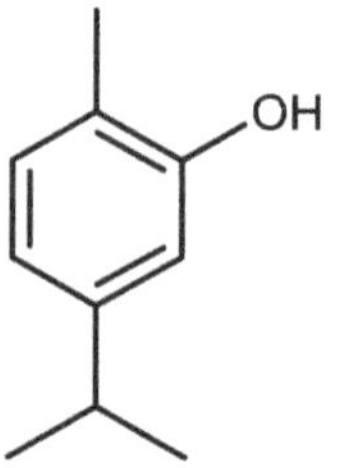

Carvracol

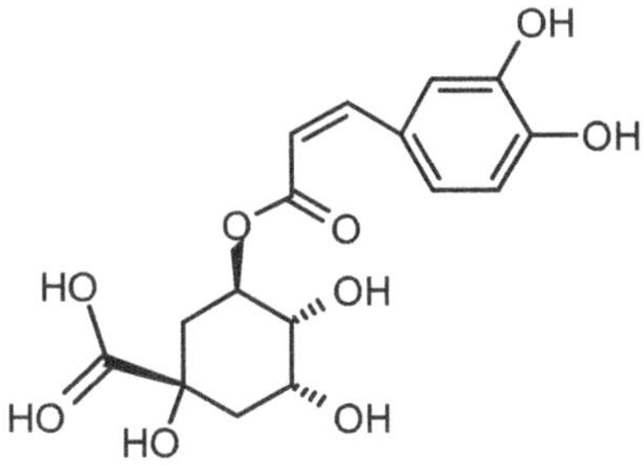

OH
OH
O
O
HO
OH
HO
HO
OH

Chlorogenic-acid

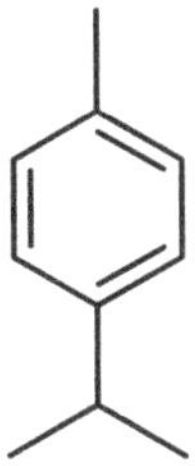

Cymene

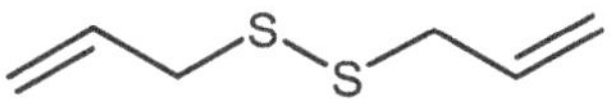

S
S

Diallyl-disulfide

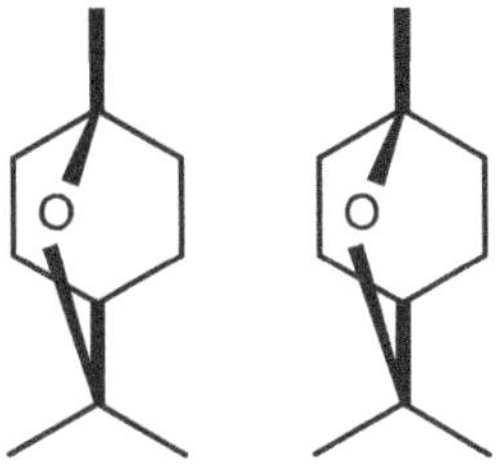

O
O

Eucalyptol (Isomers)

OH

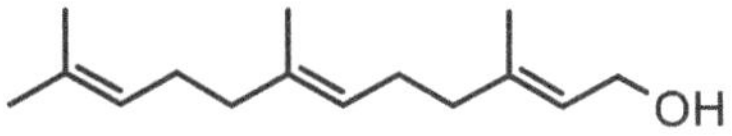

Farnesol

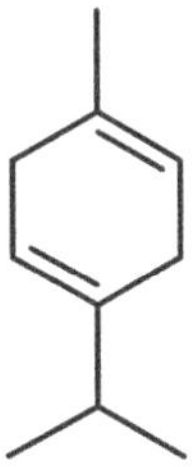

Gamma-terpinene

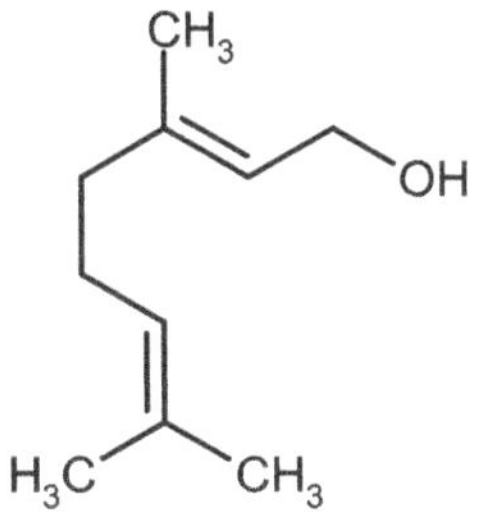

CH_3
OH
H_3C
CH_3

Geraniol

CH_3
CH_3
H_3C
O
O
O—P—O—P—O
O
O

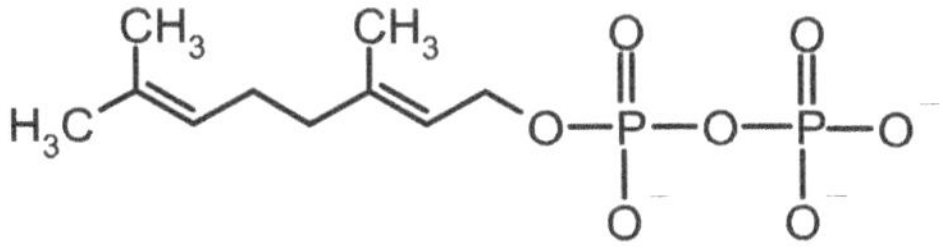

Geranyl-pyrophosphate

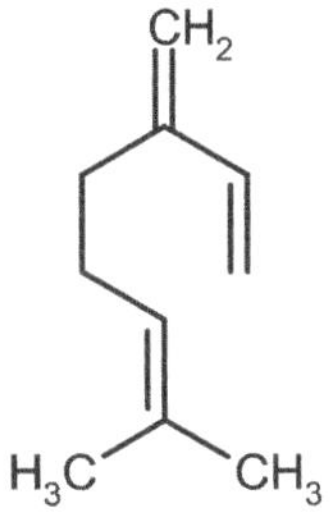

CH_2
H_3C
CH_3

Myrcen

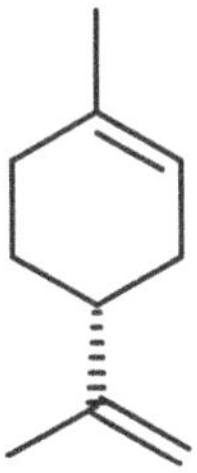

Limonene-2D-skeletal

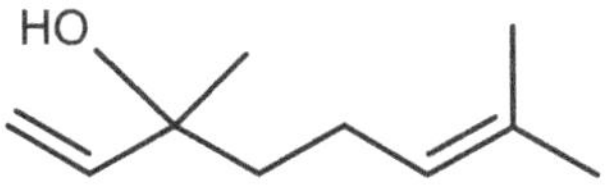

HO

Linalool-skeletal

OH
HO
O
OH
OH
O

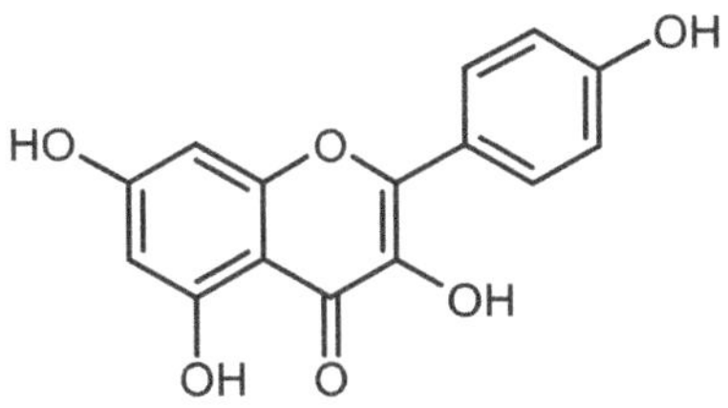

kaempferol

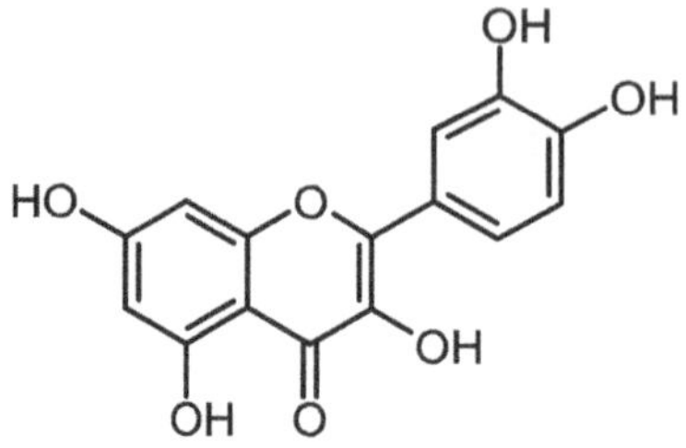

Quercetin

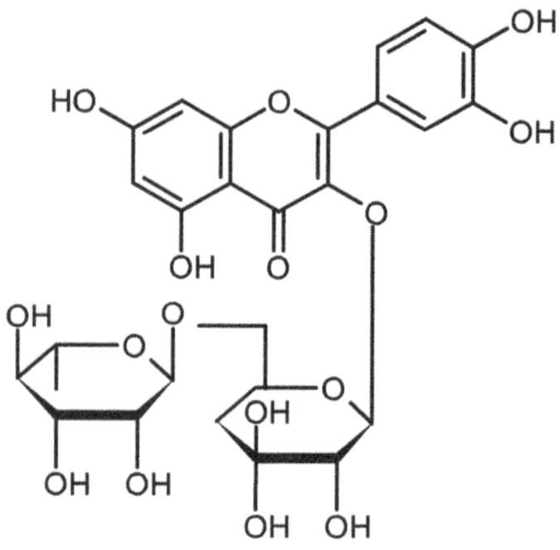

Rutin

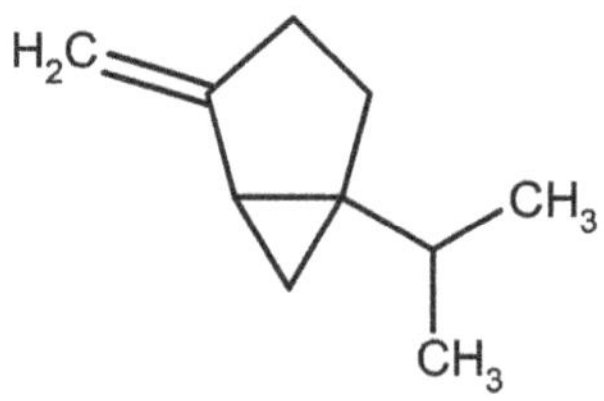

Sabinene

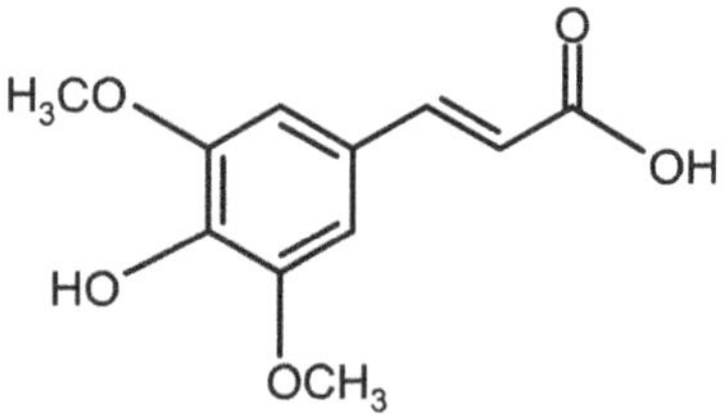

Sinapic-acid

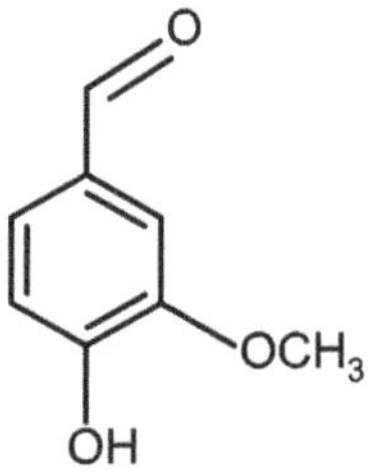

Vanillin

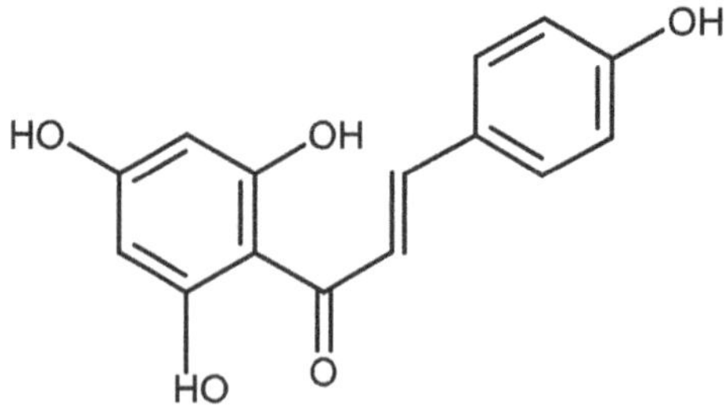

Chalcone

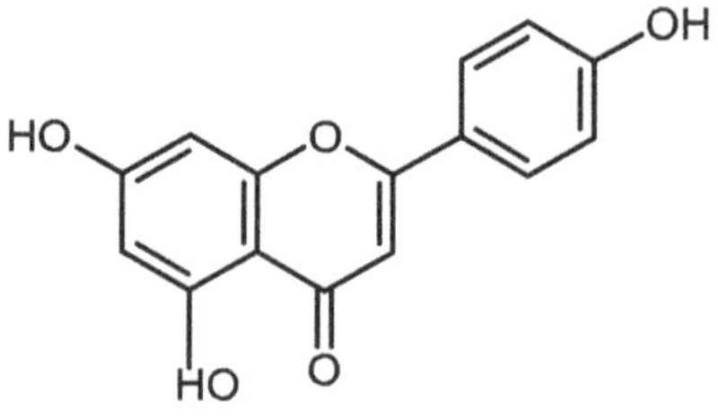

A Flavone

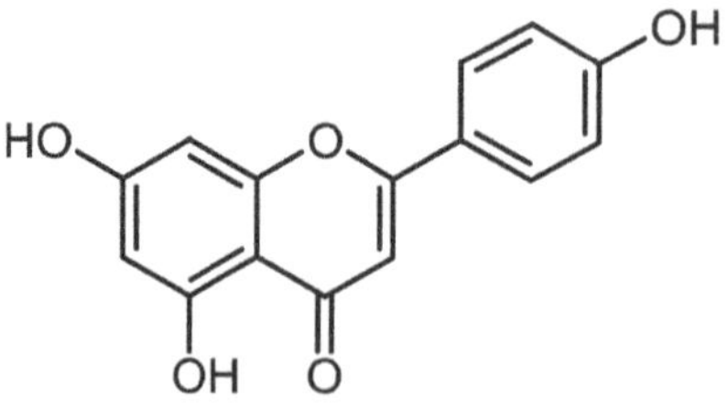

Apigenin

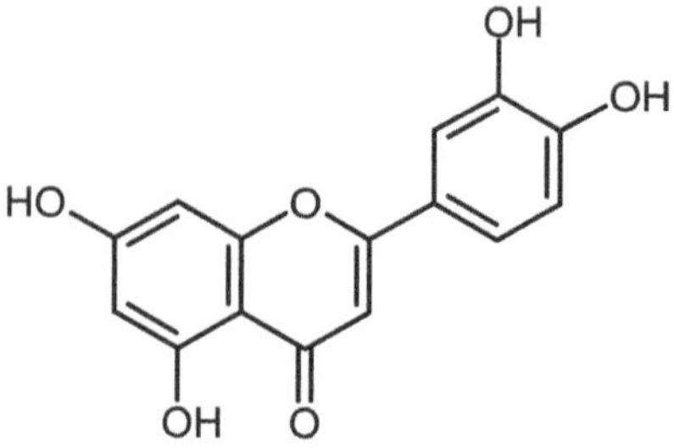

luteolin

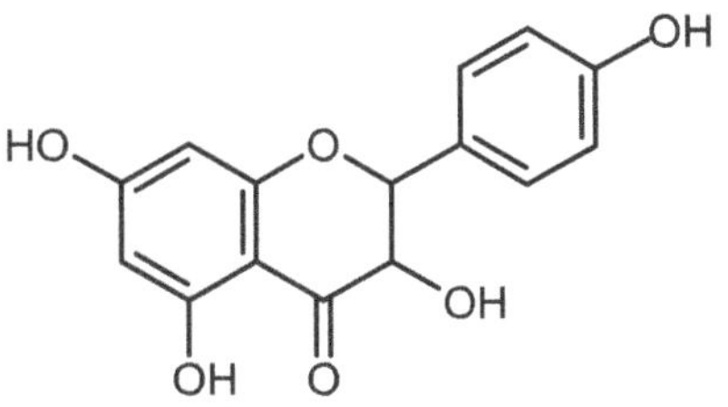

A Flavonol

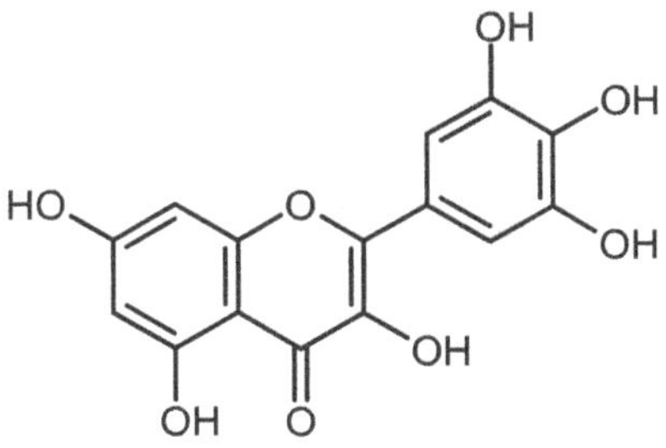

Myricetin

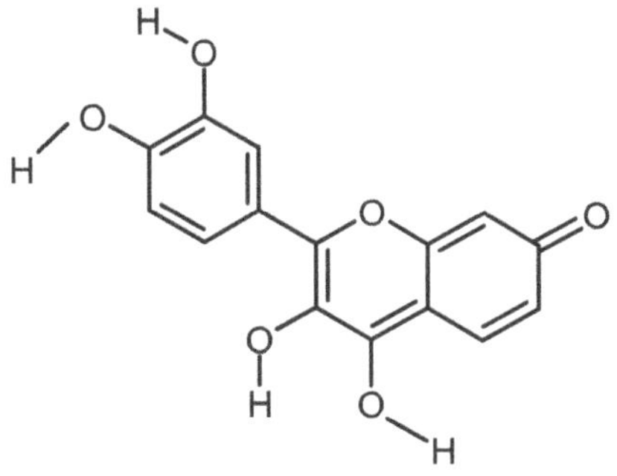

Fisetin

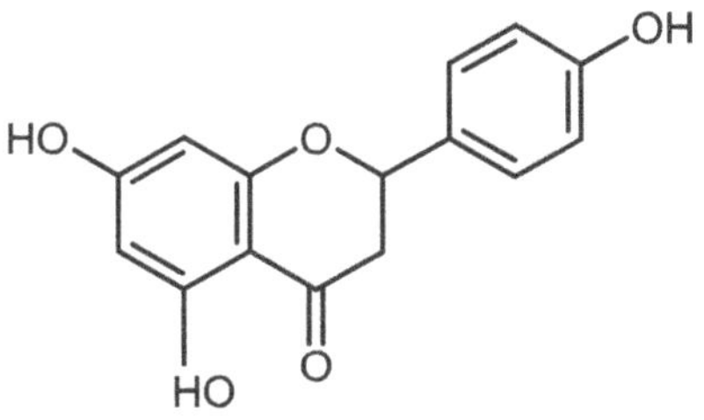

A Flavanone

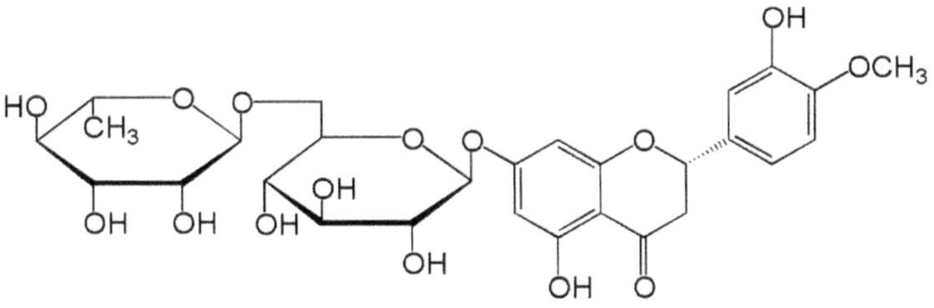

Hesperidin

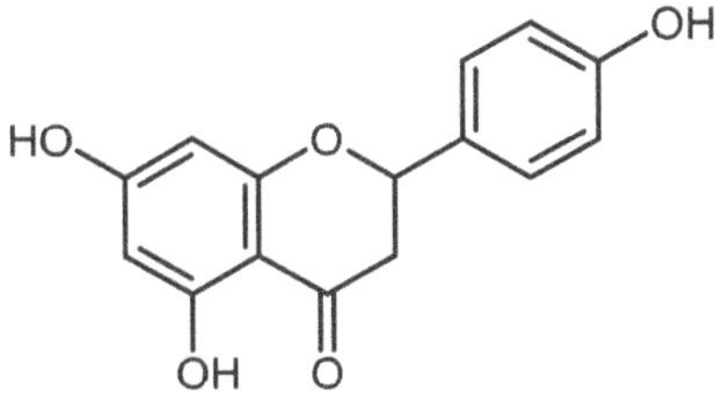

Naringenin

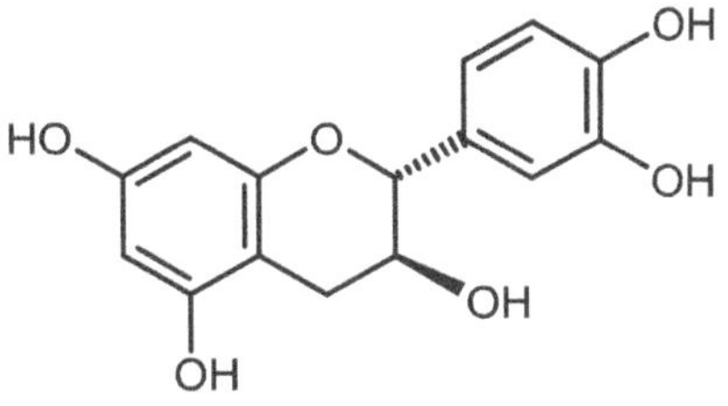

Catechin

Epicatechin

Epigallocatechin

An Isoflavonoid

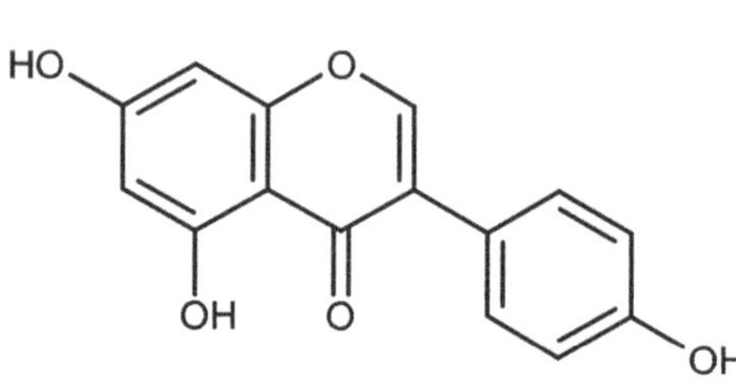

Genistein

Daidzein

An Anthocyanin

A trans form of punicic acid ('catalpic' acid). – present in pomegtanate

6 shogaol (double bond at 6th carbon)

limonene

30
COOH
21
22
18
O
H
28
H
β − D − GlcA —— β − D − GlcA —— O
H
24

Glycyrrhizic acid (1)

OH
1
OCH_3
6
2
5
3
4
1 CH_2
CH_2
3
H_2C

Eugenol

O
C
CH_2
CH_2
CH_2
CH
OH
$(CH_2)_n$
CH_3
HO
OCH3

cinnamate pathway | polyketide or acetate pathway

Gingerol

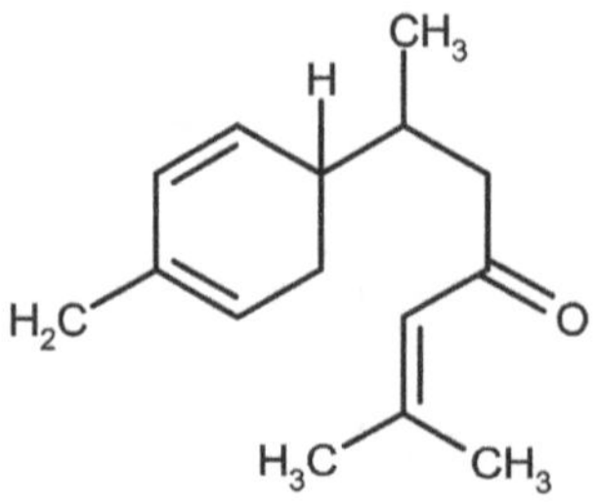

H
CH_3
H_2C
O
H_3C CH_3

α-Tumerone $C_{15}H_{22}O$

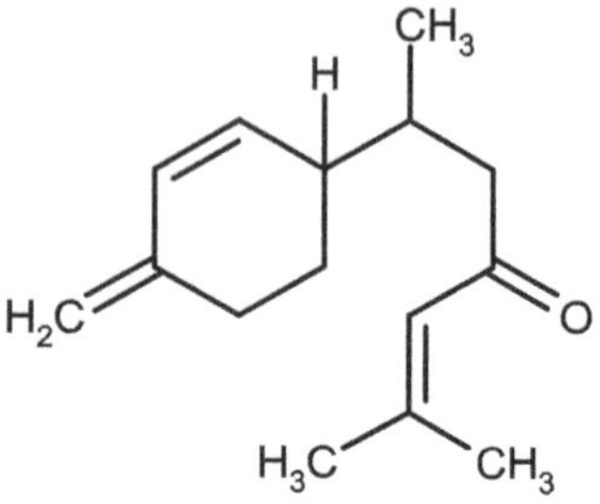

H
CH_3
H_2C
O
H_3C CH_3

β-Tumerone $C_{15}H_{22}O$

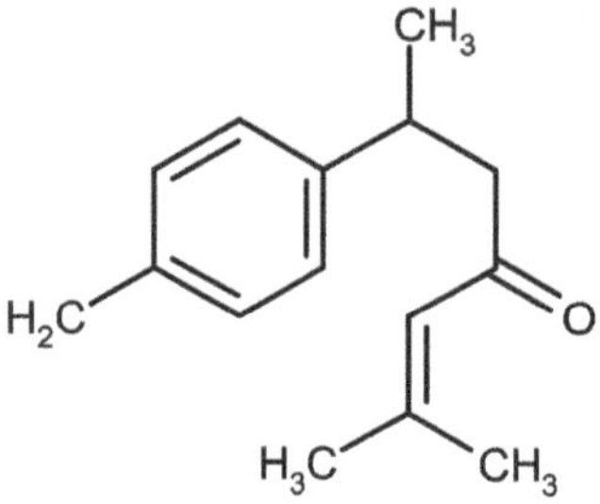

CH_3
H_2C
O
H_3C CH_3

Ar-Tumerone $C_{15}H_{20}O$

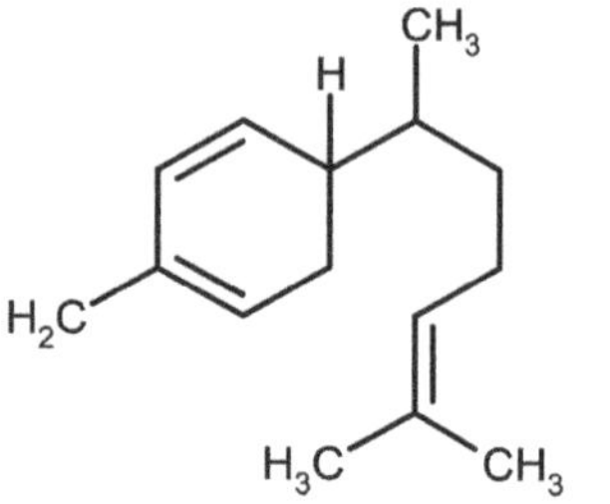

H
CH_3
H_2C
H_3C CH_3

(–)-α-Tumerone $C_{13}H_{24}$

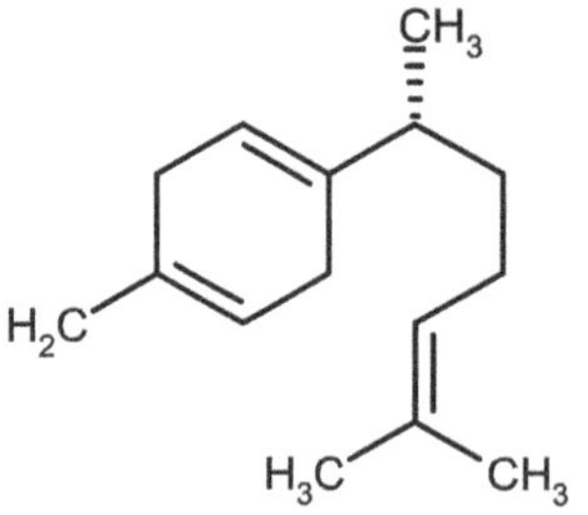

CH_3
H_2C
H_3C CH_3

β-Curcumene $C_{13}H_{24}$

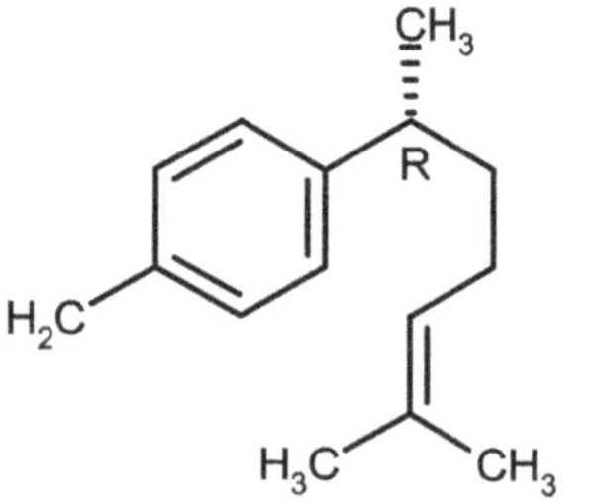

CH_3
R
H_2C
H_3C CH_3

(–)-ar-Curcumene $C_{13}H_{22}$

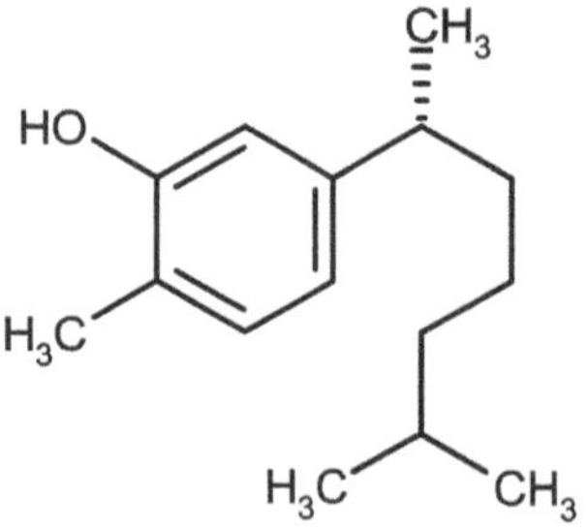

CH_3
HO
H_3C
H_3C CH_3

Xanthorrhizol $C_{15}H_{22}O$
(Hydroxy-ar-curcumene)

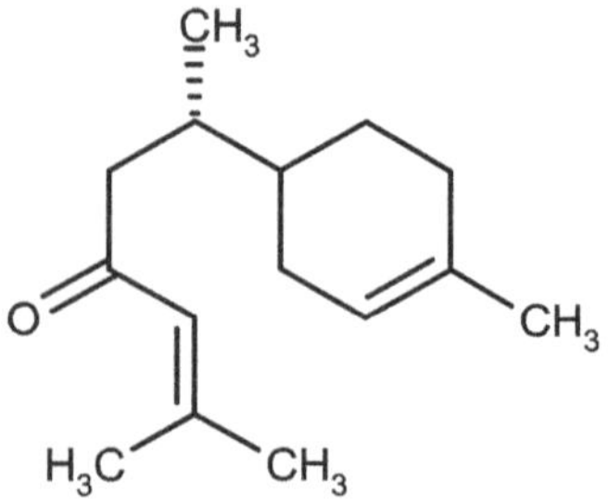

CH_3
O
CH_3
H_3C CH_3

Atlantone (α and γ).

Sesquiterpenoids of Curcuma Longa.

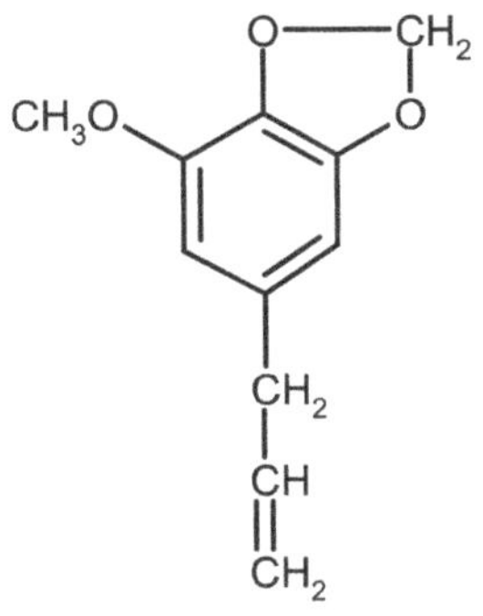

Myristicin

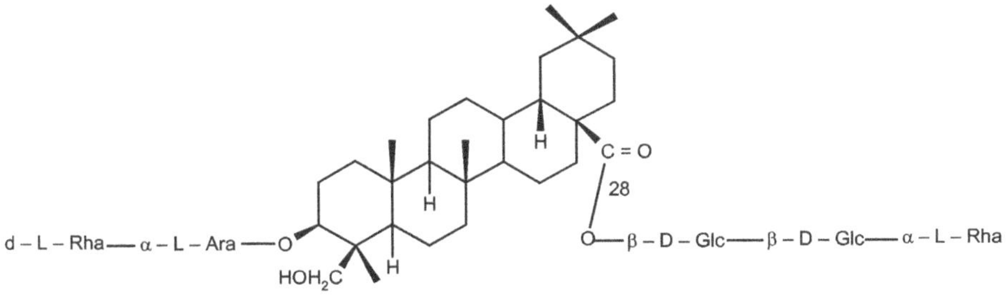

Hederasaponin C (2)

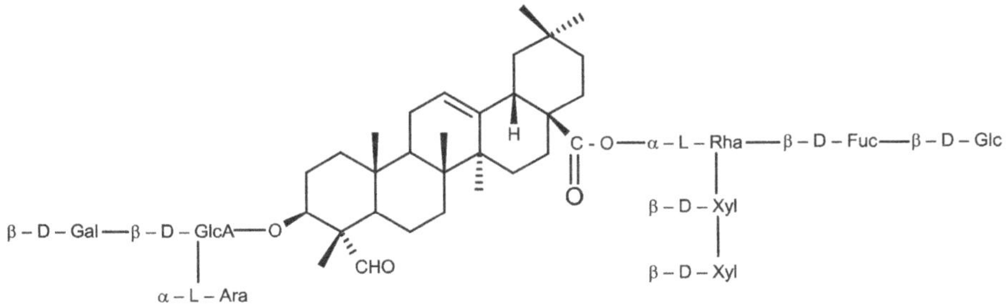

Gypsoside A (7)

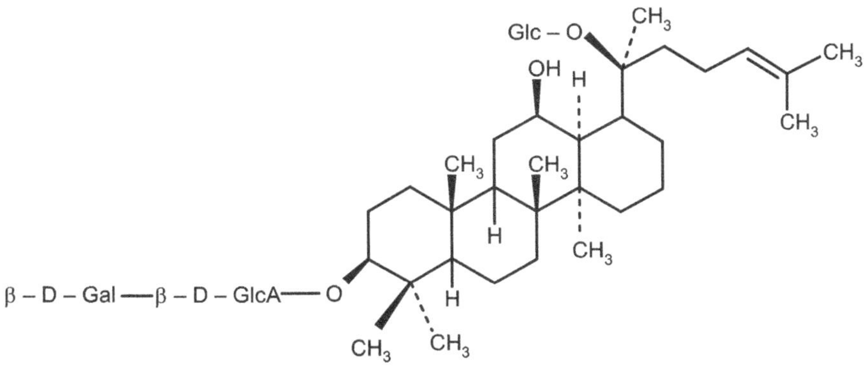

Ginsenoside Rd (5)

Beta-Sitosterol

Mangiferin

Glycyrrhizin = Ca^{2-} & K^{-} salts of Glycyrrhizinic acid

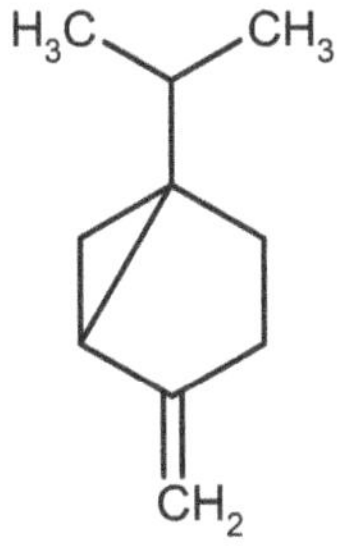

Sabinene

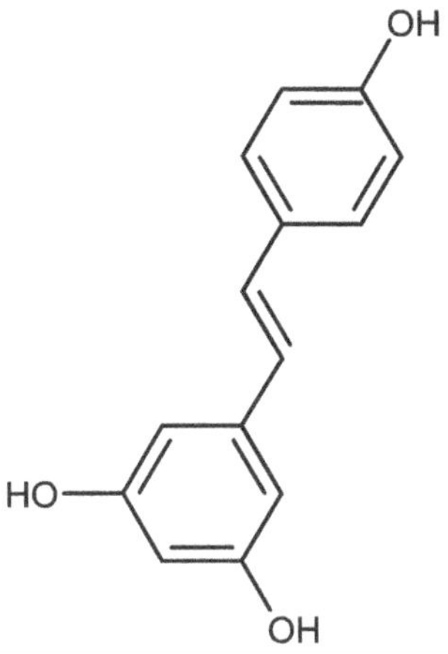

Resveratrol

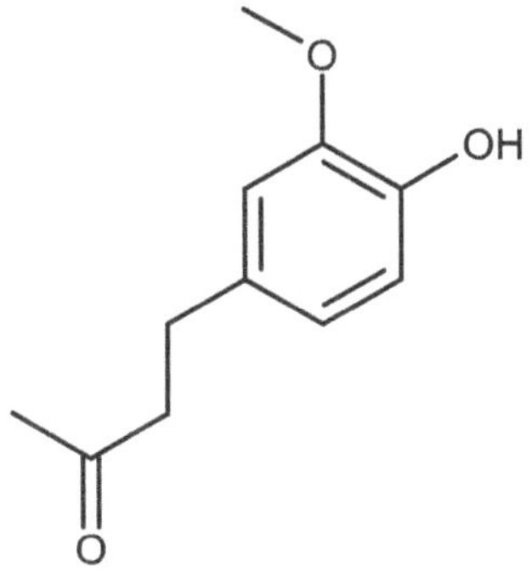

Zingerone

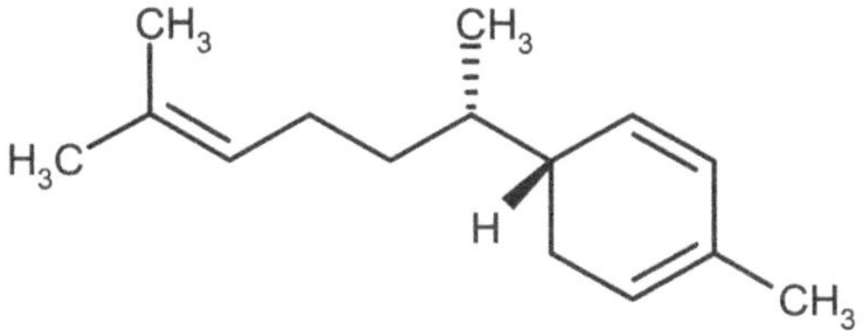

Zingiberene

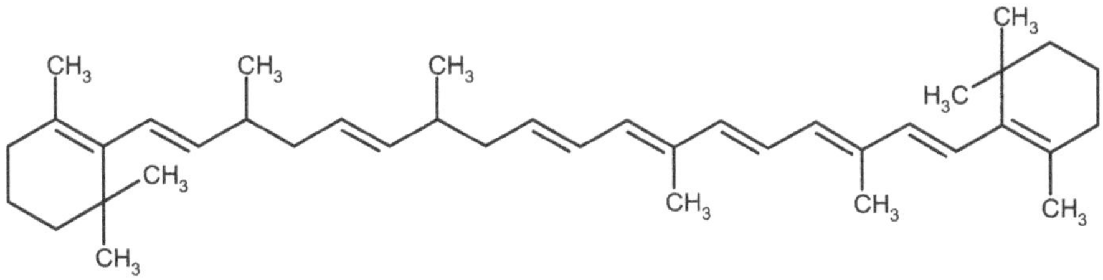

Beta Carotene

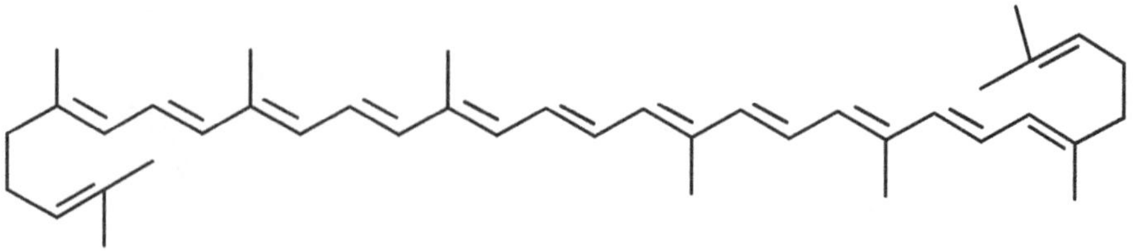

Lycopene
Molecular Weigh 536.89
Molecular Formula $C_{40}H_{56}$

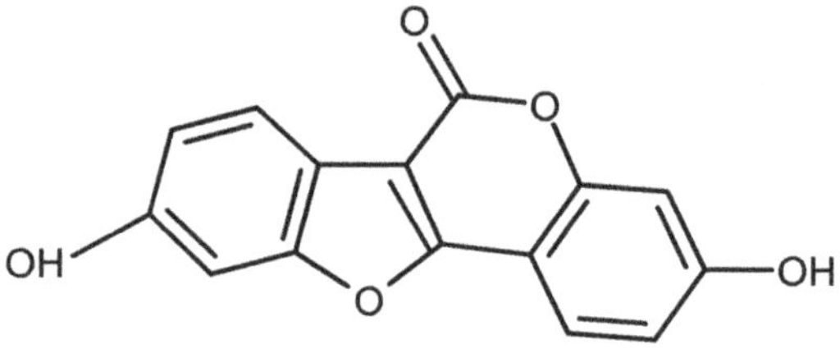

OH O OH O O OH

Coumesterol

H H O

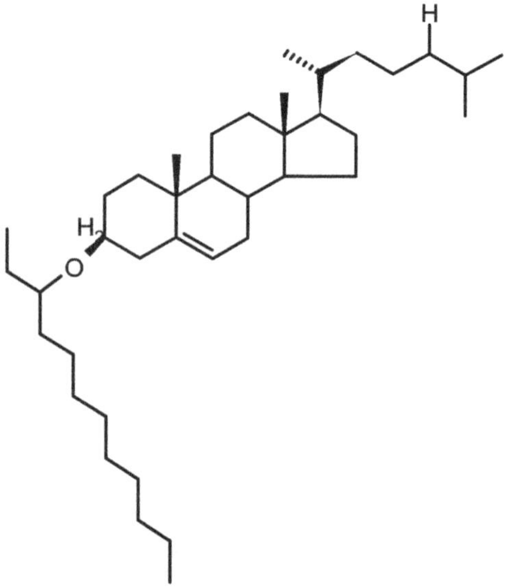

Brassicasterol

Table 1 Plant Sources of the saponins.

Saponin	Plant Source
Glycyrrhizic acid	Glycyrrhiza glabra L.
Hederasaponin C	Hedera helix L.
β-Aescin	Aesculus hippocastanum L.
Helianthoside 2	Helianthus annuus L.
Ginsenoside Rd	Panax ginseng C.A. Mey.
Quillajasaponin	Quillaja saponaria Mol.
Saponinum album	Gypsophila paniculata L.

The vevet skinned baobab Fruit:

This fruit's flesh is full of vitamin C, calcium and antioxidants. It is an elongated fruit found in Africa [e.g., Nigeria] and and is becoming a favourite more than pomegranate. The baobab jam, made from the pulp looks like honey and it is appetizing.

2.5 Free Radical Level and Life Span

Dr. K.T. Augusti,
(Presently Research Professor of Medical Bio. chem. S.H.S. Kannur University)

In elements the electrons are moving in different orbitals and different directions. For e.g: an element contains two electrons in its outermost orbit and they move in opposite directions. If one of them is lost the remaining one orbit is in a higher potential energy. Then this form of the element or its combination is called a free radical. If oxygen traps an electron then that contains an excess electron over the normal one. Then this oxygen is called a superoxide, it can part with this excess electron to a proton and make it hydrogen peroxide a precursor of hydroxy free redical ($OH^•$). Thus super oxide and H_2O_2 are precursors of free radicals. This $OH^•$, Free radical can pluck away a hydrogen atom from sugars, lipids or proteins and make a new free radical out of the attacked molecule. The removed hydrogen atom combines with attacking $OH^•$ and produces water. The newly created free radicals start the chain reaction in the system, and produce a series of free radicals which in due course damage the cellular components if they are not neutralized in time by antioxidants free radical scavengers.

The origin and production of free radicals are represented below.

$$O_2 + e^- \rightarrow O_2^{•} - \text{(superoxide)} \qquad \ldots..1$$

$$2O_2^{•} + 2H^+ \underset{SOD}{\rightarrow} H_2O_2 + O_2 \qquad \ldots..2$$

$$Fe^{2+} + H_2O_2 \rightarrow Fe^{3+} + OH^- + OH^{•} \qquad \ldots..3$$

$$\underset{\text{(Free radical)}}{OH^{•}} + RH \rightarrow \underset{\text{(New free radical)}}{R^{•}} + H_2O \qquad \ldots..4$$

SOD is super oxide dismutase that converts $O_2^{•-}$ to hydrogen peroxide. Eventhough hydrogen free radical ($H^•$) induces reduction in other compounds, oxygen generated free radicals e.g.: O_2^{*-}, $OH^•$, $ROO^•$, do more harm by inducing chain reactions. Compounds originated from oxygen free radicals e.g; H_2O_2, HClO induce oxidations. These compounds/Free radicals put together are called reactive oxygen species (ROS). As coffee contains H_2O_2 and caffeine, excess coffee may be avoided.

H_2O_2 is decomposed by the actions of catalase and glutathione peroxidase (Free radical Scavenging enzymes Reactions 5 & 6) respectively

$$2H_2O_2 \rightarrow 2H_2O + O_2 \quad \text{.....5}$$

$$2GSH + H_2O_2 \rightarrow GSSG + H_2O \quad \text{.....6}$$

Free radicals have merits and demerits. They are responsible for killing germs, i.e. ingested or extracellular bacteria. Oxidative reactions in biological systems due to oxidative stress generate free radicals under physiological conditions. For e.g; cytochrome P_{450} and cyclooxygenase generate free radical intermediates. Thus the production of free radicals would appear to be a natural part of cellular metabolism. One of the early events in normal inflammatory reaction is increased activation and migration of leucocytes into the inflamed area. Leucocytes namely macrophages and neutrophils possess the enzyme NADPH oxidase, which catalyzes the one electron reduction of O_2 to O_2^{*-} which can potentially through a series of reactions, catalyzed by metal ions generate the other oxygen free radicals (OFRs). Leucocytes also possess other enzymes, e.g; myeloperoxidase, which generates HClO from H_2O_2. Such free radicals are normally used by leucocytes to kill bacteria.

Children suffering from chronic granulomatous disease die from bacterial infections because they have a genetic defect which prevents their leucocytes from generating OFRs. However over production of free radicals lead to damages to the retina, the eye lens and many receptors on our cell surfaces. They damage β cells of the islets of Langerhans and induce diabetes mellitus. Similarly excess free radicals lead to lipid peroxidation mainly in liver and heart. The former leads to liver diseases and the latter induces CHD. Further the free radicals damages mitochondrial DNA which leads to mutation and the expression of oncogenes that produce cancer. The damage of DNA takes place because ROS convert amino groups of bases to keto groups and sugar groups attached to them to new free radicals. Another major problem with free radicals is the production of cataract and the process of ageing. Prolonged hyperglycemia as in uncontrolled diabetes mellitus may lead to autooxidation and production of superoxide. Therefore control of diabetes throughout the life of a DM patient is absolutely necessary to avoid diabetic retinopathy, neuropathy and nephropathy. Chronic DM patients suffer from massive heart attack

because of the onslaught of free radicals. Therefore you can imagine how important for good health to control b.s. level and all other sources of free radical production. Free radicals can also oxidise LDL which may lead to atherosclerosis (hardening of blood vessels) that induces CHD. As exercise enhances ATP production and expenditure, it may lessen the chances of electron escape from respiratory chain, i.e. ETC–generated electron may be less there to convert respiratory O_2 to super oxide (O_2^{*-}). Occasional fasting may also curtail the production of electrons and superoxide.

Therefore the younger generation should agree to the fact that the age old practices of lent/fasting etc. did only improve our health aspect and when we threw away this practice all the risk factors doubled up for CHD and cancer. An experiment on animals proves the advantages of less food consumption. When the food of experimental rats was reduced to 2/3 of its original and normal intake, eventhough their body weight and size were reduced considerably their life span increased by 50%. Now let us have a look at our old religious practices. Hindus in Kerala had 40 days lent prior to their piligrimage to Sabarimala. During these days they remained strict vegetarians. Similarly Christians had two lents viz: 25 days prior to X'mas and 50 days prior to Easter. They also remained strict vegetarians on both these occasions. These systems helped both the groups to take plenty of green vegetables which contained lot of free radical scavengers.

Now modernism almost discouraged both the groups to reduce the lents just to 3-5 days a year. Moslems also had a strict lent for one month during Ramadhan. Eventhough they do not stick to vegetarianism they do not eat three times a day but only once in the night with lot of fruits, nuts etc. This helped them a lot to improve their health. Many reports are there that during Ramadhan Moslem-diabetic patients get a better blood sugar control. Now they also rarely do this practice.

Antioxidants/Free Radical Scavengers

Organic sulphides, their sulphoxides, cysteine derivatives as found in onions, garlic and cabbage, β-carotene found in carrots, certain fruits and leaves, e.g; Moringa leaves, flavonoids found in many fruits and bark, polyphenols found in tea, curcumin found in curcuma longa, many terpenes found in spices and the vitamins like C and E are good antioxidants. They neutralize oxidants, i.e. ROS like hydroxy and peroxy radicals. The above vitamins, flavanoids, curcumin and polyphenols are donors of hydrogen to free radicals that can antioxidize and scavenge hydroxy and peroxy radicals ($ROO^{\bullet}$). The above antioxidants may be represented as ROH. Terpenes and β carotene have double bonds and they can easily donate the electron and nutralise the ROS. Organic sulfides and their oxides can easily absorb electrons and break into harmless free radicals and neutralize harmful ROS. These reactions can be represented as follows.

$$ROH + OH^{\bullet} \rightarrow RO^{\bullet} + H_2O \text{ and } RH + OH^{\bullet} \rightarrow R^{\bullet} + H_2O$$

$$R^{\bullet} + O_2 \rightarrow ROO^{\bullet} \text{ then } \quad ROO^{\bullet} + ROH \rightarrow ROOH + RO^{\bullet}$$

$ROO^{\bullet}$ is an intermediate in lipid per oxidation also and it is very harmful.

Vitamin C can regenerate vitamin E from its $RO^{\bullet}$ form also

$RO^{\bullet}$ + ROH (Vit. C) → ROH (Vit. E) + Dehydroascorbic acid.

$$\text{Dehydroascorbic acid} + 2GSH \xrightarrow[\text{Dehydroascorbic reductase}]{} \text{Vit. C} + GSSG$$

β carotene + $OH^{\bullet}$ → β Carotene^{+} + OH^{-} (stable hydroxy radical)

Similarly compounds with conjugated double bonds help to scavenge free radicals. Organic sulphides scavenge free radicals as follows.

$$RSSR + e^{-} \rightarrow RSSR^{-} \rightarrow RS^{\bullet} + RS^{-}$$

$$RS^{-} + OH^{\bullet} \rightarrow RS^{\bullet} + OH^{-} \text{ and } RSH + OH^{\bullet} \rightarrow RS^{\bullet} + H_2O$$

$RS^{\bullet} + RS^{\bullet} \rightarrow RSSR$ and the cycle repeats and scavenge any number of free radicals. As organic sulphides and their cysteine and oxide derivatives are available in plenty in onions, garlic, cabbage and asafetida, their additions to our diet help us to scavenge ROS regularly and spare our body from the onslaught of them. Moringa leaves contain fiber, β carotene and vitamin C. So I call it a three in one. Fiber is good to scavenge cholesterol.

According to Dr. Bordia, Moringa fruits contain ω_3FAs and Se also. Se is a good antioxidant too.

Therefore as all green vegetables, (e.g.; various leaves, beans and fruits) and onions, garlic, cabbage, carrots and tea contain antioxidants, their regular use shall help our body to scavenge all types of ROS. In addition to them all sources of vitamins C and E are also good to supply antioxidants. e.g.; germinated seeds, citrus fruits, vegetable oils, fish oils etc. There are reports that the use of above vegetables reduces the incidence of CHD and cancer. In my former department of biochemistry at Kariyavattom Campus of Kerala University, before I shifted to M.G. University my students have demonstrated the antioxidant actions of banyan tree flavanoids, onion and garlic sulphur compounds and garlic protein. We have observed the beneficial effects of these compounds in lowering the free radical levels in high fat or alcohol fed rats and also in nicotine injected rats. Dr. Vijayalekshmy demonstrated the antioxidant action of a plantane flavonoid. Dr. Vijayammal and myself worked on the benefits of antioxidants on nicotine and published the results.

Main Pathways of Free Radical Production

Free radicals and related ROS are produced mainly through four normal ways.

1. From Electron Transport Chain (ETC) that is responsible for ATP production and as hydrogen combines with respiratory oxygen some electrons escape and produce ROS e.g; $OH^{\bullet}$ (See reactions 1-3)
2. Through the activities of enzymes like Xanthine oxidase and aldehyde dehydrogenase many ROS are also produced.
3. Through NADPH oxidase system, ROS are produced in leukocytes.
4. In erythrocytes when oxygen combines with haemoglobin some ROS are produced. It is assumed that between 1 and 5% of all O_2 used in metabolism escapes as free radicals.

In addition to the above ways if our body is exposed to X-rays or U.V. rays ROS are produced enormously. In Cobalt ^{60} therapy its radiations split the water in our body fluids and produce free radicals which destroy cancer cells as well as normal cells nearby.

$$3H_2O \xrightarrow{\text{Radiation}} H_2 + H^{\bullet} + OH^{\bullet} + H_2O_2 \text{ etc.}$$

UV radiation through Ozone holes in the sky falls on animal body and produces free radicals. This may induce skin cancer. Thus radiation is a tool for cancer cure and also cancer induction. If the free radical production in our body is uncontrolled as in conditions of alcoholism, over eating and smoking, they damage many of our biological systems. For e.g; in additions to what stated earlier they oxidize many amino acids and produce harmful amines like histamine, tryptamine, terramine etc. The oxygen free radicals oxidize proline in collagens to hydroxyl prolines that hardens the skin. When wounds are healed scars appear because of the action of free radicals on collagen of our skin. Similarly on ageing our skin hardens and rinkles appear because of the actions of uncontrolled free radicals on the skin. **Age related diseases are mainly the after effects of free radicals. The ROS bring about damages to our neurons and various receptors on the cells. In aged people the defects in secretory glands, eye sight and memory are partly due to the onslaught of free radicals and partly due to metabolic defects/nutritions etc.**

Excerpts from the Presidential address of Dr. K. Madhawankutty, Former Director of Medical Education Govt. of Kerala at the National Seminar on Nutraceuticals.

Plants are the fountain – head of medicine

Plants provide us nearly 35% of the medicines and drugs that we use, so much so, that many pharmaceutical companies have collecting centres specially for plants used as drugs in many forests of the 3rd world. The list of such drugs is endless.

Neem, Opium, Olive, Iris, Sarpagandhi, Vinca rosea, Thulasi, Turmeric, Ginger, Eucalyptus, Lemon Grass, Aarogyapacha (a green plant for health used by tribes), Ginseng, Sandal wood, Cinchona, Vep, Lime, Onion, Garlic, Cashew, Tomatoes, Coccinia Indica, Black pepper, Garcinia Cambogia (Kodampuli), Bitter gourd, Ash gourd, Amla (goose berry) Sugar cane, Moringa, Pomegranate, Papaya, Betel leave and various spices are on the list (More than 200 plants).

Many of these have been our household articles of food from times immemorial and perhaps have given way for more modern (fashionable) vegetables. For as Marktwain put it humorously "Training is every thing". For many peach was once a bitter almond, a cauliflower is nothing but a cabbage with college education.

In fact the WHO is now actively encouraging developing countries to use herbal medicines, which they have been traditionally using for countries and have identified 3000 plants which come from the forest of India and other tropical countries. The active ingredients from these plants are worth nearly Rs.20000/- millions for U.S. market alone and nearly 8 times that for the world market.

The papers being presented here have great relevance for solving the problems of the present world. Let us encourage the so called functional foods viz; items of food enriched with antioxidants/nutraceuticals etc. Only when we gave up all these things and resorted to a cola, hamburger, pizza, fast food culture, did our country become the world capital for obesity/diabetes etc.

Editors comments: Many medical people slowly recognize now that functional food contains medicinally active compounds called nutraceuticals other than vitamins, minerals etc. and that they can function as antioxidants and prevent many fatal diseases like cancer, CHD, DM, Dementia etc. Mushrooms are the latest addition to the list of functional foods.

Most of the nutraceuticals are antioxidants and they are present in our functional foods viz; onions, garlic, turmeric, ginger, limes, oranges, carrots, tea, amla, papaya, pomegranate, grapes, apples, mangoes, sweet potatoes, green leaves, mushrooms etc. Therefore regular addition of one or more of these dietary components in our food shall prevent various cancers, CHD, dementia, Alzheimer's disease and ageing. These are compiled from the panel discussion on Nutraceuticals at the National Seminar on the "Evaluation of Nutraceuticals that prevent diseases," held under Kannur University at Thalassery Campus during 28th Nov. to 2nd Dec. 2006.

Panel Members

Dr. Arun Bordia, Rtd. Cardiologist of RNT Medical College, Udaipur, Rajasthan.

Dr. K. Bhaskaran, Prof. of Pharmacology, Pariyaram Medical College, Kannur

Dr. B. Nagarajan, Prof. of Oncology, Cancer Inst. Chennai-20.

Dr. P. R. Sudhakaran, Prof and head of the Dept. of Biochemistry, Kerala Univerisity.

Dr. K.T.Augusti, Prof. and Head of the Dept. of Medical Biochemistry, School of Health Sciences, Kannur University Campus at Thalassery and Organising Secretary of the Seminar.

This book is the outcome of their combined efforts to give it as a legacy for the young generation.

2.6 Role of Diet in the Prevention of Cancer & C.H.D

Dr. K Madhavan kutty, MBBS, MSc, FABMS, FAMS.
Director, Centre for Medical Education & Formerly Principal of the Calicut, Alleppey, Trichur & Trivandrum Medical College

For a very long time medical experts believed that all diseases were caused by germs. The discovery of viruses strenghthened this belief. But it became increasingly clear that this is not a problem which can be solved so easily. Take the lovely example of the common cold. We all know that cold is caused by a special virus. **But all who come into contact with this virus do not get the disease. On the other hand, the contact must be coupled with reduced immunity of the individual, the climate, the state of the individual's stress and so on.** All these have to be taken into consideration before we come to a definite conclusion.

The case of cancer is at the other end of the spectrum. We need to believe that there is a cause-effect relationship between a carcinogen and malignancy, for example inhalation of asbestos gives rise to lung cancer. Only one or two is likely to be affected out of a thousand people who are exposed to the same situation. Is it an allergic phenomenon or is there any genetic transposition that makes him a victim to cancer? We have no answer.

What is Immunity ?

The immune system is a highly complex and sophisticated system. Like an army[1], it keeps a corps of cells with specific tasks and these cells are always in a state of readiness and challenge. Some cells like monocytes act as Sentinels whereas B cell derived antibodies and T.cells act as infantry and artillery. The helper T.cells cause the alaram reaction and the suppressor T cells block it. The macrophages are scavanger cells who clean up the battlefield and remove the debris caused by the battle. Certain plant principles or Neutraceuticals help in the working of these cells[2]. It is estimated that the human organism is capable of generating upto a billion numbers of distinct antibody molecules to attack foreign cells who are invaders, and can clearly remember these invaders. That is why vaccination which is highly selective succeeds. This flurry of activity cannot be organized and co-ordinated unless they constantly send messages back and forth. A cell sends a message of squirting a small short-lived peptide. The immune cells should have receptors to receive these messages. It has been proved that immune cells also contain opiate receptors, including the brain peptides or endorphins, which can alter the mood of the individual and can in fact work like a self-made opium molecule.

Plants, The Fountain Head of Medicine

Plants provide us with nearly 30% of the medicines and drugs that we use, so much so, that many pharmaceutical companies have collection centres specifically for plants used as drugs in many areas in the developing countries from where the product is transported in bulk. The list of such drugs is endless. Opium, olive, Iris, Sarpagandhi, Vinca rosea, Thulasi, Sandalwood, Cinchona, Ginseng, Neem and various others including most of the spices are on the list. In fact, the W.H.O is now actively encouraging developing countries to use herbal medicine, which they have been traditionally for centuries and have identified 3000 plants which come from the forests of India and other tropical countries. The export market for these herbal material to the U.S. market alone is of the order of Rs.200 crores (2000 million), and 8 times that if the world market is taken into consideration. Though marginal attempts have been made by the governmental agencies, it is quite unfortunate that the Government of India is not alive to this gold mine.

Traditional herbal remedies

Today, there is a revival of interest in developing this field and many private entrepreneurs have started exploring the possibilities of manufacturing herbal remedies in a big way. There are at least reasons for this. One is the economic gain, the second is the effectiveness of these remedies and the third is the fact that it produces no after effects. The use of the herbal remedies is not only the hall mark of ayruvedic medicine, but has been used by the adivasis of our country from times immemorial. Whether it was in the Amazon valley, or the forests of Africa, West Indies, China, Indonesia, Myanmar, Srilanka, and even in European Countries like Germany, Italy, France, Russia, and Switzerland. From 1987-1990, the author of this article was the principal investigator and project director of a scheme sanctioned by the Government of India to study the use of plants for treatment of diseases by the adivasis of Kerala. We conducted a survey on behalf of the KANFED (Kerala Association for Non Formal Education and Development) especially in the adiwasi belts of Wyanad and Attappadi. We were able to publish the results in a book "Drugs used in Tribal Medicine in Kerala" where we have described about the medicinal use of more than 300 such medicinal plants.

Vegetables and Cancer

Doctors have been warning patients for centuries that they are what they eat. In fact this is one of the basic tenets of "Nature Cure Therapy". The famous Framingham study is about the relationship of food habits and Blood pressure/C.H.D.

Untill recently the link between diet and Cancer had rested on macroevidence which came primarily from population studies which showed that some societies had specific types of Cancer depending on their food habits[3,4]. For example people who traditionally eat smoked fish in the coastal districts of Kerala are prone to get oesophageal cancer. People in advanced countries like U.S.A whose food consisted of processed food, mainly of meat origin, without the necessary roughage and fibre had a higher percentage of gastrointestinal cancer, especially colon cancer. People who imbibed a special kind of beer in certain parts of France and Germany had a predilection to get Carcinoma of Liver. Several such cases have been recorded of relationship between food and cancer.

Now the focus has shifted from these population studies as they cannot be modified immediately to the study of the components of plant, and animal products that may influence the process of malignancy positively or negatively. Various workers, especially of the National Institute of Health in Bethesda, Washington, USA, and the National Institute of Nutrition Hyderabad[5] have proved that vegetables and fruits (especially of yellow or orange colour) like orange, lime, pomegranate, and especially Indian goose berry are vegetables with excellent anticancerous effects. Please note that Indian goose berry (amla) is the active ingredient of some famous ayurvedic preparations, eg: Chyavanaprasha.

In all Tribal systems of medicine, which have been studied so far, it has been found that these vegetables and fruits had a pride of place. The plants so listed include lime, onions, garlic, ginger, cashew fruits, coccinia indica, black pepper, Garcinia cambogia, betel leaves, bitter gourd, sugar cane, Ash gourd, Pine apple, turmeric, moringa oliefera, gooseberry (Nellikai; Amla), Pappaya, Tamarind....etc. Many of these have been our household items of food from time immemorial[6].

The role of vegetarian diet in the prevention of Cancer & CHD

Apart from that of Cancer, the role of diet in the prevention of diseases like obesity, hypertension, arteriosclerosis, and Coronary disease have been well-documented. The main aetiological factor in the causation of this group of diseases is the over-indulgence in food, especially of animal origin. From the sixties, a large number of scientists have been investigating a number of food groups, nutrients, mineral and food additives in the hope of pin-pointing factors causing Cancer and CHD. More recently studies have been focused on the protective effect of certain food factors that may confer protection against Cancer and CHD. It is found that vegetables contain nutraceuticals capable of inhibiting Cancer and CHD in man.

Vegetable products like seeds (Chick Pea, Soya bean, Groundnut…etc), tubers including sweet potatoes, yam and red grapes and various vegetable products contain nutraceutical antioxidants. Onions and garlic are excellent plant products. They not only act as antioxidants, but are good tumour suppressants and remember you can buy ½ a kg of these substances for the cost of an antioxidant tablet and they will at lest give you 10 times the antioxidant support.

The Call of Spices

The Arabs and Westerners came to Kerala in search of spices for time immemorial. Apart from black pepper, ginger, turmeric, coffee and tea, cardamom, cloves, nutmeg (Jathica), sandal wood, nux vomica, opium, ganja, datura, squill, santonin, hemp, phyllum seeds, aconite, saphagola, coriander, chilies and a host of other substances were freely exported from India. Most of these spices are rich sources of nutraceuticals[7] of the nature of polyphenols, terpenes, flavonoids, carotenoids & theols (Sulphur compounds).

Exploitation of Indian Dugs

We realized the real worth of Neem and turmeric only when the Westerners exploited them. We had to spend a lot of money to get the foreign patent on turmeric cancelled and even with Herculean efforts we were not able to do so in the case of Neem. Many other plants have been exploited by the Westerners in this manner. The case of Rawolfia serpentina and serpasil and the case of vinca rosea and the anticancer drugs vincrestin and vinblastin are instances which come immediately to ones's mind. Similarly sandalwood, thulasi, onions, garlic, gooseberry, red variety of sandalwood (Raktha chandanam), vep and countless other plant-based drugs have been exploited to the hilt, in the drug and cosmetic industry. The use of drugs like the extract of cheru (used as cloth marker) in the treatment of skin cancer, similarly vinca rosea is used to make very effective anticancer drugs like vinblastin & Vincrestin. In fact, this exploitation is on constant increase, and vast depots to collect these materials have been set up in India.

It is high time that we catch on to the seriousness of the problem and initiate a high-level research programme in this wonder world of medicinal plants and that the government and the Universities become interested in this programme to tap the benefits of medicinal plants. This is needed to stop the drain of our national wealth by multinational drug companies. I am happy to record that a dedicated group of research workers are working under the guidance of Dr. Bordia in Rajasthan, and a similar team is working in the drug research institute at Lucknow. Down south, good work is being done at N.I.N, Hyderabad. Nearer home in Kerala, we have dedicated teams working with Dr.R.Kuttan at Trichur, Dr.K.R.Panicker at Thiruvananthapuram, and Dr.K.T.Augusti at the Universities of Kerala, M.G and Kannur. They are indeed doing yeoman service in the field of neutraceuticals and functional foods and have produced excellents.

Even our Vedas have declared "Annam Brahma" meaning that the very soul arises from the food that we take and let us hope that our glorious traditions will be preserved in our country and not exploited by westerners.

References

1. Lau B.HS. Garlic for health. Published by Lotus Light Publications P.O.Box 2.Wilmot, WI 53192.1988.P.45-49.
2. Lau B.HS., Woolley. JL et. al. Superiority of intralesional immunotherapy with Corynebacterium parvum and Allium Sativum in control of murine transitional cell carcinoma. J.Urol.136 (1986).
3. Nagao M, Honda M et. al. Mutagenesis of smoke condensates and charred surface of fish and meat. Cancer Lett.2 (1977)221-26.
4. Bernard.E.Statland. Nutrition and Cancer.Clin.Chem.38(1992)1587-1594.

5. Krishnaswamy, K and Polasa, K. Diet, Nutrition and Cancer- the Indian Scenario. Indian J Med.Res.102 (1995)200-209.

6. Madhavankutty. Holistic Medicine. Published by Center For Medical Education and Administration, Calicut-4. 1983, P.31-37.

7. Ramachandran, H.D, Kusum, R and Raina, P.L. Modulatory effect of dietary factors on iron-induced *in vivo* lipid peroxidation in liver and serum of albino rats. Indian Jour. Exp. Biol.44 (2006)32-38.

Chapter – 3

Terpenes, Carotenoids and Phytosterols

3.1 Role of Terpenes and Terpenoids present in Functional Foods

K.V. Shahid, Senior Research Fellow,

Department of Entomology, College of Agriculture, Vellayani, Thiruvananthapuram

P. Faizal,

Lecturer in Med. Biochemistry, School of Health Science,. Thalassery Campus of Kannur University. 670661

Ayurvedic Medicines contain many plant products rich in terpenes and their derivatives. Terpenes and Terpenoids constitute one of the most important groups of biologically active compounds in plants of various nature and most of them are spices. **They are grouped as monoterpenes, sesquiterpenes, diterpenes, triterpenes and tetraterpenes with their derivatives (see the charts prepared by Minu Ann Sebastain et. al.)**

Most naturally available monoterpene oils are cineole from Eucalyptus Spp. and pinene from Pinus spp. Terpenes as a class possess antioxidant, vasodilatory and anti-inflammatory actions. Paeoniflorin is a monoterpene glucoside found in the Chinese herb Paeonia lactiflora with anti-inflammatory, sedative, antipyretic and antispasmodic actions[1]. Limonene, α-pinene, β-pinene, α and β phellandrene, sabinene etc. are monoterpenes present in various spices as described in the charts. **They have vasodilatory and anti-inflammatory actions**. Cardamom (Elettaria Cardamomum) constitutes about 5% by weight the essential oils. Miyazawa and Kameoka[2] studied the volatile oil composition of cardamom by gas chromatography and recorded 23 components in it. They are cyclic and aliphatic terpenes, terpenoxides and esters, aromatic hydrocarbons, aliphatic and cyclic alcohols and sesquiterpene alcohols. Baderi[3] analyzed 49 volatile compounds and 20 of them representing 97.14% of the cardamom oil were classified. Author of this article Mr.Shahid identified eleven compounds in a Kerala variety of cardamom volatiles by gas chromatography[4] and they were pinene, sabinene, myrcene, limonene, 1, 8-cineole, linalool, terpene-4-o1, α-terpineol, linalylacetale, geraneol and α-terpinyl acetate. The chief constituents which determine the flavour of the oil are 1, 8 ceneol, α-terpinyl acetate and linalyl acetate. The ratio of 1, 8 cineol to α- terpinyl acetate twists the flavour characteristics of the oil. Terpeneol and its acetyl ester are the active components with enhanced absorption.

The terpenoid constituents are responsible for antifungal and antibacterial effects[5]. The flavour components also showed antibacterial effects against several food borne microorganisms[6]. Al-Zuhair et. al.[7] have shown that cardamom oil has analgesic action. In Ayurveda Cardamom seeds are described as aromatic, acrid, sweet, cooling, stimulant, carminative, diuretic, cardiotonic and expectorant. **Cardamom is used as an ingredient in the preparations for the treatment of asthma, bronchitis, hemorrhoids, renal and vesicle calculi, cardiac disorders, anorexia, dyspepsia and rheumatism (see the chart in P. 492 showing diseases and ayurvedic medicines by Mohind Mohan, Ramalath et. al.).** Many spices are added to food preparations as preservatives. Cookies mixed with Cardamom, Cinnamon and Clove powders or their volatile oils are acceptable for human consumption at concentrations ranged from 1.5 to 2 times of their threshold levels viz, 1% cardamom and Cinnamon powders, 0.5% Clove powder or the volatile oils of the former two at 0.05% and for the last one at 0.075% level. Gaschromatography-mass spectrometry of Cardamom, Cinnamon, and clove volatiles showed that hydrocarbon volatiles were absent in Clove oils and the former two contained 7.6% and 21.92% of it respectively. However oxygenated volatile terpenoids were in the order 78.74%, 60.65% and 97.86% respectively. The stability of cookie lipids (against peroxidation) and consequently different cookie antioxidant treatments were studied and indicated that the antioxidant efficiency of clove, Cardamom and Cinnamone powders and their volatile oils increased by increasing their concentrations in cookies. **In addition, Clove powder and its volatile oil had the most effective antioxidant activity compared with Cinnamon and Cardamom** (http://www.ingentaconnect.com) ***content/els/0022474x12000/ 00000036/ 000000...11/10/2006)***

Antiinflammatory and Analgesic Activities of Cardamom Oil

A comparative study of the anti inflammatory activity of the oil extracted from commercial Elettaria Cardamom seeds, in doses of 175 and 280 μl/kg and indomethacin in a dose of 30 mg/kg against acute carrageenan-induced oedeme in male albino rats was performed, which proved to be marked.

Investigation on the analgesic activity of Cardamom oil using p-benzoquinone as a chemical stimulant proved that a dose of the oil at 233 μl/kg in mice produced 50% protection against the writhing (stretching syndrome) induced by intraperitoneal administration of a 0.02% solution of p-benzoquinone. In addition the antispasmodic activity was determined on a rabbit intestine preparation using acetylcholine as agonist, the results proving that Cardamom oil exerts its antispasmodic action through muscuranic receptor blockage.

Limonene and other Citrus Oils

Limonene is the precursor of the main constituents of the monoterpenes in mints, Mentha spp (Lamiaceae) including carvone and menthol[8.] Limonene is also found in citrus oils and dill, Anethum graveolens (Apiaceae). Limonene and other citrus oils have antitumour effects in mice. A study supported by the US National Cancer Institute, found that hydrocarbons from dill and caraway oils containing carvone and limonene, increased the level of the detoxifying enzyme glutathione S-transferase in mice[9]. Limonene, terpentine and other terpene hydrocarbons have been found to possess antiviral properties in low doses[10(a)]. They are also used as nasal decongestants[10(b)]. The hydrocarbons in dill oil are thought to contribute to their diuretic action[11].

α-pinene and β- pinene are widely distributed in plants, with high proportions in oil of terpentine from different species of pinus. Pinene has a pleasant aromatic odour and is an important component of many culinary spices, including black pepper. Other monoterpene hydrocarbons including α-sabinene,

P-cymene, Myrcene and α-phellandrene present in various spices (see chart) endow them with biological effects such as antioxidant and antitumour activities.

Terpenoid Alcohols

They rank with phenols as being among the most potent antimicrobial essential oil compounds without the irritant properties of the latter. Linalool is widely distributed, contributing to the flavour and biological activity of grapevine leaves, lemon, basil, tea leaves, thyme and cardamom[12]. Linalool has potent effects on the CNS *in vivo*, including sedative, spasmolytic and hypothermic activities. Linalool has also been shown to produce an inhibitory effect on acetylcholine release and on the channel opening time of the neuromuscular junction, as well as a local anaesthetic action[13.] Other terpene alcohols include geraniol and citronellol from rose oil, and scented geraniums. Nerol is a stereoisomor of geraniol. Borneol is found in rosemary oil. Santalol is a sesquiterpene alcohol from heartwood of sandalwood. The wood is used in many Ayurvedic preparations and its syrup gives a cooling effect when applied on the forehead.

Monoterpene Aldehydes

Citrus oils contain such aldehydes corresponding to the above mentioned alcohols viz; geranial and citronellal. The best quality oils come from the bitter orange, citrus aurantium and the lemon, C. lemon. Although the hydrocarbon limonene is the major constituent, the aroma of the oils is determined by the presence of aldehydes viz, the isomers of geranial (α-citral) and neral (β-citral) together known as citral and also citronellal. The oil of the lemon-scented gum-Eucalyptus citriodora (Myrtaceae)ae) consists mainly of citronellal with a small amount of the alcohol citronellol, while that of the lemon scented tea tree contains both citral and citronellal.

Apart from its pleasant aroma, citral is valued for its sedative, antiviral and antimicrobial properties. Citral rich oils derived from lemon grass and tea tree were shown to inhibit candida albicans at more than four times the rate (zone of inhibitions) of tea tree oil.

Phenolic Volatile Oils

They are the most potent and potentially irritant compounds found in essential oils. Phenols are represented in both major classes of aromatic compounds – **the monotropenes and phenyl propanoids**. The major monoterpene phenols, Thymol, and Carvacol, are found in Thyme, Thymus spp and oregano, Origanum vulgare. Other compounds present are the alcohols linalool, geraniol and α-terpineol[14]. Thymol is an expectorant, antimicrobial, anthelminthic and antispasmodic. The tincture is a safer means of administration than the oil itself. Eugenol is a phenylpropanoid with a free hydroxyl group. It is widely distributed in plants. One of the main sources being clove oil from flower buds of syzygium aromaticum. It is a major constituent of bay leaf, nutmeg and allspice. Eugenol has antimicrobial properties akin to thymol which coupled with its anesthetic properties make it an effective disinfectant and cauterizing agent in dentistry. Clove oil is an effective topical remedy for toothache and is a powerful stimulant and aromatic. Clove powder is an essential ingredient in the "composition powder" made famous by Samual Thompson. It is a food preservative with potent inhibitory effects on lipid peroxidation[15] and duel inhibition of arachidonic acid and platelet-aggregating factor (PAF) for eugenol[16]. Further studies have also confirmed in vivo anticonvulsant[17] and antiulcerogenic activity[18].

Phenolic Ehers

The majority of these phenols are also phenypropane derivatives and many are present in spices such as cloves, aniseed, celery seed, basil and tarragon. These ethers in isolated form are irritant and toxic. However the spices themselves are generally considered to be safe.

Myristicin and Safrole

They are found in nutmeg and black pepper. The former is present in carrot, Parsley and dill. Myristicin is structurally related to safrole and is toxic in high doses. Safrole is found as a minor constituent in cocoa, nutmeg and black pepper. However safrole is restricted in use due to suspected carcinogenic properties. Nutmeg exhibits narcotic and intoxicating properties though it does have medicinal uses in lower doses[19].

Pulegone, Thujone, Carvone and Camphor

They are monoterpenoid ketones with one or two cyclic structures. In high doses they are toxic. They are present in some of the more benign essential oils such as those from spearmint and fennel. Ketone volatiles are mucolytic and of benefit for respiratory congestion[10(a)]. Carvone isomers are found in spearmint and caraway seeds. Thujone was originally isolated from the Arbor Vitae, Thuja occidentalis. It is also present in worm wood, mugwort etc. Pulegone is found in the oil of pennyroyal. Both these Ketones have similar properties and both of them need same precautions for their use. Camphor is derived from the heart wood of the camphor laural and in some lavendar varieties. Camphor is a CNS stimulant, primarily used as a topical agent for its antipruritic, rubifacient and mucolytic properties. It is also toxic in high doses.

Monoterpene Oxides

Bisabolol oxide from chamomile, 1, 8 cineol and ascaridole found in essential oils are typical examples of this group. Cineol is the major constituent of eucalyptus oil and hence it has an alternative name also viz; eucalyptol. It is an expectorant and mucolytic agent and is a universal ingredient in cough lozenges and other medications. Ascaridol is highly toxic and explosive when mixed with organic acids. It is the main constituent of wormseed oil and strongly anthelmintic and its use is limited.

Esters

Lavender oil contains the alcohol linalool along with its esters linalyl acetate. Most esters are gentle, non-irritant compounds whose action is mainly sedative and antispasmodic.

Balsams

They are resinous mixtures that contain cinnamic and benzoic acids or their esters. Benzoin is a balsamic resin derived from the bark of Styrax benzoin trees. Benzoin contains cinnamic, benzoic and triterpene acids. Its action is antiseptic, stimulant, expectorant, diuretic and antifungal. It is used as a food preservative and also as an ingredient in pharmaceutical preparations. Wounded soldiers used certain drinks containing balsams as a medicine in middle age wars.

Resins

Resins are secreted by plants into special ducts often as a response to damage of the bark by woundings, wind blows etc. They are translucent and burn with a smoky flame and hence their use in incense[20]. Balsams and resins are made up of sesquiterpenes and triterpenes of varying nature.

References

1. Huang. K. The Pharmacology of Chinese Herbs (1993) CRC Press Boca Raton.
2. Miyazawa, M and Kameoka, H. The constitution of the essential oil and nonvolatile oil from cardamom seed. J.JPN, Oil Chem. Soc.24(1) (1975) 22.
3. Baderi, A.Z.M; El-Akel, A.T.M and Morsi, H.H.H. Evaluation of Chemical, Physical and antimicrobial properties of cardamom essential oil. Bull. Faculty of Agr. University Cairo 42, (1)(1991) 183-197.
4. Shahid, K.V and John Zachariah. T. Studies on Cardamom volatile oil by gas chromatography techniques Paper presented at the National Seminar on the Evaluation of Nutraceuticals that prevent diseases, Thalassery Campus of Kannur University, 29th Nov. to 2nd Dec. 2006. Abstracts pp.70-71.
5. Vijayan, K.K.; Madhusoodhanan, K.J et. al. The properties and uses of cardamom. In: Cardamom the genus Elettaria, P.N.Ravindran and K.J.Madhusoodhanan (eds) (2002) pp. 268-281.
6. Kubo, I, Hemejima, M and Murari, H. Antimicrobial activity of flavour components of cardamom. J Agri. Food Chem. 39 (1991) 1984-1986.
7. Al-Zuhair, H; El-Sayeh, B et. al. Pharmacological studies of Cardamom Oil in animals. Pharmacological Res.34 (1996). 79-92.
8. Croteau, R. Metabolism of monoterpenes in mint (Metha) Speices, Planta medica 57(1991) S10-S14.
9. Zheng, G, Kenny, P and Lam, L. 'Anethofuran, Carvone and limonene: Potential cancer chemoprotectative agents from dill weed oil and Caraway oil, Planta Medica 58 (1992) 338-341.
10. (a) Schnaubelt, K 'Friendly molecules', International Journal of Aroma Therapy 2 (1989)20-22 and Potential application of essential oils in viral diseases, ibid (1988/89) ½: 32-35

(b) Battaglia, S The complete guide to Aromatherapy, The perfect potion (Aust.) 1995 Brisbane.

11. Maharan, G; Kadry, H et. al. GC/MS analysis of volatile oil of fruits of Anethum graveolens, International Journal of Pharmacognosy 30(1992) 139-144.

12. Duke, J.A. Beckstrom-Sternberg, S.M. Phytochemicals Database, 2001) sUSDA-ARS-NGRI- Beltsville Agricultural Research Centre, Beltsville, Maryland.

13. Re, L; Barocci, S et. al. Linalool modifies the nicotinic receptor-ion channel kinetics at the mouse neuromuscular junction. Pharmacology Research. 42(2000) 177-182.

14. Stahl-Biskup, E. The Chemical Composition of 'Thymus oils', Journal of Essential oil Research, 3(1991) 61-82.

15. Toda, S; Ohnishi, M; Kimura, M and Toda, T. Inhibitory effects of eugenol and related compounds on lipid peroxidation induced by reactive oxygen. Planta Medica 60(1994)282.

16. Saeed, S. Simjee, R; Shamin, G and Gilani, A. Eugenol: a dual inhibitor of platelet–activating factor and arachidonic acid metabolism, Phytomedicine 2(1995) 23-28.

17. Sayyah, M; Valizadeh, J and Kamalinejad, M Anticonvulsant activity of the leaf essential oil of Laurus nobilis against pentylene tetrazole-and maximal electroshock-induced seizures'. Phytomedicine 9(2002) 212-216.

18. Capasso, R; Pinto, L; et. al. Preventative effect of eugenol on PAF and ethanol – induced gastric mucosal damage. Fitoterapia 71(2000) S131-S137.

19. Hall, R. Toxicants Occurring Naturally in Foods. 1973. National Academy of Sciences, Washington DC.

20. Andrew Pengelly. The constituents of medicinal Plants CABI Publishing (2004) Walling Ford. Oxon, OX 108DE UK pp. 85-109.

3.2 Sources and Health Improving effects of Terpenes

Minu Sebastian, Aparna. G.S, Merlin M., Sajna.K.P., Deepa Mol & Anjana

Department of Medical Biochemistry & Medical Microbiology School of Health Sciences, Thalassery Campus of Kannur University

Terpenes

Terpenes are volatile organic compounds that are usually derived from natural sources such as pine trees or citrus fruits. They generally have strong characteristic odors. Terpenes are strong antioxidants and the essential oil group are vaso diabetes with pain relieving effects.

Terpenes, their Sources and Derivatives

All the following terpenes form derivatives like lactones, alcohols and acids.

1. **Monoterpenes contain two isoprene units ($C_{10} H_{16}$)**	Essential oils. Menthol, Iridoids, Pinene, Nerol, Citral. etc.
2. **Sesquiterpenes- ($C_{15} H_{24}$).**	Bitter principles and balsams. e.g; Bisabolol, Nirolidol Farnesol and a lactone Parthenolide.
3. **Diterpenes –($C_{20} H_{32}$).**	Resin acids, bitter principles, balsams, gibberellin, and related derivatives, e.g; Vitamin A, Phytol, Forskolin, and taxol
4. **Triterpenes-($C_{30} H_{48}$).**	Saponins, Steroids, e.g; Phytosterols like withanolides, guggulsterones, glycyrrhetic acid, squalen

5. Tetraterpenes-(C_{40} H_{64}),.	Carotenoids and Xanthophylls. e.g; Beta Carotene, Lycopene etc
1. a. Monoterpene acyclics.	Many of them are present in grapes and cardamam. e.g; Muscatgrapes and wines like White Riesling, Myrcene, trans-Ocimene, cis-Ocimene, Linalool, Geraniol, Nerol, Citronellol, Hoterenol etc.
b. Cyclic derivatives.	Neroloxide, Roseoxide etc
c. Monocyclic terpenes.	Limonene, alpha-Terpenene, alpha-Phellandrene, Beta-Phellandrine, gamma- Terpinene, Menthol, Pulegol, Pulegone, Carveol, Carvone, 1,3, Menthadien-7-al 1,8-Cineol, 1,4-Cineol etc.
d. Bicyclic terpenes.	Sabinene, Thugone, alpha-Pinene, bete-Pinene Camphene, delta 3 Carene, Camphor, Fenchone etc.
2. a. Sesquiterpene alycyclics.	Trans-alpha-Farnesene, Cis –alpha Farnesene, beta-Farnesene, Farnesol, All-trans-alpha-Sinesal, beta-Bisabolene, (-)-Zingiberene, (-)-Sesquiphellandrene, Humulene etc.
b. Bicyclic sesquiterpenes.	beta-Cadinene, Valencene, (+)-Nootkatone, beta-Selinene, beta-Caryophyllene.

Contents of Terpenes in some Sources as Volatile Components

Black Pepper.	alpha-Pinene (1-16 %), Sabinene (0.2-19 %), beta caryophyllene (9-30 %), Delta 3-carene (0-20 %), Limonene(16-24 %), beta-Pinene (5-14 %).
Vanilla.	Vanillin (1.3-3.8 %).

Allspice.	Eugenol (50-80 %), beta-Caryophyllene (4-7 %), Methyleugenol (3-28 %), 1,8-Cineole & alpha Phellandrene (in traces).
Caraway.	Carvone (55 %), Limonene (44 %).
Coriander.	Linalool, Linalyl acetate, Citral, alpha-Alkenates.
Fenugreek.	Stolon.
Nutmeg.	alpha-Pinene (27 %), beta- Pinene (21 %), Sabinene (15 %), Limonene (9 %), Safrole (3.3 %), Myristicin(0.5-14 %), 1,8 Cineole (1.5-4.2 %).
Cardamom.	1, 8 Cineole (20-40 %), alpha- Terpenyl acetate (28-34 %), Limonene (2-14 %), Sabinene (3-5%)
Clove.	Eugenol (73-85 %), beta-Caryophyllene (7-12 %), Eugenol acetate (1.5-11 %), Safranal (47 %) 2, 6, 6, Trimethyl –4-hydroxy- l-cyclohexen-L-formaldehyde (14 %).

Terpene Related Volatile and Nonvolatile Compounds

Ginger.	(-)-Zingiberene (30 %), beta- Bisabolene (10-15 %), Sesquiphellandrene (15-20%), Traces of Curcumene, Citral, Citronellyl acetate etc.
Turmeric.	Turmerone (30%), ar-Turmerone (25 %), Zingiberene (25%)
Carotenes.	They are present in oranges, tomatoes, turnips, corn, and apricot. e.g; alpha-carotene-of carrots and pumpkins; beta-carotene of leafy greens, red orange and yellow fruits, gamma and delta carotenes of various colored vegetables. Lycopene- of tomatoes, grape fruits etc. Phytofluene of star fruit, sweet potatoes, Phytone –of sweet potato and orange.
Xanthophylls.	They are present in various yellow pigmented vegetables.
Canthaxanthin	Paprika, Cryptoxanthin-Mango, tangerine, orange;
Zeaxanthin	Spinach, kale, egg yolk, red pepper; Astaxanthin-Yeast, krill, salmon;
Lutein-	Spinach, turnip greens, egg yolk, pumpkin, mango and papaya.

Polyterpenes. They are composed of more than eight isoprene units. Not edible and found in plant latex. e.g; gutta-percha, rubber etc.

Ginko Biloba. The active constituents of this plant are flavone glycosides and the terpene lactones (Ginkolides and bilobalide). They increase blood circulation to brain and inhibit platelet activating factors (PAF) and protect cells of nerve system.

Uses of Terpenes

(a) The addition of terpene/terpene mixture or liposome terpene combination to the diet or drinking water (e.g; Putting Thulasi leaves in drinking water) will improve one's health, body weight, and efficiency of food consumption because of the reduced microbial load in G.I.T. due to the action of terpenes.

(b) Terpene combination will reduce bacterial contamination in chilled drinks. It will reduce the pathogenic bacteria like Salmonella, E. Coli etc present in water and also in our intestine.

(c) Consumption of food or drinks rich in terpenes shall protect our body from the perils of carcinogens, radiation and oxidative stress.

(d) Terpenes have anti-inflammatory, antiseptic, anti-viral, bactericidal, and anti-fungal activity.

3.3 Radioprotective, Antimetastatic, Antidiabetic and Nephro protective Actions of certain Terpenes

A. Andrews and K.G. Ajantha.

Dept. of Medical Biochemistry, School of Medical Education Gandhi Nagar M.G. University Kottayam

K. Krishna Kumar,

Dept. of Biochemistry University of Kerala Kariavattom, Thiruvananthapuram.

Monoterpenes are the class of compounds widely distributed in a variety of fruits and essential oils[1,2]. Terpenoid compounds are one of the promising groups of chemicals in the field of cancer preventions[3]. Certain monoterpenoids are found to induce activity of detoxifying glutathione-S-transferase[4]. Limonene present in citrus fruits and perillic acid were used and evaluated in phase I clinical trials in cancer[5]. Some studies at Amala Cancer Research Centre at Thrissur, Kerala showed earlier that the above monoterpenes are good immunomodulaters[6] and possess antimetastatic activities[7].

Radioprotective Effects

In a recent study Raphael and Kuttan[8] of the above research centre showed the protective effects of some of the monoterpenes against a sublethal dose γ radiation-induced damages in experimental mice. These terpenes were purchased from Sigma Chemicals St. Luis MO USA.

Five groups of mice were used in this experiment with 10 animals in each group. Groups 1, 2 and 3 were treated with carvone, limonene and perillic acid respectively at a dose of 100 μ moles/kg body weight for the former two and half a dose for the last group by i.p. Group 4 was treated with vehicle - control, paraffin oil daily. Group 5 was kept as radiation treated control. All groups were treated with a single sublethal dose of radiation (6 Gy) from ^{60}Co. Drugs were intraperitonially administered from the same day of radiation and were continued for ten consecutive days for all the experiments. Blood was collected from tail vein and parameters such as total WBC count, differential count, body weight and Hb content were recorded prior to the radiation exposure and continued every third day for 30 days. Liver, intestine, bone marrow samples and blood from 6 animals of each group were collected after 48th hour, 7th day, and 10th day of radiation. ALP, ALT and TBARS values of blood, GSH and TBARS values of liver and GSH values of intestinal mucosa were estimated. Histopathological examination of small intestine was also conducted. Bone marrow cell count was determined using hemocytometer. The number of α-esterase positive cells were determined by azodye coupling method.

Administration of terpenes was found to increase the total WBC count, bone marrow cellularity and α -esterase positive cells, which were lowered after the radiation exposure. Elevated levels of liver and serum lipid peroxidation and serum ALP in the irradiated animals were significantly lowerd by the treatment. Differential count and Hb levels were not altered significantly in any group during tests. GSH levels in liver as well as in intestine were raised by treatment which were very low after irradiation. Histopathological studies showed some damages to the intestine and liver of irradiated animals after 48 hours. The maximum liver toxicity and increased numbers of globlet and dead cells were also observed in these animals. Terpenoid treatment ameliorated these effects. Among the terpenes carvone was least active and the other two were more or less equally active in ameliorating the damages induced by radiation in the body Limonene>Perillic acid>carvone.

Monoterpenes used in this study clearly proved their immuno modulatory as well as stem cell proliferative activity as repoted earlier also[6]. Protection to the body was assured through an elevation of GSH in the tissues on treatment by the monoterpenes. GSH is a good free radical scavenger. In irradiated animals free radical production is increased by the split of water ($H_2O \xrightarrow{\gamma} H^{\bullet} + H_3O^{+} + OH^{\bullet}$ etc) and this leads to all types of tissue damages in the body. GSH very efficiently terminates the onslaught of free radicals in the body, viz; $2GSH + 2OH^{\bullet} \rightarrow 2H_2O + GSSG$.

These studies elucidate the role of monotepenes as nutraceuticals. These compounds are nontoxic nutritive ingredients present in various fruits (e.g; citrus fruits) and essential oils consumed by man. Therefore importance of these compounds as dietary components is very high.

In another work the above team[9] also studied the beneficial effects of limonene on lung metastasis induced by B_{16} F_{10} melanoma cells in $C_{57}BL/6$ mice. Administration of lemonene (100 μ moles/kg body weight/day) i.p for 10 days remarkably reduced the metastatic tumor nodule formation by 65%. The results correlated with the biochemical parameters such as serum sialic acid, lung collagen hydroxy proline and uronic acid contents. Serum sialic acid level in control group was as high as 126.8 μg/ml serum which was significantly lowered in limonene treated group to a level of 49.3 μg/ml serum. Uronic acid level was also inhibited to 56 % in the treated group. Histopathological studies also correlated with these above results.

These findings indicate that limonene could inhibit the metastatic progression of B_{16} F-10 melanoma cells in mice with a concomitant decrease of lung fibrosis, its glycosaminoglycans and serum sialic acid. GGT a marker enzyme for metastatic tumor was increased in the control, but it was significantly reduced by limonene treatment (See the figures of terpenes in the chart PP 41-42).

The chemopreventive activity of limonene during initiation can be attributed to the induction of phase I and II enzymes with resulting carcinogen detoxification[10]. The chemopreventive activity of limonene during promotion/progression may be partly due to inhibition of the post translational isoprenylation (transfer of isoprene units) of growth controlling small G proteins[11]. Both limonene and perillic alchohol (reduced form of perillic acid) are being evaluated in phase I clinical trials in advanced patients[12]. Some earlier studies showed that metastasis could be inhibited by phenolic nutraceuticals such as catechin and curcumin[13] which were found to produce artificial cross links with collagen[14]. Viscum album[15] and various allium principles such as DAS, DADS and AMS (Allyl methyl sulfide)[16] have shown to possess antimetastatic activity.

Mechanism of Actions

Just like theols (Organo sulfur compounds), mono terpenes are one of the most promisig group of compounds of plant origin and they have shown to possess anticarcinogenic activity[17]. Most of them are used as chemopreventive agents[3]. The exact mechanism of action of monoterpenes like limonene in the inhibition of metastatsis could be the inhibition of farnelysation of 'ras' oncoproteins[18]. In metastasis secretion of glyco proteins[19] and shedding of gangliodes[20] have been reported. Sialic acid usually occurs as a terminal component of carbohydrate chains of glyco proteins and glycolipids. Sialic acid elevation has a direct relation with tumor metastasis[21]. Similarly γ glutamyl transpeptidase (GGT) which is a glutathionase is increased in the serum of tumor bearing animals. Glutathione (GSH) is an antioxidant as it is being a scavenger of hydroxyl radicals, and singlet oxygen[22]. The elevations of the above parameters (GGT & sialic acid) marking the severity of tumors are being significantly lowered by the nutraceuticals[23] of alliums, viz; DADS, AMS etc. and citrus fruits viz; limonene as observed earlier and in this study. Uronic acid and hexosamines being the parts of sialic acid are also decreased in the treated animals, where as GSH being an antioxidant is raised in the treated groups. All these changes observed in the treated groups may explain the mechanism of action of the nutraceuticals to a certain extent.

Antidiabetic effects of a Terpenoid from Salacia Oblonga Wall

Krishna Kumar, Augusti, and Vijayammal[24] of Kerala University isolated a terpenoid from Salacia oblonga Wall, a plant widely used as an ingredient in Ayurvedic Drugs for treating diabetes. S.ob. terpenoid is very strong as a hypoglycemic and antioxidant agent but weak as a hypolipdemic. It is a stimulant for pancreatic secretion of insulin at a dose of 250 mg/kg/day S.ob. terpenoid lowered the blood sugar by 40% and cholesterol by 18% in streptozotocin diabetic rats after one month treatment. It also improved serum insulin by 21% and GTT significantly. Liver hexokinase activity was raised by 11% and glucose-6-pase activity was lowered by 18%. Lipid peroxidation was also lowered by 16% and activities of antioxidant enzymes viz; SOD and catalase were raised by 18% and 35% respectively. Body weight was raised by 25% and the treated animals appeared smart and cheerful as the untreated group remained weak and dozing.

Nephroprotective action of Terpenes present in Ganoderma Lucidum (Fr) P. Krast.

A medicinal mushroom called Ganoderma lucidum, commonly known as Reishi in Japan and Ling zhi in China is well known for its medicinal properties. Ganoderma is a rich source of bitter principles called triterpenes. At present about 130 triterpenes are reported to occur in G. lucidum alone[25]. The vast majority are ganoderic acids and lucidenic acids[26]. The biological activities reported for oxygenated triterpenes include bitterness, hepato protection and cytotoxicity to hepatoma cells, inhibition of histamine release, angiotensin converting enzyme, cholesterol absorption, cholesterol biosynthesis and thrombin induced platelet aggregation[27]. The immunomodulating property of the mushroom provides a promising approach for cancer prevention and their administration is found useful alone or in combination with chemotherapy and radiotherapy[25]. G. lucidum occurring in South India has been reported to possess significant antio-oxidant activity[28]. This indicated its capacity to prevent oxidative stress and the consequent damage caused by free radicals. The major chemical constituents of Ganoderma are polysaccharides and terpenes. Methanolic extract of G. lucidum has been found to possess significant nephro protective activity when administered at a high dose[29].

Thulasi G. Pillai et. al[30]. extracted total terpenes of G. lucidum by chloroform in a soxhlet apparatus for 8-10 hrs. and the residue left on evaporation of chloroform extract yielded 2 g/100g mushroom. It was further purified by using silica gel column chromatography and TLC. The chloroform:methanol (9/10) solvent elution gave pure terpene fraction. The terpene fractions were detected by anisaldehyde-sulfuric acid and antimony trichloride reagents and observed under U.V. The yield was 5% of the original crude extract.

The above workers further tested the nephro protective action of this fraction against cisplatin induced renal toxicity. Cisplatinum (II) diamine dichloride (cisplatin) is a potent antineoplastic agent containing the heavy metal platinum, but one of the undesirable property of cisplatin is its toxicity profile which includes severe nephrotoxicity and neurotoxicity. Four groups of mice were used to test the nephro protective activity of the terpenes. One group was kept as normal control. Group 2 was given cisplatin (16 mg/kg). Groups 3 & 4 were given terpene (50 & 100 mg/kg respectively) which was dissolved in olive oil, 1hr before the cisplatin injection. 72 hrs after that all groups were sacrificed and blood was collected for serum samples. The kidneys were dissected and stored at –70°C until analysis was completed. A homogenate was prepared in 50 mM phosphate buffer (pH = 7) to get a 10% concentration of the sample. This homogenate was centrifuged at 1000 rpm for 10 mts in cold centrifuge at 0°C and supernatant was used for enzyme assays and protein determination. In cisplatin treated mice serum creatinine, urea and alkaline phosphatase were increased three fold and all of which were significantly reduced in G. lucidum terpene treated groups. Similarly LPO was increased in the control cisplatin treated group 2 which was also reduced by G.L. terpene treatment significantly and that too to the normal level. On the contrary renal superoxide dismutase activity was significantly discreased in the control group 2 and it was also restored to the normal level in the G.L. treated groups 3 & 4.

In China and Japan the fruiting bodies of G. lucidum are considered as a panacea and are extensively used for treatment of a number of disease conditions. The results of Thulasi G. Pillai et al suggest that the terpenes of G. lucidum could help to prevent nephrotoxicity consequent to cisplatin chemotherapy. This is due to the antioxidant actions of the terpenes present in the drug preparation. G. lucidum terpenes may therefore be useful in adjuvant therapy of cancer.

References

1. Zheng, G; Kenny, P and Lan, L. Anethofuran, Carvone and limonene; Potential cancer chemopreventive agents from dill weed oil and caraway oil. Planta Medica. 58 (1992) 338-341.
2. Steinmez K.A. and Potter, J.D. Epidemiol cancer causes control 2(1991) 325
3. Gould, M.N. Cancer chemoprevention and therapy by monoterpenes. Environ. Health Perspect 105 (1997) 977-979.

4. Lam, L.K.T. and Hasegawa, S. Nutr. Cancer 12 (1989)43

5. MC Namee. Lancet 342 (1993) 801.

6. Raphael, T.J. and Kuttan, G. Immunomodulatory activity of naturally occurring monoterpenes carvone, limonene and perillic acid. Immunopharmacology and Immunotoxicology 25(2) (20030 285-294.

7. Raphael T.J, and Kuttan, G. Effect of naturally occurring monoterpenes carvone, limonene and perillic acid in the inhibition of experimental lung metastatsis induced by $B_{16}F_{10}$. J. Exp.Clin.Res. 22(3) (2003) 419-424.

8. Raphael, T.J. and Kuttan G. Ameliorative effect of monoterpenes on radiation induced toxicity. Amala Research Bulletin 25(2005) 204-212.

9. Raphael T.J. and Kuttan G. Preliminary study of antimetastatic activity of naturally occurring monoterpene limonene Amala Res. Bulletin 23(2003)99-106

10. Crowell, P.L. and Gould, M.N. Chemoprevention and therapy of cancer by Limonene. Crit Rev. oncology 5 (1994) 1-22.

11. Ren, Z and Gould, M.N. Modulation of small G protein iso prenylation by anticancer monoterpenes in insitu mammary gland pithelial cells. Carcinogenesis 19(1998) 827-832.

12. Crowell, P.L. Prevention and therapy of cancer by dietary monoterpenes. J. Nutrition 129 (1999) 7758-88.

13. Menon, L.G; Kuttan, R and Kuttan, G. Inhibition of lung metastasis in mice induced by B_{16} F_{10} melanoma cells by polyphenolic compounds. Cancer Lett. 95 (1995) 221-225.

14. Menon, L.G.; Kuttan, R; Muraleedharan, N.R. et. al. Effect of isoflavones-genitesin and Diazen in the inhibition of lung metastasis in mice induced by B_{16} F_{10} melanoma cells. Nutrition and Cancer. 30(1998) 74-77.

15. Antony, S; Kuttan, R; Kuttan, G. Effect of viscum album, in the inhibition of lung metastasis in mice induced by $B_{16}F_{10}$ melanoma cells. J. Clin Cancer Res. 16(1997) 157-162

16. Kuttan, G and Kuttan, R. Effect of Diallyl sulphide, diallyl disuplide and allyl methyl sulphide on the inhibition of lung metastasis of $B_{16}F_{10}$ melanoma cells J. Clin. Biochem. Nutr. 27(1999) 131-139

17. Wattenberg W, Vetta, L et. al. Inhibition of N-nitrosodiethylamine carcinogenesis in mice by naturally occurring organosulphur compounds and monoterpenes, Cancer Res. 49(1989) 2689-2692

18. Acrowell, R.R; Chang. Z et. al. Selective inhibition of isoprenylation of 21-26 K.D. Protein by anticarcinogen-d-limonene and its metabolites. J. Biol. Chem. 266 (1991) 17679-17685.

19. Bizik, J; Grofova, M and Sevec, J. Release of a Mr. 14,000 glycoprotein in the culture media of certain human sarcoma and melanoma cell lines. Eur. J. Cancer Clin. Oncol. 21 (1985) 311-324

20. Hersey, P. Review of melanoma antigens recognized by monoclonal antibodies. Their functional significance and applications in diagnosis and treatment of melanoma, Pathology II, (1985) 346-345

21. Bhavanandan, V.P., Kallic, A.W. et. al. Partial characterization of sialoglycopeptides produced by cultured human melanoma cells and melanocytes. Biochemistry 20(1981) 3586-3594

22. Barry Halliwell and John H, Gutteridge N C : Free radicals in biology and medicine, Oxford (1985) 104.

23. Haripriya Muralidharan and Kuttan, G. Effect of naturally occurring sulfur containing compounds in the inhibition of lung metastasis induced by B_{16} F_{10} melanoma cells in mice. Amala Res. Bulletin 18(1998) 99-108.

24. Krishna Kumar K, Augusti, K.T. and Vijayammal, P.L. Antiperoxidative and hypoglycemic activity of Salacia oblonga extract in diabetic rats. Pharm. Biol. 37(1999)1-5

25. Gao Y and Zhou, S. Cancer prevention and treatment by Ganoderma, a mushroom with medicinal properties. Food Reviews International 19(2003) 275-325.

26. Nishitoba, T; Sato, H et. al. New bitter C_{27} and C_{20} terpenoids from the fungus G. lucidum. Ag. Biol. Chemistry 48(1984) 2905-2907.

27. Shiao, M, Lee, K.R. et. al. Natural products and biological activities of the Chinese medicinal fungus G. lucidum in Food Phytochemicals. II, Teas, spices and Herbs. American Chemical Soc.1994 pp 342-354.

28. Jones, S and Janardhanan, K.K. Antioxidant and antitumor activity of Ganoderma lucidum (curt. Fr) P. Karst-Reish (Aphy llophoromycetideae) from South India. Int. J. Med. Mushroom. 2(2000) 195-200.

29. Sheena, N; Ajith, T. A. and Janardhanan, K.K. Prevention of nephrotoxicity induced by the anticancer drug cisplatin, using G. lucidum occurring in South India. Curr. Sci. 85(4) 2003. 478-482.

30. Thulasi. G. Pillai, Thomas, G.S and Janardhanan, K-K Protective effect of terpenes isolated from Ganoderma lucidum against cisplatin induced renal toxicity. Amala Research Bulletin 26(2006) 152-157.

3.4 Medicinal Effects of Zingiber Officinale Rosc. (Ginger)

K. Suneesh and A.V. Archana
Dept. of Medical Biochemistry, and Microbiology
SHS, Thalassery Campus of Kannur University
E-Mail:suneesh_k39@yahoo.com

Introduction

Ginger, the rhizome of Zingiber officinale, is one of the most widely used species of the ginger family (Zingiberaceae) and is a common condiment for various foods and beverages. Ginger has a long history of medicinal use dating back 2,500 years in China and India for conditions such as headaches, nausea, rheumatism, and colds[(1)] Characterized in traditional Chinese medicine as spicy and hot, ginger is claimed to warm the body and treat cold extremities, improve a weak and tardy pulse, address a pale complexion, and strengthen the body after blood loss[2].

Active Constituents

Ginger contains a number of pungent constituents and active ingredients. Steam distillation of powdered ginger produces ginger oil, which contains a high proportion of sesquiterpene hydrocarbons, predominantly zingiberene[3]. The major pungent compounds in ginger, from studies of the lipophilic rhizome extracts, have yielded potentially active gingerols, which can be converted to shogaols, zingerone, and paradol[4]. In addition, ginger contains up to 3 percent of essential oils that cause fragrance of the spice. The main constituents are sesquiterpenoids with (-) zingiberene as the main component. Lesser amounts of other sesquiterpenoids are beta-sesqui phellandrene, bisabolene, and farnesene. The pungency of ginger is due to nonvolatile phenylpropanoids particularly gingerol and zingerone and diarylheptanoids viz., gingeroles and shogaoles. The latter are more pungent and formed from the former when ginger is dried.

The compound 6-gingerol appears to be responsible for its characteristic taste. Zingerone and shogaols are found in small amounts in fresh ginger and in larger amounts in dried or extracted products. This may be a reason that in Ayurvedic medicines dry ginger is used rather than raw fresh ginger

Mechanisms of Action

The mechanism underlying ginger's anti-emetic activity is not clearly understood, but the aromatic, spasmolytic, carminative, and absorbent properties of ginger suggest it has direct effects on the gastrointestinal tract[5].

Studies do not indicate ginger has any influence within the vestibular or oculomotor system[6]. A mechanism involving the central nervous system cannot be ruled out, considering several of ginger's components antagonize serotonin type-3 receptors: however, this has not been clearly demonstrated[7-9].

The compounds 6-gingerol and 6-shogaol have been shown to have a number of pharmacological activities, including antipyretic, analgesic, antitussive, and hypotensive effects[10]. Ginger extracts exhibit inhibition of platelet aggregation and thromboxane synthesis *in vitro*[11-15], which has led to concerns that ginger extracts may prolong bleeding; however, several European studies using ginger orally did not find any significant anticoagulant effects *in vivo*[16]. Daily consumption of 15 g raw ginger rhizome or 40 g cooked rhizome by [18] healthy volunteers for two weeks failed to decrease platelet cyclooxygenase activity[17,18]. Similarly, differences were not found in bleeding time, platelet count, and platelet functioning when eight healthy volunteers were given a single 2 gram dose of the dried rhizome or placebo[18]. *In vitro* studies suggest ginger may produce anti-inflammatory effects by inhibiting arachidonic acid metabolism in both the cyclooxygenase and lipoxygenase pathways[19-21].

Clinical Indications, Motion Sickness

Ginger has long been used as a remedy to decrease nausea and vomiting associated with several conditions. A randomized, double-blind, placebo-controlled study was performed to assess the effects of ginger extracts on motion sickness and gastric slow-wave dysrhythmias induced by circular vection[22]. Volunteers with a history of motion sickness were pre-treated with ginger (1,000 mg and 2,000 mg). Individuals then underwent circular vection during which nausea, tachygastria, and vasopressin were assessed. Ginger improved each of the above parameters, significantly prolonging the latency period before nausea onset and shortening the recovery time after vection cessation.

Five other double-blind studies have been performed that demonstrated a positive effect of ginger oil on motion sickness[23-27]. These studies show ginger to be as effective as many traditional antiemetic pharmaceuticals such as dimenhydrinate, domperidone, scopolamine, cyclizine, and meclizine. One double-blind study found no benefit with ginger (0.5-1.0 g) when compared to scopolamine, d-amphetamine, or placebo[28]. Therefore more evaluation of the aspects are needed.

Nausea and Vomiting in Pregnancy

Ginger is used to ameliorate symptoms of nausea in pregnancy. Most recently, a double-blind, placebo-controlled, randomized clinical trial was conducted on 26 women in the first trimester of pregnancy[29]. Subjects ingested one tablespoon of ginger syrup (containing 1 g ginger) or placebo in 4-8 ounces of water four times daily. Duration and severity of nausea was evaluated over a two-week period. Daily vomiting ceased in eight of 12 women in the ginger group by the sixth day, while only two of 12 in the placebo group reported a cessation of vomiting. At the end of the study, 20 women (77 percent) consuming the ginger syrup reported a significant decrease in nausea, while 20 percent in the placebo group reported improvement.

Other double-blind, placebo-controlled studies have been performed evaluating the effectiveness of ginger on morning sickness[30]. In one study of 70 pregnant women, participants received either 250 mg freshly prepared ginger powder or a placebo. Results indicated a significant reduction in nausea and number of vomiting episodes[31].

Post-surgical Nausea

Two double-blind studies were performed on women following major gynecological surgery[32,33]. In both studies there were three parallel groups comparing efficacy of ginger to placebo or 10 g metoclopramide. Women were dosed one hour before anesthesia was administered. In the study by Bone et. al.[32], nausea in the placebo group was observed throughout the duration of the study, while only 28 percent in the ginger group and 30 percent in the metoclopramide group experienced nausea. In the study by Phillips et. al. ginger also significantly reduced nausea and vomiting when compared to placebo and metoclopramide.

In a recent double-blind study, ginger failed to demonstrate an anti-emetic effect following laparoscopic surgery[34]. Pre-operative doses of 100 or 200 mg were administered and followed by repetitive 100 or 200 mg doses. An earlier double-blind study on the effect of ginger on postoperative nausea also failed to demonstrate beneficial effects compared to placebo[35]. Doses of ginger in this study ranged from 0.5-1.0 g ginger extract.

Chemotherapy-induced Nausea

Cancer chemotherapy can cause severe nausea, vomiting, and abdominal discomfort, which can limit therapy. Anticancer agents such as cisplatin, cyclophosphamide, and methotrexate slow gastric emptying[36,37]. In a double-blind study of chemotherapy-induced nausea, 41 patients with leukemia received either ginger or a placebo after administration of compazine[38]. The results showed a significantly greater symptomatic benefit from ginger compared to placebo. In a study on rats, following cisplatin administration, significant inhibition of gastric emptying occurred. The inhibitory effects of gastric emptying were partially reversed by pretreatment with ginger extract and ginger juice[39]. Similar efficacy of these ginger preparations was also observed in antiemetic studies against cisplatin-induced emesis in dogs[40].

Osteoarthritis

Ginger extract has been studied as an alternative to NSAID therapy for arthritic conditions. A randomized, placebo-controlled, crossover study comparing ginger extracts and ibuprofen was performed on 75 individuals with osteoarthritis of the hip or knee[41]. Patients received either 170 mg ginger extract, 400 mg ibuprofen, or placebo three times per day and were followed for three weeks. The study revealed significant improvement in symptoms for both the ginger and ibuprofen groups before crossover: however, at the study's end there was no difference between ginger and placebo. No side effects were noted in the ginger group; however, side effects prompting removal from the study occurred in the ibuprofen group. More studies are recommended using different doses and duration of treatment to assess the efficacy of ginger extract for this condition

Ginger Chemistry, Technology, and Quality Evaluation

Ginger is used in more ways than any other spice. Derived products such as ginger powder, syruped ginger, volatile oil and oleoresin are described by various scientists in great detail. The increasing world demand for quality products of added value such as the oleoresin and volatile oil show prospects for their production in the growing countries. The chemistry of the components which contribute aroma and pungency that characterize ginger is critically reviewed. The physico-chemical parameters prescribed as a measure of quality for ginger and its products in the existing standards can assure only hygienic quality and purity, and possibly the source, when new parameters such as GC-fingerprints are included. Other important properties such as functional, physiological, toxicological and biosynthetic aspects of the components stimulating flavor are described as a monograph.

The lipid lowering and antioxidant potentional of ethanolic extract of Zingiber officinale was evaluated in steptozotocin (stz) induced diabetes in rats. Ethanolic extract of Zingiber officinale (200 mg/kg) fed orally for 20 days produced, significant anti hyperglycemic effect ($P<0.01$) in diabetic rats. Further, the extract treatment also produced statistically significant decrease of lipids in liver and pancreas ($P<0.01$) as compared to diabetic control rats. Zingiber officinale extract treatment also lowered the liver and pancreas thiobarbituric acid reactive substances (TBARS) values ($P<0.01$) as compared to pathogenic diabetic rats. The results of test drug were comparable to gliclazide (25 mg/kg, orally) a standard anti hyperglycemic agent. The results indicate that ethanolic extact of Zingiber officinale Roscoe can protect the tissues from lipid peroxidation. The extract also exhibit significant lipid lowering activity in diabetic rats. The present study is the first pilot study to assess the potential of Zingiber officinale in diabetic dyslipidaemia. (U, Bhandari, Raman Kanojia and K, K Pillai. Available online 14 January 2005. Hamdard University, New Delhi-62)

Drug-Botanical Interactions, Side Effects, and Toxicity

No drug interactions are known: however, due to ginger's apparent effect on platelets, it should be used cautiously in individuals using anticoagulants.

Side Effects and Toxicity

Ginger is on the U.S. Food and Drug Administration's GRAS (generally recognized as sale) list. The British Herbal Compendium documents no adverse effects of ginger[42].

Dosage

For most purposes a typical dose of dry ginger is 1-4 g daily, taken in divided doses. To prevent motion sickness, it is best to begin treatment 1-2 days before the scheduled trip and continue dosing throughout the duration of travel. For nausea and vomiting during pregnancy, ginger tea made from fresh ginger root, boiled and diluted to taste, appears to work best.

Warnings and Contraindications

Despite widespread use of ginger by pregnant women, the safety of this herb has not been formally established. The Complete German Commission E Monographs recommends against the use of ginger root for nausea and vomiting of pregnancy: however, American editors, citing thousands of years of use and no pertinent scientific validity for this contraindication, refute this recommendation.

The German Commission E also mentions gall stones as a relative contraindication for ginger, without citing a rational[43].

Experiments on ginger extract as a protective agent in ISO induced myocardial injury

The British Herbal compendium reported its actions as carmanative, antiemetic, spasmolytic, circulatory stimulated and anti inflammatory[44]. Limited *in vitro* studies have shown that water and organic solvents extracts of Zinger officinale Rosc (Z.O) possess antioxidant properties[45,46(a&b)]. A combination of ginger and garlic has been reported to produce hypoglycemic and hypolipidemic[47] effects. Banerjee[48] and Seth et. al.[49] showed that dietary ginger protected the tissues from oxidative stress induced by organophosphate pesticide (malathion) in rats. Srivastava[13] and Bhandari et. al.[50] showed cholesterol lowering and antiplatelet aggregation activities of ginger. Protective effects of Z.O are reported, however there is no experimental evidence regarding its biochemical role in the prevention of myocardial damage. Therefore Nazam, Bandari[51] and Pillai have conducted a study to elucidate the role of Z.O in maintaining the myocardial integrity in ISO induced damages observed in rats.

(a) Ethanolic extract of Z.O (200 mg/kg) was used to treat rats for 20 days prior to ISO injection subcutaneously (80 mg/kg) in two divided doses at 24 hr intervals in order to study its protective effects against ISO induced myocardial infarction. One group of rat was kept as control, another group was injected with ISO at the above dose without any pre-treatment with Z.O. A fourth group was simply treated with Z.O for 20 days at the above dose without ISO injection.

In the ISO injected control group of rats there was a significant elevation in serum marker enzymes viz, LDH, CK, AST, and ALT. Similarly serum TBARS also increased significantly marking sever myocardial infarction, in this group. In the Z.O pretreated group these values were corrected significantly and it indicates that Z.O contains some active principles that protect heart from ISO induced infarction. On the contrary endogenous antioxidant enzymes viz, SOD and catalase, and tissue GSH levels decreased significantly in the ISO injected rats. Net weight of the myocardium increased significantly. Pretreatment of ISO injected rats with Z.O reversed these values towards normal. Treatment with Z.O didn't change these parameters in normal animals to a significant level. Histopathological examination of rat's heart section confirmed myocardial injury with ISO injection, and it was significantly reversed by Z.O pretreatment in them. Inflammation/edema etc., are after effects of tissue injuries and this condition might have led to an increase in the weight of myocardium of ISO injected rats. Z.O pretreatment ameliorated this condition as well as the leak of marker enzymes from the myocardium. Pharmacological augumentation of endogenous myocardial antioxidants has been identified as a promising therapeutic approach in diseases associated with increased oxidative stress[52,53]. Increased SOD activity has been reported to be beneficial in the event of increased free radical generation[54]. However a simultaneous increase in catalase and/ or tissue improvement of glutathione level which is a free radical scavenger as well as a participant in glutathione peroxidase is essential for an overall beneficial effect of an increase in SOD activity[55,56].

Nazam's group[51] found that pretreatment with ethanolic extract of ginger protected the myocardium against infiltration and also to decrease the water content of the heart tissues in isoproterenol injected rats

Further experiments by others[57,58] showed the biochemical role of ginger extract against myocardial damage and protective effect on atherosclerosis

(i) Guh et. al.[59] reported on the antiplatelet effects of gingerol. It also inhibited at a concentration of 10 µm thromboxane B_2 and prostaglandin D_2 formation and abolished completely phosphoinositides breakdown induced by arachidonic acid. Z.O has pronounced antioxidant activity comparable to that of synthetic antioxidant preservatives[60]. Research has found ginger to be a powerful antioxidant, antiinflammatory, antiulcer, antiemetic, antimotion sickness, antiatherogenic, anticlotting of blood, anticarcinogenic, hypocholestrelomic and promoter of circulatory system[13-16,61-65]. There are several studies that demonstrate very positive results on minimizing joint pain from arthritis and other inflammatory diseases due to various infections. It may have also blood thinning and antiatherogenic property making it effective in the treatment of heart diseases. Further the gingeroles have analgesic, sedative, antipyretic, antibacterial, and GIT motility effects. Ginger can also be used to prevent scurvy. However people suffering from gall stones or allergic to ginger and pregnant women should avoid its use. Gingerols have been found to be potent inhibitors of prostaglandins and leukotrienes that on oversupply enhance inflammation. Paul Schulick who established the anti inflammatory effects of ginger states literally hundreds of thousands of lives can be saved by ginger, emphasizes that it should be in every ones daily supplement routine[66]. As many other inhibitors of lipoxygenase are strong antioxidants, the above compounds from ginger having such property are also an attribute to these vegetables as a source of nutraceuticals. Z.O extracts were shown to have significant super oxide[64] and OH$^\bullet$ scavanging activity[62] *in vitro* with a concomitant inhibitory action on lipid peroxidation[63,65]. The combined effects of the ginger terpenoids may therefore offer cardio protective action against ISO injection as well as in stress full conditions that a busy person may bear from day to day affairs. Therefore dietary use of Z.O may help us to protect our body from cardiovascular diseases.

It may be noted that aryl heptenone compound with anti fungal properties was identified in ginger in 1990. It has 3 isomers, A, B and e with the name ginger e none.[67]

References

1. Grant KL, Lutz RB. Ginger. Am J Health Syst Pharm 2000;57:945-947.
2. Chang CP, Chang JY, Wang FY, Chang JG. The effect of Chinese medicinal herb Zingiberis rhizoma extract on cytokine secretion by human peripheral blood mononuclear cells. J Ethnopharmacol 1995:48:13-19.
3. Govindarajan VS. Ginger--chemistry, technology, and quality evaluation: part 1. Crit Rev Food Sci Nutr 1982; 17:1-96.
4. Govindarajan VS. Ginger--chemistry, technology, and quality evaluation: part 2. Crit Rev Food Sci Nutr 1982; 17:189-258.
5. Tyler VE. Some recent advances in herbal medicine. Pharm Int 1986:7:203-207.
6. Holtmann S, Clarke AH, Scherer H, Hohn M. The anti-motion sickness mechanism of ginger. A comparative study with placebo and dimenhydrinate. Acta Otolaryngol 1989:108:168-174.
7. Phillips S, Hutchinson S, Ruggier R. Zingiber officinale does not effect gastric emptying rate. A randomised, placebo controlled, crossover trial. Anaesthesia 1993:48:393-395.
8. Micklefield GH, Redeker Y, Meister V, et. al. Effects of ginger on gastroduodenal motility. Int J Clin Pharmacol Ther 1999:37:341-346.
9. Lumb AB. Mechanism of antiemetic effect of ginger. Anaesthesia 1993; 48:1118.
10. Suekawa M, Ishige A, Yuasa K. et. al. Pharmacological studies on ginger. I. Pharmacological actions of pungent constituents, (6)-gingerol and (6)-shogaol. J Pharmacobiodyn 1984:7:836-848.
11. Kiuchi K Shibuya M, Sankawa U. Inhibitors of prostaglandin biosynthesis from ginger. Chem Pharm Bull (Tokyo) 1982; 30:754-757.

12. Kiuchi F, Iwakami S, Shibuya M, et. al. Inhibition of prostaglandin and leukotriene biosynthesis by gingerols and diarylheptanoids. Chem Pharm Bull (Tokyo) 1992; 40:387-391.

13. Srivastava KC [Srivas KC on Medline]. Effects of aqueous extracts of onions, garlic and ginger on platelet aggregation and metabolism of arachidonic acid in the blood vascular system: in vitro study. Prostaglandins Leukot Med 1984; 13:227-235.

14. Srivastava KC. Isolation and effects of some ginger components of platelet aggregation and eicosanoid biosynthesis. Prostaglandins Leukot Med 1986; 25:187-198.

15. Srivastava KC. Effect of onion and ginger consumption on platelet thromboxane production in humans. Prostaglandins Leukot Essent Fatty Acids 1989; 35:183-185.

16. Bordia A, Verma SK, Srivastava KC. Effect of ginger (Zingiber officinale Rosc.) and fenugreek (Trigonella foenumgraecum L.) on blood lipids, blood sugar and platelet aggregation in patients with coronary artery disease. Prostaglandins Leukot Essent Fatty Acids 1997; 56:379-384.

17. Janssen PL, Meyboom S, van Staveren WA, et. al. Consumption of ginger (Zingiber officinale roscoe) does not affect ex vivo platelet thromboxane production in humans. Eur J Clin Nutr 1996; 50:772-774.

18. Lumb AB. Effect of dried ginger on human platelet function. Thromb Haemost 1994; 71:110-111.

19. Srivastava KC. Aqueous extracts of onion, garlic and ginger inhibit platelet aggregation and alter arachidonic acid metabolism. Biomed Biochim Acta 1984; 43:S335-S346.

20. Srivastava KC, Mustafa T. Ginger (Zingiber officinale) in rheumatism and musculoskeletal disorders. Med Hypotheses 1992; 39:342-348.

21. Backon J. Ginger: inhibition of thromboxane synthetase and stimulation of prostacyclin: relevance for medicine and psychiatry. Med Hypotheses 1986; 20:271-278.

22. Lien HC, Sun WM, Chen YH, et. al. Effects of ginger on motion sickness and gastric slow-wave dysrhythmias induced by circular vection. Am J Physiol Gastrointest Liver Physiol 2003:284:G481-G489.

23. Grontved A, Brask T, Kambskard J, Hentzer E. Ginger root against seasickness. A controlled trial on the open sea. Acta Otolaryngol 1988; 105:45-49.

24. Riebenfeld D, Borzone L. Randomized double-blind study comparing ginger (Zintona,) and dimenhydrinate in motion sickness. Healthnotes Rev 1999; 6:98-101.

25. Careddu P. Motion sickness in children: results of a double-blind study with ginger (Zintona,) and dimenhydrinate. Healthnotes Rev 1999; 6:102-107.

26. Mowrey DB, Clayson DE. Motion sickness, ginger, and psychophysics. Lancet 1982; 1:655-657.

27. Schmid R, Schick T, Steffen R, et. al. Comparison of seven commonly used agents for prophylaxis of seasickness. J Travel Med 1994; 1:203-206.

28. Wood CD, Manno JE, Wood MJ, et. al. Comparison of efficacy of ginger with various antimotion sickness drugs. Clin Res Pr Drug Regul Aff 1988; 6:129-136.

29. Blumenthal M. Ginger as an antiemetic during pregnancy. Altern Ther Health Med 2003; 9:19-21.

30. Fischer-Rasmussen W, Kjaer SK, Dahl C, Asping U. Ginger treatment of hyperemesis gravidarum. Eur J Obstet Gynecol Reprod Biol 1991; 38:19-24.

31. Vutyavanich T, Kraisarin T, Ruangsri R. Ginger for nausea and vomiting in pregnancy: randomized, double-masked, placebo-controlled trial. Obstet Gynecol 2001; 97:577-582.

32. Bone ME, Wilkinson DJ, Young JR, et. al. Ginger root--a new antiemetic. The effect of ginger root on postoperative nausea and vomiting after major gynaecological surgery. Anaesthesia 1990; 45:669-671.

33. Phillips S, Ruggier R, Hutchinson SE. Zingiber officinale (Ginger)--an antiemetic for day case surgery. Anaesthesia 1993; 48:715-717.

34. Eberhart LH, Mayer R, Betz O, et. al. Ginger does not prevent postoperative nausea and vomiting after laparoscopic surgery. Anesth Analg 2003; 96:995-998.

35. Arfeen Z, Owen H, Plummer JL, et. al. A double-blind randomized controlled trial of ginger for the prevention of postoperative nausea and vomiting. Anaesth Intensive Care 1995; 23:449-452.

36. Kishibayashi N, Ichikawa S, Yokoyama T, et. al. Pharmacological properties KF18259, a novel 5-HT3-receptor antagonist, in rats: inhibition of the distal colonic function. Jpn J Pharmacol 1993; 63:495-502.

37. Visnovsky P. The effect of cyclophosphamide and methotrexate on gastric emptying and secretion in rats. Bratisl Lek Listy 1992; 93:9092. [Article in Slovak]

38. Pace JC. Oral ingestion of encapsulated ginger and reported self-care actions for the relief of chemotherapy associated nausea and vomiting. Diss Abstr Int 1987;47:3297-B.

39. Sharma SS, Gupta YK. Reversal of cisplatin-induced delay in gastric emptying in rats by ginger (Zingiber officinale). J Ethnopharmacol 1998;62:49-55.

40. Sharma SS, Kochupillai V, Gupta SK, et. al. Antiemetic efficacy of ginger (Zingiber officinale) against cisplatin-induced emesis in dogs. J Ethnopharmacol 1997;57:93-96.

41. Bliddal H, Rosetzsky A, Schlichting P, et. al. A randomized, placebo controlled, cross-over study of ginger extracts and ibuprofen in osteoarthritis. Osteoarthritis Cartilage 2000;8:9-12.

42. Bradley P, ed. British Herbal Compendium. Bournemouth: British Herbal Medical Association; 1990.

43. Blumenthal M, ed. The Complete German Commission E Monographs. Austin, TX: American Botanical Council; 1998:62:135-136.

44. Bradly, P.R. British Herbal Compendium Bournemouth (UK) (British Herbal Medical Association,U.K) (1992)190

45. Jitoe, A; Masuda T, et. al. Anti oxidant activity of tropical ginger extract and analysis of the contained curcuminoids, J. Agri Food Chem. 40(1992)1337

46. (a) Krishanakanth, T.P and Lokesh, B.R. Scavanging of super oxide anions by spice principles, Indian. J. Biochem. Biophys. 30(1990)133

    (b) Reddy, A.C and Lokesh, B.R .Studies on Spice principles as antioxidant in the inhibition of lipid peroxide in rat liver microsomes Mol Cell Biochem.111(1992)117

47. Ahmed R.S and Sharma, S.B. Biochemical Studies on Combined effect Garlic and Ginger in albino rats. Indian J Exp Biol, 30(1997)122

48. Banerjee, B.D. The influence of various factors on immune toxicity assessment of pesticide chemicals. Toxicol Lett;107(1999) 21

49. Seth, V; Ahmed, R.S, et. al. Malathion induced oxidative stress in rats: Modulation by Z. Officinale Rose(Ginger). Proceedings 67th Annual meeting Society of Biological Chemists, New Delhi; India.1999

50. Bhandari, U; Sharma, J.N and Zafar R. The protective action of ethanolic ginger extract in cholesterol fed rabbits. J.Ethanopharmacol 61(1998)167

51. Nazam Ansari, M. Bhandari, U and Pillai; K.K. Ethanolic Zingiber Officinale R.extract pretreatment alleviates isoproterenol induced oxidative stress myocardial necrosis in rats. Indian Jour. Exp. Biol 44(2006)892-897

52. Lawson, C.S; Cottart, D.J ans Herase, D.J. The anti arrhythmic action of ischemic pre conditioning in rat hearts does not involve functional Gi protein.Cardiovasc.Res, 27(1993)681

53. Siveski –Iliskovic N, Hill et. al. Probucol protects against adriamycin Cardio myopathy without interfering with its antitumour effect. Circulation, 91(1995)10

54. Yen, H.C; Oberley, T.D et. al. The protective role of manganese superoxide dismutase against adriamycin –induced acute cardiac toxicity in transgenic mice.J.Clin.Investigation.98(1996)1253

55. Engelman. D.T, Watanbe, M et. al. Hypoxic preconditioning preserves antioxidant reserve in the working rat heart. Cardiovasc Res.29(1995)133

56. Schacfer, J; Peters T, Neirhause, K.H et. al. Mechanism of anti protection and the role of stress protein in natural defences, auto protection and Salutogenesis, Med Hypothesis 51(1998)153

57. Verma. S.K, Singh, M and Bordia, A, Protective effect of ginger, Zingiber officinale Rosc on experimental atherosclerosis in rabbits. Indian. J. Exp. Biol .42(2004)736

58. Sheela S.C. and Shyamala Devi. C.S protective effect of Abana, A polyherbal formulation on isoproterenol induced myocardial infarction in rats.Indian.J.Pharmacol.,32(2000)198

59. Guh, J.H, KO F.N et. al. Anti platelet effect of gingerol isolated from Zingiber officinale. J.Pharm. Pharmacol47(1995)329

60. Govindaraja, V, S. Ginger-Chemistry, technology, and quality evaluation: Part 2. Critical Reviews Food Science Nutrition. 17(1982)258.

61. Aeschbach, R; Loliger J. Scott, B.C et. al. Antioxidant actions of thymol, carvacrol, gingerol, Zingerone and hydroxy tyrosol. Food Chem Toxicol. 32(1994)31

62. Krishnakanth, T.P and Lokesh, B.R. Scavanging of super oxide anions by spice principles. Indian J. Biochem Biophys. 30(1993)133

63. Reddy, A.C and Lokesh B.R. Sudies on spice principles as antioxidant in the inhibition of lipid peroxide in rat liver microsomes. Mol.Gel.Biochem, 111(1992)117

64. Cao, Z.F, Chen, Z.G et. al. Scavanging effects of ginger on superoxide anions and hydroxyl radicle. Zhonggua Zhong Yao. Za Zhi 18(1993)750

65. Lin, N; Huo, G et. al. Efeects of Zingiber Officinale Rose on lipid per oxidation in hyperlipidemia rats Weisheng Yan Jiu32(2003)22. (Chinese article)

66. Schulick, P. Common Spice or wonder drug? Ginger Herbal Free Press, Brattleboro, Vermont, USA.1993.

67. Endo, K; Kanno, E and Oshima, Y. Structures of antifungal diaryl heptenones, gingerenones, isolated from the rhizomes of zingiber officinale. Phyto chemistry, 29 (1990) 797.

3.5 Phytosterols and Carotenoids Present in Functional Foods

Suneesh, K
Lecturer, Dept. Medical Biochem. SHS. Kannur University

Phytosterols (PS) or plant sterols are structurally similar to cholesterol. The most common PS are β-sitosterol, campesterol and stigmasterol. Epidemiologic and experimental studies suggest that dietary PS may offer protection from the most common cancers in Western societies, such as colon, breast and prostate cancer. This review summarizes the findings of these studies and the possible mechanisms by which PS offer this protection. These include the effect of PS on membrane structure and function of tumor and host tissue, signal transduction pathways that regulate tumor growth and apoptosis, immune function of the host and cholesterol metabolism by the host. In addition, suggestions for future studies to fill the gaps in our knowledge have been given.

Phytosterols (plant sterols, PS) are the counterparts of cholesterol in animal products. They have a structure similar to that of cholesterol but with some modifications. These modifications involve the side chain and include the addition of a double bond and/or methyl or ethyl group. The most common dietary PS are β-sitosterol (SIT), campesterol and stigmasterol (Fig. 1). The Western diet contains 80 mg PS/d, whereas vegetarian and Japanese diets contain 345 and 400 mg/d, respectively[1]. The best dietary sources of PS are unrefined plant oils, seeds, nuts and legumes[2,3]. Processing of plant oils (such as refining and deodorization) reduces PS content, but the loss varies with the type of oil and hydrogenation of refined oils, however, has little effect on PS content[3].

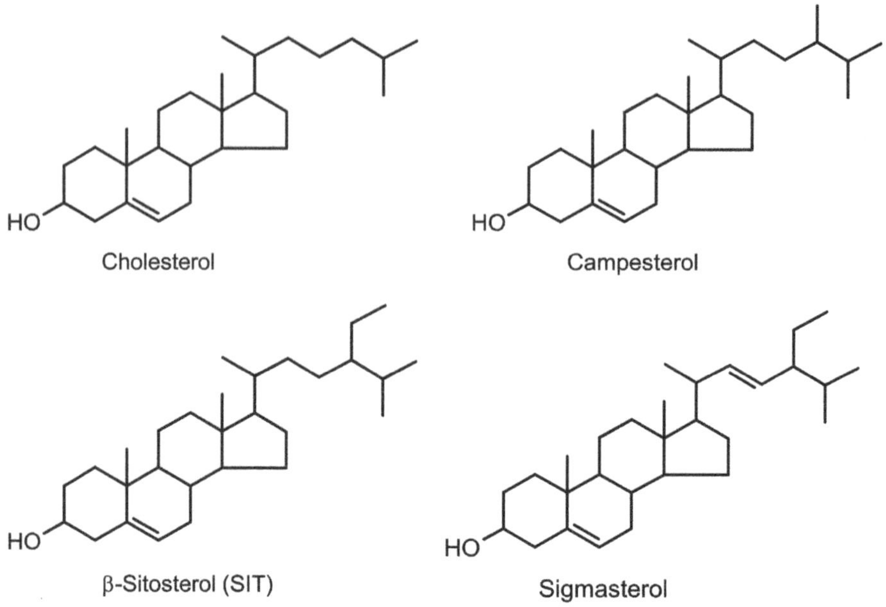

HO Cholesterol

HO Campesterol

HO β-Sitosterol (SIT)

HO Sigmasterol

Fig.1 Structures of cholesterol and phytosteroles.

The interest in studying PS was due initially to their effectiveness in reducing the absorption of dietary cholesterol and thus offering protection from cardiovascular diseases[4,5]. Several review articles on this subject have appeared in the literature[6,7] and thus will not be addressed here. β-sitosterol is present in saw palmeto, pumpkin seeds, rice bran, wheat gem, corn oils and soy beans.

Anticancer Properties of Phytosterols

In recent years, a great deal of interest has been given to the role of PS in the protection from cancer. Raicht et al.[8] suggested that dietary SIT may offer protection from chemically induced colon cancer. These authors examined the growth of methyl nitrosourea-induced tumor in rats fed 0.2% SIT in the diet for 28 wk. There was a 39% reduction in the number of rats that developed the tumor and a 60% reduction in the number of tumors per rat with SIT feeding.

Usually, the development of colon cancer is preceded by an increase in cell proliferation in the colonic mucosa, i.e., hyperplasia. Accordingly, this condition is considered to be a risk factor for the development of colon cancer[9]. Several investigators examined the effect of dietary PS on colonocyte proliferation in mice[10] and rats[11]. In these studies, cell proliferation was stimulated by including cholic acid in the diet and monitored by using labeled ^{3}H-thymidine or bromodeoxy uridine. Feeding a 1–2% PS mixture, which was made up of 56% SIT, 28% campesterol, 10% stigmasterol and 6% dihydrobrassicasterol by weight, for 22 days resulted in normalizing the cholic acid-induced hyperproliferation of colonocytes[11]. In rats fed colon cancer-inducing chemical carcinogens, such as methylnitrosourea, treatment with SIT resulted in reduction of the proliferative compartment of the crypt and cell proliferation[12].

In vitro studies using established human tumor cell lines have revealed an inhibitory effect of SIT on tumor growth of HT-29 cells (a human colon cancer cell line) with 16 μmol/L of SIT supplementation for 5 days[13]. SIT concentration used was the maximum dose within its solubility range and within the physiologic range (4-70 μmol/L) in the blood[7]. However, this concentration is lower than that available to colonocytes *in vivo* because we absorb only 5% of dietary intake[7]. Similar results to those obtained in HT-29 cells, but at a lower magnitude, were also observed using 16 μmol/L of SIT in LNCaP, a human prostate cancer cell line[14]. LNCaP preserves most of the *in vivo* characteristics of prostate cancer[15]. The tumor cells produce prostate-specific antigen (PSA) and acid phosphatase in culture[15] and grow and metastasize in nude[16] and SCID mice[17]. Thus, it offers a unique model to study human prostate cancer *in vitro*. SIT (16 μmol/L) has been shown to be effective in reducing tumor growth as judged by reduction in cell number and PSA production in the media[14]. The effect of SIT and campesterol compared with cholesterol on the growth and apoptosis of MDA-MB-231, a human breast cancer cell line, has been investigated[18]. SIT and campesterol were the only two PS detected in the blood[19, 20]. In these studies, 16 μmol/L of both cholesterol and campesterol was found to be without effect on tumor growth, whereas 16 μmol/L of SIT inhibited the growth of the tumor by 66-80% after 3-5 days of supplementation. The results obtained support the epidemiologic studies that suggest a protective role of PS in the development of cancer[1].

Very little *in vivo* work has been done on the effect of PS on tumor growth and metastasis. To examine the effect of PS on the growth of human tumors in SCID mice, these mice were fed a diet supplemented with 2% of either a PS mixture or cholesterol and 0.2% cholic acid to stimulate sterol absorption. Mice were xenographed with MDA-MB-231 cells after 15 days of consuming the diets and the growth of the tumor was monitored weekly[21]. After 8 weeks, mice fed the PS had 33% smaller tumors ($P < 0.03$) and 20% lower metastasis than those fed the cholesterol diet.

Dietary supplementation of SIT at 60 mg/d for 6 months has been shown to improve the clinical symptoms of prostatic hyperplasia in humans[22]. This disorder, which is benign and does not lead to prostate cancer, is common among older men and results in restricted urinary flow and polyuria due to the enlargement of the gland. In Europe, prostatic hyperplasia is treated clinically with SIT-containing products[22], but these products have not been approved by the Food and Drug Administration in the U.S.

Mechanism of Action of SIT on Tumor Development

The exact mechanism by which SIT offers protection from cancer is not known. However, several theories have been proposed and the findings in these areas are summarized in the following.

Effect of SIT on Membrane Structure

Because SIT has a structure similar to cholesterol, an integral lipid component of biological membranes, its incorporation into membranes has been investigated. SIT incorporation into HT-29 cell membranes did not affect total phospholipid concentration or the cholesterol/phospholipid ratio and had very little effect on the fatty acid composition[13]. However, the incorporation of SIT resulted in a significant effect on the concentration of two phospholipids, i.e., a 50% decrease in sphingomyelin and an 8% increase in phosphatidylcholine. This suggests alteration in some signal transduction pathways, which will be discussed later.

Recently, the incorporation of SIT and campesterol into several tissues of rats was investigated[19]. Rats were fed a diet containing 2% PS mixture, containing by weight, 56% SIT, 28% campesterol, 10% stigmasterol and 6% dihydrobrassicasterol, plus 0.2% cholic acid to enhance the absorption of PS, for 22 days. There was a fivefold increase in plasma PS compared with controls. PS was found to accumulate in adipose tissue and liver microsomes. There was no effect of PS incorporation on microsomal cholesterol concentration of the liver. However, PS reduced the cholesterol concentration by 25% in the testis. There was an increase in some polyunsaturated fatty acids and a decrease in 16:1 fatty acid with PS accumulation in membranes of the liver, testis and prostate. There was no effect of PS incorporation on phospholipid composition of membranes studied.

Effect of PS on Membrane Fluidity

Membrane fluidity has been shown to be influenced by the lipid composition of membranes[23]. For proper function of membranes, fluidity should be maintained at a very narrow range. Incorporation of SIT into liver membranes by feeding rats 5% PS for 21 days decreased the fluidity[24].

There was an increase in the activities of several hepatic fatty acid desaturases (Δ9, Δ6 and Δ5) with SIT incorporation, probably as a compensatory mechanism for the decreased fluidity. The significance of these functional alterations in terms of tumor development has not been investigated.

Effect of PS on Membrane-bound Enzymes

As mentioned above, the incorporation of PS into membranes results in increases in the activities of some fatty acid desaturases in the liver[24]. Recent work indicates that there was a 33–44% decrease in the activities of hepatic and prostatic 5 α-reductase and 55% in prostatic aromatase in rats fed a 2% PS mixture in the diet[25]. These two membrane-bound enzymes are involved in the metabolism of testosterone. Higher levels of both androgens and estrogens, the end products of the action of these two enzymes, respectively, on testosterone, have been implicated in the development of prostate hyperplasia and prostate cancer[26,27]. These results may support the epidemiologic studies that suggest an association between lower levels of prostatic cancer in Asians and vegetarians with diets high in PS compared with the Western diet[28].

Hirano et. al.[29] demonstrated that *in vitro* incubation of some PS with prostatic membranes of benign prostatic hyperplasia patients at concentrations from 10^{-3} to 10^{-6} mol/L inhibited Na^+, K^+-ATPase activity by 23-67%. These authors suggested that PS may suppress prostate metabolism and growth through this mechanism.

Effect of PS on Signal Transduction Pathways

Two pathways have been investigated to explain the inhibition of tumor growth by SIT, protein kinase C (PKC)[30] and the sphingomyelin cycle[31]. *In vivo* work demonstrated the lack of effect of SIT incorporation on the activity of PKC in rat mucosa[11]. Moreover, *in vitro* work on HT-29 cells demonstrated the lack of effect of SIT on phospholipase C, a key enzyme in the PKC pathway, which catalyzes the generation of the two second messengers, inositol trisphosphate and diacylglycerol[32]. These *in vitro* results confirm the in vivo observations on the lack of effect of SIT on the PKC pathway.

The observed changes in membrane phospholipid pattern in HT-29 cells supplemented with SIT, mainly in sphingomyelin, suggest an effect of SIT on the sphingomyelin cycle (**Fig. 2**). Investigating this pathway in HT-29 cells and LNCaP cells revealed the activation of the cycle and increased production of ceramide, the second messenger[14]. Several studies suggest activation of protein phosphatase 2A (PP2A) by ceramide as an intermediate step for the action of ceramide on cell growth and apoptosis[33]. SIT supplementation increased the activity but not the amount of PP2A in LNCaP cells[3]. The effect of SIT on other signal transduction pathways has not been investigated.

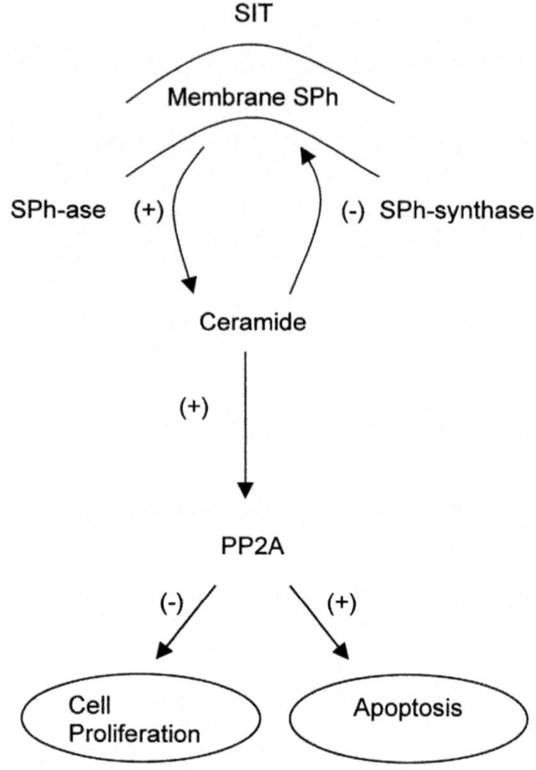

Fig. 2 Proposed mechanism by which β-sitosterol inhibits tumor growth and stimulates apoptosis. Abbreviations: SIT, β -sitosterol; SPh, sphingomyelin; PP2A, protein phosphatase 2A; SPh-ase, sphingomyelinase; SPh-synthase, sphingomyelin synthase.

Effect of PS on Apoptosis

The rate of tumor growth is dependent upon a balance between the rates of cell proliferation and apoptosis. Apoptosis or programmed cell death, as influenced by PS, has been investigated in two tumor cell lines, MDA-MB-231 and LNCaP cells[34,35]. In both cell lines, 16 μmol/L of SIT was found to stimulate apoptosis by four- to six fold above control levels after 3-5 days of treatment[34,35]. Apoptosis was assessed by measuring the release of nucleosomes into the cytoplasm. SIT treatment elevated PP2A activity only in the LNCaP line[35]. This suggests that activation of PP2A may not be a unified mechanism for the action of SIT on apoptosis. The mechanism by which SIT stimulates apoptosis requires further investigation.

Effect of PS on Membrane Integrity

Recent studies demonstrated the lack of cytotoxicity of PS at physiologic levels on cells[34]. Treatment of a breast cancer cell line with SIT and campesterol at the highest concentration within the solubility range (16 μmol/L) had no effect on the release of lactic dehydrogenase from cells in culture. Lactic dehydrogenase release is used as an index for membrane integrity.

Effect of PS on Immune Function

In a recent publication[36], a mixture of SIT and its glucoside at a mass ratio of 100:1 was shown to stimulate human peripheral blood lymphocyte proliferation *in vitro*. In addition, the ingestion of 60 mg/d of this mixture by volunteers for 4 weeks resulted in enhancement of T-cell proliferation upon stimulation *in vitro*. The specific contribution of the SIT glucoside component in this supplement was not clear. Additional studies are required to examine the mechanism by which PS may stimulate immune system function.

Effect of PS on Tissue Esterogenic Properties

Because estrogen receptors play a role in the development of sex organ tumors, estrogenic properties of PS were assessed. It has been shown that fish develop infertility when exposed to high levels of wood pulp, which is rich in SIT, in the water[37]. However, studies in mammals such as rats using plant sterols or stanols did not demonstrate any estrogenic effect *in vivo* or *in vitro*[38]. These studies showed that PS do not bind to estrogen receptors and do not affect uterine wet weight of immature rats. Furthermore, PS did not stimulate transcriptional activity of human estrogen receptors in yeast[39].

Free or esterified stanols at high levels (100 μmmol/L) did not stimulate the growth of estrogen-responsive MCF-7 cells in culture nor increase uterine wet weight of rats when fed at 8.3% in the diet for 4 days[39]. Accordingly, the reported results on fish could be due to some other components in wood pulp.

Effect of PS on Neutral and Acidic Sterols in the Colon

Cholesterol and primary bile acids are converted in the large intestine by bacterial action to coprostanol and secondary bile acids, respectively. The presence of high levels of these modified sterols in the colonic content has been suggested to play a role in the development of colon cancer[40]. Dietary

PS have been shown to alter the level of fecal sterols[41,42]. The mechanisms by which PS influence colonic fecal sterols may include the action of PS on colonic bacteria and alteration of cholesterol absorption[43].

The mechanisms by which PS influence cell growth and apoptosis of tumor cells require additional study. This is especially urgent because the public has been advised concerning the effectiveness of dietary PS in reducing blood cholesterol and encouraged to consume PS-enriched products such as margarine and salad dressing. It is intriguing to mention that the added protection from several types of cancer afforded by PS treatment occurs at the same levels of PS used to lower blood cholesterol. The interaction between PS and other phytochemicals such as phytoestrogen, vitamin E and antioxidants, which have also been shown to protect from cancer, should be explored.

CAROTENOIDS: They are tetra terpenes and over 600 types of carotenoids are found in nature providing red, orange and yellow pigments to fruits and vegetables. Some in particular are alpha and beta carotenes-act as provitamins, converted to vitamin by human digestive system. Carotenoids are long chain hydrocarbons with conjugated double bonds.

Lycopene is a deep red pigment, found in tomatoes and other pink red fruits and vegetables. It has a simple acyclic structure and is considered as the prototype of carotenoids. They are a group of lipid soluble antioxidants based around an isoprenoid carbon skeleton. The most important of these is beta carotene, although at least 20 others may be present in membranes and lipoproteins. They are particularly efficient scavengers of singlet oxygen[44], but can also trap peroxy radicals at low oxygen pressure with an efficiency at least as great as that of alpha tocopherol. Because of these conditions prevailing in many biological tissues, the carotenoids might play a role in preventing *in vivo* lipid peroxidation[45]. The other important role of certain carotenoids is as precursors of vitamin A (retinol). Vitamin A also has antioxidant properties[46] which do not however show any dependency on oxygen concentration

Despite having no provitamin A function, carotenoids such as lycopene and lutein, are still biologically active. High serum lycopene concentrations have been linked to a reduced risk of atherosclerosis, while preventive effects against heart disease and cancer have also been reported[44]. As an antioxidant it is a powerful quencher of oxygen free radicals compared to other carotenoids. Lycopene also appears to play a particular role in reducing the risk of postrate cancer[47].

Beta Carotene

When it comes to nutritional supplementation, and antioxidants in particular, **beta carotene** is an antiaging micronutrient of the highest order, standing firmly alongside Vitamin C, Vitamin E, and the mineral Selenium in its ability to reduce illness, improve overall health, and increase longevity.

What can beta carotene do for you? Studies conducted over several years indicate that beta carotene may play a significant role in reducing the effects of certain illnesses (such as heart disease, decreased immune function, cataracts, and forms of cancer) and, in certain cases, perhaps even prevent them.

Beta-carotene acts as a precursor of vitamin A, and is therefore called a provitamin A compound. Foods or supplements containing beta-carotene are converted to vitamin A for the maintenance of healthy skin, good vision, and a robust immune system.

Beta-carotene is also a powerful antioxidant, and has been shown to help guard against cancer and heart disease.

Beta-carotene is a member of the carotenoid family, a group of powerful antioxidants that also includes alpha-carotene, lycopene, zeaxanthin, and lutein. However, of all the carotenoids, only alpha-carotene and beta-carotene are converted to significant amounts of vitamin A in the body, and beta-carotene is by far the most plentiful carotenoid found in fruits and vegetables.

Along with Beta-carotene flavonoids are also found which are antioxidant substances that give color and flavor to many orange and red colored fruits and vegetables. Foods such as carrots, tomatoes, sweet potatoes, cantaloupe, watermelon, apricots, and mangoes are good sources of beta-carotene; romaine lettuce, spinach, kale, and broccoli are also rich in carotenoids (the yellow color is covered up by chlorophyll in green leafy plants).

Here's a tip regarding flavonoids: Many flavonoids in fruits and vegetables are in the skin, so it's best not to peel them before eating. However, grilling or lightly steaming some foods, such as carrots and spinach, can actually improve the body's ability to absorb the flavonoids in them.

Beta-carotene, derived from the Latin name for carrot, belongs to a family of natural chemicals known as carotenes or carotenoids. Members of this family include lycopene, astaxanthin, and zeaxanthin. Widely found in plants, carotenes give yellow and orange fruits and vegetables their rich colors. Beta-carotene is also used as a coloring agent for foods such as margarine.

Beta-carotene is converted to vitamin A (retinol) by the body. While excessive amounts of vitamin A in supplement form can be toxic, the body will convert only as much vitamin A from beta-carotene as it needs. This feature makes beta-carotene a safe source of vitamin A.

Like all other carotenoids, beta-carotene is an antioxidant. Consuming foods rich in beta-carotene appears to protect the body from damaging molecules called free radicals. Free radicals cause damage to cells through a process known as oxidation. Over time, this damage can lead to a variety of chronic illnesses. Some studies suggest that dietary intake of beta-carotene may reduce the risk of two types of chronic illness – heart disease and cancer. Supplementation, however, is more controversial. See discussion in the section that follows.

Therapeutic Uses

Prevention

Population-based studies suggest that groups of people who eat 4 or more daily servings of fruits and vegetables rich in beta-carotene may have less of a chance of developing heart disease or cancer. Foods rich in beta-carotene include those that are orange or yellow, such as peppers, squashes, and carrots.

Interestingly, however, a few studies indicate that people who take beta-carotene supplements may actually be at an increased risk for such conditions as cancer and heart disease. Researchers speculate that multiple nutrients consumed in a healthy, balanced diet may be more protective than beta-carotene supplements alone.

Treatment

Sun Sensitivity

Studies suggest that high doses of beta-carotene may decrease sensitivity to the sun. This is particularly helpful for people with skin conditions caused by sunlight exposure, such as erythropoietic protoporphyria, a condition characterized, in part, by development of hives or eczema upon exposure to the sun. Under the guidance of an appropriate health care provider, the oral supplement dose of beta-carotene is slowly adjusted over a period of weeks, and exposure to sunlight gradually increased.

Scleroderma

Because people with scleroderma, a connective-tissue disorder characterized by hardened skin, have low levels of beta-carotene in their blood, some researchers speculate that beta-carotene supplements may be beneficial for those with the condition. Due to methodological flaws in the studies that have been conducted to date, however, research has not confirmed this theory. At this time, it is best to obtain beta-carotene from dietary sources and avoid supplementation until more information is available.

Dietary Sources

The richest sources of beta-carotene are yellow, orange, and green leafy fruits and vegetables (such as carrots, spinach, lettuce, tomatoes, sweet potatoes, broccoli, cantaloupe, and winter squash). In general, the greater the intensity of the color of the fruit or vegetable, the more beta-carotene it contains.

Dosage and Administration

Beta-carotene supplements are available in both capsule and gel forms. Beta-carotene is fat-soluble and, therefore, should be taken with meals containing at least 3 g of fat to ensure absorption.

Pediatric

- For children younger than 14 with erythropoietic protoporphyria (see Treatment section for brief description of this condition), 30-150 mg per day (50,000-250,000 IU) in single or divided oral doses for 2-6 weeks is recommended. The supplement may be mixed with orange or tomato juice to facilitate administration. In the case of this sun-sensitive condition, a doctor can measure blood levels of beta-carotene and adjust the dose accordingly.

Adult

- For general health, 15-50 mg (25,000-83,000 IU) per day is recommended.
- For adults with erythropoietic protoporphyria, 30-300 mg (50,000-500,000 IU) per day for 2-6 weeks is recommended. A health care provider can measure blood levels of beta-carotene and adjust the dose accordingly.
- It is recommended to eat five or more servings of fruits and vegetable every day. This level of intake of fruits and vegetables provides approximately 3-6 mg of beta-carotene.

Precautions

Beta-carotene offers protection from cancer only when other important antioxidants, including vitamins C and E, are present in the diet. Since beta-carotene may increase the risk of heart disease and cancer in those who smoke or drink heavily, this supplement should be used with caution, if at all, by heavy smokers or drinkers.

Although beta-carotene affords protection from sunlight for people with certain skin sensitivities, it does not protect against sunburn.

Side Effects

Side effects from beta-carotene include:

- Skin discoloration (yellowing that eventually goes away)
- Loose stools
- Bruising
- Joint pain

Pregnancy and Breastfeeding

While animal studies indicate beta-carotene is not toxic to a fetus or a newborn, there are no human studies to confirm these findings. The supplement may pass into breast milk, but no information on the safety of its use during breastfeeding has been reported. Therefore, while pregnant or breastfeeding, beta-carotene supplements should only be used under the guidance of a physician or other appropriately trained specialist.

Pediatric Use

Side effects in children are the same as those seen in adults.

Geriatric Use

Side effects in older adults are the same as younger adults.

Interactions and Depletions

People taking the following medications should avoid beta-carotene supplements:

Cholestyramine, Colestipol

Cholestyramine, a medication used to lower cholesterol, can lower blood concentrations of dietary beta carotene by 30-40 %, according to a 3-year study in Sweden. Colestipol, a cholesterol-lowering medication similar to cholestyramin, may also reduce beta-carotene levels.

Orlistat

You should not take beta-carotene with orlistat, a weight loss medication, because orlistat can reduce the absorption of beta-carotene by as much as 30 %, thereby reducing the amount of this nutrient in the body. If you must take both orlistat and beta-carotene supplements, you should separate the time between taking the medication and the supplements by at least 2 hours.

Other

In addition to these medications, mineral oil (used to treat constipation) may lower blood concentrations of beta-carotene and ongoing use of alcohol may interact with beta-carotene, increasing the likelihood of liver damage.

Additional Information on the use of Phytosterols

- Plant sterols and plant stanols are collectively known as phytosterols. Plant sterols are plant compounds with chemical structures similar to that of cholesterol. Especially high sterol levels are found in rice bran, wheat germ, corn oils, and soybeans. In a more concentrated form, these substances are called plant stanols. Structurally these compounds are chemically similar to cholesterol. However, unlike cholesterol derived from animal sources–which absorbs easily and raises the body's own cholesterol levels–phytosterols are present only at very low levels in the body because they are difficult to absorb.

  Interestingly, phytosterols so closely resemble cholesterol that they can actually block food-based cholesterol from being absorbed into the bloodstream. The result is that both phytosterols and dietary cholesterol end up excreted in waste matter.

  Recently food manufacturers have begun to incorporate plant sterols and stanols into such "functional foods" as vegetable oil spreads (Benecol or Take Control, for example). Nutritional supplement manufacturers also offer phytosterols in tablet form for those individuals who don't want the extra calories of cholesterol-lowering margarine.

  Concentrated extracts of another phytosterol called beta sistosterol have been tested for lessening such discomforts of benign prostatic hyperplasia (BPH) as frequent and painful urination.

Health Benefits

Because of their ability to block dietary cholesterol absorption, phytosterols can help lower your cholesterol levels. In the last few years, clinical research has also discovered other effects, including reducing symptoms of an enlarged prostate, improving the control of blood sugar among people with diabetes, and reducing inflammation among patients with autoimmune diseases such as rheumatoid arthritis and lupus.

Because much of this research is still in a preliminary phase, nutritionally oriented physicians are currently recommending phytosterols only for prostate disorders and cholesterol-lowering.

Specifically, phytosterols may help to:

- **Prevent heart disease.** By lowering total and LDL cholesterol levels, plant sterols and stanols may reduce your risk of heart disease. Studies have shown that daily phytosterols can lower these cholesterol measurements by an average of 10% to 14%. Because of these strong findings, the National Cholesterol Education Panel issued a new recommendation in 2001 that plant stanols and sterols be added to cholesterol-lowering regimens, along with the more traditional cholesterol-fighting tools, such as regular exercise, weight loss, and a low-fat diet. Phytosterols do not appear to lower triglycerides, another blood lipid that is harmful in excess, or to raise levels of HDL, the "good" cholesterol.
- **Ease enlarged prostate.** For the last 20 years, an herbal preparation containing phytosterols has been available in Germany for treatment of benign prostate hypertrophy (BPH). More recently, two six-month studies on 350 men with BPH given the phytosterol beta-sitosterol showed an increase in their urinary flow rate and a decrease in pain and burning.
- **Calm inflammation in rheumatoid arthritis (RA).** Most traditional treatments for RA involve drugs that suppress the body's immune response, which can often cause troubling side effects. A mixture of the phytosterols beta-sitosterol and beta-sistosterolin has shown promise in helping to decrease inflammation and calm the overactive immune response that characterizes RA and other autoimmune diseases. More research is needed, however.
- **Control blood sugar in diabetes.** Some phytosterols stimulate insulin secretion and may contribute to better blood sugar control, a problem in people with diabetes. Animal studies have suggested that beta-sitosterol and beta-sistosterolin might be beneficial for people with diabetic and pre-diabetic conditions. More research is necessary before these findings are recommended to people with diabetes.

Dosage Information

Special Tips: The cholesterol-controlling margarines such as Benecol and Take Control suggest a dose of 2 tablespoons daily to help lower total and LDL cholesterol levels.

For lowering cholesterol: Take 200-250 mg three times a day, with meals. **For enlarged prostate (BPH):** Take 125-250 mg a day, on an empty stomach.

[Guidelines for Use]

- Because phytosterols help block dietary cholesterol adsorption, they should be taken with meals.
- Beta-sitosterol, when used for prostate enlargement, is generally taken on an empty stomach to enhance its absorption into the bloodstream.
- Some research has shown that phytosterols can slightly lower concentrations of fat-soluble vitamins such as beta-carotene, but other studies show no such effect. Although carotene levels normally vary with the seasons, it may be a reasonable precaution to increase your intake of beta-carotene (or carotene-containing foods such as carrots, yellow squash, and sweet potatoes) while taking phytosterol supplements.
- If you are taking phytosterols in the margarine form, simply replace your usual spread. You may need to eat somewhat larger amounts than you are accustomed to in order to achieve an effective dose.

General Interaction

- There are no known drug or nutrient interactions associated with phytosterols in typical doses. There may be some reduction in the body's levels of carotenoids, but this finding is under debate.

Possible Side Effects

- At typical doses, there are no known side effects or adverse reactions. However, in one study in which participants took three to four times the suggested dose, some gastrointestinal upset occurred.

High Cholesterol Patients

Take 200-250 mg three times a day, with meals.

Prostate Problems

Take 125-250 mg a day.

Abbreviations used: PKC, protein kinase C; PP2A, protein phosphatate 2A; PS, phytosterols; PSA prostate-specific antigen; SIT, β-sitosterol.)

References

1. Messina M., Barnes S. The role of soy products in reducing the risk of cancer. J. Natl. Cancer Inst. 1991;83:541-546.
2. Weihrauch J. L., Gardner J. M. Sterol contents of foods of plant origin. J. Am. Diet. Assoc. 1978;73:39-47.
3. Awad A. B., Chan K. C., Downie A. C., Fink C. S. Peanuts as a source of β-sitosterol, a sterol with anticancer properties. Nutr. Cancer 2000;36:238-241.
4. Vahouny G. V., Connor W. E., Subramanian S., Lin D. S., Gallo L. L. Comparative lymphatic absorption of sitosterol, stigmasterol and frucosterol, and differential inhibition of cholesterol absorption. Am. J. Clin. Nutr. 1983;37:805-809.
5. Ikeda I., Tanaka K., Sugano M., Vahouny G. V., Gall L. L. Inhibition of cholesterol absorption in rats by plant sterols. J. Lipid Res. 1988;29:1573-1582.
6. Nguyen T. T. The cholesterol-lowering action of plant stanol esters. J. Nutr. 1999;129:2109-2112.
7. Ling W. H., Jones P.J.H. Dietary phytosterols: a review of metabolism, benefits and side effects. Life Sci 1995;57:195-206.
8. Raicht R. F., Cohen L. I., Fazzini E. P., Sarwal A. N., Takahashi M. Protective effect of plant sterols against chemically induced colon tumors in rats. Cancer Res 1980;40:403-405.
9. Lipkin M., Uehara K., Winawer S., Sanchez A., Bauer C., Phillips R., Lynch H. T., Blattner W. A., Fraumeni J, Jr. Seventh-day Adventist vegetarians have a quiescent proliferative activity in colonic mucosa. Cancer Lett 1985;26:139-144.
10. Janezic S. A., Rao A. V. Dose-dependent effect of dietary phytosterols on epithelial cell proliferation of the murine colon. Food Chem. Toxicicol. 1992;30:611-616.
11. Awad A. B., Henandez A.Y.T., Fink C. S., Mendel S. L. Effect of dietary phytosterols on cell proliferation and protein kinase C activity in rat colonic mucosa. Nutr. Cancer 1997;27:210-215.
12. Dreshner E. E., Cohen B. J., Raicht R. F. The kinetics of the protective effect of β-sitosterol against MNU-induced colonic neoplasia. J. Cancer Res. Clin. Oncol. 1982;103:49-54.
13. Awad A. B., Chen Y. C., Fink C. S., Hennessey T. β-Sitosterol inhibits HT-29 human colon cancer cell growth and alters membrane lipids. Anticancer Res 1996;16:2797-2804.

14. Von Holtz R. L., Fink C. S., Awad A. B. β-Sitosterol activates the sphingomyelin cycle and induces apoptosis in LNCaP human prostate cancer cells. Nutr. Cancer 1998;32:8-12.

15. Horoszewicz J. S., Leong S. S., Kawinski E., Karr J. P., Rosenthal H., Chu T. M., Mirand E. A., Murphy G. P. LNCaP model of human prostatic carcinoma. Cancer Res 1983;43:1809-1818.

16. Wang Y., Corr J. G., Thaler H. T., Tao Y., Fair W. R., Heston W. D. Decreased growth of established human prostate LNCaP tumors in nude mice fed a low-fat diet. J. Natl. Cancer Inst. 1995; 87:1456-1462.

17. Zhou J. R., Gugger E. T., Tanaka T., Guo Y., Blackburn G. L., Clinton S. K. Soybean phytochemicals inhibit the growth of transplantable human prostate carcinoma and tumor angiogenesis in mice. J. Nutr. 1999;129:1628-1635.

18. Downie A., Fink S. C., Awad A. B. Effect of phytosterols on MDA-MB-231 human breast cancer cell growth. FASEB J 1999;13:A333(abs.)

19. Awad A. B., Garcia M. D., Fink C. S. Effects of dietary phytosterols on rat tissue lipids. Nutr. Cancer 1997;29:212-216.

20. Westrate J. A., Meijer G. W. Plant sterol-enriched margarines and reduction of plasma total- and LDL-cholesterol concentrations in normocholesterolemic and mildly hypercholesterolemic subjects. Eur. J. Clin. Nutr. 1998;52:334-343.

21. Awad A. B., Downie A., Fink C. S., Kim U. Dietary phytosterol inhibits the growth and metastasis of MDA-MB-231 human breast cancer cells grown in SCID mice. Anticancer Res 2000;20:821-824.

22. Berges R. R., Windeler J., Trampisch J. H., Senge T. Randomized, placebo-controlled, double-blind clinical trial of β-sitosterol in patients with benign prostatic hyperplasia. Lancet 1995;345:1529-1532.

23. Spector A. A., Yorek M. A. Membrane lipid composition and cellular function. J. Lipid Res. 1985;26:1015-1035.

24. Leikin A. I., Brenner R. R. Fatty acid desaturase activities are modulated by phytosterol incorporation in microsomes. Biochim. Biophys. Acta 1989;1005:187-191.

25. Awad A. B., Hartati M. S., Fink C. S. Phytosterol feeding induces alteration in testosterone metabolism in rat tissues. J. Nutr. Biochem. 1998;9:712-717.

26. Howie B. J., Shultz T. D. Dietary and hormonal interrelationships among vegetarian Seventh-Day Adventists and non-vegetarian men. Am. J. Clin. Nutr. 1985;42:127-134.

27. Schweikert H. U., Tunn U. W., Habenicht U. F., Arnold J., Senge T., Schulze H., Schroder F. H., Blom J. H., Ennenoser O., Horniger W., Bartsch G. Effects of estrogen deprivation on human benign prostatic hyperplasia. J. Steroid Biochem. Mol. Biol 1993;44:573-576.

28. Mettlin C. Clinical oncology update: prostate cancer. Recent developments in the epidemiology of prostate cancer. Eur. J. Cancer 1997;33:340-347.

29. Hirano T., Homma M., Oka K. Effects of stinging nettle root extracts and their steroidal components on the NA^+, K^+-ATPase of the benign prostatic hyperplasia. Planta Med 1994;60:30-33.

30. Nishizuka Y. Intracellular signaling by hydrolysis of phospholipids and activation of protein kinase C. Science (Washington, DC) 1992;258:607-614.

31. Hannun Y. A., Linardic C. M. Sphingomyelin breakdown products: antiproliferative and tumor suppressor lipids. Biochim. Biophys. Acta 1994;1154:223-236.

32. Awad A. B., von Holtz R. L., Cone J. P., Fink C. S., Chen Y.-C. ß-Sitosterol inhibits the growth of HT-29 human colon cancer cells by activating the sphingomyelin cycle. Anticancer Res 1998;18:471-479.

33. Wolff R. A., Dobrowsky R. T., Bielawski A., Obeid L. M., Hannun Y. A. Role of ceramide-activated protein phosphatase in ceramide-mediated signal transduction. J. Biol. Chem. 1994;269:19607-19609.

34. Awad A. B., Downie D., Fink C. S. Inhibition of growth and stimulation of apoptosis by β-sitosterol treatment of human breast cancer MDA-MB-231 cells in culture. Int. J. Mol. Med. 2000;5:541-545.

35. Awad A. B., Gan Y., Fink C. S. Effect of β-sitosterol, a plant sterol, on growth, protein phosphatase 2A and phospholipid D in LNCaP cells. Nutr. Cancer 2000;36:74-78.

36. Bouic P.J.D., Estebeth S., Leibenberg R. W., Albrecht C. F., Pegel K., Van Jaarsveld P. P. Beta-sitosterol and beta-sitosterol glucoside stimulate human peripheral blood lymphocyte proliferation: implications for their use as an immunomodulatory vitamin combination. Int. J. Immunopharmacol. 1996; 18:693-700.

37. Mellanen P., Petanen T., Lehtimaki J., Makela S., Bylund G., Holmbom B., Mannila E., Okari A., Santti R. Wood-derived estrogens: studies in vitro with breast cancer cell line and in vivo in trout. Toxicol. Appl. Pharmacol. 1996; 136:381-388.

38. Baker V. A., Hepburn P. A., Kennedy S. J., Jones P. A., Lea L. J., Sumpter J. P., Ashby J. Safety evaluation of phytosterol esters. Part 1. Assessment of estrogenicity using a combination of in vivo and in vitro assays. Food Chem. Toxicol. 1999; 37:13-22.

39. Turnbull D., Frankos V. H., Leeman W. R., Jonker D. Short-term tests of estrogenic potential of plant stanols and plant stanol esters. Regul. Toxicol. Pharmacol. 1999; 29:211-215.

40. Dwyer J. T. Health aspects of vegetarian diets. Am. J. Clin. Nutr. 1988; 48:712-738.

41. Cohen B. I., Mosbach E. H., Raicht R. F. Effect of dietary bile acids, cholesterol and β-sitosterol upon formation of coprosterol and 7-dehydroxylation of bile acids by rats. Lipids 1974; 9:1024-1029.

42. Andriamiarina R., Laraki L., Pelletier X., Debry A. Effects of stigmasterol-supplemented diets on fecal neutral sterols and bile acid excretion in rats. Ann. Nutr. Metab. 1989; 33:297-303.

43. Rao A. V., Janezic S. A. The role of dietary phytosterols in colon carcinogenesis. Nutr. Cancer 1992; 18:43-52.

44. Pukuzawa, K; Inokami, Y; Tokumura, A. Rate constants for quenching singlet oxygen and activities for inhibiting lipid per oxidation of carotenoids and alpha-tocopherol in liposomes. Lipid, 1998; 33:751-756.

45. Chaudiere, J and Ferrari-Illiou, R. Intracellular antioxidants from chemical to biochemical mechanisms. Food Chem. Toxicol.1999; 37: 949-962.

46. Keys, S.A and Zimmerman, W.F. Antioxidant action of retinol, glutathione and bovine photoreceptor cell membranes. Exp. Eve. Re.1999; 68:693-702.

47. Criston, A; Di Pierro, F and Bombardelli, E. Botanical derivatives for the prostate. Fitoterpia, 2000; 71:S21-S28.

3.6 Phytosterols

Dr. K.T. Augusti & K. Suneesh
Dept. Med. Biochem. SHS. Kannur University.

Phytesterols are characterized by a (OH) group attached to C_3 of a steroid nucleus with an extra methyl or ethyl substituent in the side chain (on C_{24}) not present in animal sterols. Phytosterols are minor but beneficial components of the human diet (e.g. yams, cereals, soyabeans, mushrooms etc), since they may inhibit growth of tumors and help in the regulation of blood cholesterol. Therapeutically they are important constituents of the following herbs.

(i) The active hypoglycemic principle isolated from the seeds of momordica charantia: which is a mixture of steroidal glycosides (Beta sitosterol – D – Glucoside and 5, 25 - stigmasten-3- beta- ol -D-glucoside). Considerable amount of work has been done in this regard by many viz; Day et. al[1]. Karananayake et. al.[2], Shihib et. al[3]. John et. al[4]. and Miura et. al[5].

(ii) Steroidal compounds including stigmast – 4-en-3-one are thought to be present in stinging nettle root (urtice dioica) extracts and responsible for potent inhibitory action on enzymes in benign prostatic hyperplasia[6].

(iii) Withania someniferum (Solanaceae), known as ashwaganda contains steroidal lactones called withanolides which exhibit antitumor and hepatoprotective action[7].

(iv) Commiphora mukul – myrrh (guggal in Ayurveda) contains steroids, which lower blood cholesterol and triglycerides via stimulation of thyroid function[8].

(v) Another group of steroidal compounds are saponins[7] and they are present in cereals, soyabeans, yams, potatoes, ginseng, spinach, tomatoes, asparagus as well as legumes. They are endowed with anticancer, anti-inflammatory, antiallergic, antiviral, immuno modulatory, anti hepatotoxic, antidiabetic, hypocholesterolemic, antistress and diuretic activities.

Due to detergent effects noted earlier for saponins, they are capable of increasing permeability of membranes. Therefore their excessive use may lead to hemolysis. The slow rate of absorption significantly slows down the rate of haemolysis and associated toxicity[9]. Saponins are regularly consumed by humans as they are present in cereals[10], and they rarely demonstrate side effects. Some saponins present in ginseng and soyabeans have been found to reduce inflammation[11]. The carboxylic group at C_{28} or C_{3O} in the sterioid nucleus is responsible for the anti-inflammatory action[12].

Phytosterols including saponins reduce serum cholesterol concentrations probably due to the structural similarity with cholesterol that enable them to reduce absorption of cholesterol from intestine[9]. Probably the saponins present in many vegetables like spinach, tomatoes, soyabeans and asparagus as well as many legumes may play such a role and protect the heart and liver from hypercholesterol related diseases. The medicinal property of panax ginseng may be due to its saponin components. The detergent property of saponins enable them to lower surface tension. The triterpenoid saponins include glycyrrhetic acid from liquorice root, ursane and lupines represented by ginsenoids from Panax ginseng and jujubosides from zizuphus jujuba[7]. Numerous triterpenoid saponins have been shown to inhibit pathogenic fungi, e.g., monodesmosides α and β hederin from common ivy (Hedera helix)[7]. Antifungal activity appears to be influenced by the number and kinds of sugar residues in each glucoside[13]. Non-glycosidic triterpenes are found in some mushrooms viz, reishi (ganoderma lucidum) and poria coccus.

A Standard Phytosterol used for the Study of its Health Promoting Effects

Withaperuvin E is a trihydroxy, steroidal lactone (14, 17, 20 trihydroxy withanolide) isolated from the roots of physalisperuvianna Linn. It belongs to the class of withasteroids[14]. It showed antilipid peroxidation activity in rats.

Lipid peroxidations was induced in rats by cumene hydroxide. The inhibition of malon dialdehyde (MDA) production by withaperuvin E (WPE) has been comparable to that with a synthetic antioxidant parabenzoquinone[15]. WPE compound has an α, β - unsaturated δ lactone chain in the side chain of a steroidal 1, 4- quinone A ring with an epoxide in the 5, 6 position of B ring, in addition to three tertiary hydroxyl groups at 14, 17 and 20 positions. The antioxidant activity of WPE was assayed by estimating its protective effect against cumine hydroxide induced lipid peroxidation[16]. Predominant TBARS Viz. MDA was estimated by the standard method using Thiobarbituric acid as substrate[17]. Rats were maintained on normal diet and water. Overnight fasted rats were anaesthetized by I.P. injection of pentobarbitone (3mg/100g b.w.). Liver was perfused with normal saline before taking it out. It was homogenized in glass teflon homogenizer in cold condition. 5% rat liver homogenate was incubated at 37^{0}C with different concentrations of WPE, Parabenzo quinone and drug vehicle (Tween 80:water 1:9) for 20 min, and cumene hydroxide (1.5 mM) was added to each plate. The mixture was further incubated for 20 min. at the end of which 100 μl aliquot was withdrawn from each plate and mixed with 1.5 ml tri chloroacetic acid (10%). TCA soluble fraction was transferred to a separate tube and mixed with 1.5 ml TBA (0.67% aqueous TBA in 50% TCA, 1:1). The reaction mixture was boiled in water both for 30 min, cooled and absorbance was recorded at 535 nm. The protective effect was proportional to the compounds concentration (30-180 μg/ml). At about 180 μg/ml withaperuvin E, the degree of protection was 53% when compared to the control value of TBARS. Changes were highly significant[15] as per students t-test. WPE as an antioxidant adds to the growing list of phytosterols with free readical scavenging action[18]. Quinones act as electron acceptor for flavoprotein NADPH - Cytochrome C reductase[19] and that property may be attributed to the function of WPE.

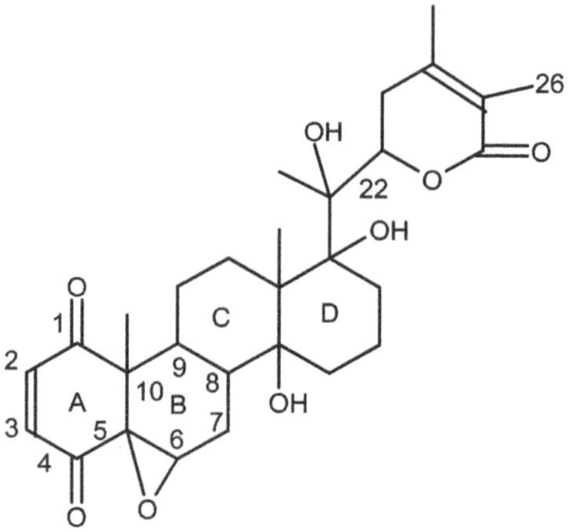

Withaperuvin E

Phytoestrogens

They are of plant origin and have structural similarities to oestrogens, so they are classified as phytoestrogens. They bind to oestrogen receptors but whose oestrogen activity is relatively low. Isoflavone such as genistein of soyabean and lignan derivatives such as schizandrins from Schisandra sinensis belong to this class. **They have oestrogenic, antitumor and antioxidant properties**. Schizandrins reverse destruction of liver cells[20] by inducement of cytochrome P-450, while other lignans are antimicrobial, antiviral and antineoplastic. Recent Studies on lignans have focused on a range of compounds demonstrating cardiovascular activities such as inhibition of cyclic AMP phosphodiesterase, PAF antagonism, calcium channel and antihypertensive and antioxidant effects[21]. Lignans are also present in grains and pulses and their regular consumption has been shown to affect oestrogen levels in humans[22].

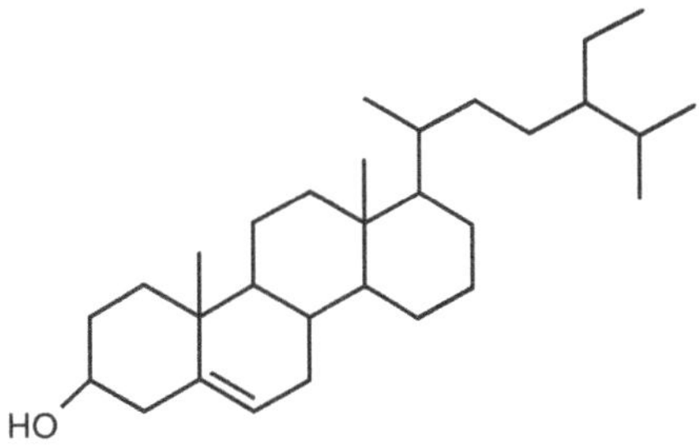

β Sitosterol

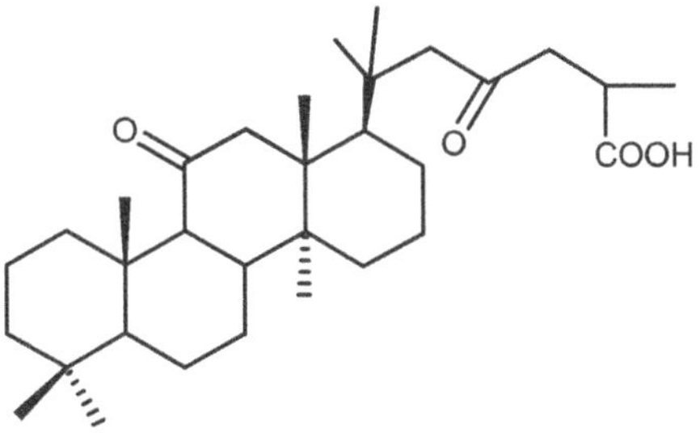

Ganoderic acid

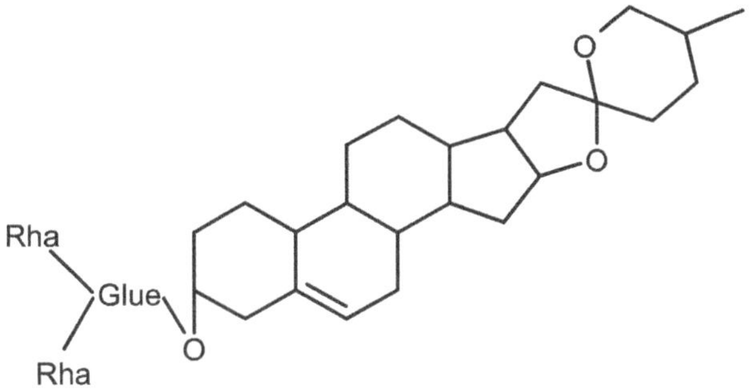

Dioscin from Dioscorea Villosa (a variety of yam)

Steroidal Saponin

Ganoderma

An Immune Booster

The miraculous king of herbs has got highest ranking in the world of fungi. It is an exceptional mushroom with remarkable medicinal properties. Botanically it is a highly–evolved genus belonging to the family of fungi called polyporaceae. It has been immortalized through out Chinese history and culture. The various species of ganoderma contain more than 200 active elements having specific medicinal properties. Extensive international modern research on ganoderma is showing evidences of its ability to promote over all health and longevity both in health and diseases.

The most significant phytosterols found in reishi (ganoderma lucidum) and poria coccus are non-glycosidic triterpenes, e.g. ganoderals and ganoderic acids from reishi. Kim et. al[23]. reported on the isolation of well over 100 triterpenes from the fruit and mycelium of ganoderma lucidum. These compounds inhibit histamine release, ACE and cholesterol synthesis[24] and some were proved to have cytotoxicity against hepatoma cells *in vitro*[25]. Ten of those lanostane triterpenes have been found to be ACE inhibitors and antihypertensive[26]. Several of the terpenes inhibit HIV-1 *in vitro*[23]. **Poriatin another triterpene isolated from Poria coccus showed immunomodulating properties, viz; demonstrated antiviral activity and increased production of macrophages and other immune cells.** It has also demonstrated immuno suppressive activity and reduced the severity of induced autoimmune encephalitis in conjuction with a standard autoimmune drug. Poriatin is an aldosterone antagonist[27]. *Mushrooms are claimed to possess antiviral, antibiotic, anti-inflammatory, hypoglycemic, hypocholesterolemic and hypotensive activities*[28]. Many health claims are made on the effect of ganodoma on the immune system. These claims are based primarily on the presence of high MW polysaccharides and free radical scavengers like triterpenes present in the mushroom. In an experiment conducted by Lakshmi, Sneha Mathew et. al[29], 5 days prior feeding of the methanolic extract of this mushroom gave significant protection to mice later irradiated with 4.5 Gy of gamma rays. G.lucidum extract was found to delimit the metabolic changes to a great extent in the liver of irradiated mice. The effects of the extract were evident from the restoration of the activities of GSH, GPX, SOD, CAT and inhibition of lipid peroxidation. Currently more than hundred different triterpenoids are known to occur in G. lucidum alone. Majority are various ganoderic acids and lucidenic acids[30]. The ganoderic acids, C, A and D appear to have antiallergic activity and inhibiting histamine release[31] and reduce hypertension respectively. In Chinese medicine fruiting bodies of G.lucidum is considered as a Panacea because of its proven ability to treat a number of diseases.

The biological activities of oxygenated triterpenes include bitterness, hepatoprotection and cytotoxicity to hepatoma cells, inhibition of histamine release, angiotensin converting enzyme, cholesterol biosynthesis and stimulation as well as inhibition of thrombin induced platelet aggregation[32].

References

1. Day C; Cartwright T; Provost J and Bailey C.J. Hypoglycemic effect of Momordica charantia extracts. Planta Med. 56(5) (1990) 426-429.

2. Karunanayake E.H; Jeevathayaparan S and Tennekoon K.H. Effect of Momordica charantia fruit juice on streptozotocin – induced diabetes in rats. J. Ethanopharmacol 30(2) (1990) 199-204.

3. Shibib B.A; Khan L.A and Rahman R. Hypoglycemic activity of Coccinia indica and momordica charantia in diabetic rats: depression of the hepatic gluconeogenic enzymes, glucose – 6- phosphatase and fructose -1, 6 bisphostase and elevation of both liver and red cell shunt enzyme glucose – 6 – phosphate dehydrogenase. Biochem.J. 292(1993) 267-270.

4. John AJ; Cherian, R; Subhash, H.S and Cherian, A.M. Evaluation of the efficacy of bitter gourd (Momordica charantia) as an oral hypoglycemic agent – a randomized controlled clinical trial. Ind.J.Physiol. Pharmacol. 47(3) (2003): 363-365.

5. Miura, T.; Itoh, C; Iwamoto, N; Kato,M; Kawai M; Park, S.R and Suzuki, I; Hypoglycemic activity of the fruit of the Momordica charantia in type 2 diabetic mice. J. Nutr. Sci. Vitaminol (Tokyo)- 47(5)(2001) 340-344.

6. Hirano, T; Homa, M and Oka, K. Effects of stinging nettle root extracts and their steroidal components on the Na^+, K^+ ATPase of the beningn prostatic hyperplasia Planta Medica 60(1999) 2055-2061.

7. Andrew Pengelly, Triterpenoids and Saponins in: The Constituents of Medicinal Plants pp 74-79. CAIB Publishing. 875 Massachusetts Ave.7th Floor, Cambridge, MAO 2139.USA.

8. Bruneton, J; Pharmacognosy Phytochemistry Medicinal Plants Lavoisier Pubs. 1995. Paris.

9. Mills. S and Bone, K. Principles and Practice of Phytotherapy Churchill Livingstone (2000) Edinburgh.

10. Osbourn, A.E. Saponins in cereals. Phytochemistry 62(2003) 1-4.

11. Oh, S.R; Kinjo, J. et. al. Effects of triterpenoids from Pueroria lobata on immunohemolysis. Planta Medica 66(2000) 506-510.

12. Recio, M.C; Giner, R.M; Manez and Rios, J.L. Structural requirements for the anti-inflammatory activity of natural terpenoids. Planta Medica 61(1995) 182-185.

13. Favel, A; Steinmetz, M.D. et. al. In vitro antifungal activity of triterpenoid saponins. Planta Medica 60(1994) 50-53.

14. Ray, A.B and Gupta. M; Progress in Chemistry of Organic Natural Products 63(1994)1-106. Springer – Verlag. Vienna.

15. Tripathi, Y.B and Shukla, S. Withaperuvin E a new free radical scavenger isolated from Physalis peruviana. Indian Jour. Biochem & Biophys. 32 (1995) 308-309.

16. Pandey. S; Sharma M, Chaturvedi, P and Tripathi, Y.B. Indian J.Exp. Biol. 32(1994) 180-183.

17. Ohkawa,H; Ohishi, N & Yagi, K. Anal. Biochem 95(1979) 351-358.

18. Shin-ya, K; Hayakawa, Y and Seto, H. J Nat.Prod. 56(1993), 1255-1258.

19. Hogberg, J; Moldeus P et. al. Eur. J.Biol.Chem, 59(1975)457-462.

20. Huang, K.C. The pharmacology of Chinese herbs (1993) CRS, Press, Boca Raton.

21. Ghisalberti, E.L. Cardiovascular activity of naturally occurring lignans. Phytomedicines 4(1997) 151-166.

22. Beckham, N. Phytoestrogens and compounds that affect oestrogen metabolism – pt, 1, Australian Journal of Medical Herbalism 7(1995)11-16.

23. Kim, H; Shim, M and Kim, B. Biologicaly active lanostane – type triterpenoids from ganoderma lucidum, Proceedings, International Journal of Ganoderma Science (2001), Auckland.

24. Komoda, Yasu; Sonada, Y and Sate, Y. Ganoderic acid and its derivatives as cholesterol synthesis inhibitors. Chemical Pharmaceutical Bulletin 37(1989) 531-533.

25. Hirotani, M; Tsutomu, F and Shiro, M. Lanostane derivatives from Ganoderma Lucidum. Phyto chemistry 24(1985) 2055-2061.

26. Morigiwa, A; Kitabatake, K; Fujimoto, Y and Ikehaura, N Angiotensin converting enzyme – inhibiting triterpenes from Ganoderma lucidum, Chemical Pharmaceutical Bulletin 34(1986) 3025-3028.

27. Hobbs, Christopher. Medicinal Mushrooms. An Exploration of Tradition, Healing and Culture, Botanica Press (1995) Santacruz.

28. Andrae, T; Borchers Stern, J.S; Hackeman RM, Keen CL; Gershwin, M.E. Mushroom, tumors and immunity PSE BM. Vol. 221(1999).

29. Lakshmi, B; Sneha Mathew; Nitha, B; Devasagayam, TPA and Janardhan, K.K. Methanolic extract of a Medicinal Mushroom Ganodarma Lucidum Protects radiation induced oxidation damage in Mice. Amala Research Bulletin Vol.23 (2003) 32-46

30. Khoda, H; Tokumoto, W; Sakamoto. K; Hirai, Y; Yamasaki, K; Komoda, Y Chem. Pharm.Bull.33(1985) 1367.

31. Jong,SC; Birmingam, JM. Medical benefits of Mushroom, Ganoderma. Adv. Appl Microbiology 37(1992)101-134.

32. Shino, M. S; Lee, LJ; Wang, CT, Natural products and biological activities of the Chinese medicinal fungus G.Lucidum. Food Phytochemicals II, Teas, spices and herbs. Am.chemical society. 1994. 342-354.

Chapter – 4

Phenolics of the Functional Foods

4.1 Role of Polyphenols as Nutraceuticals

By G.R. Sajitha,

Lecturer, Dept. Biochemistry, Sree Mookambika Institute of Medical Science, Padanilam, Kulasekharam, T.N. 629161

Any naturally occurring active principle that controls blood and tissue parameters e.g. B.P and immune responses of the body is a nutraceutical. Let us now discuss on polyphenols here. Among the nutraceuticals this group has a unique position in our functional foods such as rhizomes, fruits, bark, leaves etc of various plants[1]. Tannins represent the largest group of polyphenols. They are widely distributed in the bark of trees, insect galls, leaves, stems and fruits. They were originally isolated from the bark and insect galls of oak trees[2]. They are the chief plant constituents responsible for astringency. Tannins are high molecular weight compounds (500-5000 Daltons) containing sufficient phenolic hydroxyl groups to permit the formation of stable cross links with proteins and as a result of this cross linking, enzymes may be inhibited. Tannins are of two types viz; hydrolyzable and condensed types.

Hydrolyzable Tannins

They are derived from simple phenolic acids, particularly gallic acid which is linked to a sugar by esterification. The gallic acid groups are normally bonded to form dimmers such as ellagic acid. Ellagic acid is found in grapes, nuts, goose berries (amla), straw berries etc. Hydrolyzable tannins break down on hydrolysis to give gallic acid and glucose or ellagic acid and glucose, known as gallotannins and ellagotannins respectively. They are readily soluble in water and alcohol.

Actions of Hydrolyzable Tannins

They protect inflammed mucous membrane, reduce hypersecretions from them, reduce inflammations and swelling due to infections, prevent bleeding from wounds, uterus e.g. menorrhagia, metrorrhagia, relieves diarrhoea, dysentery etc[2]. PP (see section B. PP 140-151).

Gallotannic acid and agrimonin isolated from Quercus spp. and agrimon eupatoria respectively have different biological actions. The former has antihaemorrhagic and the latter has antidiarrhoeic activities. Both are astringents also.

Condensed Tannins or Phlobotannins

They are polymers of flavanols (catechins) and flavan-3, 4- diols (leucoanthocyanins). Upon hydrolysis they form insoluble red residues or phlobaphenes and in addition cyanin chloride (a purple pigment of rose petals) from the latter on hydrochloric acid hydrolysis. Rose flower gets its colour due to cyanin chloride. Condensed tannins are partially soluble in water and alcohol. The basic catechin type molecules are of low astringency.

Oligomeric Procyanidins (OPC_S)

They are a major subcategory of condensed tannins in which two or more molecules of catechin are linked by simple carbon atoms of A and B, rings. They are present **in green and black teas and redwine**. Grape seeds contain a trimeric procyanidin. They and another polyphenol resveratrol are responsible for many of the benefits associated with red wines including findings of lower mortality from cardiovascular and cerebrovascular diseases among low to moderate wine drinkers[3]. Green tea is especially rich in the beneficial epigallocatechin, which is a potent antioxidant and vascular protective too. According to the findings of Bombardelli and Morazzoni[4] and Bone[5], the grape seed extract show the following activities.

(a) 20 times stronger than ascorbic acid as an antioxidant.

(b) Vascular protective and antiatherogenic in action.

(c) Free radical scavenging action and inhibitory on lipid peroxidation and enzymes, responsible for degradation of collagens.

According to Johnes[6] consumption of tannins may lead to reduce absorption of proteins and other nutrients. Therefore it is advisable to avoid tea along with meals.

Experiments with Ellagic Acid

According to the work of Thresiamma and Kuttan[7] oral administration of ellagic acid (100 μmole/kg) daily for seven weeks in animals ameliorated the damages induced by intraperitonial injection of carbon tetrachloride (0.15ml) thrice weekly for the above period, viz; condition of liver fibrosis and elevated activities of ALT, ALP and LPO were significantly reduced. $CC1_4$ produces free radicals such as $CCl_3^{\cdot}$ and $Cl^{\cdot}$ ($CCl_4 \rightarrow CCl_3^{\cdot} + Cl^{\cdot}$) which are responsible for liver damages and they are significantly scavenged by a strong antioxidant such as ellagic acid (such protection is also offered by leucopelargonin, see the article by Annuradha). Ashoori et. al[8]. reported that ellagic acid was found to be a stronger inhibitor of LPO than Vitamin.E.

Experiments with Virgin Coconut Oil (VCO)

Nevin and Rajmohan[9] carried out some experiments with Virgin Coconut oil (8% of diet) in normal rats for 45 days and reported on its beneficial effects as compared to ground nut and mature coconut oils with respect to serum and tissue lipid parameters and LPO. Lipid parameters and LPO were least in the virgin coconut oil treated rats as compared to others. Besides this HDL cholesterol level increased and LDL cholesterol level decreased significantly with VCO as against the other two oil treated groups. Polyphenol fraction (PF) isolated from VCO by methanol significantly reduced oxidation of LDL *in vitro* as compared to the other two oils' fractions. These workers attributed the beneficial effects of VCO to its polyphenols. Besides this, tender coconut is a good health promoter as it is a good source of Vit. E like polyphenols.

Experiments with Green Tea Polyphenols (GTP)

Sabu et. al[10]. showed the antidiabetic and related effects of green tea polyphenol fraction in alloxan diabetic rats. GTP was found to reduce serum glucose levels by 44% at a dose of 100 mg/kg for 15 days in these rats. Elevated hepatic enzymes (ALP and ALT) and serum LPO were significantly reduced by GTP administration. On the contrary liver glycogen level and the antioxidant potential of the treated animals increased significantly. However their catalase and glutathione peroxidase levels were unchanged. GTP contains the polyphenols especially gallocatechin (GC), epigallocatechin (EGC), epicatechin(EC), epigallocatechin gallate (EGCG) and epicatechin gallate (ECG). The last one is the major polyphenol in tea. Tea components possess antioxidant, antimutagenic and anticarcinogenic effects. Black tea is lesser active than green tea. Chinese consume 3 to 4 cups of green tea daily and that may be one reason that Chinese suffer the least from CHD and cancer. Many more workers proved the beneficial effects of tea as a beverage for human health. Many references are given by Sabu et. al[10]. Polyphenols are more active in green tea than in black tea as the polyphenols in the latter are partly oxidized and inactivated. EGCG inhibits LPO and intestinal glucose uptake by sodium dependent glucose transporter and there by it controls blood glucose.

Triphala is Three in One

Triphala means a combination of three fruits used in Ayurvedic medicine, viz, Terminalia bellerica, Terminalia chebula and Emblica officinalis. They are taken in equal amounts for each preparation of the medicine. Among them the last one is amla which is edible and people in India use it as a pickle. Their Sanskrit names are bibhitaki, harithaki and amalaki respectively and which are prescribed by most health care practitioners in

India[11,12]. Thriphala strengthens the different tissues of the body, prevents aging, promotes health and immunity[13]. It corrects constipation, cleanses and tonifies the gastrointestinal tract and also detoxifies the whole body, and improves digestion and assimilations[14]. It exhibits anti-viral, anti-bacterial, anti-fungal and anti-allergic properties[15,16]. Triphala and its constituents act as cardio-tonic, control blood pressure, improve blood circulation and reduce cholesterol levels[17,18]. Triphala also shows immunomodulatory properties and helps in improving the body's defence system[19].

Accending to recent studies triphala shows antimutagenic[20-22] radio protecting[23-25] and antioxidant activities[26-28]. Naik et. al[29]. and other groups further studied the antioxidant properties of other herbs as well as of amla[30] and chebula[31]. Oxidative stress and exposure to radiation cause damage to biomolecules[32,33]. Jagetia et. al[23] showed that triphala scavenges free redicals and protects mice from radiation-induced damage when administered intraperitoneally and exposed to 10 Gy of γ-radiation. Kumar et. al[25] confirmed the radioprotective effect of a triphala rasayna. Naik et. al[31] observed that an aqueous extract of Terminalia chebula can act as a potent antioxidant and a probable radioprotective agent. Free radicals have one or more unpaired elections and therefore they act with substrate either by electron transfer or by transfer of hydrogen atom[34]. Among the several free radicals hydroxyl radical ($OH^{\cdot}$) is the most potent oxidant, produced during radiation exposure as well as Fenton reactions.[32-34]. It is a highly oxidizing radical with standard reduction potential of 1.9V vs NHE at pH 7.

Super oxide ($O_2^{\cdot-}$) radical is one of the most important reactive oxygen free radicals constantly produced in living cells[33,35]. One of the methods of generating superoxide radicals is observed in xanthine oxidase (XO) assay, where XO enzyme catalyzes the oxidation of xanthine to uric acid. During this conversion it produces superoxide by the reduction of moleculr oxygen[36,37], which is detected by 2,6 dichlorophenol indophenol (DCIP)[28,31]. In order to understand the factors responsible for the potent antioxidant and radio protecting ability of triphala it has been evaluated for radical scavenging ability.

Determination of Xanthine Oxidase Inhibitory Action and Phenolic Content

The radical scavenging experiments were carried out by Naik et al[36] using fast reaction kinetic tools and the reactivity of triphala towards different radicals such as ($OH^{\cdot}$), ($O_2^{\cdot-}$), DPPH ($2,2^1$-diphenyl-1-Pierylhydrazyl) and $ABTS^{\cdot-}$ ($2_1 2^1$ azinobis (3-thylbenzthiazoline-6- sulfonic acid). When triphala was tested by the above team for super oxide radical scavenging activity using xanthine and its oxidase assay, it was observed that in addition to reacting with superoxide radical, it also inhibited uric acid formation[36], indicative of xanthine oxidase enzyme inhibitory activity.

Phenolic Contents

Naik et. al[36]. estimated the total phenolic content (phenolic acids, flavonoids and tannins) in triphala using spectrophotometric methods. The Folin-ciocaltue method, which is based on the principle of reduction of phosphomolybdic acid by phenols in the presence of aqueous alkali was employed to determine the total phenolic content. Gallic acid was used as a standard and the results were expressed as % gallic acid equivalents, gave a mean value of 38 ± 3%. Tannins are usually subdivided into two groups, hydrolyzable tannins and condensed tannins. The total tannin content present in triphala was measured using Folin-Dennis Colorimetri method. The measurements were compared in terms of % tamic acid equivalents. The tannin content in triphala was found to be 35 ± 3%. Analysis of total flavononid content in triphala has been done using colorimetric method and quercetin as standard flavonoid. The results showed that triphala did not contain any significant amount of flavonoids.

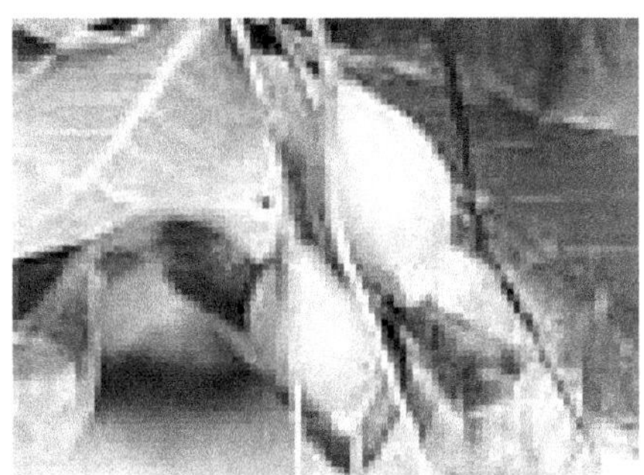

Terminalia Bellerica

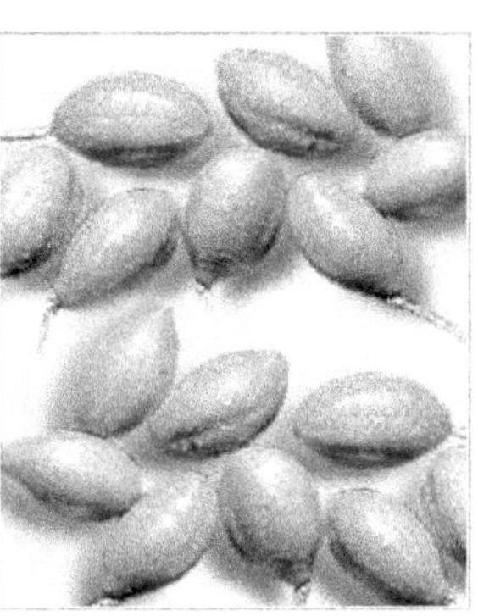

Terminalia Chebula

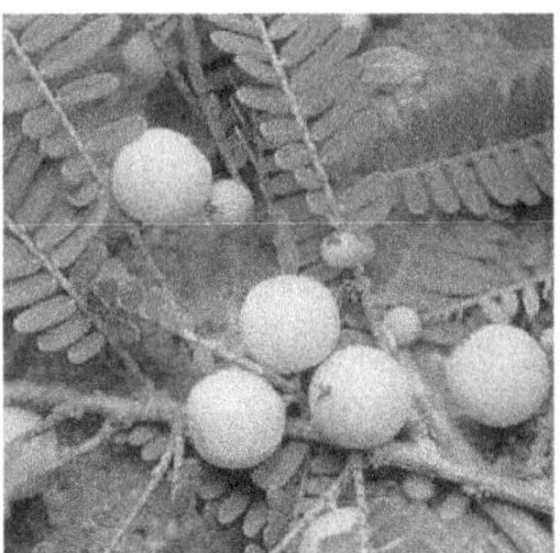

Emblica officinalis

During the extraction process, tannins may get hydrolyzed to give free gallic acid or they may remain in bound form. HPLC method was used for the estimation of gallic acid in triphala (column C_{18}PC x 500; mobile phase, aqueous acetonitrile [10%-HCl (0.05m)-KCl(0.1M); detection by absorbance at 260 mm]. The chromatogram of triphala showed several prominent peaks having retention time of 8.30, 9.44; 10.88 and 14.38 min. The peak at 14.33 min corresponds to gallic acid as determined by comparison with the standard. The amount of gallic acid in triphala was quantified by a calibration curve. It was found to be 73 mg/g, i.e. about 7% of the total phenolics estimated earlier. It is possible that some of the polyphenols in the extract are present in either glycosylated/esterified form or in some other bound form that does not allow estimation as free acids / phenolics. Therefore Naik et. al[26]. subjected the aqueous solution of triphala to acid hydrolysis by boiling it with 0.IN HCl for 2 hrs. The hydrolyzate on examination by HPLC showed significantly increased amount of gallic acid (150 mg/g) which is about 15% but still less than the total percentage of phenolics present in triphala. This shows that tannins also significantly contributed to the overall free radical activity of triphala and most of them may be in bound form. The above findings of Naik et. al. confirm that the anti-oxidant and radio protecting ability of triphala arise from the polyphenols, which reduce oxidative stress by converting the reactive oxygen free radicals to non-reactive products. Studies elsewhere also indicate the presence of gallic acid in the fruit of E officinalis, T.chebula and T.bellerica[21,31,38]. In these fruits gallic acid is present either in free form or bound tannin form (gallotannins and ellagotannins).

Antioxidants have a Sparing Action on Vitamin C and E in the Body

Major chemical compounds in T.bellerica are ellagic and gallic acids, in T.chebula it is gallic acid and in E.officinalis it is epigallocatechin gallate (EGCG) in addition to several derivatives of gallic acid. EGCG is found in tea[39] also which is a very good health tonic according to Chinese traditions. Free radicals cause several diseases viz; liver Cirrhosis, atherosclerosis, Cancer, diabetes etc, and compounds that scavenge free radicals have great potential in ameliorating these diseases. Antioxidant vitamins C and E reduce oxidative stress in diabetes and these Vitamins in turn are maintained in by antioxidants such as S-allyl cysteine sulfoxide[40]. **Therefore the earlier ideas that Vitamins C and E shall take care of all the functions of the antioxidant system in our body need a through revaluation.** Pomegranate flavanoids and garlic oil showed improvement in serum Vitamin C level. [Personal communication from Andrews A, SME. M.G.University, Kottayam.]

Medicinal Uses with Individual Members of Triphala

1. **Terminalia Bellerica Gaertn Roxb**

   Local name: Baheda, Bibhitaki (Sanskrit), Tannika (Mal)

Medicinal uses: Fruits are bitter astringent. Contains Beta-sitosterol, gallic acid, ellagic acid, chebulagic acid and many free sugars and derivatives, e.g. galactose, fructose, mannitol and a glucoside (Belericannin)[41]. Seeds contain proteins and oxalic acid. Due to the presence of these compounds, fruits have got astringent, laxative, bronchial, sedative, analgesic, anti-inflammatory and nutritive effects. Antidiabetic action of a methanolic extract of this fruit was reported by Sabu and Kuttan[38]. Dry powder of the fruits, when mixed with water and applied locally, then it relieves pain and swelling. Baked fruits are useful in cough and bronchitis. Powdered fruit, with 5 g honey, is given orally for the treatment of bronchial asthma. Powder of baked fruits when given with cold water is said to be useful for the treatment of diarrhoea. Fresh paste of the fruits is applied locally for the treatment of leprosy. Pulp of half ripe fruits is used as purgative. Fruits are reported to have antibiotic activity against a wide variety of microorganisms. Phyllembin (ethyl gallate) was isolated from this fruit[42] as well as from Embilica officinalis[43].

2. **Terminalia Chebula Retz**

   Local names: Harithaki (Sanskrit), Kadukka(Mal)

   Medicinal uses: This fruit is also a component of Triphala. It contains about 30% of astringent substances, Viz; chebulinic acid, tannic acid, gallic acid etc. Resins and a purgative principle of nature of anthraquinone and sennoside are also present[44,45]. Various extracts of the fruit contains a constituent which has wide antibacterial and antifungal spectrum[45]. It also inhibits growth of E.coli, the most common organism responsible for urinary tract infection. Sabu and Kuttan[28] reported on the antidiabetic action of a methanolic of T.chbula also. Suchalata and Srinivasalu[46] observed antioxidant activity of the several polyphenols such as querectin, gallic acid, catechins, catechol and epigallo catechin which are potent antioxidants[47]. These compounds could scavenge the supreoxide ($O^{\cdot -}_2$) and hydroxyl radicals generated after myocardial infarction (MI) induced by iosproterenol as observed in the former groups study[46]. T.Chebula was advocated earlier also as a component of herbal formulations for the disorders of heart[48].

3. **Emblica Officinalis Gaertn**

   Local names: Goose berry, Amla. Nellikka (Mal)

Medicinal use: The fruit is a rich souce of Vitamin C. The other constituents are tannins, alkaloid etc[49]. The fruit pulp is being used in several indigenous medical preparations against a variety of conditions such as liver injury[50], atherosclerosis[51] and diabetes[52]. The preparation of E. officinalis with other medicinal plants called chavanaprasha is a healthy drug and has been used in India from time immemorial to rejuvenate the body[53]. It is claimed to reduce aging and age related ailments such as dementia, loss of complexion and digestive power, weakeness of sense organs etc. The presence of ascorbic acid[54], galactopectins and ellagic acid[55] was confirmed in the fruits. Jeena and Kuttan[53] evaluated the antioxidant potential of this fruit. According to them an aqueous extract of amla was found to be a potent inhibitor of lipid peroxidation and very good scavenger of hydroxyl and super oxide radicals *in vitro.* The antioxidants present in the fruits are aqueous soluble, but extractable with ether and heat stable. The active fraction contains epigallocatechin gallate (EGCG) and gallic acid derivatives.

E. officinalis has been shown to reduce liver injury caused by administration of xenobiotics in animals. It reduces serum, aortic and hepatic level of cholesterol in animals fed with high cholesterol diet[56]. It is also antimutagenic as tested in Salmonella typhimuriam assays against polycylclic aromatic hydrocarbons[57]. Apart from the tannins[58], the fruit contains trigalloyl glucose and polyphenols such as ellagic acid[55], flavonoids[59] and phyllemblic acid[43]. The antioxidant activity of the fruit is mainly associated with the aqueous extract and is partially extractable with diethyl ether. The active fraction is dialysable which indicates that the antioxidant compounds are probably polyphenols. Praveen Kumar et. al[60,61] showed that a rasayana of this fruit viz; Brahmarasayana is capable of stimulating bone marrow cells and the proliferation of WBC in normal and cyclophosphamide treated animals.

Methanolic extracts of triphala were studied individually and also in combination by Sabu and Kuttan[38]. Lipid peroxidation and hydroxyl radical formation were better inhibited by T. bellerical as compared to the other three is shown below. However suproxide generation was inhibited maximally by E.O. followed by triphala (T.P). The order was as follows. E.O > T.P > T.C > T.B. Blood sugar control was better by T.B than by other three at 2nd hr. after their administration to alloxan diabetic rats at a dose level of 100 mg/kg. However continuous treatment of the diabetic rats with FBS range 350-400 mg/dl at a fixed dose of T.C, T.B, E.O and T.P(triphala) i.e. 100 mg/kg/day, showed the blood glucose level (mg/dl) as follows on the eleventh day. Control=321.3±18.3; T.C.=239.3 ± 22.9; T.B.=240.6 ± 50; E.O=228 ± 14; T.P=183.5 ± 10.4 respectively for each. Here triphala showed the maximum hypoglycemic effect followed by E.O Free radicals cause several diseases viz; liver cirrhosis, atherosclerosis, cancer, diabetes, etc and compounds that scavenge free radicals have a great potential in ameliorating these diseases[62]. Antioxidants and Vitamins C and E reduce oxidative stress in diabetes and nutraceutcals such as allium oils and their precursor amino acids maintain the levels of the above Vitamins in the body[40,63]. Therefore many firmly believe that plant sources may help humanity to tide over the problems of diabetes, cancer, CHD and even Alzheimer's disease if selected vegetables/fruits are used regularly for a prophylactic treatment. According to a report in the September 1 issue of Am.Jour Med (2006) the benefits of fruit juices were highlighted, i.e. Researchers in Japan and the U.S. followed almost 2000 dimentia free volunteers for up to ten years while monitoring their consumption of fruit and vegetable juices. The risk of Alzhemer's disease was reduced by 76% who drank juices more than thrice a week compared with those who drank them less than once a week. These effects of the juices were definitely due to the antioxidant actions of the nutraceuticals present in them. PP (see PP 26-30).

Polyphenols of Two Edible Plants

Cassia tora Linn and Eclipta alba Linn are two other plants which are edible and also that contain certain unknown polyphenols. Annie Abraham et. al[64]. of Kerala University reported on the antioxidant effects of the methanolic extract of the leaves of the former in an *in vitro* experiment using rat liver and brain homogenates. The antioxidant action was assayed by the degree of inhibition of lipid per oxidation and enhancement in superoxide scavenging action. The total phenolic content in the methanolic extract of Cassia tora leaves was found to be 4.6 mg/g, however the nature of the phenols are yet to be determined.

Annie's group also found the beneficial effects of an aqueous extract of Eclipta alba Linn against selenite cataract formation in rats[64]. Experiemntal cataract was induced by a single subcutaneens injection of sodium selenite (4 mg/kg) on the 10th post partu day in rats. Aqueous extract of E. alba was administered as intraperitoneal injections in the treated group from 8th to 15th day at a concentration of 2.5 mg/kg to test the antioxidant effect of the extract. After the treatment period rats were sacrificed and the activities of lens superoxide dismutase (SOD), catalase, Ca^{2+} - ATPase, concentratons of Ca^{2+}, LPO and GSH content were evaluated. Selenite induced cataract is characterized by the production of free radicals causing oxidative stress in the lens. In the treated rats the activities of SOD, catalase, Ca^{2+} -ATPase and glutathione content were found to be significantly increased and the concentrations of Ca^{2+} and TBARS were found to be decreased significantly as compared to the cataract induced control group. These results demonstrate the protective effects of the extract of E.alba which is rich in poly phenol antioxidants against selenite cataract formation

References

1. Bors, W; Michael. C and Stettmair, K Structure activity relationship governing antioxidant capacities of plant polyphenols. Methods of Enzymolgoy 335 (2001)166-180.
2. Andrew Pengally, constituents of medicinal plants (2004) P.30 CABI Publishing 875 Masschusetts Avenue 7th floor, Cambridge, MAO 2139. U.S.A.
3. Jones, F. The save your heart wine guide (1995), Head Line Pubs. London
4. Bombardelli, E and Morazzoni, P. Vitis Vinifera L; Fitoterapia LXVI (1995) 291-317.
5. Bone, K. Oestrogen modulation. The modern phytotherapist 1(1995) 8-10
6. Johns, T. The Origins, Human Diet and medicine (1990), University of Arizona Press, Tucson.
7. Thresiamma, K.C. and Kuttan R. Inhibition of liver Fibrosis by ellagic acid. Indian J. Physiol. Pharmacol 40(4) (1996) 363-366.
8. Ashoori. F, Nishigaki et. al. Suppression by ellagic acid of carbon tetrachloride or ^{60}Co irradiation-induced lipid peroxidation in rats. J. Clin. Biochem. Nutr 8(1990) 209-216.
9. Nevin, K.G. and Rajmohan T. Beneficial effects of virigin coconut oil on lipid parameters and in vitro LDL oxidation. Clinical Biochemistry. 37(2004)830-835.
10. Sabu, M.C; Smitha, K and Kuttan, R. Antidiabetic activity of green tea polyphenols and their role in reducing oxidative stress in experimental diabetes. Jour. Ethno pharmacology 83(2002) 109-116.
11. Kulkarni, P.H; Clinical Assessment of the effect of Sookshma Triphala in Lipoma, Ayurvedic Research papers II. Pune 1995, PP66-71

12. Rege, N.N, Thatte, U.M and Dahanukar, S.A; Adaptogenic proerties of six rasayana herbs used in Ayurvedic medicine. Phytother. Res. 13(1999) 275-291.

13. Juss, S.S; Triphala-the wonder drug. Indian Med. Gaz. 131(1997) 194-196.

14. Nadkarni, A.K; Indian Materia Medica, Popular Press Ltd. Mumbai 1976. 3rd edn. Pp 1308-1315.

15. Singh, P.K, Micotoxin elaboration in Triphala and its constituents. Indian Phytopathol; 56(2003) 380-383.

16. Mehta, B.K; Shitu, S and Wankada, H; In vitro antimicrobial efficiency of Triphala. Fitoterapia, 64 (1999) 371-372.

17. Thakur, C.P; Thakur B et. al. The Ayurvedic medicines, haritaki, amla and bahira reduced cholesterol induced atherosclerosis in rabbits. Int. J.Cardiol. 21 (1998) 167-175.

18. Tariq. M; Hassian, S.J; Asif. M and Jahan, M. Protective effects of fruits extracts of Emblica officinalis Gaertn and Terminalia bellerica Roxb. In experimental myocardial necrosis in rats. Indian J.Exp.Biol. 15(1977)488-486.

19. Srikumar, R; Parthasarathy, N.J and Devi, R.S; Immunomodulatory activity of Triphala on neutrophile functions. Biol.Pharm.Bull 28(2005) 1398-1403.

20. Kaur; S; Michael, H; Arora, S et. al. The in vitro cytotoxic and apoptotic activity of triphala – an Indian herbat drug. J.Ethnopharmacol, 97(2005)15-20.

21. Kaur, S; Arora, S et. al. The in vitro antimutagenic activity of Triphala an Indian herbal drug. Food Chem. Toxicol; 40(2002) 527-534.

22. Arrora, S; Kaur, K and Kaur S; Indian Medicinal plants as a resorvoir of protective phytochemicals. Teratogen carcinogen mutagen suppl. 1(2003) 295-300.

23. Jegetia. G.C; Baliga, M.S. et. al. The evaluation of the radioprotective effect of Triphala (an ayurvedic rejuvenating drug) in the mice exposed to gamma radiation. Phytomedicine, 9(2002)99-108.

24. Jagetia, G.C., Matagi, K.J et. al. Triphala, an ayurvedic rasayana drug, protects mice against radiation-induced lethality by free radical scavenging. J. Attern. Complement Med. 10(2004)971-978.

25. Kumar, P.V; Kuttan, R and Kuttan, G Radioprotective effects of Rasayanas. Ind.J.Exp.Biol. 34(1996)848-850.

26. Vani, T; Rajani, M; Sarkar, S and Shishoo, C.J. Antioxidant properties of the Ayurvedic formulation Triphala and its constituents. Ind.J.Pharmacology 35(1997)313-317.

27. Jagetia, G.C; Rao, S.K. et. al. The evaluation of nitric oxide scavenging activity of certain herbal formulations in vitro a preliminary study. Phytother. Res; 18(2004) 561-565.

28. Naik, G.H; Priyadarsini, K.I. et. al. In vitro antioxidant studies and free radical reactions of Triphala an ayurvedic formulation and its constituents phytother. Res. 19(2005)582-586.

29. Naik, G.H; Priyadarsini, K. I. et. al. Comparative antioxidant activity of individual herbal components used in ayurvedic medicines. Phytochemistry 63(2003)97-104.

30. Khopde, S.M. et. al. Characterizing the antioxidant activity of amla (Phyllanthus emblica) extract Curr. Sci. 81(2001) 185-190.

31. Naik.G.H; Priyadarsini, K.I et. al. Studies on the aqueous extracts of Terminalia chebula as a potent antioxidant and a probable radioprotection. Phytomedicine 11(2004) 530-538.

32. Von. Sonntag, C. The chemical basis of Radiation biology, Taylor and Francis, London 1987. PP 65-84.

33. Halliwell, B and Gutteridge, J.M.C Free radicals in Biology and Medicine, Clarendon Press, Oxford, 1993, PP 22-81.

34. Spinks, J.W.T. and Woods, R.J. Introduction to radiation chemistry. John Wiley, New York, 1991, 1991. P243.

35. Winterbourn, C.C. and Kettle, A.J. Radical-radical reactions of superoxide: a potential route to toxicity. Biochem. Biophys Res. Comm. 305(2003) 729-736.

36. Naik, G.H; Priyadarsini, K.I and Harimohan Current Science 90(8) (2006) 1100-1105.

37. Muraoka, S and Miura, T; Inhibition of Xanthine oxidase by phytic acid and its antioxidant action. Life Sci 74(2004) 1691-1700.

38. Sabu, M.C and Kuttan, R Antidiabetic activity of medicinal plants and its relationship with their antioxidant property. Jour. Ethnopharmacology 81(2002) 155-160.

39. Sabu, MC; Smitha, K and Kuttan R. Antidiabetic activity of green tea polyphenols and their role in reducing oxidative stress in experimental diabetes. Jour Ethnopharmacology 83(2000)109-116.

40. Helen, A; Krishnakumar, K; Vijayammal, P.L and Augusti, K.T. A comparative study of antioxidants, S-allyl cysteine sulfoxide and vitamin E on the damages induced by nicotine. Pharmacology 67(2003)113-117.

41. Sharma, N.K Medicinal plants of Hadoti plateu (Rajasthan) uses and conservation. In: Medicinal plants Tradition knowledge. P.C. Trivedi(ed). P.185 (2006), published by I.K. International publishing house Pvt. Ltd. New Delhi.

42. Antarkar, D.S and Vaidya. A.B. Therapautic approach to Malaria in Ayurveda. Symposium on recent advances in protozoan diseases. Hundustan Ciba Geigy Research Centre. Goregaon, Bombay. India. 1983.

43. Pillay, P.P. and Iyer, M.K. A chemical examination of Emblica officinalis. Curr. Sci. 27(1968)266-267.

44. Augusti, K.T., Rajesh, P.R and Divya Rani. S Beneficial effects of Kolstrahlin-An Ayurvedic Drug. Ind.Jour.Multi.Res. 1(2) 2005. 193-201

45. Patel N.B et. al. Tetraredron 8(1987)234

46. Suchalatha, S, Srinivasalu, C and Shyamala Devi. Indian Jour. Biochem. & Biophysics. 42(2005)246-249.

47. Roginsky. V. Arch Biochem. Biophys 414(2003)261-270.

48. Suchalatha, S; Thirugnana Sambantham, P et. al. Ind.Jour.Exp.Biol. 42(2004) 224-226.

49. Dahnukar, S. et. al. Ind.Drugs 19(1982)271.

50. De, S; Ravishankar, B and Bhavsar, G.C. Plants with hepatoprotective activity. A review. Indian Drugs 30(1993) 306-308.

51. Thakur, C.P; Thakur, B et. al. The Ayurvedic medicines Harithaki, Amla and Bahira reduce cholesterol induced atherosclerosis in rabbits. Indian.J.Cardiol 21(1988) 167-175.

52. Tripathi, S.N; Tiwari, C.M, et. al. Screening of hypoglymic action in certain indigenous drugs. J.Res. Indian Med.Yoga Homoep. 14(1979)159-169.

53. Jeena. K. Jose and Kuttan R, Antioxidant activity of Emblica officinalis. J.Clin. Biochem.Nutr. 19(1995) 63-70.

54. Mitra, K and Ghose, A.K; Ascorbic acid value of Indian Gooseberry (Phyllanthus emblica) Ann.Biochem. Exp.Med; 2(1942) 205-210.

55. Damodaran, M and Nair, K.R; A tannin from Indian gooseberry (Phyllanthus emblica) with protective action on ascorbic acid. Biochem. J. 30(1936) 1014-1020.

56. Thakur, C.P Emblica officinalis reduces serum, aortic and hepatic cholesterol in rabbits. Experientia 41(1985) 423-424.

57. Grover, I.S. and Kaur, S. Effect of Emblica officinalis Gaertn (Indian gooseberry), fruit extract on sodium azide and 4-nitro-O-phenylene induced mutagenesis in Salmonella typhimurium. Indian.J.Exp. Biol, 27(1989)207-209.

58. Brahmachari, H.D and Gupta, V.S. Studies on Phyllanthus emblica(Amla) Part III-Role of tannins in stabilizing the ascorbic acid of the fruit. Indian J.Appl. Chem.. 21(1958) 173-174.

59. Khanna, P; Taparia, R and Jain, S.C. Flavonoids from Emblica officinalis Gaertn, tissue cultures. Indian J.Bot. 5(1982)43-44.

60. Praveen Kumar, V; Kuttan, R and Kuttan, G. Effect of Rasayana in normal and tumor bearing mice. J.Exp.Clin.Cancer. Res. 13(1994)67-70.

61. Praveen Kumar, V; Kuttan, R and Kuttan, G Chemoprotective action of Rasayana against cyclophosphomide toxicity. Tumori, 80(1994) 306-308.

62. Wilson, R.L. Free radicals and tissue damage, mechanistic evidence from radiation studies in: Biochemical Mechanisms of liver injury. Academic press, New York (1998) 123.

63. Helen, A; Krishna Kumar, K; Vijayammal, P.L and Augusti. K.T. Antioxidant effect of onion oil (Allium cepa. Linn) on the damages induced by nicotine in rats as compared to alpha tocopherol, Toxicology Letters. 116(2000) 61-68.

64. Annie Abraham, Rajiva C.S, Cibin, T.R. et. al. Antioxidant properties of Cassia tora Linn and Eclipta alba Linn. Papers presented at the Symposium on Drugs affecting Lipid metabolism, Organized by the Dept. of Biochem. Kerala University. Feb. 27-28. 2007. Trivandrum P.P. 25 and 27-28.

4.2 Flavonoids and some related Polyphenols from Natural Sources

Prof (Dr). Jose Padikkala*, and P.V. Fijesh.

Amala Cancer Research Centre, Amala Nagar, Thrissur, 680555

* Associate Director, Amala Cancer Research Centre,

e-mail: jpadikkala@rediffmail.com.

Introduction

Polyphenols form one of the major classes of secondary metabolites. They possess a large range of structures and contribute to organoleptic and nutritional qualities of fruits, vegetables and beverages. Interest in nutritional attributes of polyphenols has significantly increased, particularly in flavonoids, are even more so, now we have been made aware of the possible relation between their consumption, and their relevance for health in protection against degenerative diseases and aging.

Flavonoids have important effects in plant biochemistry and physiology, acting as antioxidants, enzyme inhibitors, precursors of toxic substances and pigments and light screens (Harborne et. al. 1975); McClure, 1986). They are typically phenolic compounds and, therefore act as potent metal chelators and free radical scavengers (Hughes and Wilson 1977; Torel et. al. 1986; Clemetson, 1989). They are powerful chain breaking antioxidants. Flavonoids occur as yellow and white plant pigments. These are found free as well in bound forms, viz; glycosides.

Major Functional Foods that contain Flavonoids

Many fruits and vegetables viz; pomegranate, onions, apples, brocolli, tomatoe, green tea, celery, olives, soyabean, etc contain flavonoids, or their isomers. Therefore all these items are termed functional foods. Extensive studies have been done on some of them, especially the former eight items. Flavonoids display a remarkable array of biochemical and pharmacological actions. Some of which suggests that certain members of this group of compounds may significantly affect the function of mammalian celluar systems. Anti-inflammatory, antioxidant, antiallergic, hepatoprotective, antithrombotic, antiviral and anticarcinogenic activities of various flavonoids were discussed separately by various workers (Gabor, 1979; 1986; Havstein, 1984; Cody et. al. 1986, 1988; Farkas et. al. 1986; Selway,

1986; Welton et. al. 1988; Middeltas and Kandaswami, 1993; Carroll et. al. 1998). Oxidative damage is caused by reactive oxygen (ROS) and nitrogen (RNS) species. Flavonoids are described as the important natural products from plants which play a protective effect against reactive oxygen species (ROS) such as the hydroxyl and superoxide radicals (Husain et. al. 1987; Bors et. al. 1987). Antioxidant agents of natural origin have attracted special interest because they can protect human body from free radicals.

Diagram of Oxidative Stress and its after effects

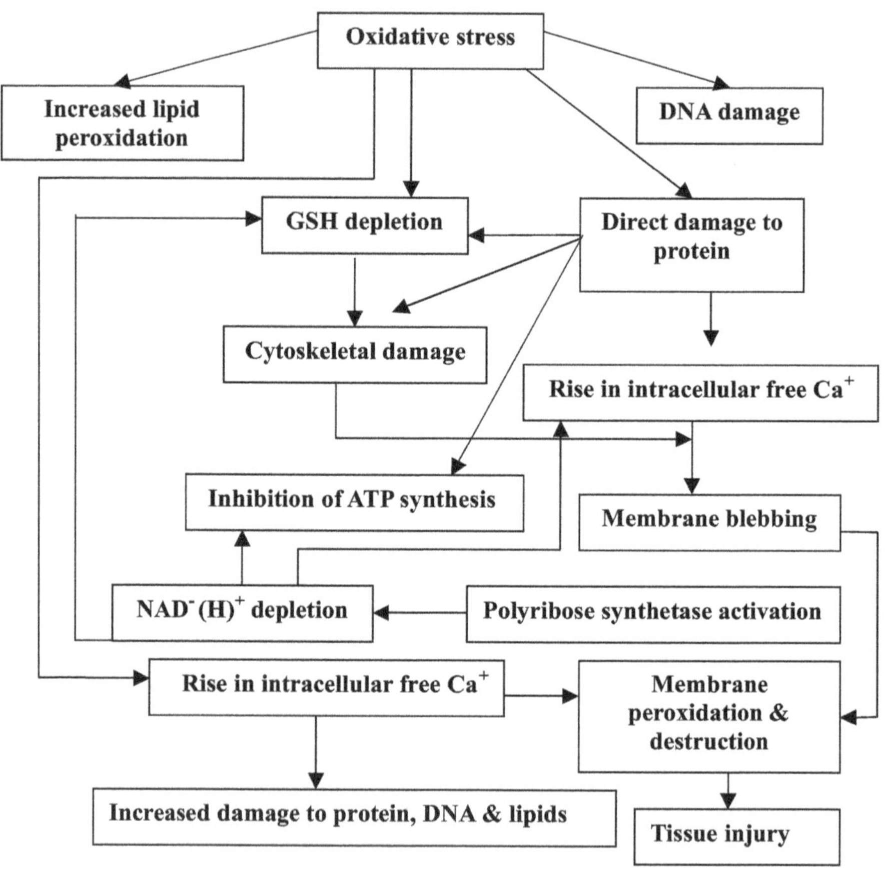

The evaluation of their direct free radical-scavenging activity revealed them as hydrogen or electron-donating compounds or antioxidants by virtue of the reducing properties of the multiple hydroxyl groups attached to aromatic ring systems, along with their ability to delocalize the resulting phenoxyl radical within the structure.

Flavonoids also can increase the intracellular reduced glutathione during oxidative stress, which in turn reduce the level of reactive oxygen species, decrease malonayldialdehyde formation and prevent the influx of Ca+. Their antioxidant activity has been claimed to be more than the Vit-C, Vit-E, Selenium and Zinc. They prevent the formation of oxidized cholesterol through antioxidant effect. They are also beneficial in a large number of human diseases like stroke, trauma, Alzheimer's and Parkinson's syndrome.

Flavonoids of Various Structure and Nature

Flavonoids are widely distributed in plant kingdom and more than 4000 varieties of flavonoids are known and about 100 flavonoids are known to be biologically active in humans. Certain plant species containing flavonoids have been used for thousand of years in traditional medicines. Flavonoids are also highly unstable compounds which undergo numerous enzymatic and chemical reactions during post harvest food storage and processing thus adding to the complexity of plant polyphenol composition.

Flavonoid structures are characterized by a 15-carbon (C6-C3-C6) backbone consisting of oxygenated and two aromatic rings (Fig. 1a). The chemical structure of flavonoids are based on a C_{15} skeleton with a chromane ring bearing a second aromatic ring B in position 2 (flavanones, flavones, flavonols, and anthocyanins), 3 (isoflavonoids) or 4 (Fig. 1b). In a few cases, the six-membered heterocyclic ring C occurs in an isomeric open form or is replaced by a five-membered ring (Fig. 1c). The oxygen bridge involving the central carbon atom (C_2) of the 3C - chain occurs in a rather limited number of cases, where the resulting heterocyclic is of the furan type.

Various subgroups of flavonoids are classified according to the substitution patterns of ring C. Both the oxidation state of the heterocyclic ring and the position of ring B are important in the classification. Based on their basic chemical structure: the most common forms of flavonoids are flavones, flavonols, flavanones, isoflavones, anthocyanins and proanthocyanidins. However the major classes are flavones (e.g; apigenin) and flavonols (e.g; kaempferol & quercetin).

Flavonoids are synthesised by the phenylpropanoid metabolic pathway in which the aminoacid phenylalanine is used to produce 4-coumaroyl-CoA. This can be combined with malonyl-CoA to yeild the true backbone of flavonoids containing two phenyl rings. Conjugate ring closure structure of this primary structure results in the familiar form of flavonoids, the three ringed structure of flavone. The metabolic pathway continues through a series of enzymatic modifications to yeild flavanones to dihyroflavonols to anthocyanins. Along this pathway many products can be formed, including the flavonols, flavan-3ols, proanthocyanidins (condensed tannins) and a host of other polyphenols.

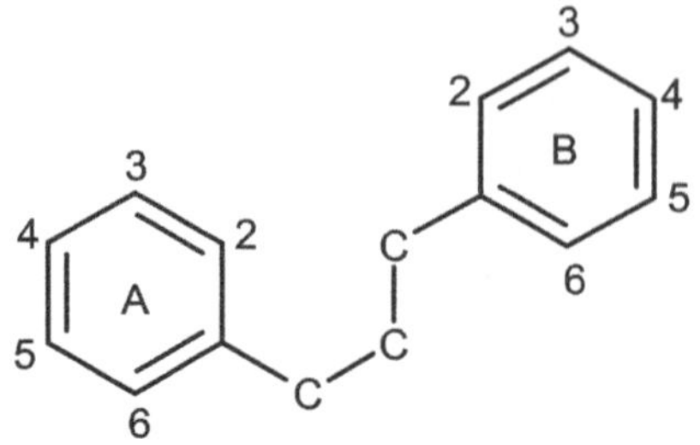

Fig. 1a

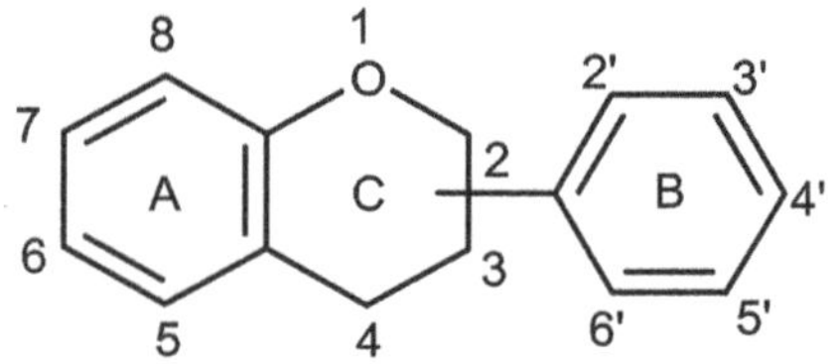

Fig 1b

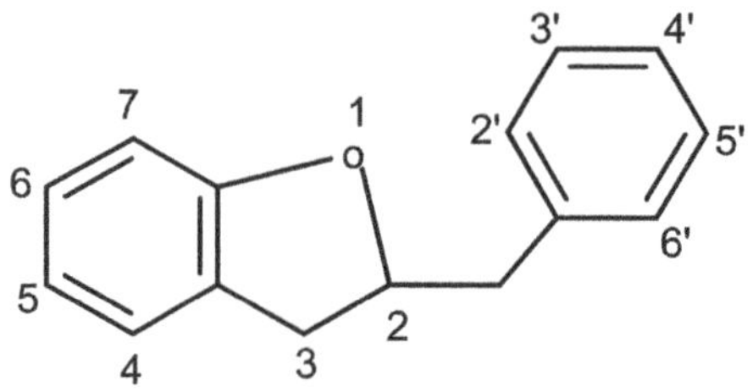

Fig. 1c

Fig: 1a,b,c; Showing variations among flavonoids skeleton.

Chalcones

Chalcone is an important aromatic ketone that forms the central core for a variety of important biological compounds, which are known collectively as chalcones. They are also intermediates in the biosynthesis of flavonoids, which are substances widespread in plants (Table: 1) and with an array of biological activities. They show antibacterial (Li et. al. 1995); antifungal (Jayasinge et. al. 2004); antitumour (Miranda et. al. 1999) and anti-inflammatory (Zdzislawa et. al. 2007) properties.

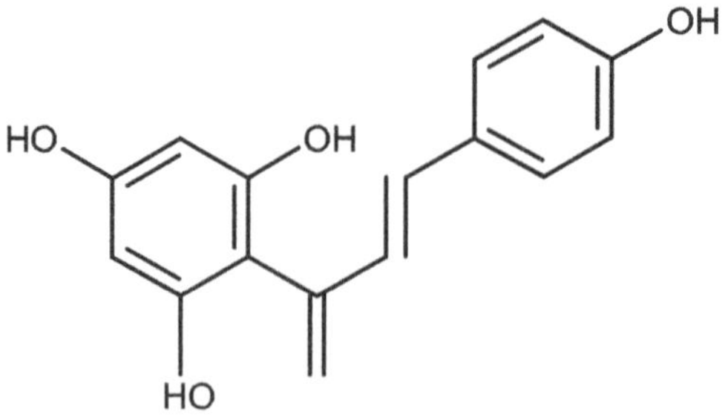

Chalcone

Major Flavonoids and their Health Benefits

Flavone

Flavones define one of the largest subgroup of flavonoids based on the backbone of 2-phenylchromen-4one (2-Phenyl-1-benzopyran-4-one). The natural distribution is demonstrated for almost all the plant and plant tissues. It is a colourless crystalline compound and the precursor for a number of white and yellow pigments. Flavones function as copigments in flowers, as antioxidants to protect plants from UV damage, and as phytoalexins with antimicrobial potentials (Schmelzer et. al. 1988; Yu et. al. 2006). These diverse functions of flavones in plants as well as their various roles in the interactions with other organisms offer many potential application, in agriculture, human nutrition and pharmacology. The antioxidant activity of flavones has increased their use in cancer prevention and coronary heart diseases. Various flavone aglyca and their O- or C-glycosides have been identified so far.

Natural flavones include apigenin, luteolin and tangeritin, echioidinin and the flavone glycosides include; luteolin 7-O-glycoside, apigenin 4'-O-β-glycopyranoside, echiodinin 5-glycoside etc.

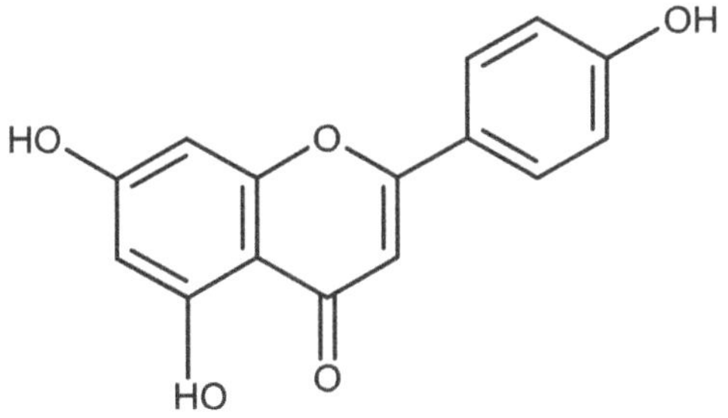

Flavones

Biological activity studies on flavones have showed their potent antioxidant nature. Oxidative tension is a potent yet non-specific metabolic trigger for inflammation, cancer, coronary heart diseases, diabetes and other neurodegenerative diseases. Examples of *in vivo* and *in vitro* studies on beneficial effects of flavones include:

***Luteolin*:** (3′,4′,5,7-tetrahydroxyflavone), an important member of the flavonoid family, is present in various fruits and vegetables and has contributed to the antioxidant activity (Shimoi et. al. 1994), on reactive oxygen species in human leucocytes (Perez-Garcia et. al. 2000). Luteolin is also reported to have anti-inflammatory properties and mediates its action by inhibiting nitric oxide production (Kim et. al. 1999). Luteolin has anti-allergic properties (Kimata et. al. 2000), antitumorigenic (Yasukawa et. al.

1989), and to be an inhibitor of protein kinase C (Ferriola et. al. 1989) and lipoxygenase (Yamamoto et. al. 1998). And a recent report (Kimata et. al. 2000) establishes luteolin as a potent inhibitor of human mast cell activation through the inhibition of protein kinase C activation and Ca^{2+} influx. Luteolin exerts growth inhibitory effects on NK/Ly ascites-tumour-cell cultures *in vitro* (Molnar et. al. 1981). The growth and metabolism of human leukaemic CEM-C1 and CEM-C7 cell lines are also inhibited by luteolin (Post et. al. 1992). The flavonoids luteolin and quercetin are also reported to arrest cell cycle in the G-phase of human melanoma cells (Casagrande and Darbon, 2001). It has been previously established that luteolin and quercetin inhibit DNA topoisomerase II of *Leishmania* and that they can induce cell-cycle arrest leading apoptosis of *Leishmania donoäani* promastigotes (Mittra et. al. 2000).

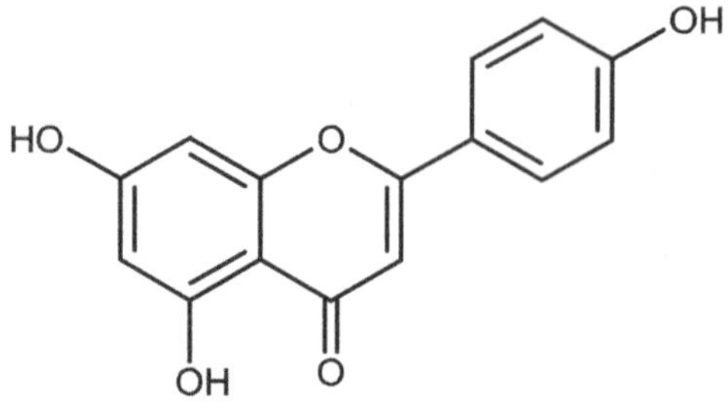

Apigenin

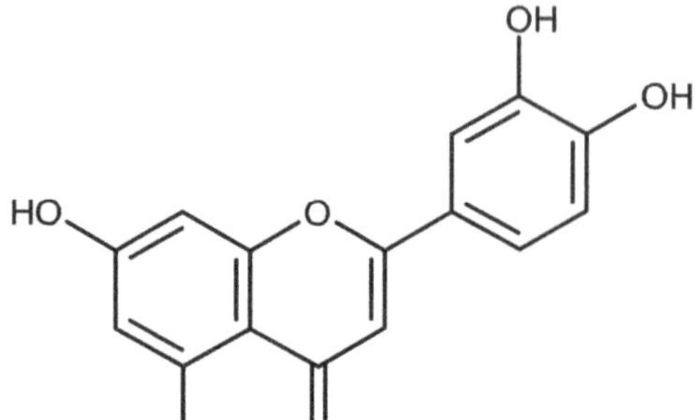

Luteolin

The experimental studies on apegenin led to an inhibition of protein kinase CK2 activity (Hessenauer et. al. 2003); activity of MAPK and PI(3)K (Zhu et. al. 2003); TNF-induced transactivation in prostate cell lines (Kobayashi et. al. 2002); breast cancer cell lines MDAMB231 (Lindenmeyer et. al. 2001); UV-induced skin tumorigenesis in mice when topically applied; proliferation and migration of endothelial cells and capillary formation *in vitro* (Trochon et. al. 2000); human anaplastic thyroid carcinoma (Yin et. al. 1999); aromatase activity (Jeong et. al. 1999); inhibited the growth of HL60 cells (Wang et. al. 1999; Takahashi et. al. 1998) and in preventing LDL oxidation and has an important role in ameliorating atherosclerosis (Naderi et. al. 2003).

Flavonols

Flavonols are polyphenolic secondary metabolites that are presenting varying levels in commonly consumed fruits, vegetables and beverages with a 3-hydroxyflavone backbone. Flavonols have long held an interest for nutritionists, which has increased following a Dutch study in the early 1990's and later that of others, showing that dietary intake of flavonols was inversely correlated with the incidence of coronary heart disease, cancer etc (Hertog 1993, Rice-Evans2001). Among the most recent candidates that have drawn important attention are the flavonoids; flavanols has attracted increasing interest as a result of recent epidemiological, mechanistic and human intervention studies. The main factors that have hindered workers in the field of flavonol research are (i) the accurate measurement of these compounds in foods and biological samples, and (ii) a dearth of information on their absorption and metabolism. Several studies using flavanols have revealed their protective effects in cardiovascular diseases by exerting systemic and coronary vasodilator effects by reducing blood pressure, cardiac hypertrophy. They also inhibit low density lipoprotein peroxidation, and reduce the progression of atherosclerosis *in vivo* (Hayek et. al. 1997). They also inhibit proinflammatory mediator release, intracellular calcium ion levels and protein kinase C phosphorylation in human mast cells (Kempuraj et. al. 2005).

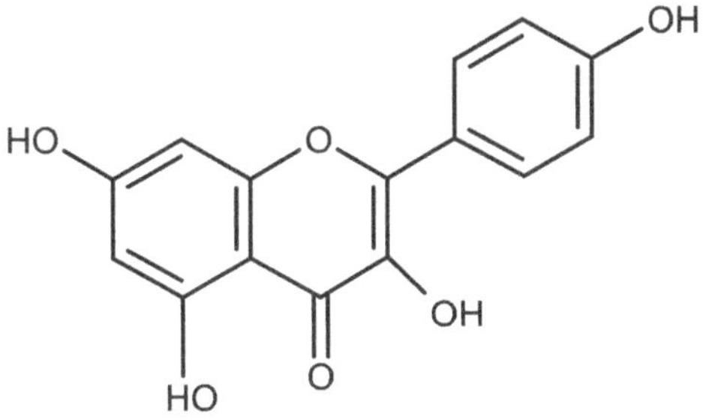

Flavonols

Some of the major flavanols include quercetin (3,3',4',5,7-pentahydroxy-2-phenylchromen-4-one), kaempferol (3,4',5,7-tetrahydroxy-2-phenylchromen-4-one), myricetin (3,,3',4',5',5,7-hexahydroxy-2-phenylchromen-4-one), fisetin (3,3',4',7-tetrahydroxy-2-phenylchromen-4-one), galangin.

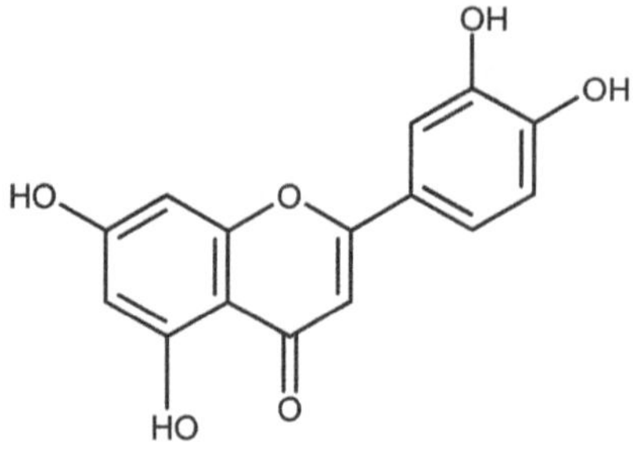

Quercetin 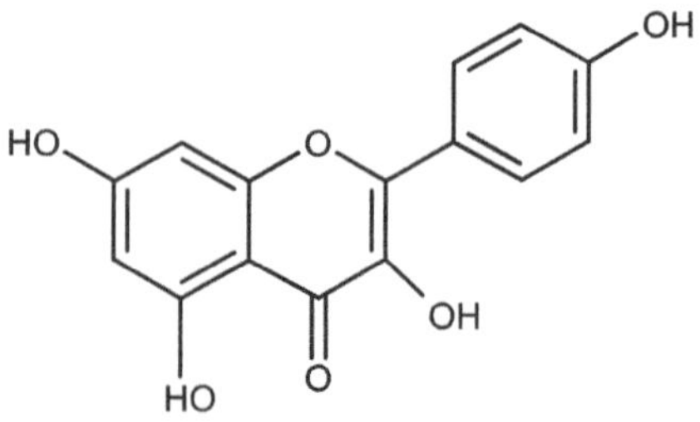 **Kaempferol**

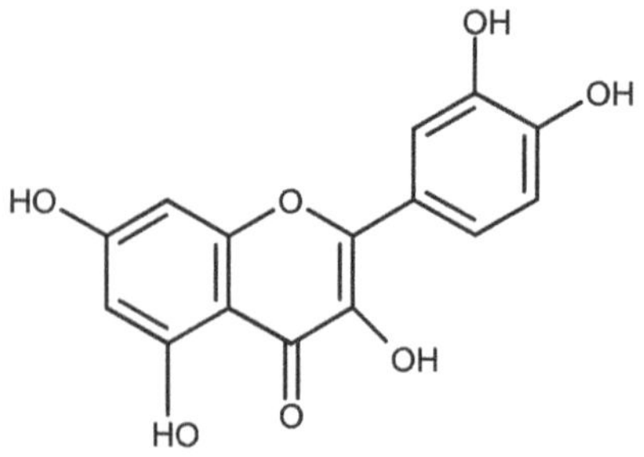

Myricetin 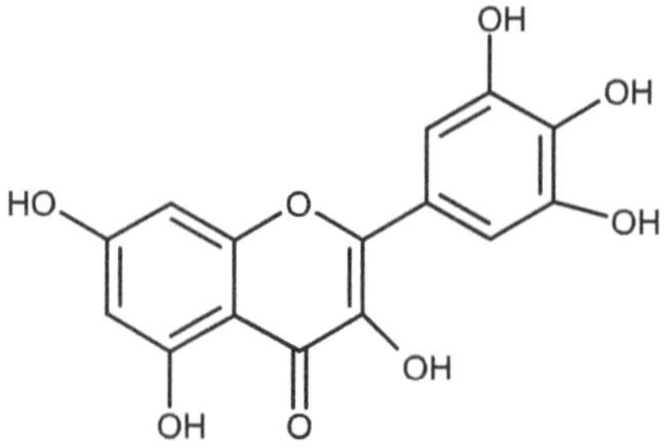 **Fisetin**

The bilogical activity of some of the flavanols: Quercetin is an important flavonol which is found in many fruits and vegetables, as well as in olive oil, red wine and tea (Havsteen, 1983; Xiao et. al. 1987; Levy et. al. 1984; Tan et. al. 2003). Quercetin, in addition to having antioxidant properties, has been suggested to prevent atherosclerosis and chronic inflammation (Havsteen, 1983), to modulate cell-cycle regulation, to interact with type II estrogen binding sites and to induce tumor cell apoptosis (Xiao et. al. 1987; Levy et. al. 1984) and are effective inhibitor of human breast cancer cell proliferation *in vitro*. Glycosides of quercetin are capable of inhibiting lipoxygenase induced LDL oxidation.

Kaempferol is widely present in broccoli (Nijveldt et. al. 2001), Ginkgo biloba (Chin et. al. 2003), fruits and vegetables (Herrmann, 1976; Justesen et. al. 1988; Karakaya et. al. 1999). Several biological activities have been attributed to kaempferol, including inhibition of lipoxygenase and cyclooxygenase (Moriyama et. al. 2003; Della Loggia et. al. 1988). It also possesses antiaggregatory (Chang et. al. 1998), antibacterial (Kataoka et. al. 2001) and anticancer (Dimas et. al. 2000) activities. Kaemferol can also induce apoptosis in glioma cells by elevating intracellular oxidative stress (Vivek et. al. 2007). It can also inhibit IL-4 is involved in several human diseases including allergies, autoimmunity, and cancer.

Myricetin flavonols are present in a large number of plants (Ong et. al. 1997), including tea, berries, fruits, vegetables and medicinal herbs (Hertog et. al. 1993). It is an effective scavenger of free radicals generated by both enzymatic and nonenzymatic systems (Furuno et. al. 2002). It inhibits cancer development induced by polycyclic aromatic hydrocarbons (Mukhtar et. al. 1988) in SENCAR mice. In addition, it has been shown to have antiviral activity by inhibiting the reverse transcriptase (Ono et. al. 1990), antiaggregatory effects on blood platelets (Robak et. al. 1988) and antiatherosclerotic effect via inhibition of oxidative modification of low-density lipoprotein by macrophages (de Whalley et. al. 1990).

Galangin, is another member of the flavonols and is present in high concentrations of honey and *Alpinia officinarum*, a spice plant that has also been used as an herbal medicine for a variety of ailments in Asia. Galangin is also present in propolis, which is a resinous material made by bees and is used in many Asian countries for the management of numerous diseases, including respiratory, subcutaneo-mucosal and viral infections (Amoros et. al. 1994; Park et. al. 1995). Galangin has been demonstrated to possess several biological actions such as antioxidative and radical scavenging activities (Cholbi et. al. 1991; Imamura et. al. 2000), antimutagenic (So et. al. 1997; Wall et. al. 1988), anticlastogenic effect (Heo et. al. 1992; 1994), anti-inflammatory activity (Gabor et. al. 1991; Kang et. al. 2000), as well as an inhibitory effect on cytochrome P450 hydroxylase in human liver microsomes (Buening et. al. 1981; Ciolino et. al. 1999). Galangin has been recently proposed as a candidate agent for cancer chemoprevention (Heo et. al. 2001).

Flavanones

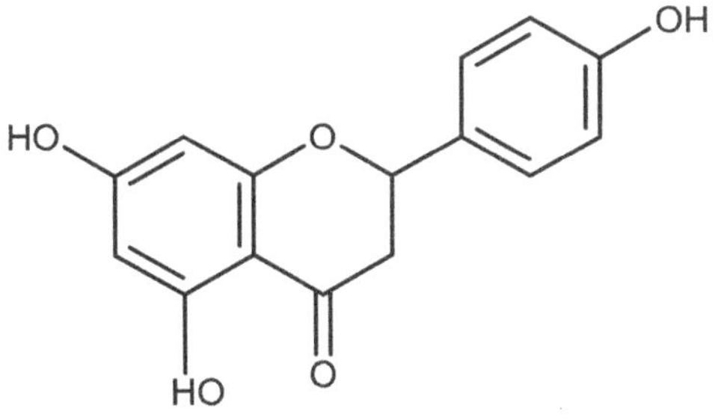

Flavanone

Flavanones constitute the majority of flavanoids in citrus fruits, grape fruits and limes. These groups of compounds share 2,3-dihydro-2-phenylchromen-4-one skeleton. Flavanones also exist in their aglycon or glycosidic form. The biomedical interest in flavanones appears to be associated with low risk for various cancers; antiviral activity; anti-inflammatory activity (Rotelli et. al. 2003); lowering of blood pressure; antioxidant; anti-estrogenic and cholesterol lowering ability. The major flavanones includes: hesperidin, naringenin, eriocetrin etc.

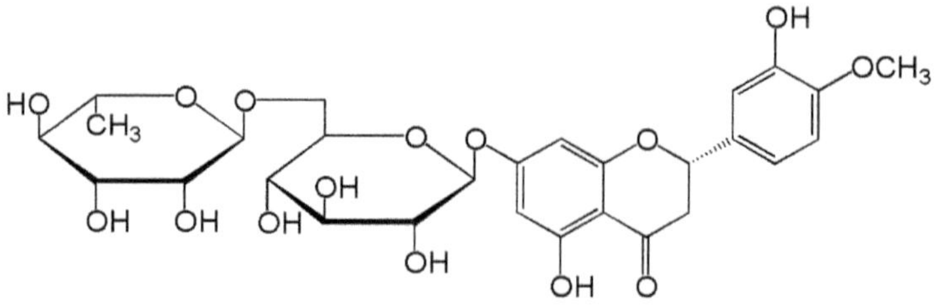

Hesperidin

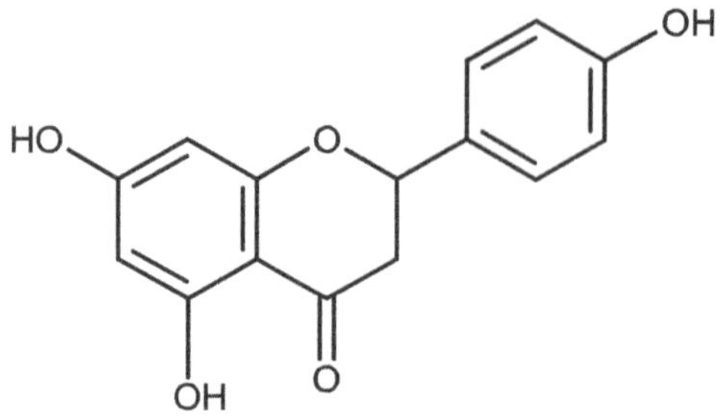

Naringenin

Naringenin is a flavonoid that has been shown in lab and animal studies to have antioxidant, anti-hormone (anti-estrogen), and cholesterol-lowering abilities.

Hesperidin, the most important flavanone of Citrus sp., significantly increases HDL cholesterol and lowers LDL cholesterol, total lipid and triglyceride plasma levels in normolipidemic rats and in rats with diet- and triton-induced hyperlipidemia (Monforte et. al. 1995).

Anthocyanins

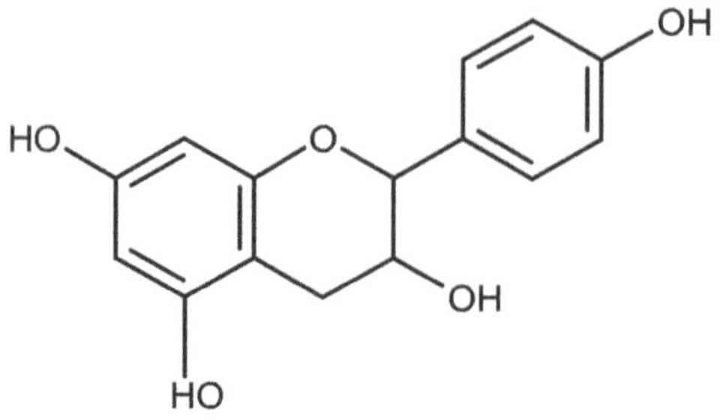

Anthocyanins are water soluble vacoular flavonoid pigments and widely found in many berries, in dark grapes, cabbages and other pigmented foods, plants and vegetables. The anthocyanins are subdivided into the sugar free anthocyanidin aglycosides and the anthocyanin glycosides. The differences between individual **anthocyanins** are related to the number of hydroxyl groups, the nature, number of sugars and the position of these attachments (Kong et. al. 2003). The anthocyanodins constitute a large family of differently coloured compounds and occur in countless mixtures in practically all parts of higher plants. They are of great economic importance as fruit pigments and thus are used to colour fruit juices, wine and some beverages. The moderate consumption of such compounds is associated with a lower risk of coronary heart disease, it has been proposed that **anthocyanins** may exert therapeutic activities on human diseases associated with oxidative stress, e.g. coronary heart disease and cancer (Duthie et. al. 2000). The antioxidant properties of **anthocyanins** have been demonstrated by both *in vitro* and *in vivo* experiments (Lazze et. al. 2003; Kahkonen & Heinonen, 2003; Tsuda et. al. 1999, 2000). It has also been suggested that **anthocyanins** play an important role in the prevention against mutagenesis and carcinogenesis mediating some physiological functions related to cancer suppression (Kamei et. al. 1995). **Anthocyanins** show inhibitory effects on the growth of some cancer cells and also inhibit cell transformation (Hou et. al. 2004). The major naturally occurring anthocyanins include, cyanidin, delphinidin, malvidin, pelargonidin, peonidin and petunidin etc.

As mentioned earlier their functions include protection of plants from damaging U.V radiation, environmental pollutions, and various oxidative stresses. Further they also act as enzyme inhibitors, pigment and light screens. In the Bhopal gas tragedy in 1984 due to poisonous gas "Methyl isocyanate" leakage from an industry, only the trees enriched with flavonoids in the bark, e.g; banyan tree survived. This is because the poisonous gas CH_3NCO was neutralized by the flavonoids in the bark. ArOH represents phenolic groups in flavonoids. $ArOH + CH_3NCO \rightarrow ArOCONHCH_3$ (Urethane derivative). The flavanols present in the banyan tree are leucocyanidin, leucopelargonidin, leucodelphinidin etc. Most of them occur as their glycosides. Flavonoid metabolites produced after bacterial action in the intestine are readily absorbed and some are known to possess therapeutic benefits in their own rights (Bone, 1997). Due to the process of enterohepatic circulation, the therapeutic benefits of flavanoid metabolites are sustained over a relatively long duration. Flavonoids were once ascribed with vitamin P activity by Szent Gyorgi as they decreased the permeability of cell membranes. However later vitamin status was not bestowed upon flavonoids. Now their importance as an antioxidant and membrane stabilizing factor are well recognized (Basakar and Nath 1981; Andrew P, 2004).

Leucocyanins and anthocyanins: Former are precursors of the latter which are the coloring substances of flowers, fruits etc. Both of them are mostly present as their glycosides in nature. The aglycon parts are leucocyanidin, leucopelargonidin, leucodelphinidin etc. Their glycosides were isolated from the bark of banyan tree and they demonstrated antidiabetic action on feeding (250 mg/kg body weight) for some days to alloxan diabetic rats, rabbits and dogs. Their blood sugar, serum cholesterol etc. were well controlled and their body weights and general health improved significantly (Brahmachari & Augusti, 1964, Vinod Kumar 1989, Geetha et. al. 1994). Further leucopelargonin imparted protection to rats from CCl4 induced injury to liver. (PP 456-467). Bilberry anthocyanin have effects on microcirculation and are used in diabetic neuropathy, and ophthalmology. They have showed a super oxide an ion scavenging effect *in vitro* and *in vivo* (Martin-Argon, Basabe et. al. 1999). Similarly several anthocyanin rich berries showed superoxide radical scavenging and antilipoperoxidative activities. (Constantino, Rastelli et. al. 1994)

Flavon-3-Ols

These are polyphenolic compounds found in green and black teas, and red wines. The major flavon-3-ols include catechin, epicatechin, epigallocatechin, epigallocatechingallate etc. These exert diverse physiological effects against proliferative diseases and cardiovascular diseases.

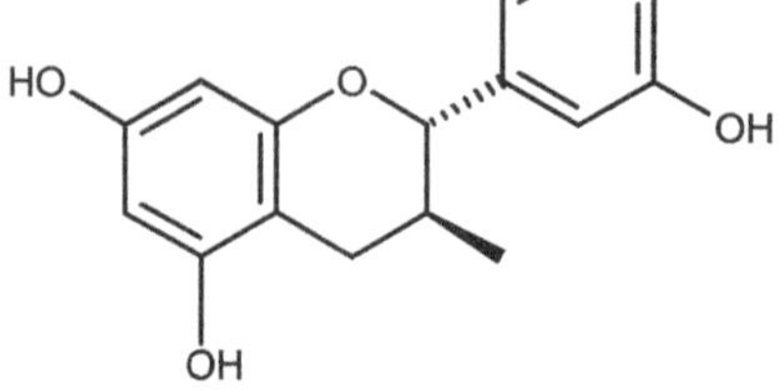

HO OH OH OH

Catechin

HO OH OH OH OH

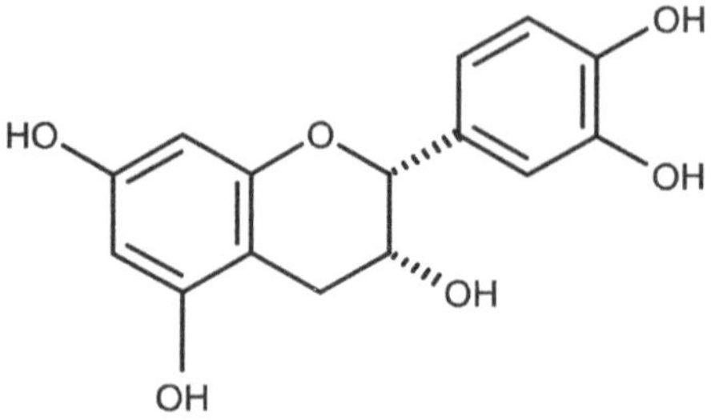

Epicatechin

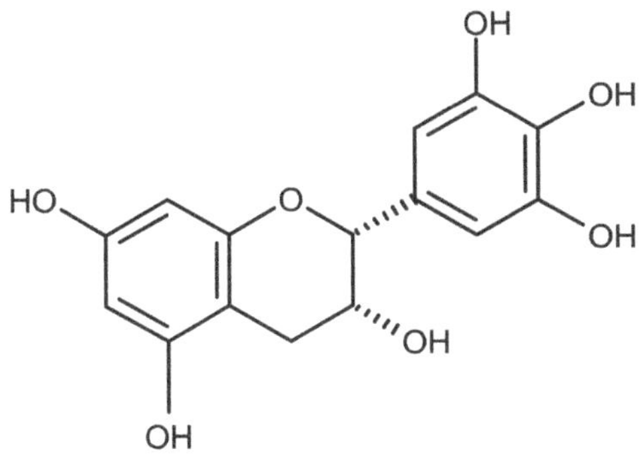

Epigallocatechin

In vitro and *in vivo* animal experiments have shown that catechins have antimutagenic and anticarcinogenic properties, and that they may play a role in the prevention of cardiovascular diseases. Proposed mechanisms for these potential human health promoting properties include inhibition of the metabolic activation of procarcinogens to DNA-reactive substances. Catechins, also referred *in vitro* and *in vivo* animal experiments have shown that they have antimutagenic, anticarcinogenic and antimetastatic (Menon et. al. 1999) properties, and that they may play a role in the prevention of cardiovascular diseaes, induction of enzyme systems involved in detoxification, and protection against DNA damaging free radicals through their antioxidant activity (Middleton & Kandaswami, 1994). Catechins may help prevent low-density lipoprotein (LDL) from oxidative damage through their free radical quenching and metal chelating abilities (Wiseman et. al. 1997), or play a role in the inflammatory and thrombotic processes involved in atherosclerosis (Middleton, 1998; Wollny et. al. 1999). Basakar and Nath (1981) studied the hypocholesterolemic effects of epicatechin, hesperidin and quercetin at a dose of 500 mg/kg b.w in 2% cholesterol rich diet fed rats for a period of three months. These drugs produced a significant reduction ($p<0.001$) both in serum and liver cholesterol levels.

Their order of activity was epicatechin > quercetin > hesperidin. Their mechanism of action is related to the antioxidant and enzyme regulatory functions of the flavonoids. Other benefits noted are maintenance of body weight and non toxicity of the drugs. Francis et. al. (1989) tested 18 flavonoids isolated mostly from functional foods for their ability to inhibit the mutagenicity of aflatoxin B1(AFB1) towards strains TA 100 and TA 98 of Salmonella typhimurium provided with a rat liver activation system. Flavonols in general were more reactive in this regard, while flavanones showed a strain specific response. The flavanol group compounds did not display any activity. The most effective flavonoids were kaempferol, morin, fisetin, biochanin A1 and the glycoside rutin, all of which exhibited a dose dependent inhibition pattern (Concentration 0.1-0.5 μ mol/ml medium). The results indicated that the active flavonoids may be interacting with some components of the microsomal enzyme systems, thus interfering with the bioactivation of AFB1 which is necessary for DNA-adduct formation and mutation. Flavonoids also possess collagen stabilizing activity and they protect the body's connective tissue from degeneration (Mills and Bone 2000).

Isoflavonoids

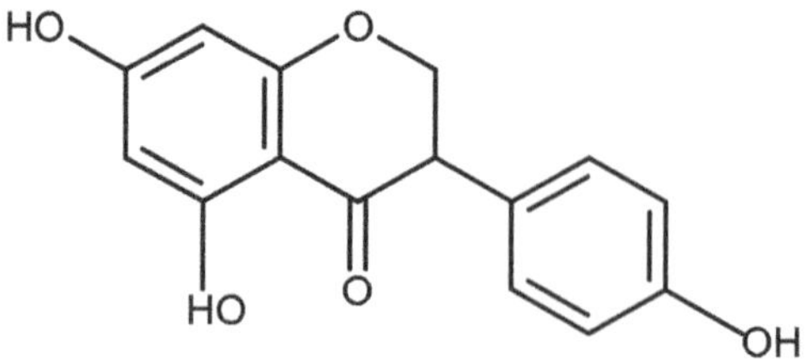

HO O HO O OH

The isoflavonoids are all colourless compounds and are a subgroup of flavonoids which have the second phenol ring in the C3 position. Isoflavonoids are structurally similar to estrogens and are weakly estrogenic, with a potency of one thousand to one hundred thousand when compared to estradiol. Many epidemiological and experimental studies suggest that isoflavonoids prevent some kinds of cancers, osteoporosis, and atherosclerosis. Isoflavonoids also possess antioxidant activity to keep the low density lipoprotein (LDL) in an unoxidated form. Major isoflavone includes: genistein, daidzen, formononetin, biochanin, coumestrol. They are present in soybeans and legumes. These phytoestrogens bind to oestrogen receptors, but whose oestrogen activity is relatively low. Efficacy of genistein isolated from soybeans and its product as preventive drugs of breast tumors and other cancers as well as for alleviating hot flushes and other symptoms associated with menopaus has been reported in clinical trials (Albert, Attabre et. al. 2002). Isoflavones are also found in liquorice (Glycyrrhiza glabra), alfalfa, black cohosh and red clover (Andrew, P, 2004).

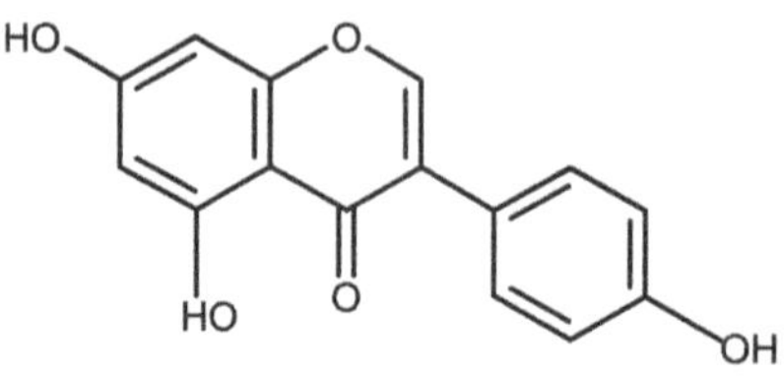

HO O HO O OH

Genistein

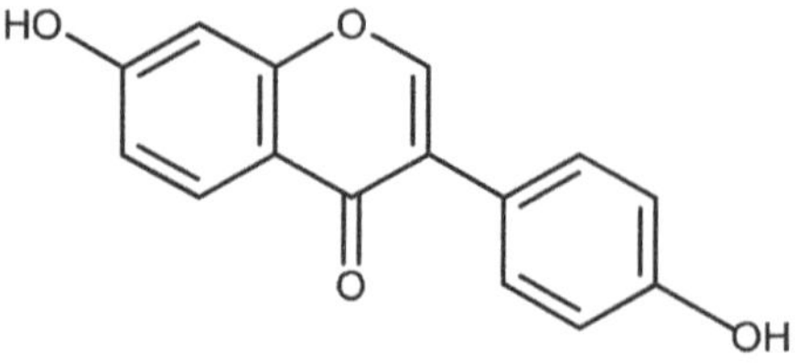

HO O O OH

Daidzein

The biological effects of genistein include tyrosine kinase inhibition (Akiyama et. al. 1987), topoisomerase inhibition, induction of cell cycle arrest (Chen et. al. 2004; Hedlund et. al. 2002; Shen et. al. 2002), apoptosis (Davis et. al. 1998), and increased antioxidant activity (Wei et. al. 1995). Genistein can also modulate growth factor signaling in the transgenic adenocarcinoma mouse prostrate model (Wang et. al. 2004) and can reduce the incidence and number of poorly differentiated tumors *in vivo* (Aronson et al, 1999; Lamartiniere et al. 2002). The biological effects of genistein, as well as of daidzein, appear to be primarily mediated via sex hormone (i.e. androgen and estrogen) signaling (Wang et. al. 2006; Zava et. al. 1997; Allred et. al. 2001; Lund et. al. 2004) and also in the inhibition of lung metastasis in mice by B16F10 melanoma cells (Menon et. al. 1998).

Proanthocyanidins

Proanthocyanidins, also known as condensed tannins, are flavonoid polymers that have a long history of use as tanning agents for animal skins, and are determinants of flavor and astringency in teas, wines and fruit juices. Proanthocyanidin structures vary depending upon the nature (stereochemistry and hydroxylation pattern) of the flavan-3-ol starter and extension units, the position and stereochemistry of the linkage to the 'lower' unit, the degree of polymerization, and the presence or absence of modifications such as esterification of the 3-hydroxyl group. The building blocks of most proanthocyanidins are the flavan-3-ols (+)-catechin and (–)-epicatechin.

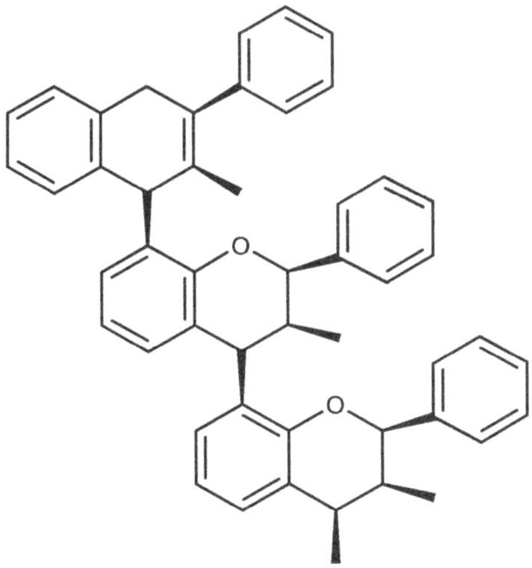

O

O

Proanthocyanidins (Condensed tannins)

Proanthocyanidins and their derivatives are present in the fruits, bark, leaves and seeds of many plants, where their major function is to provide protection against microbial pathogens, insect pests and larger herbivores. The deposition of proanthocyanidins in the endothelial layer of the seed coat in many species would appear to be a classic example of a pre-formed protective barrier. Proanthocyanidins health protective effects includes: antioxidant (Bagchi et. al. 2000; Serafini et. al. 2003), anti-inflammatory (Subarnas & Wagner, 2000), anticancer (Ahamad et. al. 2000; Kandil et. al. 2002) antibacterial (Foo et. al. 2000), antimutagenic (Daver et. al. 2003), immunomodulatory (Lin et. al. 2002) against atherosclerosis (Vinson et. al. 2002) and also in the protection of heart (Pataki et. al. 2002) and kidney (Avramovic et. al. 1999).

Bioavailability of Flavonoids

Flavonoids and their polymers constitute a large class of food constituents, many of which alter metabolic products and have a positive impact on health (Table.1). Fruits and vegetables have been conferred the term 'functional foods' because apart from providing taste, aroma and nutritive value, they provide additional physiological benefits. The consumption of fruits and vegetables has been associated with lower incidence and lower mortality rates of cancer. There is a highly significant negative correlation between intake of total fruits and vegetables and cardio and cerebro-vascular disease mortality. The risk of vascular degeneration, high blood pressure and stroke is diminished in people consuming large amount of fruits and vegetables.

The protective effect of fruits and vegetables has been attributed to the presence of antioxidant, specially vitamins, ascorbic acid, ά-tocophenol and β carotene. However an array of studies has shown that the majority of antioxidant activity may be from phenolics compounds such as flavonoids incliuding isoflavones, anthocyanin, flavon -3-ols and proanthocyanidins.

Table 1 Major dietary sources of commonly occurring flavonoids

Flavonoid Subgroup	Representative Flavonoids	Biological Source
Flavones	Luteolin, Apigenin, Chysin	Capsicum, pepper, Celery, Parsley
Flavanones	Naringenin, Hesperidin Eriodictyol	Orange, other citrus fruits Grape fruit.
Flavonols	Quercetin, Myricetin Kaempferol, Rutin	Onion, apple, cherry, broccoli, tomato, berries, tea, red wine.
Isoflavonoids	Genistein, Diadzein Glycetin, Formononetin	Soya beans, legumes
Flavan-3-ols	Catechin, Epicatechin Epigallocatechin Gallocatechin	Chocolate, beans, tea, red wine, apple, cherry, apricot. Red grapes
Anthocyanins	Pelargonidin, Cyanidin Malvidin, Petunidin Peonidin	Cherry, strawberry, red wine.
Proanthocyanidins	B2-3-O-gallate (Catechin-catechin-gallic-acid dimmer)	Grape seed, pine bark extract.

Epidemiological studies have shown that consumption of food and beverages rich in phenolic content (especially flavonoids) can reduce the risk of heart disease by showing the progression of atherosclerosis by acting as antioxidant towards low density lipoprotein.

Phenolic compounds are a group of secondary metabolites in edible plants. They have many potent biological properties. The antioxidant properties of phenolics are mainly because of their redox properties, which allow them to act as reducing agents, hydrogen or electron donators and singlet oxygen quenchers. Much interest has been focused on flavonoids that are found in many food products of plant origin such as vegetables, fruits, berries, tea and wine. Flavonol (Quercetin and Kaempferol) and flavons (apigenin and buteolin) are abundantly found in various plant based foods. Flavonones are present in citrus fruits, catechin in green tea and anthocynin in red berries. Almost all plant foods such as pomegranate, cocoa, strawberries, rasberries, blackberries, pineapples, apples, pears, plums, citrus fruits, grape fruits, carrots, tomatoes, broccoli, cabbage, brinjals, parslay, peppers, onion, walnuts and whole grains contain phenolic acids. The flavonoids present in different foods are given in the table.

Flavonoids comprise a vast array of biologically active compounds ubiquitous in medicinal plants, many of which have been used in traditional and folklore medicine for thousands of years. Of the many actions of flavonoids, antioxidant and antiproliferative, antiallergic, anti-inflammatory effects and against cardiovascular diseases appears to surpass any other clinically available compound. Herbal medicines are known for centuries to be protectant against one or the other diseases, the use of medicinal plants in Indian systems of medicine like Ayurveda, Siddha, and Unanni is one such case. Punica granatum or pomegranate is one of such plant that possesses vast ethnomedical history and represents a phytochemical (Lansky and Newmann, 2007) reservoir of heuristic medicinal value. These phytochemicals mainly polyphenols are associated with plant based anti-inflammatory (Balkwill et. al. 2005; Simmons and Buckely, 2005, Gosser et. al. 2006) activity, antioxidant; *in vivo* antiulcer activity in ethanol and aspirin induced toxicity (Ajaikumar et. al. 2005); anticancer (Lansky et. al. 2005; Kano et. al. 2005; Fang et. al. 2005; Zheng et. al. 2005) activities. Pomegranate fruit contains the following polyphenols and flavonoids which make it a wonderful gift of nature. It contains anthocyanins of the nature, glycosides of delphinidin, cyanidin, and pelargonidin and hydrolysable tannins such as punicalin, pedunculagin, punicalagin, ellagic tannins like gallagic and ellagic acid esters of glucose, phenolic acids such as caffeic acid, chlorogenic acid etc. which account for 92% of the antioxidant activity of the fruit. Punicalagin an ellagictannin is the most abundant polyphenol responsible for greater than 50% of the fruit juice's potent antioxidant activity (Aviram and Rosenblat 2004 and Wang, Xei et. al. 2004). Peel extract contains sugar bound flavonoids like luteolin, quercetin, kaempferol, naringenin etc. which exhibit strong antioxidant activity. Pomegranate juice has shown to exert anti proliferative, anti invasive, anti eicosanoid and proapoptic actions in breast and prostate cancer cells and other solid malignancies (Sukiki 2001). Pomegranate juice (PJ) and seed extract are inhibitors of lipooxygenase and cyclooxygenase which play a role in arterial plaque formation and inflammation (Polograto 2003). PJ has also protective effects on SOD, Catalase and peroxidase enzymes and it inhibits foam cell formation, B.P, Carotid intima media thickness and atherosclerosis (Aviram 2002).

Available evidence suggests that the bioavailability of many flavanoids is poor and plasma values are very low. (Hollman, Vries et. al. 1995), although there is some evidence that augumenting the intake of flavonoids might improve biochemical indices that retard oxidative damages (Stein, Keevil et. al. 1999).

Experiments on Therapeutic Effects

As flavonoids have polyphenolic groups, they act as antioxidants and maintain the heart circulatory system very well by strengthening the blood vessels including various capillaries. They can protect the body from stress as biological modifiers (Middleton & Kandaswami 1994). They demonstrate synergistic effects with vitamin C and also reduce the membrane permeability as once ascribed to vitamin P by Szent Gyorgi. Rutin and related flavonoids are effective in reducing permeability of blood capillaries and are widely used for peripheral vascular disorders (Basakar and Nath 1981).

A study in Holland (Zutphen Elderly Study) carried out on several aged men showed that dietary intake of flavanoids for five years decreased mortality from coronary artery disease very considerably (Andrew P 2004). Their functional food consisted of Tea, Onions, and Apples enriched with various flavonoids and poly phenols. The interscales of onions contain quercetin. Tea contains catechin type of condensed tannins and apple is rich in quercetin, kaempferol, myricitin etc (Jones, 1995, Hertog, Feskens et al 1993)

Citrus fruit flavonoid nomilin induces Glutathione-S-transferase that enhances detoxification and others viz; tangeretin and nobiletin inhibit bacterial mutagenesis (Calomme, Pieters et al 1996). Silymarine, a flavonolignin complex from Silybum mariani is an inducer of phase 1 detoxification and it protects liver mitochondria and microsomes from lipid per oxidation. It causes hepatic regeneration and increase in glutathione level. Flavonoids regulate certain enymes e.g. Nepetrin and its glycoside nepitin from Rosinarin officinalis and glycosides of luteolin and kaempferol inhibit the action of aldose reductase that causes diabetic cataract (Pathak and Gingla 1991). Certain other flavonoids, control the activities of

1. Xanthine oxidase that causes hyperuricemia leading to gout
2. Tyrosine protein kinase that produces premalignant cells
3. Lipooxygenase and cyclooxygenase that produce inflammatory prostaglandins, leukotriens and thromboxanes and
4. cyclic nucleotide phosphodiesterase that promotes platelet aggregation.

Quercetin and some other flavonoids are effective inhibitors on the release of histamine, induced by various agents. They also inhibit a number of stages of inflammation in chronic arthritis (Middleton and Drzewiecki 1984). They offer the advantage of a high margin of safety and lack of side effects over the classical anti-inflammatory drugs. Treatment with 180 mg of rutin isolated from Fagopyrum esculentum (buck wheat herb) for a month flushed out induced oedema plaques in cornea and conjunctiva (Schilcher & Muller 1981). Certain other flavonoids exert protective action against lipid per oxidation stimulated by a variety of toxins (Pathak and Gingla 1991).

Experiments conducted by Andrews, Ajantha et. al. (2006) on rats have shown that the damages induced by feeding alcohol or lead acetate separately or their combination for a month were significantly decreased by a simultaneous feeding of an ethyl acetate fraction of pomegranate fruit extract (100 mg/Kg /day) as effectively as garlic oil or vitamin E. viz; alterations of certain enzyme activities, e.g. AST, ALT, Catalase and lipid profile were prevented. The protective action of the PF extract (250 mg/kg) on gastric mucosa subjected to alcohol or aspirin toxicity was reported by Ajaikumar, Asheef et. al. (2005) and that from certain oxidants by Yasuko, Takao et. al. (2002). All these findings high light the importance of flavonoids and related phenols as a major class of nutraceuticals that prevent diseases like diabetes, CHD, cancer, dementia, aging etc.

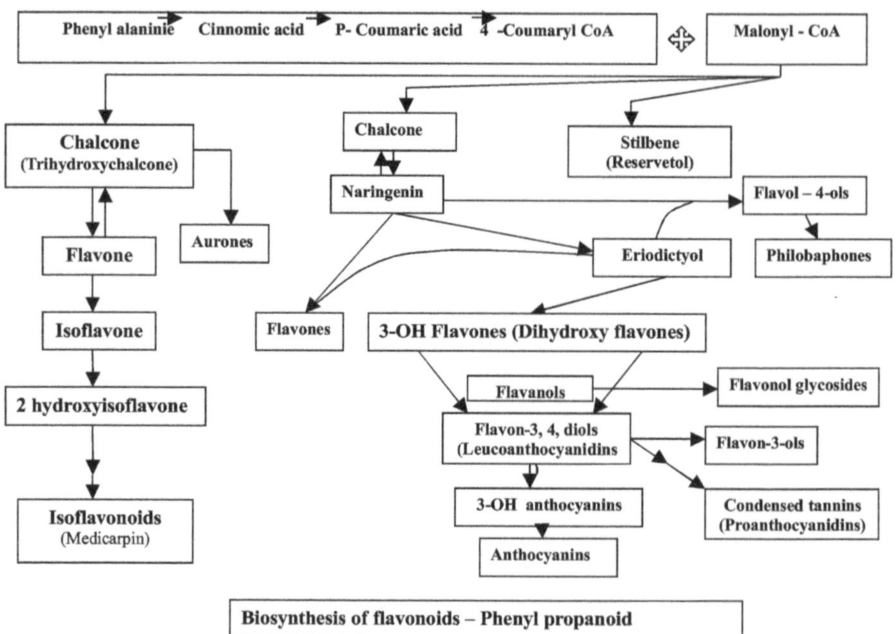

Biosynthesis of flavonoids – Phenyl propanoid

Acknowledgement

The authors acknowledge with thanks the authorites of Amala Cancer Research center Thrissur and also our colleagues especially V.K. Jaimsha, V.R.Vineesh and K.S.Sudha for their cooperation in the preparion of this article.

Reference

1. Ahmad N, Gupta S, Mukhtar H. 2000. Green tea polyphenol epigallocatechin- 3-gallate differentially modulates nuclear factor kB in cancer cells versus normal cells. *Archives of Biochemistry and Biophysics* 376: 338–346.

2. Ajaikumar, K.B., Asheef, M., Babu, B.H., Padikkala, J., 2005. The inhibition of gastric mucosal injury by *Punica granatum* L. (pomegranate) methanolic extract. Journal of Ethnopharmacology 96, 171–176.

3. Akiyama T, Ishida J, Nakagawa S, Ogawara H, Watanabe S, Itoh N, et. al. Genistein, a specific inhibitor of tyrosine-specific protein kinases. J Bio Chem 1987; 262:5592– 95.

4. Albert, A; Attabre,C, et. al. (2002). Efficacy and safety of a phytoestrogen preparation derived from glycin max(L) in Climacteric symptomatology, Phytomedicine 9: 85-92.

5. Allred CD, Ju YH, Allred KF, Chang J, Helferich WG. Dietary genistin stimulates growth of estrogen-dependent breast cancer tumors similar to that observed with genistein. Carcino 2001; 22: 1667– 73.

6. Amoros M, Lurton E, Boustie J, Girre L, Sauvager F, Cormier M. Comparison of the anti-herpes simplex virus activities of propolis and 3-methyl-but-2-enyl caffeate. J Nat Prod 1994; 57:644– 47.

7. Andrews, A; Augusti, K.T. Ajantha, K.G. et. al. (2006). Antioxidant and related effects of nutraceuticals present in pomegranate fruit extract and garlic oil in lead salt and alcohol administered rats for a month. 2006.in: Proceedings of the National Seminar on the Evaluation of Nutraceuticals that prevent diseases. 29 Nov. Thalassery Campus of Kannur Uty.

8. Andrew Pengally(2004) Constituents of Medicinal plants. p,30. CABI Publishing 875 Massachusetts Avenue. 7th Floor, Cambridge, MAO 2139. U.S.A

9. Aronson WJ, Tymchuk CN, Elashoff RM, McBride WH, McLean C, Wang H, et. al. Decreased growth of human prostate LNCaP tumors in SCID mice fed a low-fat, soy protein diet with isoflavones. Nutr Cancer 1999;35:130– 36.

10. (a) Aviram, M; Rosenblat, M; Gaitini, D; et. al. (2004) Pomegranate juice consumption for 3 years by patients with carotid artery stenosis reduces common carotid intima-media thickness, blood pressure and LDL oxidation. Clinical Nutrition.23(3)423-33.

    (b) Aviram, M(2002)Pomegranate juice as a major source of polyphenolic flavonoids and it is a most potent antioxidant against LDL oxidation and atherosclerosis. Free Radic. Res. 36: 71.

11. Avramovic V, Vlahovic P, Mihailovic D, Stefanovic V. 1999. Protective effect of a bioflavonoid proanthocyanidin-BP1 in glycerol-induced acute renal failure in the rat: renal stereological study. *Renal Failure* 21: 627–634.

12. Augusti, K.T; Regi, S.D. et. al. (1994) Effect of leucopelargonin derivative from Ficus bengalensis Linn on diabetic dogs. Ind.J.Med. Res. 99:82-86.

13. Bagchi D, Bagchi M, Stohs SJ, Das DK, Ray SD, Kuszynski CA, Joshi SS, Pruess HG. 2000. Free radicals and grape seed proanthocyanidn extract: importance in human health and disease prevention. *Toxicology* 148: 187–197.

14. Balkwill, F., Charles, K.A., Mantovani, A., 2005. Smoldering inflammation in the initiation and promotion of malignant disease. Cancer Cell 7, 211–217.

15. Basakar, P.W and Nath, N(1981) Cholesterol lowering action of Vitamin P-like compounds in rats. Ind.Jour.Exp. Biol. 19:787-789.

16. Bors W and Saran M (1987) Radical scavenging by flavonoid antioxidants. *Free Radical Res Commun* 2:289–294.

17. Brahmachari, H.D and Augusti, K.T.(1964) Isolation of orally effective hypoglycemic compounds from Ficus bengalensis Linn. Ind.J.Physiol. Pharmacol. 8:60-64.

18. Buening MK, Chang RL, Huang MT, Fortner JG, Wood AW, Conney AH. Activation and inhibition of benzo(a)pyrene and aflatoxin B1 metabolism in human liver microsomes by naturally occurring flavonoids. Cancer Res 1981;41:67– 72.

19. Bone, K(1997) Grape seed extract : The facts, the fiction and the future. Mediherb's Conference, Sydney.

20. Calomme, M; Pieters, L. et. al. (1996) Inhibition of bacterial mutagenesis by citrus flavonoids. Planta Medica, 62:222-226.

21. Carroll KK, Guthrie N, So FV and Chambers AF (1998) Anticancer properties of flavonoids, with emphasis on citrus flavonoids, in *Flavonoids in Health and Disease* (Rice-Evans CA and Packer L eds) pp 437–446, Marcel Dekker Inc., New York

22. Casagrande, F. and Darbon, J. (2001) Effects of structurally related flavonoids on cell cycle progression of human melanoma cells : regulation of cyclin-dependent kinases CDK2 and CDK1. Biochem. Pharmacol. *61*, 1205-1215.

23. Chang FR, Wei, JL, Teng CM, Wu YC. Antiplatelet aggregation constituents from Annona purpurea. J Nat Prod 1998;61:1457– 61.

24. Chen, A.C. Donovan, SM, Genistein at a concentration present in soy infant formula inhibits Caco-2BBe cell proliferation by causing G2/M cell cycle arrest. J Nutr 2004;134:1303– 38

25. Chin L, Lin Y, Huang C, Wen K. Evaluation of quantitative analysis of flavonoid aglycones in Ginkgo biloba extract and its products. J Food Drug Anal 2000;8:289– 96.

26. Cholbi MR, Paya M, Alcaraz MJ. Inhibitory effects of phenolic compounds on CCl4-induced microsomal lipid peroxidation. Experientia 1991;47:195– 99.

27. Ciolino HP, Yeh GC. The flavonoid galangin is an inhibitor of CYP1A1 activity and an agonist/antagonist of the aryl hydrocarbon receptor. Br J Cancer 1999;79:1340– 46.

28. Clemetson CAB (1989) Bioflavonoids, in *Vitamin C* (Clemetson CAB ed) pp 101–128, RC Press, Inc., Boca Raton, FL.

29. Cody V, Middleton E and Harborne JB, eds (1986) *Plant Flavonoids in Biology and Medicine: Biochemical, Pharmacological, and Structure-Activity Relationships*. Alan R. Liss, Inc., New York.

30. Cody V, Middleton E, Harborne JB and Beretz A, eds (1988) *Plant Flavonoids in Biology and Medicine II: Biochemical, Cellular and Medicinal Properties*. Alan R. Liss, Inc., New York.

31. Constantino, L;Rastelli, G. et. el. Composition, superoxide radicals, scavenging and antilipoperoxidant activity of some edible fruits. Fitoterapia LXV (1994)44-47

32. Cortes JR, Perez-G M, Rivas MD, Zamorano J. Kaempferol inhibits IL-5 induced STST6 activation by specially targeting JAK3. J Immunol. 2007; 179(6): 3881-87.

33. Dauer A, Hensel A, Lhoste E, Knasmueller S, Mersch SV. 2003. Genotoxic and antigenotoxic effects of catechin and tannins from the bark of *Hamamelis virginiana* L. in metabolically competent, human hepatoma cells (Hep G2) using single cell gel electrophoresis. *Phytochemistry* 63: 199–207.

34. Davis JN, Singh B, Bhuiyan M, Sarkar FH. Genistein-induced upregulation of p21WAF1, downregulation of cyclin B, and induction of apoptosis in prostate cancer cells. Nutr Cancer 1998; 32:123– 31.

35. de Whalley CV, Rankin SM, Hoult JR, Jessup W, Leake DS. Flavonoids inhibit the oxidative modification of low density lipoproteins by macrophages. Biochem Pharmacol 1990;39:1743–50.

36. Della Loggia R, Ragazzi E, Tubaro A, Fassina G, Vertua R. Antiinflammatory activity of benzopyrenes that are inhibitors of cyclo and lipo-oxygenase. Pharmacol Res Commun 1988;20 (Suppl 5): 91–9 4.

37. Dimas K, Demetzos C, Mitaku S, Marselos M, Tzavaras T, Kokkinopoulos D. Cytotoxic activity of kaempferol glycosides against human leukaemic cell lines in vitro. Pharmacol Res 2000;41:85 –88.

38. Duthie, G.G., Duthie, S.J. and Kyle, J.A.M. (2000) Plant polyphenols in cancer and heart disease: implications as nutritional antioxidants. Nutr. Res. Rev., 13, 79--106.

39. Elliott Middleton JR, Chithan Kandaswami and Theohais C Theohardies. The effects of plant flavonoids on mammalian cells: implication for inflammation, heart diseases and cancer. Pharmacological reviews. 2000; 52: 673 – 751

40. Ephraim P Lannsky, Robert A Newman. *Punica garanatum* (pomegranate) and its potential for prevention of inflammation and cancer. Journal of ethnopharmacology. 2007; 109: 177-206.

41. Fang, J., Xia, C., Cao, Z., Zheng, J.Z., Reed, E., Jiang, B.H.H., 2005. Apigenin inhibits VEGF and HIF-1 expression via PI3K/AKT/p70S6K1 and HDM2/p53 pathways. FASEB Journal: Official Publication of The Federation of American Societies for Experimental Biology 19, 342–353.

42. Farkas L, Gabor M and Kallay F (1986) in *Flavonoids and Bioflavonoids,* Akademiai Kiado, Budapest.

43. Ferriola PC, Cody V, Middleton E. Jr. protein kinase C inhibition by plants flavonoids. Kinetic mechanisms and structure-activity relationships. Biochem Pharmacol. 1989; 38(10): 1617-1624.

44. Foo LY, Lu Y, Howell AB, Vorsa N. 2000. The structure of cranberry proanthocyanidins which inhibit adherence of uropathogenic P-fimbriated *Escherichia coli in vitro. Phytochemistry* 54: 173–181.

45. Francis, AR;Shetty, TK and Battacharya, RK(1981) Modifying role of dietary factors on the mutagenicity of aflatoxinB1: in vitro effect of plant flavonoids. Mutation Research.222:393-401.

46. Furuno K, Akasako T, Sugihara N. The contribution of the pyrogallol moiety to the superoxide radical scavenging activity of flavonoids. Biol Pharm Bull 2002;25:19–23.

47. Gabor M (1979) Anti-inflammatory substances of plant origin, in Handbook of Experimental Pharmacology: Anti-Inflammatory Drugs (Vane JR and Ferreira SH eds) pp 698–739, Springer-Verlag, New York.

48. Gabor M (1986) The Pharmacology of Benzopyrone Derivatives and Related Compounds, Akademiai Kiad, Budapest.

49. Gabor M, Razga Z. Effect of benzopyrene derivatives on simultaneously induced croton oil ear oedema and carrageenin paw oedema in rats. Acta Physiol Hung 1991;77:197– 207.

50. Gao S, Liu GZ, Wang Z. Modulation of androgen receptor-dependent transcription by resveratrol and genistein in prostate cancer cells. Prostate 2004;59:214– 25.

51. Geetha, BS, Mathew, BC and Augusti, KT(1994)Hypoglycemic effects of leucodelphinidin derivative isolated from Ficus bengalensis Linn. Indian J. Physiol. Pharmacol.38(3):220-222.

52. Grosser, T., Fries, S., FitzGerald, G.A., 2006. Biological basis for the cardiovascular consequences of COX-2 inhibition: therapeutic challenges and opportunities. The Journal of Clinical Investigation 116, 4–15.

53. Harborne JB, Mabry TJ and Mabry H (1975) *The Flavonoids*. Academic Press, New York.

54. Havsteen B (1984) Flavonoids: A class of natural products of high pharmacological potency. *Biochem Pharmacol* 32:1141–1148.

55. Havsteen B. Flavonoids, a class of natural products of high pharmacological potency. Biochem Pharmacol 1983;32:1141– 48.

56. Hayek T, Fuhrman B, Vaya J, Rosenbalt M, Benlinky P, Coleman R, Elis A, Aviram M. Reduced progression of atherosclerosis in apolipoprotein E-deficient mice following consumption of red wine, or its polyphenols quercetin or catechin, is associated with reduced susceptibility of LDL to oxidation and aggregation. Arterioscler Thromb Vasc Biol. 1997 Nov; 17(11):2744-52.

57. Hedlund TE, Johannes WU, Miller GJ. Soy isoflavonoid equol modulates the growth of benign and malignant prostatic epithelial cells in vitro. Prostate 2002; 54:68 –78.

58. Heo MY, Lee SJ, Kwon CH, Kim SW, Sohn DH, Au WW. Anticlastogenic effects of galangin against bleomycin-induced chromosomal aberrations in mouse spleen lymphocytes. Mutat Res 1994; 311:225–2 9.

59. Heo MY, Sohn SJ, Au WW. Anti-genotoxicity of galangin as a cancer chemopreventive agent candidate. Mutat Res 2001;488:135–50.

60. Heo MY, Yu KS, Kim KH, Kim HP, Au WW. Anticlastogenic effect of flavonoids against mutagen-induced micronuclei in mice. Mutat Res 1992; 284:243–49.

61. Herrmann K. Flavonols and flavones in food plants. J Food Technol 1976; 11:433– 48.

62. Hertog MG, Feskens EJ, Hollman PC, Katan MB, Kromhout D. Dietary antioxidant flavonoids and risk of coronary heart disease: the Zutphen Elderly Study. Lancet 1993; 342: 1007 – 1011.

63. Hertog MGL, Hollman PCH, Katan MB and Kromhout D (1993b) Intake of potentially anticarcinogenic flavonoids and their determinants in adults in the Netherlands. *Nutr Cancer* 20:21–29.

64. Hessenauer A, Montenarh M, Gotz C. Medizinische .Inhibition of CK2 activity provokes different responses in hormonesensitive and hormonerefractory prostate cancer cells. Int J Oncol. 2003 Jun; 22(6):126370.

65. Hollman, PCH; Vries, JHM; Leeuwen, SD(1995) Absorption of dietary quercetin glycosides and quercetin in healthy illeostomy volunteers .Am.J.Clin. Nutr.62:1276-1282.

66. Hou, D.X., Kai, K., Li, J.J., Lin, S., Terahara, N., Wakamatsu, M., Fujii, M., Young, M.R. and Colburn, N. (2004) Anthocyanidins inhibit activator protein 1 activity and cell transformation: structure--activity relationship and molecular mechanisms. Carcinogenesis, 25, 29--36.

67. Hughes RE and Wilson HK (1977) Flavonoids: Some physiological and nutritional consideration. *Prog Med Chem* 14:285–301.

68. Husain SR, Cillard J and Cillard P (1987a) Hydroxyl radical scavenging activity of flavonoids. *Phytochemistry* 26:2489–2491.

69. Imamura Y, Migita T, Uriu Y, Otagiri M, Okawara T. Inhibitory effects of flavonoids on rabbit heart carbonyl reductase. J Biochem (Tokyo) 2000;127:653–58.

70. Jeong HJ, Shin YG, Kim IH, Pezzuto JM. Inhibition of aromatase activity by flavonoids. Arch Pharm Res 1999 Jun; 22(3):30912

71. Jones, F. The save your heart wine guide.(1995).Headline Pubs.London.

72. Justesen U, Knuthsen P, Leth T. Quantitative analysis of flavonols, flavones, and flavanones in fruits, vegetables and beverages by highperformance liquid chromatography with photo-diode array and mass spectrometric detection. J Chromatogr A 1998;799:101– 10.

73. Kahkonen, M.P. and Heinonen, M. (2003) Antioxidant activity of anthocyanins and their aglycons. J. Agric. Food Chem., 51, 628--633.

74. Kamei, H., Kojima, T., Hasegawa, M., Koide, T., Umeda, T., Yukawa, T. and Terabe, K. (1995) Suppression of tumor cell growth by anthocyanins in vitro. Cancer Invest., 13, 590--594.

75. Kandil FE, Smith MAL, Rogers RB, Pepin MF, Song LL, Pezzuto JM, Seigler DS. 2002. Composition of a chemopreventive proanthocyanidinrich fraction from cranberry fruits responsible for the inhibition of 12-Otetradecanoyl phorbol-13-acetate (TPA)-induced ornithine decarboxylase (ODC) activity. *Journal of Agricultural and Food Chemistry* 50: 1063– 1069.

76. Kang SS, Kim JS, Son KM, Kim HP, Chang HW. Isolation of COX-2 inhibitors from Alpinia officinarum. Korean J Pharmacogn 2000; 31:57 – 62.

77. Kanno, S., Tomizawa, A., Hiura, T., Osanai, Y., Shouji, A., Ujibe, M., Ohtake, T., Kimura, K., Ishikawa, M., 2005. Inhibitory effects of naringenin on tumor growth in human cancer cell lines and sarcoma S-180-implanted mice. Biological and Pharmaceutical Bulletin 28, 527–530.

78. Karakaya S, El SN. Quercetin, luteolin, apigenin and kaempferol contents of some foods. Food Chem 1999;66:289– 92.

79. Kataoka M, Hirata K, Kunikata T, Ushio S, Iwaki K, Ohashi K, et. al. Antibacterial action of tryptanthrin and kaempferol, isolated from the indigo plant (Polygonum tinctorium Lour.), against Helicobacter pylori-infected Mongolian gerbils. J Gastroenterol 2001;36:5– 9.

80. Kempuraj D, Madhappan B, Christodoulou S, Boucher W, Cao J, Papadopoulou N, Cetrulo, CN, Theoharidas. Br. J. Pharmacol. 2005; 145(7): 934-944.

81. Kim, H. K., Cheon, B. S., Kim, S. Y. and Kim, H. P. (1999) Effects of naturally occurring flavonoids on nitric oxide production in the macrophage cell line RAW 264.7 and their structure and activity relationships. Biochem. Pharmacol. *58*, 759-765.

82. Kimata, M., Inagaki, N. and Nagai, H. (2000) Effects of luteolin and other flavonoids on IgE-mediated allergic reactions. Planta Med. *66*, 25-29.

83. Kobayashi T, Nakata T, Kuzumaki T. Effect of flavonoids on cell cycle progression in prostate cancer cells. Cancer Lett. 2002 Feb 8;176(1):1723.

84. Koga T, Meydani M. Effect of plasma metabolites of (+)-catechin and quercetin on monocyte adhesion to human aortic endothelial cells. Am J Clin Nutr 2001;73:941–48.

85. Kong, J.M., Chia, L.S., Goh, N.K., Chia, T.F. and Brouillard, R. (2003) Analysis and biological activities of anthocyanins. Phytochemistry, 64, 923--933.

86. Lalith Jayasinghe, B A I S Balasooriya, W. Chintha Padmini, Noriyuki Hara and Yoshinori Fujimoto. Geranyl chalcone derivatives with antifungal and radical scavenging properties from the leaves of Artocarpus nobilis. Phytochemistry. 2004; 9: 1287-1290.

87. Lamartiniere CA, Cotroneo MS, Fritz WA, Wang J, Mentor-Marcel R, Elgavish A. Genistein chemoprevention: timing and mechanisms of action in murine mammary and prostate. J Nutr 2002;132:552S–58S.

88. Lansky, E.P., Harrison, G., Froom, P., Jiang, W.G., (2005). Pomegranate (*Punica granatum*) pure chemicals show possible synergistic inhibition of human PC-3 prostate cancer cell invasion across Matrigel. Investigational New Drugs 23, 121-2. Erratum in: Investigational New Drugs 2005, 23, 379.

89. Lazze, M.C., Pizzala, R., Savio, M., Stivala, L.A., Prosperi, E. and Bianchi, L. (2003) Anthocyanins protect against DNA damage induced by tert-butylhydroperoxide in rat smooth muscle and hepatoma cells. Mutat. Res., 535, 103--115.

90. Li R, Kenyon GL, Cohen FE, Chen X, Gong B, Dominguez JN, Davison E, Kurban G, Miller RE, Nuzum EO, et al. invitro antimalarial activity of chalcones and their derivatives. J Med Chem. 1995; 38 (26): 5031-5037.

91. Lin LC, Kuo YC, Chou CJ. 2002. Immunomodulatory proanthocyanidins from *Ecdysanthera utilis*. *Journal of Natural Products* 65: 505–508.

92. Lindenmeyer F, Li H, Menashi S, Soria C, Lu H. Institut National de la Sante et. de la Recherche. Apigenin acts on the tumor cell invasion process and regulates protease production. Nutr Cancer. 2001;39(1):13947.

93. Lund TD, Munson DJ, Haldy ME, Setchell KDR, Lephart ED, Handa RJ. Equol is a novel anti-androgen that inhibits prostate growth and hormone feedback. Biol Reprod 2004;70:1188– 95.

94. Martin-Argon, S; Basabe, B, et. al. (1999) In vitro and in vivo antioxidant properties of Vaccinium myrtillus. Pharmaceutical Biol. 37:109-113.

95. McClure JW (1986) Physiology of flavonoids in plants, in *Plant Flavonoids in Biology and Medicine: Biochemical, Pharmacological, and Structure-Activity Relationships* (Cody V, Middleton E and Harborne JB eds) pp 77–85, Alan R. Liss, Inc., New York.

96. Menon LG, Kuttan R, Kuttan G. Antimetastatic activity of Curcumin and Catechin. *Cancer Letters 1999, 141(1-2), 159-165.*

97. Menon LG, Kuttan R, Muraleedharan G Nair, Yu-Chen Chang, Kuttan G. Effect of isoflavones-Genistein and Daidzein in the inhibition of lung metastasis in mice induced by B16F10 melanoma cells. *Nutrition and Cancer 1998, 30(1), 74 -77.*

98. Middleton E & Kandaswami C (1994): The impact of plant flavonoids on mammalian biology: implications for immunity, inflammation and cancer. In The Flavonoids: Advances in Research Since 1986, ed. JB Harborne, pp 619-652. London: Chapman & Hall.

99. Middleton, E and Drzewiecki,G (1984) Flavonoid inhibition of human basophil histamine release stimulated by various agents. Biochemical Pharmacology 33:3333-38

100. Middleton E (1998): Effect of plant flavonoids on immune and inflammatory cell function. Adv. Exp. Med. Biol. 439, 175- 182.

101. Middleton E and Kandaswami C (1993) The impact of plant flavonoids on mammalian biology: Implications for immunity, inflammation and cancer, in *The Flavonoids: Advances in Research Since 1986* (Harborne IR ed) pp 619–645, Chapman and Hall, London.

102. Mills, S and Bone, K(2000). Principles and Practice of Phytotherapy. Churchill, Livingstone, Edinburgh.

103. Miranda CL. Stevens JF, Helmrich A, Henderson MC, Rodriguez J, Yang H, Deinzer ML, Barnes DW and Buhler DR. Antiproliferative and cytotoxic effects of prenylated flavonoids from hops (*Humulus lupulus*) in human cancer cell lines. Food and chemical toxicology. 1999; 4: 271-285.

104. Mittra, B., Saha, A., Chowdhury, A. R., Pal, C., Mandal, S., Mukhopadhyay, S., Bandopadhyay, S. and Majumder, H. K. (2000) Luteolin, an abundant dietary component is a potent anti-leishmanial agent that acts by inducing topoisomerase II-mediated kinetoplast DNA cleavage leading to apoptosis. Mol. Med. *6*, 527-41.

105. Molnar, J., Beladi, I., Domonker, K., Foldeak, S., Boda, K. and Veckenstedt, A. (1981) Antitumor activity of flavonoids on NK/Ly ascites tumor cells. Neoplasma *28*, 11-18.

106. Monforte MT, Trovato A, Kirjavainen S, Forestieri AM, Galati FM, Lo Curto RB. Biological effects of hesperidin, a citrus flavonoid: hypolipidemic activity on experimental hypercholesterolemia in rat. Farmaco. 1995; 50(9):595-99

107. Moriyama H, Iizuka T, Nagai M, Miyataka H, Satoh T. Antiinflammatory activity of heat-treated Cassia alata leaf extract and its flavonoid glycoside. Yakugaku Zasshi 2003;123:607– 11.

108. Mukhtar H, Das M, Khan WA, Wang ZY, Bik DP, Bickers DR. Exceptional activity of tannic acid among naturally occurring plant phenols in protecting against 7,12-dimethylbenz (a)anthracene-, benzo(a)pyrene-, 3-methylcholanthrene-, and N-methyl-N-nitrosoureainduced skin tumorigenesis in mice. Cancer Res 1988; 48:2361–65.

109. Naderi GA, Asqary S, Sarraf-Zadegan N, Shirvany H. Anti-oxidant effect of flavonoids on the susceptibility of LDL oxidation. Mol Cell Biochem. 2003; 246(1-2): 193-96.

110. Nijveldt RJ, van Nood E, van Hoorn DE, Boelens PG, van Norren K, van Leeuwen PA. Flavonoids: a review of probable mechanisms of action and potential applications. Am J Clin Nutr 2001; 74:418– 25.

111. Nowakowska zdzislawa. A review of anti-infective and anti-inflammatory chalcones. European journal of medicinal chemistry. 2007; 42: 125-137.

112. Ong KC, Khoo HE. Biological effects of myricetin. Gen Pharmacol 1997; 29:121–26.

113. Ono K, Nakane H, Fukushima M, Chermann JC, Barre-Sinoussi F. Differential inhibitory effects of various flavonoids on the activities of reverse transcriptase and cellular DNA and RNA polymerases. Eur J Biochem 1990; 190:469–76.

114. Park YK, Koo MH, Sato HH, Contado JL. Survey of some components of propolis which were collected by Apis mellifera in Brazil. Arch Biol Technol 1995; 38:1253–59.

115. Pataki T, Bak I, Kovacs P, Bagchi D, Das DK, Toskai A. 2002. Grape seed proanthocyanidins improved cardiac recovery during reperfusion after ischemia in isolated rat hearts. *American Journal of Clinical Nutrition* 75: 894–899.

116. Pathak, D; Pathak, K and Gangla, A.K(1991) Flavonoids as medicinal agents-recent advances:Fitoterapia LXII.371-389.

117. Perez-Garcia, F., Adzet, T. and Canigueral, S. (2000) Activity of artichoke leaf extract on reactive oxygen species in human leukocytes. Free Radical Res. *33*, 661-665.

118. Polograto, JA(2003) Effects of flavonoid rich 6 beverages on prostacyclin synthesis in humans and human aortic endothelial cells.Assoc. with invivo platelet function.J.Med.Food. 6.301.

119. Post, J. F. and Varma, R. S. (1992) Growth inhibitory effects of bioflavonoids and related compounds on human leukemic CEM-C1 and CEM-C7 cells. Cancer Lett. *24*, 207-213.

120. Rice-Evans, C (2001) Flavonoid antioxidants; Current Medicinal Chemistry, 8:797-807.

121. Robak J, Korbut R, Shridi F, Swies J, Rzadkowska-Bodalska H. On the mechanism of antiaggregatory effect of myricetin. Pol J Pharmacol Pharm 1988;40:337–40.

122. Rotelli AE, Guardia T, Juarez AO, de la Rocha NE, Peizer LE. Comparative study of flavonoids in experimental models of inflammation. Pharmacol Res. 2003: 48(6):601-606.

123. Schilcher, H and Muller, A (1981) ":Fagopyrum esculentum Moench-a new pharmaceutically useful flavonoid plant" Proceedings of the International Bioflavonoid symposium, Munich..

124. Schmelzer E, Jahnen W, Hahlbrock K (1988) In situ localization of lightinduced chalcone synthase mRNA, chalcone synthase, and flavonoid endproducts in epidermal cells of parsley leaves. Proc Natl Acad Sci USA 85: 2989–93

125. Selway JWT (1986) Antiviral activity of flavones and flavans, in *Plant Flavonoids in Biology and Medicine: Biochemical, Pharmacological, and Structure-Activity Relationships* (Cody V, Middleton E and Harborne JB eds) pp 521–536, Alan R. Liss, Inc., New York.

126. Serafini M, Bugianesi R, Maiani G, Valtuena S, De Santis S, Crozier A. 2003. Plasma antioxidants from chocolate. *Nature* 424: 1013.

127. Shen JC, Klein RD, Wei Q, Guan Y, Contois JH, Wang TTY, et. al. Low-dose genistein induces cyclin-dependent kinase inhibitors and G1 cell cycle arrest in human prostate cancer cells. Mol Carcinog 2002; 29:92 – 102.

128. Shimoi K, Masuda S, Furugori M, Esaki S, and Kinae N (1994) Radioprotective effect of antioxidative flavonoids in x-ray irradiated mice. *Carcinogenesis* 15:2669–2672.

129. Simmons, D.L., Buckley, C.D., 2005. Some new, and not so new, anti-inflammatory targets. Current Opinion in Pharmacology 5, 394–397.

130. So FV, Guthrie N, Chambers AF, Carroll KK. Inhibition of proliferation of estrogen receptor-positive MCF-7 human breast cancer cells by flavonoids in the presence and absence of excess estrogen. Cancer Lett 1997;112:127– 33.

131. Stein, J; Keevil, JG; Wieb, DA(1999) Purple grape juice improves endothelial function and reduces the susceptibility of LDL cholesterol to oxidation in patients with coronary artery disease. Circulation, 100:1050-55.

132. Subarnas A, Wagner H. 2000. Analgesic and anti-flammatory activity of the proanthocyanidin shellegueain A from *Polypodium feei* METT. *Phytomedicine* 7: 401–405.

133. Sukuki, R (2001), Cytotoxic effect of conjugated trienoic fatty acid on mouse tumor human monocytic leukemic cells. Lipids.36(5)477-82.

134. Takahashi T, Kobori M, Shinmoto H, Tsushida T. Structure activity relationships of flavonoids and the induction of granulocytic or monocytic differentiation in HL60 human myeloid leukemia cells. Biosci Biotechnol Biochem 1998; 62(11).

135. Tan WF, Lin LP, Li MH, Zhang YX, Tong YG, Xiao D, et. al. Quercetin, a dietary-derived flavonoid, possesses antiangiogenic potential. Eur J Pharmacol 2003; 459:255– 62.

136. Torel J, Cillard J and Cillard P (1986) Antioxidant activity of flavonoids and reactivity with peroxy radical. *Phytochemistry* 25:383–385.

137. Trochon V, Blot E, Cymbalista F, Engelmann C, Tang RP, Thomaidis A, Vasse M, Soria J, Lu H, Soria C. Apigenin inhibits endothelialcell proliferation in G(2)/M phase whereas it stimulates smoothmuscle cells by inhibiting P21 and P27 expression. Int J Cancer 2000 Mar 1;85(5):6916

138. Tsuda, T., Horio, F., Kitoh, J. and Osawa, T. (1999) Protective effects of dietary cyanidin 3-O-b-D-glucoside on liver ischemia-reperfusion injury in rats. Arch. Biochem. Biophys., 368, 361--366.

139. Vinod Kumar, R and Augusti, KT (1989) Antidiabetic Effect of a leucocyanidin derivative isolated from the bark of Ficus bengalensis Linn.26:400-404.

140. Tsuda, T., Kato, Y. and Osawa, T. (2000) Mechanism for the peroxynitrite scavenging activity by anthocyanins. FEBS Lett., 484, 207—210

141. Vinson JA, Mandarano MA, Shuta DL, Bagchi M, Bagchi D. 2002. Beneficial effects of a novel IH636 grape seed proanthocyanidin extract and a niacin-bound chromium in a hamster atherosclerosis model. *Molecular and Cellular Biochemistry* 240: 99–103.

142. Vivek Sharma, Christy Joseph, Soumya Ghosh, Anindita Agarwal, Manoj Kumar Mishra and Ellora Sen. Kaempferol induces apoptosis in glioblastoma cells through oxidative stress. Molecular Cancer Therapeutics. 2007; 6:2544-2553.

143. Wall ME, Wani MC, Manikumar G, Abraham P, Taylor H, Hughes TJ, et. al. Plant antimutagenic agents: 2. Flavonoids. J Nat Prod 1988; 51:1084– 91.

144. Wang IK, LinShiau SY, Lin JK. Induction of apoptosis by apigenin and related flavonoids through cytochrome c release and activation of caspase9 and caspase3 in leukaemia HL60 cells. Eur J Cancer 1999 Oct; 35(10):151725.

145. Wang J, Eltoum IE, Lamartiniere CA. Genistein alters growth factor signaling in transgenic prostate model (TRAMP). Mol Cell Endocrinol 2004; 219:171– 80.

146. Wang, RF; Xei, WD; Zhang, Z, et. al. (2004). Bioactive compounds from seeds of punica granatum . J. Nat.Prod..67(12) 2096.

147. Wang X, Clubbs EA, Bomser JA. Genistein modulates prostate epithelial cell proliferation via estrogen- and extracellular signal regulated kinase-dependent pathways. J Nutr Biochem 2006; 17: 204– 10.

148. Wei H, Bowen R, Cai Q, Barnes S, Wang Y. Antioxidant and antipromotional effects of the soybean isoflavone genistein. Proc Soc Exp Biol Med 1995; 208:124– 30.

149. Wiseman SA, Balentine DA & Frei B (1997): Antioxidants in tea. Crit. Rev. Food Sci. Nutr. 37, 705- 718.

150. Wollny T, Aiello L, Di Tommaso D, Bellavia V, Rotilio D, Donati MB, De Gaetano G & lacoviello L (1999): Modulation of haemostatic function and prevention of experimental thrombosis by red wine in rats: a role for increased nitric oxide production. Br. J. Pharmac. 127, 747- 755.

151. Xiao D, Zhu SP, Gu ZL. Quercetin induced apoptosis in human leukemia HL-60 cells. Zhongguo Yao Li Xue Bao 1997; 18:280– 83.

152. Yamamoto H, Sakakibara J, Nagatsu A, and Sekiya K (1998) Inhibitors of arachidonate lipoxygenase from defatted perilla seed. *J Agric Food Chem* 46:862–865.

153. Yasukawa K, Takido M, Takeuchi M, and Nakagawa S (1989) Effect of chemical constituents from plants on 12-*O*-tetradecanoylphorbol-13-acetate-induced inflammation in mice. *Chem Pharm Bull* 37:1071–1073.

154. Yasuko, N; Takao, K; Akitane, M; Loster, P (2002) Antioxidant activities of pomegranate fruit extract and its anthocyanidins. Jour. Agric and Food Chem. 50:166-167.

155. Yin F, Giuliano AE, Van Herle AJ. Signal pathways involved in apigenin inhibition of growth and induction of apoptosis of human anaplastic thyroid cancer cells (ARO). Anticancer Res 1999 SepOct; 19(5B):4297303.

156. Yu O, Matsuno M, Subramanian S (2006) Flavonoids in flowers: genetics and biochemistry. In JA Teixeira da Silva, ed, Floriculture, Ornamental and Plant Biotechnology: Advances and Topical Issues, Ed 1. Global Science Books, London, pp 283–293

157. Zava D, Duwe G. Estrogenic and antiproliferative properties of genistein and other flavonoids in human breast cancer cells in vitro. Nutr Cancer 1997; 27:31–40.

158. Zheng, P.W., Chiang, L.C., Lin, C.C., 2005. Apigenin induced apoptosis through p53-dependent pathway in human cervical carcinoma cells. Life Sciences 76, 1367–1379.

159. Zhu F, Liu XG, Liang NC. Effect of emodin and apigenin on invasion of human ovarian carcinoma HO 8910PM cells in Vitro. Ai Zheng. 2003 Apr; 22(4):35862.

4.3 Uses of Curcumin as a Nutraceutical Agent

Drs. Girija Kuttan, Chandrasekharan Guruvayoorappan and Ramadasan Kuttan*

Amala Cancer Research Centre, Amala Nagar, Thrissur 680 555, Kerala, India
E-Mail:amalaresearch@rediffmail.com
Fax:914872307968.

***Corresponding author;** Dr. Ramadasan Kuttan, Director, ACRC.

Introduction

The herbal renaissance has produced a profound effect on the Western medicine which is now trying to acknowledge methods of healing that have existed for millennia in the traditional medicine throughout the world, especially Asia. The surge in research on drugs from natural sources is now moving out of the herbalists' shop away from the core texts into the drugs research laboratories. **India's herbal tradition is as old as China's.**

We have rich resources but we have been complacent. In the modern era, much interest has been given to revisit and revive these herbal drugs for the welfare of mankind.

Cucuma longa Linn., an indigenous plant of the ginger family (Zingiberaceae), grows widely all over India. It is known by different names in different languages viz., *Haridra* (Sanskrit), *Haldi* (Bengali, Oriya and Hindi), *Manjal* (Malayalam, Tamil), *Paspu* (Telegu), *Aurukesthur Kurcum* (Arabic) and *Turmeric* (English). The name "Turmeric" derives from the Latin *terra merita* meaning "*meritorious earth*" referring to the color of ground turmeric which resembles a mineral pigment. In many languages turmeric is simply named as "yellow root". It is a perennial herb, 2-3 ft high with short stem and tufted leaves. The rhizomes are short and thick. The rhizomes of turmeric are rich in pharmacologically active components. For a last few decades, extensive work has been done to establish the biological and pharmacological actions of turmeric and its active components. One such compound which has extensively been studied is curcumin. In this present chapter, we describe the pharmacological activities of curcumin with emphasis on its use as a nutraceutical agent.

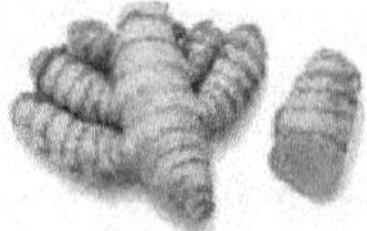

Fig. 1 Turmeric. Curcumin is present in turmeric to the extent of 77% of the curcuminoids.

Curcumin 1 (diferuloyl methane)

Cyclocurcumin

Fig. 2 Curcumins.

Demethoxy curcumin

Bis demethoxy curcumin

Fig. 3 Other curcuminoids.

(i) **Demethoxy curcumin (curcumin II), present to the extent of 18% in curcuminoids**

(ii) **Bisdemethoxy curcumin (curcumin III), present to the extent of 5% in curcuminoids. This is the most potent curcuminoids.**

(iii) **Cyclocurcumin, present to about 0.8% in chloroform extract.**

Turmeric and its uses in Traditional Medicine

The rhizome of *Curcuma longa* (Turmeric) has been used in Asian medicine since the second millennium BC (Brouk, 1975). Its use dates back nearly 4000 years, to the Vedic culture in India where it was used as a culinary spice and had some religious significance. Its utility is referred to in the ancient Indian system of medicine – Ayurveda, Unani, and Siddha.

Turmeric has been widely used as a spice and coloring agent in many foods. It is a spice commonly used in Asian cultures, where it is considered to be a magical plant because of its organoleptic properties and undoubted therapeutic and protective effects, especially for the skin and liver (Toda, 1985). Consumption of turmeric has been associated with various beneficial effects on human health (Ammon and Wahl, 1991). In **Chinese system of medicine, it is used for diseases associated with abdominal pains. In Ayurvedic and Unani systems of medicine it has been used for the treatment for different gastro-intestinal disorders and diseases of skin and joints (Srimal and Dhawan, 1985). Turmeric powder significantly increases the mucus content in gastric juices and Indian cuisine lays emphasis on turmeric's therapeutic effect against gastric disorders. In traditional medicine, it has been used in the treatment of intestinal parasites and as a remedy for poisoning, snakebites and various other complaints (Srimal, 1997).** ***In addition to its aromatic, stimulant and coloring properties in the diet, turmeric is mixed with other natural compounds such as slaked lime applied locally, is an ancient household remedy for sprains, muscular pain and inflamed joints. Turmeric in combination with other plant products has been reported for purification of blood and for menstrual and abdominal problems (Chattopadhyay et. al. 2004).*** Traditionally, it has been used in poultices to relieve pain and inflammation (Araujo and Leon, 2001; Huang et. al. 1991; Kohli et. al. 2005). Turmeric has been used in the preparation of medicinal oils and ointments. It is used as a carminative and stomachic in the treatment of digestive disorders such as flatulence, bloating and appetite loss. Turmeric roots are known to be antiseptic and aromatic. Its paste is used in cleansing and disinfecting the skin and skin ulcers without drying out its natural oils. This yellow spice has been extensively used in Indian medicine as a remedy for the healing of wounds and ulcers (Gujral et. al. 1953).

Chemical Constituents of Turmeric

Turmeric contains carbohydrates (69.4%), proteins (6.3%), fat (5.1%), minerals (3.5%) and moisture (13.1%). Turmeric contains a wide variety of phytochemicals, including curcumin, demethoxycurcumin, bisdemethoxycurcumin, zingiberene, curcumenol, curcumol, eugenol, α-phellandrene, sabinene, cineol, borneol, santonin, ferulic acid, turmerin, turmerones, and turmeronols (Chattopadhyay et. al. 2004). Curcumin (diferuloylmethane/curcumin I) is responsible for the yellow color and was first isolated in 1815, and the structure was derived in 1910.

Chemical Properties

Curcumin (Fig. 2) is a low molecular weight polyphenol, first chemically characterized in 1910 and has been the subject of hundreds of published papers. Curcumin is hydrophobic in nature and frequently soluble in dimethylsulfoxide, acetone, ethanol and oils. It has a molecular weight of 368.37 and a melting point of 183°C. It has an absorption maximum around 420 nm. Curcumin is unstable at basic pH, and degrades within 30 min to *trans*-6-(4'-hydroxy-3'-methoxyphenyl)-2,4-dioxo-5-hexanal, ferulic acid, feruloylmethane and vanillin (Lin et. al. 2000). Under acidic conditions, the color of curcumin turns yellow to deep red and the degradation of curcumin is much slower under these conditions (Wang et. al. 1997).

Analogues of Curcumin

Turmeric contains three different analogues of curcumin namely, diferuloylmethane, demethoxycurcumin and bismethoxycurcumin (Fig. 2 & 3). Most available preparations of curcumin contain approximately 77% diferuloylmethane (curcumin I), 18% demethoxycurcumin (curcumin II) and 5% bismethoxycurcumin (curcumin III). Biological activities of curcumin have been reported. Curcumin III was found to be most potent. Some reports suggest that the mixture of all three is more potent than individual ones (Huang et. al. 1998; Sreejayan and Rao, 1997).

Nutraceutical Properties of Curcumin

The great prevalence of curcumin in the vegetable kingdom is not accidental; not only do they act as the coloured pigments, but also as enzyme inhibitors, precursors of toxic substances, a defence against ultraviolet radiation exposure, chelating agents of metals and reducing agents. There is much data concerning a wide range of biological activities of curcumin in humans. Some of the biological effects of curcumin are listed in detail.

Antioxidant Effects

Numerous studies have demonstrated the effect of curcumin on various measures of oxidative cellular damage (Maheshwari et. al. 2006). Curcumin has been shown to be a potent scavenger of a variety of reactive oxygen species including superoxide anion radicals, hydroxyl radicals (Reddy and Lokesh, 1994) and nitrogen dioxide radicals (Unnikrishnan and Rao, 1995; Sreejayan and rao, 1997). It is also known to inhibit lipid peroxidation in different animal models (Reddy and Lokesh, 1992; Sreejayan and Rao, 1994). **Recent studies conducted by Priyadarshini et. al. (2003) report that the presence of phenolic group renders its free-radical-scavenging activity and that the presence of methoxy group further increased their antioxidant activity.**

Anti-inflammatory Effects

Cyclooxygenase and lipoxygenase (enzymes) play an important role as inflammatory mediators. They are involved in the release of arachidonic acid, which is a starting point for a general inflammatory response. Neutrophils containing lipoxygenase create chemotactic compounds from arachidonic acid. They also provoke the release of proinflammatory cytokines. Curcumin has shown to inhibit both cyclooxygenase and 5-lipoxygenase pathways (Zhang et. al. 1999; Skrzypczak-Jankun et. al. 2000; Wallace et. al. 2002; Huang et. al. 1991; Hong et. al. 2004; Kohli et. al. 2005). This inhibition reduces the release of arachidonic acid (Hong et. al. 2004). Curcumin inhibits both cytosolic and membranal tyrosine kinase (Rao et. al. 1993). **Intergral membrane proteins, such as tyrosine 3-monooxygenase kinase, are involved in a variety of functions, such as enzyme catalysis, transport across membranes, transduction of signals that function as receptors of hormones and growth factors, and energy transfer in ATP synthesis. Inhibition of these proteins results in inhibition of uncontrolled cell growth and proliferation. Another anti-inflammatory property of curcumins is their suggested ability to inhibit neutrophil degranulation. This is a direct way to diminish the release of arachidonic acid by neutrophils and other immune cells (Srivastava, 1989).**

Antiarthritic Effect

The antiarthritic effect of curcumin has been first demonstrated in human models by Deodhar et. al. (1980). This study showed that curcumin administration could improve morning stiffness, walking time and joint swelling and was comparatively as effective as phenylbutazone. Another clinical trial by Satoskar et. al. (1986) has proved that curcumin treatment could inhibit postoperative inflammation. **Some studies reveal that**

curcumin exhibits its potential effect in rheumatoid arthritis by inhibiting the expression of collagenase and stromelysin as well as the proliferation of synoviocytes (Funk et. al. 2006; Jackson et al., 2006).

Table 1 Biological Effects of Curcumin

Biological Activity	References
Anti-atherosclerotic	Olszanecki et. al. 2005; Sinha et. al. 2003
Antibacterial	Negi et. al. 1999; Kumar et. al. 2001; Mahady et. al. 2002; Sivalingam et. al. 2007.
Anticoagulant	Srivastava et. al. 1985
Antifibrotic	Punithavathi et. al. 2000.
Antifungal	Tantaoui-Elaraki and Beraoud, 1994; Wuthi-udomlert et. al. 2000; Kim et. al. 2003.
Anti-inflammatory	Deodhar et. al. 1980; Srihari Rao et. al. 1982; Brouet and Ohshima, 1995; Zhang et. al. 1999; Skrzypczak-Jankun et. al. 2000; Wallace et. al. 2002; Huang et. al. 1991; Hong et. al. 2004; Kohli et. al. 2005.
Antimalarial	Roth et. al. 1998; Reddy et. al. 2005; Nandakumar et. al. 2006.
Antiosteoporotic	Antunes et. al. 2000; Naganuma et. al. 2000; Ozaki et. al. 2000; Notoya et. al. 2006.
Antioxidant	Sharma et. al. 1976; Subramaniam et. al. 1994.
Antiparasitic	Kiuchi et. al. 1993; Nose et. al. 1998; Koide et. al. 2002; Saleheen et. al. 2002; Chan et. al. 2005; Perez-Arriaga et. al. 2006.
Antiprotozoan	Rasmussen et. al. 2000; Koide et. al. 2002; Gomes Dde et. al. 2002.
Antispasmodic	Itthipanichpong et. al. 2003.
Antitumor	Nagabhushan and Bhide, 1992; Ruby et. al. 1995; Aggarwal et. al. 2003; Barcerek and Matlawsa, 2005; Mosley et. al. 2007; Kuttan et. al. 2007.
Antivenomic	Arujo and Leon, 2001; Ferreira et. al. 1992; Girish and Kempraju, 2005.
Antiviral	Herganhahn et. al. 2002; Li et. al. 1993; Mazumdar et. al. 1994; De Clercq, 2000; Mazumdar 1995b; Mazumdar et. al. 1996 Liu et. al. 2005; Vajragupta et. al. 2005.

Table 1 contd...

Biological Activity	References
Cardioprotective	Nirmala and Puvanakrishnan, 1996; Sumbilla et. al. 2002.
Hepatoprotective	Park et. al. 2000; Rajakrishnan et. al. 2000; Nanji et. al. 2003; Naik et. Al. 2004; padmaja and Raju, 2005.
Hypoglycemic	Sajithlal et. al. 1998; Arun and Nalini, 2002; Suryanarayana et. al. 2003.
Hypolipemic	Babu and Srinivasan, 1997.
Immunomodulatory	South et. al. 1997; Antony et. al. 1999; Gao et. al. 2004; Ilsley et. al. 2005; Li and Liu, 2005.

Antitumor Effects

It has been stated that curcumin, as antioxidants, can inhibit carcinogenesis (Nagabhushan and Bhide, 1992; Ruby et. al. 1995; Nakamura et. al. 1998). Curcumin has been stated to be potent inhibitors of cell proliferation (Aggarwal, 2006). A large clinical study suggested the presence of an inverse association between curcumin intake and the subsequent incidence of lung cancer (Barcerek and Matlawska, 2005; Sen et. al. 2005). Curcumin inhibited melanoma growth and influenced the invasive and metastatic potential in mice (Menon et. al. 1999; Kuttan et. al. 2007). Recently curcumin, when administered in combination with paclitaxel (taxol) has been shown to inhibit metastasis of breast tumors (Aggarwal et. al. 2003). This finding may offer new insights about possible therapies for metastatic disease. *Further more, it has been speculated that curcumin can inhibit angiogenesis (Gururaj et. al. 2002). Angiogenesis is normally a strictly controlled process in the human body. The process of angiogenesis is regulated by a variety of endogenous angiogenic and angiostatic factors. It is switched on, for example, during wound healing. Pathologic, unregulated angiogenesis occurs in cancer (Fan et. al. 1995). Angiogenic inhibitors can interfere with various steps in angiogenesis, such as the proliferation and migration of endothelial cells and lumen formation. Among the known angiogenesis inhibitors, curcumin seem to play an important role (Arbiser et. al. 1998; Thaloor et. al. 1998; Mohan et. al. 2000).* However the mechanism behind the antiangiogenic effect of curcumin is unclear. A possible mechanism could be inhibition of protein kinases (Oikawa et. al. 1992), which are implicated to play an important role in signal transduction and are known for their effects in angiogenesis. *Chen and Huang (1998) had reported that curcumin could induce apoptosis in vascular smooth cells by inhibiting protein tyrosine kinase, protein kinase C,* *c-myc, mRNA expression and bcl-2 mRNA expression. Curcumin has been shown to cause apoptosis in human cancer cell lines, TK-10, MCF-7 and UACC-62 by acting as topoisomerase II poison (Martin-Cordero et. al. 2003). Recent studies using SW480, a human colon cancer cell line suggest that silencing the expression of heat shock protein, hsp70 could serve as an effective approach to augment curcumin-based therapy in cancers that are resistant due to hsp70 expression (Rashmi et. al. 2004)*. **The mechanism of curcumin-induced apoptosis has been studied by Deeb et. al. (2003) in LNCaP prostate cancer cells, where curcumin induces apoptosis by enhancing tumor necrosis factor-related apoptosis-inducing ligand (TRAIL). Another study by Woo et. al. (2003) using Caki cells indicates that curcumin induces apoptosis through down regulation of Bcl-xL and IAP, release of cytochrome *c* and inhibition of Akt, which are markedly blocked by N-acetyl cysteine, indicating the role of ROS in curcumin induced cell death. Curcumin has been shown to inhibit the activation of NF-κB by inhibiting the phosphorylation and degradation of IκBα (Singh and Aggarwal, 1995; Shishodia et. al. 2005).**

Antithrombogenic Efects

Platelet aggregation continues to the development of both atherosclerosis and acute platelet thrombus formation, followed by embolization of stenosed arteries. Activated platelets adhering to vascular endothelium generate lipid peroxides and oxygen free radicals, which inhibit the endothelial formation of prostacyclin and nitrous oxide. Curcumin can be antithrombotic because they directly scavenge free radicals, thereby maintaining proper concentrations of endothelial prostacyclin and nitric oxide (Srivastava et. al. 1985). *One study showed that curcumin can serve as a powerful antithrombotic agent in vitro and in vivo because of their inhibition of the activity of cyclooxygenase and lipoxygenase pathways (Kohli et. al. 2005). It is well known that arachidonic acid, which is released in inflammatory conditions, is metabolized by platelets to form prostaglandin, endoperoxides and thromboxane* A_2*, leading to platelet activation and aggregation (Shah et. al. 1999). The main antiaggregatory effect of curcumin is thought to be by inhibition of thromboxane* A_2 *formation. In vitro studies showed that curcumin bind to platelet membranes and may therefore have an accumulative effect over time (Srivastava et. al. 1995).*

Antiatherosclerotic Effects

Because of their antioxidative properties, curcumins are likely to have a major influence on the vascular system. Oxygen radicals can oxidize LDL, which injures the endothelial wall and thereby promotes atherosclerotic changes. A few studies have pointed out that curcumin intake protect against coronary heart disease (Olszanecki et. al. 2005). Sinha et. al. (2003) stated that curcumin, when regularly consumed might reduce the risk of death from coronary heart disease in elderly men. Furthermore, another study reported an inverse correlation between curcumin intake and total plasma cholesterol concentrations (Soni and Kuttan, 1992). Oxidative stress and vascular damages are postulated to play a key role in dementia, and the intake of curcumin is reported to prevent the development of dementia (Ringman et. al. 2005; Jefremov et. al. 2007).

Antibacterial, Antifungal and Antiviral Effects

The antibacterial effects of curcumin has been reported in various bacteria such as *Streptococcus, Staphylococcus, Lactobacillus*, and *Helicobacter pylori* (Kumar et. al. 2001; Mahady et. al. 2002). Eventhough there are various reports which shows that turmeric oil possess antifungal activity against *Aspergillus flavus, A. parasiticus, Penicillium digitatum* and *Fusarium moniliforme*, very few authors had reported about the antifungal activity of curcumin (Tantaoui-Elaraki and Beraoud, 1994; Wuthiudomlert et. al. 2000; Kim et. al. 2003). Several studies report that curcumin could inhibit aflatoxin induced liver damage in various animal models (Soni et. al. 1992; Firozi et. al. 1996; Soni et. al. 1997; Mathuria and Verma, 2007)

The antiviral activity of curcumin was shown in a study by Herganhahn et. al. (2002). The interaction of curcumin with the different stages in the replication cycle of virus was previously described (Li et. al. 1993; Mazumdar et. al. 1995a; Hergenhahn et. al. 2002). By far, most studies of the effects on viruses were performed *in vitro* and little is known about the antiviral effect of curcumin *in vivo*.

Because of the world wide spread of HIV since the 1980s, investigations of the antiviral activity of curcumin have mainly focused on HIV. Studies using curcumin as anti-HIV agents have expanded in the past 2 decades. Most of these studies focused on the inhibitory activity of reverse transcriptase, or RNA-directed DNA polymerase (De Clercq, 2000), but antiintegrase and antiprotese activities were also described (Mazumdar et. al. 1995b; Mazumdar et. al. 1996; Vajragupta et. al. 2005). Again, curcumin have mainly been studied in *in vitro* experiments; therefore, no clear contribution of curcumin to the treatment of HIV-infected patients has yet been shown (Liu et. al. 2005).

Gastroprotective Effect

One of the most important side effects of conventional anti-inflammatory drugs is their ulcerogenic activity. Curcumin was found to be a good anti-inflammatory compound and was also able to protect the gastric mucosa against a variety of ulcerogenic agents (Dasgupta et. al. 1969; Sinha et. al.

1974; Kim et. al. 2005). Recent studies indicate that curcumin can block indomethacin, ethanol and stress-induced gastric ulcer and can also protect pylorus-ligation-induced acid secretion (Sivalingam et. al. 2007). Mahady et. al. (2002) reported that curcumin could inhibit the growth of Helicobacter pylori *in vitro*. ***More recently, Di Mario et. al. (2007) have shown that clinical trials using curcumin could eradicate H.pylori infection as well as modulate the immune response in H.pylori positive patients. In relation to their low toxicity and to the properties reported (antisecretory action, stimulation of prostaglandins, inhibition of H.pylori), that curcumin could have a therapeutic potential ideal for treatment of gastrointestinal diseases associated with H.pylori infection, i.e. type B gastritis and duodenal cancer.***

Hypothesis of the links between the working mechanisms of curcumin in various diseases is given in Fig. 4. (See P 181).

Toxicity of Curcumin

There is much controversy regarding the purported toxic or even mutagenic properties of curcumin. Studies of curcumin in animals have shown a lack of significant toxicity since an early report in which doses upto 5 g/kg were administered orally to Sprague-Dawley rats (Wahlstrom and Blennow, 1978). Systematic preclinical studies funded by the prevention division of the US National Cancer Institute did not discover adverse effects in rats, dogs or monkeys of doses up to 3.5 g/kg body weight administered for up to 3 months (NCI, 1996). **Gupta et. al. (1980) reported that curcumin possess ulcerogenic activity in the stomach of the albino rat, but this finding has not been confirmed in subsequent studies. In contrast with the potential mutagenic effects of curcumin in earlier studies, several more recent reports indicate that curcumin, seem to be antimutagenic in vivo (Surh et. al. 2000; De Flora et. al. 1994). A clinical study by Aggarwal et. al. (2003), showed an inverse relation between the intake of curcumin and cancer. One possible explanation for these conflicting data is that curcumin is toxic to cancer cells or to immortalized cells, but are not toxic or are less toxic to normal cells. If this is true, curcumin might play a role in the prevention of cancer that is worthy for further investigation.**

Future Implications

Some epidemiological studies suggest a protective role of curcumin against inflammation and cancer. One clinical trial indicated that tropical treatment of curcumin may reduce oral cancers and leukoplakia (Kuttan et. al. 1987). Various cohort studies indicated an inverse association between curcumin intakes and inflammatory diseases (Lal et. al. 1999; Lal et. al. 2000; Holt et. al. 2005). Recent years have seen an increased enthusiasm in preventing various diseases with nutraceutical agents. Curcumin have received much attention in the literature over the past 20 years and a variety of potential beneficial effects have been evaluated. It is expected that curcumin may find application as a nutraceutical agent in the near future to prevent various diseases, including inflammatory disorders, carcinogenesis and oxidative stress-induced pathogenesis. Currently, the intake of rhizomes containing curcumin is recommended, although it is too early to make recommendations on daily curcumin intakes.

Effects of Curcumins on Diseases

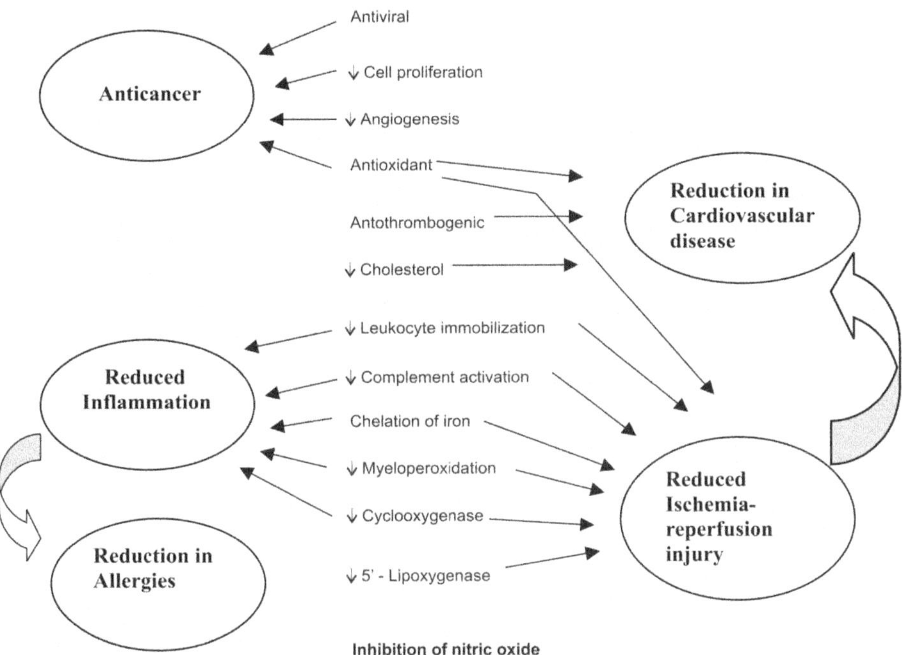

Fig. 4 Hypothesis of the links between the working mechanisms of curcumins and their effects on disease.

References

1. Aggarwal BB, Kumar A, Bharti AC. Anticancer potential of curcumin: preclinical and clinical studies. *Anticancer Res* 2003; 23: 363-398.

2. Aggarwal S, Ichikawa H, Takada Y, Sandur SK, Shishodia S, Aggarwal BB. Curcumin (diferuloylmethane) down-regulates expression of cell proliferation and antiapoptotic and antimetastatic

gene products through suppression of IκB kinase and Akt activation. *Mol Pharmacol* 2006; 69: 195-206.

3. Ammon HP, Wahl MA. Pharmacology of *Curcuma longa*. *Planta Med* 1991; 57: 1-7.
4. Antony S, Kuttan R, Kuttan G. Immunomodulatory activity of curcumin. *Immunol Invest* 1999; 28: 291-303.
5. Antunes LM, Araujo MC, Darin JD, Bianchi ML. Effects of antioxidants curcumin and vitamin C on cisplatin-induced clastogenesis in Wistar rat bone marrow cells. *Mutat Res* 2000; 465: 131-137.
6. Araujo CAC and Leon LL. Biological activities of *Curcuma longa* L. *Mem Inst Oswaldo Cruz* 2001; 96: 723-728.
7. Arbiser JL, Klauber N, Rohan R, van Leeuwen R, Huang MT, Fischer C, Flynn E, Byers HR. Curcumin as an in vitro inhibitor of angiogenesis. *Mol Med* 1998; 4: 376-383.
8. Arun N, Nalini N. Efficacy of turmeric on blood sugar and polyol pathway in diabetic albino rats. *Plant Foods Hum Nutr* 2002; 57: 41-52.
9. Babu PS, Srinivasan K. Hypolipidemic action of curcumin, the active principle of turmeric (*Curcuma longa*) in streptozotocin induced diabetic rats. *Mol Cell Biochem* 1997; 166: 169-175.
10. Balcerek M, Matlawska I. Preventive role of curcumin in lung cancer. *Przegl Lek* 2005; 62(10): 1180-1181.
11. Brouet I, Ohshima H. Curcumin, an antitumor promoter and anti-inflammatory agent, inhibits induction of nitric oxide synthase in activated macrophages. *Biochem Biophys Res Commun* 1995; 206: 533-540.
12. Brouk B. *Plants consumed by man*. New York, Academic Press, 1975; pp 331.
13. Chan MM, Adapala NS, Fong D. Curcumin overcomes the inhibitory effect of nitric oxide in Leishmania. *Parasitol Res* 2005; 96: 49-56.
14. Chattopadhyay I, Biswas K, Bandyopadhyay U, Banerjee RK. Turmeric and curcumin: Biological actions and medical applications. *Curr Sci* 2004; 87(1): 44-53.
15. Chen HW, Huang HC. Effect of curcumin on cell cycle progression and apoptosis in vascular smooth cells. *Br J Pharmacol* 1998; 124: 1029-1040.

16. Dasgupta SR, Sinha M, Sahana CC, Mukherjee BP. A study of the effect of an extract of *Curcuma longa* Linn. on experimental gastric ulcers in animals. *Indian J Pharmacol* 1969; 1: 49-54.

17. De Clercq E, Current lead natural products for the chemotherapy of human immunodeficiency virus (HIV) infection. *Med Res Rev* 2000; 20: 323-349.

18. De Flora S, Rosenkranz HS, Klopman G. Structural basis of antimutagenicity of chemicals towards 4-nitroquinoline 1-oxide in *Salmonella typhimurium*. *Mutagenesis* 1994; 9(1):39-45.

19. Deeb D, Xu YX, Jiang H, Gao X, Janakiram N, Chapman RA, Gautam SC. Curcumin (diferuloyl-methane) enhances tumor necrosis factor-related apoptosis-inducing ligand-induced apoptosis in LNCaP prostate cancer cells. *Mol Cancer Ther* 2003; 2: 95-103.

20. Deodhar SD, Sethi R, Srimal RC, Preliminary study on antirheumatic activity of curcumin (Diferuloyl methane). *Ind J Med Res* 1980; 71: 632-643.

21. Di Mario F, Cavallaro LG, Nouvenne A, Stefani N, Cavestro GM, Iori V, Maino M, Comparato G, Fanigliulo L, Morana E, Pilatto A, Martelli L, Martelli M, Leandro G, Franze A. A curcumin-based 1-week triple therapy for eradication of *Helicobacter pylori* infection: something to learn from failure? *Helicobacter* 2007; 12(3): 238-243.

22. Firozi PF, Aboobaker VS, Bhattacharya RK. Action of curcumin on the cytochrome p450-system catalyzing the activation of aflatoxin B1. *Chem Biol Interact* 1996; 100(1): 41-51.

23. Funk JL, Oyarzo JN, Frye JB, Chen G, Lantz RC, Jolad SD, Solyom AM, Timmermann BN. Turmeric extracts containing curcuminoids prevent experimental rheumatoid arthritis. *J Nat Prod* 2006; 69: 351-355.

24. Gao X, Kuo J, Jiang H, Deeb D, Liu Y, Divine G, Chapman RA, Dulchavsky SA, Gautam SC. Immunomodulatory activity of curcumin: suppression of lymphocyte proliferation, development of cell mediated cytotoxicity, and cytokine production in vitro. *Biochem Pharmacol* 2004; 68: 51-61.

25. Girish KS, Kemparaju K. Inhibition of *Naja naja* venom hyaluronidase by plant-derived bioactive components and polysachharides. *Biochemistry (Mosc)* 2005; 70: 948-952.

26. Gomes Dde C, Alegrio LV, de Lima ME, Leon LL, Araujo CA. Synthetic derivatives of curcumin and their activity against *Leishmania amazonensis*. *Arzneimittelforschung* 2002; 52: 120-124.

27. Gujral ML, Chowdhury NK, Saxena PN. The effect of certain indigenous remedies on the handling of wounds and ulcers. J Indian State Med. Assoc. 1953; 22: 273-276.

28. Gupta B, Kulshrestha CK, Sristava RK, et. al. Mechanisms of curcumin induced gastric ulcer in rats. *Indian J Med Res* 1980; 71: 806-814.

29. Gururaj AE, Belskavadi M, Venkatesh DA, Marme D, Salimath BP. Molecular mechanisms of anti-angiogenic effect of curcumin. *Biochem Biophys Res Commun* 2002; 297: 934-942.

30. Hergenhahn M, Soto U, Weninger A, Polack A, Hsu CH, Cheng AL, Rosl F. The chemopreventive compound curcumin is an efficient inhibitor of Epstein-Barr virus BLZF1 transcription in Raji DR-LUC cells. *Mol Carcinogen* 2002; 33: 137-145.

31. Holt PR, Katz, S, Kirshoff R. Curcumin therapy in inflammatory bowel disease: A pilot study. *Dig Dis Sci* 2005; 50(11): 2191-2193.

32. Hong J, Bose M, Ju J, Ryu H, Chen X, Sang S. Modulation of arachidonic acid metabolism by curcumin and related beta-diketone derivatives: Effects on cytosolic phospholipase A(2), cyclooxygenases and 5-lipoxygenase. *Carcinogenesis* 2004; 25(9): 1671-1679.

33. Huang MT, Lou YR, Xie JG, Ma W, Lu YP, Yen P, Zhu BT, Newmark H, Ho CT. Effect of dietary curcumin and dibenzoylmethane on formation of 7, 12-dimethylbenz[a]anthracene-induced mammary tumors and lymphoma/leukemias in Sencar mice. *Carcinogenesis* 1998; 19: 1697-1700.

34. Huang MT, Lysz T, Ferraro T, Abidi TF, Laskin JD, Conney AH. Inhibitory effects of curcumin on in vitro lipoxygenase and cyclooxygenase activities in mouse epidermis. *Cancer Res* 1991; 51: 813-819.

35. Ilsley SE, Miller HM, Kamel C. Effects of dietary quillaja saponin and curcumin on the performance and immune status of weaned piglets. *J Ani Sci* 2005; 83: 82-88.

36. Itthipanichpong C, Ruangrungsi N, Kemsri W, Sawasdipanich A. Antispasmodic effects of curcuminoids on isolated guinea-pig ileum and rat uterus. *J Med Assoc Thai* 2003; 86 (Suppl 2): S299-S309.

37. Jackson JK, Higo T, Hunter WL, Burt HM. The antioxidants curcumin and quercetin inhibit inflammatory processes associated with arthritis. *Inflamm Res* 2006; 55: 168-175.

38. Jefremov V, Zilmer M, Zilmer K, Bogdanavic N, Karelson E. Antioxidative effects of plant polyphenols from protection of G protein signaling to prevention of age-related pathologies. *Ann NY Acad Sci* 2007; 1095: 449-457.

39. Kim DC, Kim SH, Choi BH, Baek NI, Kim D, Kim MJ, Kim KT. Curcuma longa extract protects gastric ulcers by blocking H2 histamine receptors. *Biol Pharm Bull* 2005; 28: 2220 – 2224.

40. Kim MK, Choi GJ, Lee HS. Fungicidal property of *Curcuma longa* L. rhizome-derived curcumin against phytopathogenic fungi in a greenhouse. *J Agric Food Chem* 2003; 51: 1578-1581.

41. Kiuchi F, Goto Y, Sugimoto N, Akao K, Tsuda Y. Nematocidal activity of turmeric: Synergistic action of curcuminoids. *Chem Pharm Bull (Tokyo)* 1993; 41: 1640-1643.

42. Kohli K, Ali J, Ansari MJ, Raheman Z. Curcumin: A natural anti-inflammatory agent. *Indian J Pharmacol* 2005; 37(3): 141-147.

43. Koide T, Nose M, Ogihara Y, Yabu Y, Ohta N. Leishmanicidal effect of curcumin in vitro. *Biol Pharm Bull* 2002; 25: 131-133.

44. Kumar S, Narain U, Tripathi S, Misra K. Synthesis of curcumin bioconjugates and study of their antibacterial activities against beta-lactamase-producing microorganisms. *Bioconjug Chem* 2001; 12: 464-469.

45. Kuttan G, Kumar KB, Guruvayoorappan C, Kuttan R. Antitumor, antiinvasion and antimetastatic effects of curcumin. *Adv Exp Med Biol* 2007; 595: 173-184.

46. Kuttan R, Sudheeran PC, Joseph CD. Turmeric and curcumin as topical agents in cancer therapy. *Tumori* 1987; 73(1): 29-31.

47. Lal B, Kapoor AK, Agarwal PK, Asthana OP, Srimal RC. Role of curcumin in idiopathic inflammatory orbital pseudotumors. *Phytother Res* 2000; 14(6): 443-447.

48. Lal B, Kapoor AK, Asthana OP, Agarwal PK, Prasad R, Kumar P, Srimal RC. Efficacy of curcumin in the management of chronic anterior uveitis. *Phytother Res* 1999; 13(4): 318-322.

49. Li CJ, Zhang LJ, Dezube BJ, Crumpacker CS, Pardee AB. Three inhibitors of type 1 human immunodeficiency virus long terminal repeat-directed gene expression and virus replication. *Proc Natl Acad Sci USA* 1993; 90: 1839-1842.

50. Li X, Liu X. Effect of curcumin on immune function of mice. *J Huazhong Univ Sci Technolog Med Sci* 2005; 25: 137-140.

51. Lin JK, Pan MH, Shiau SYL. Recent studies on the biofunctions and biotransformations of curcumin. *Biofactors* 2000; 13: 153-158.

52. Liu JP, Manheimer E, Yang M. Herbal medicines for treating HIV infection and AIDS. *Cochrane Database Syst Rev* 2005(3): CD 003937.

53. Mahady GB, Pendland SL, Yun G, Lu ZZ. Turmeric (Curcuma longa) and curcumin inhibit the growth of *Helicobacter pylori*, of group I carcinogen. *Anticancer Res* 2002; 22, 4179-4181.

54. Martin-Cordero C, Lopez-Lazaro M, Galvez M, Ayuso MJ. Curcumin as a DNA topoisomerase II poison. *J Enzyme Inhib Med Chem* 2003; 18: 505-509.

55. Mathuria N, Verma RJ. Aflatoxin induced hemolysis and its amelioration by turmeric extracts and curcumin in vitro. *Acta Pol Pharm* 2007; 64(2): 165-168.

56. Mazumdar A, Raghavan K, Weinstein J, Kohn KW, Pommer Y. Inhibition of human immunodeficiency virus type-1 integrase by curcumin. *Biochem Pharmacol* 1995a; 49: 1165-1170.

57. Mazumder A, Gazit A, Levitzki M, Nicklaus J, Yung G, Kohlhagen G, Pommier Y. Effect of tyrphostins, protein kinase inhibitors, on human immunodeficiency virus type 1 integrase. *Biochemistry* 1995b; 34: 15,111-15,122.

58. Mazumder A, Wang S, Neamati N, Nicklaus M, Sunder S, Chen J, Milne GW, Rice WG, Jr. Burke TR, Pommier Y. Antiretroviral agents as inhibitors of both human immunodeficiency virus type 1 integrase and protease. *J Med Chem* 1996; 39: 2472-2481.

59. Mohan R, Sivak J, Ashton P, Russo LA, Pham BQ, Kasahara N, Raizman MB, Fini ME, Curcuminoids inhibit the angiogenic response stimulated by fibroblast growth factor-2, including expression of matrix metalloproteinase and gelatinase B. *J Biol Chem* 2000; 275: 10405-10412.

60. Mosley CA, Liotta DC, Snyder JP. Highly active anticancer curcumin analogues. *Adv Exp Med Biol* 2007; 595: 77-104.

61. Nagabhushan M, Bhide SV. Curcumin as an inhibitor of cancer. *J Am Coll Nutr* 1992; 11: 192-198.

62. Naganuma K, Amano S, Takeda H, Kitano S, Hanazawa S. Role of transcriptional factor activation protein-1 in endogenous expression of the interleukin-1 beta gene involved in Porphyromonas gingivalis fimbria-stimulated bone resorption in the mouse calvarial system. *Oral Microbiol Immunol* 2000; 15: 53-57.

63. Naik RS, Mujumdar AM, Ghaskadbi S. Protection of liver cells from ethanol cytotoxicity by curcumin in liver slice culture in vitro. *J Ethnopharmacol* 2004; 95: 31-37.

64. Nakamura Y, Ohto Y. Murakami A, Osawa T, Ohigashi H. Inhibitory effects of curcumin and tetrahydrocurcuminoids on the tumor promoter-induced reactive oxygen species generation in leukocytes in vitro and in vivo. *Jpn J Cancer Res* 1998; 89: 361-370.

65. Nandakumar DN, Nagaraj VA, Vatsala PG, Rangarajan P, Padmanabhan G, Curcumin-artemisinin combination therapy for malaria. *Antimicrob Agents Chemother* 2006; 50: 1859-1860.

66. Nanji AA, Jokelainen K, Tipoe GL, Rahemtulla A, Thomas P, Dannenberg AJ. Curcumin prevents alcohol-induced liver disease in rats by inhibiting the expression of NF-kappa B-dependent genes. *Am J Physiol Gastrointest Liver Physiol* 2003; 284: G321-G327.

67. NCI, DCPC. Clinical development plan: curcumin. *J Cell Biochem* 1996; 26S: 72-85.

68. Negi PS, Jayaprakasha GK, Jagan Mohan Rao L, Sakariah KK. Antibacterial activity of turmeric oil: A byproduct from curcumin manufacture. *J Agri Food Chem* 1999; 47: 4297-4300.

69. Nirmala C, Puvanakrishnan R. Protective role of curcumin against isoproterenol-induced myocardial infraction in rats. *Mol Cell Biochem* 1996; 159: 85-93.

70. Nose M, Koide T, Ogihara Y, Yabu Y, Ohta N. Trypanocidal effects of curcumin in vitro. *Biol Pharm Bull* 2002; 25: 131-133.

71. Notoya M, Nishimura J, Woo JT, Nagai K, Ishihara Y, Hagiwara H. Curcumin inhibits the proliferation and mineralization of cultured osteoblasts. *Eur J Pharmacol* 2006; 534: 55-62.

72. Oikawa T, Shimamura M, Ashino H, Nakamura O, Kanayasu T, Morita I, Murota S. Inhibition of angiogenesis by staurosporine, a potent protein kinase inhibitor. *J Antibiot (Tokyo)* 1992; 45(7): 1155-1160.

73. Olszanecki R, Jawien J, Gajda M, Mateuszuk L, Gebska A, Korabiowska M, Chlopicki S, Korbut R. Effect of curcumin on atherosclerosis in apoE/LDLR-double knockout mice. *J Physiol Pharmacol* 2005; 56(4): 627-635.

74. Ozaki K, Kawata Y, Amano S, Hanazawa S. Stimulatory effect of curcumin on osteoclast apoptosis. *Biochem Pharmacol* 2000; 59: 1577-1581.

75. Padmaja S, Raju TN. Protective effect of curcumin during selenium induced toxicity on dehydrogenases in hepatic tissue. *Indian J Physiol Pharmacol* 2005; 49: 111-114.

76. Parez-Arriaga L, Mendoza-Magana ML, Cores-Zarate R, Corona-Rivera A, Bobadilla-Morales L, Troyo-Sanroman R, Ramirez-Herrera MA. Cytotoxic effect of curcumin on *Giardia lambila* trophozoites. *Acta Trop* 2006; 98(2): 152-161.

77. Park EJ, Jeon CH, Ko G, Kim J, Sohn DH. Protective effect of curcumin in rat liver injury induced by carbon tetrachloride. *J Pharm Pharmacol* 2000; 52: 437-440.

78. Priyadarsini KI, Maity DK, Naik GH, Kumar MS, Unnikrishnan MK, Satav JG, et. al. Role of phenolic OH and methylene hydrogen on the free radical reactions and antioxidant activity of curcumin. *Free Radic Biol Med* 2003; 35: 475-484.

79. Punithavathi D, Venkatesan N, Babu M. Curcumin inhibition of bleomycin induced pulmonary fibrosis in rats. *Br J Pharmacol* 2000; 131: 169-172.

80. Rajakrishnan V, Jayadeep A, Arun OS, Sudhakaran PR, Menon VP. Changes in the prostaglandin levels in alcohol toxicity: Effect of curcumin and N-acetylcysteine. *J Nutr Biochem* 2000; 11: 509-514.

81. Rao CV, Simi B, Reddy BS. Inhibition of dietary curcumin of azoxymethane-induced ornithine decarboxylase, tyrosine protein kinase, arachidonic acid metabolism and abberrant crypt foci formation in the rat colon. *Carcinogenesis* 1993; 14: 2219-2225.

82. Rashmi R, Kumar S, Karunagaran D. Ectopic expression of Hsp70 confers resistance and silencing its expression sensitizes human colon cancer cells to curcumin-induced apoptosis. *Carcinogenesis* 2004; 25: 179-187.

83. Rasmussen HB, Christensen SB, Kuist LP, Karazmi A. A simple and effective separation of the curcumins, the antiprotozoal constituents of *Curcuma longa*. *Planta Med* 2000; 66: 296-298.

84. Reddy AC, Lokesh BR. Studies on spice principles as antioxidants in the inhibition of lipid peroxidation of rat liver microsomes. *Mol Cell Biochem* 1992; 111(1-2): 117-124.

85. Reddy AC, Lokesh BR. Studies on the inhibitory effects of curcumin and eugenol on the formation of reactive oxygen species and the oxidation of ferrous iron. *Mol Cell Biochem* 1994; 137(1): 1-8.

86. Reddy RC, Vatsala PG, Keshamouni VG, Padmanabhan G, Rangarajan PN. Curcumin for malaria therapy. *Biochem Biophys Res Commun* 2005; 472-474.

87. Ringman JM, Frautschy SA, Cole GM, Masterman DL, Cummings JL. A potential role of the curry spice curcumin in Alzheimer's disease. *Curr Alzheimer Res* 2005; 2(2): 131-136.

88. Roth GN, Chandra A, Nair MG. Novel bioactivities of *Curcuma longa* constituents. *J Nat Prod* 1998; 61: 542-545.

89. Ruby AJ, Kuttan G, Babu KD, Rajasekharan KN, Kuttan R. Antitumor and antioxidant activity of natural curcuminoids. *Cancer Lett* 1995; 94(1): 79-83.

90. Sajithlal GB, Chittra P, Chandrakasan G. Effect of curcumin on the advanced glycation and cross-linking of collagen in diabetic rats. *Biochem Pharmacol* 1998; 56: 1607- 1614.

91. Saleheen D, Ali SA, Ashfaq K, Siddiqui AA, Agha A, Yasinzai MM. Latent activity of curcumin against leishmaniasis in vitro. *Biol Pharm Bull* 2002; 25: 386-389.

92. Satoskar RR, Shah SJ, Shenoy SG, Evaluation of anti-inflammatory property of curcumin in patients with post operative inflammation. *Int J Clin Pharmacol Ther Toxicol* 1986; 24: 651-654.

93. Sen S, Sharma H, Singh N. Curcumin enhances vinorelbine mediated apoptosis in NSCLC cells by mitochondrial pathway. *Biochem Biophys Res Commun* 2005; 331(4): 1245-1252.

94. Shah BH, Nawaz Z, Pertani SA, Roomi A, Mahmood H, et. al. Inhibitory effect of curcumin, a food spice from turmeric, on platelet-activating factor- and arachidonic acid-mediated platelet aggregation through inhibition of thromboxane formation and Ca^{2+} signaling. *Biochem Pharmacol* 1999; 58: 1167-1172.

95. Sharma OP. Antioxidant activity of curcumin and related compounds. *Biochem Pharmacol* 1976; 25: 1811-1812.

96. Shishodia S, Amin HM, Lai R, Aggarwal BB. Curcumin (diferuloylmethane) inhibits constitutive NF-kappa B actvation, induces G1/S arrest, suppresses proliferation, and induces apoptosis in mantle cell lymphoma. *Biochem Pharmacol* 2005; 70(5): 700-713.

97. Singh S, Aggarwal BB. Activation of transcription factor NF-κB is suppressed by curcumin (diferuloylmethane). *J Biol Chem* 1995; 270: 24,995-25000.

98. Sinha M, Mukherjee BP, Mukherjee B, Dasgupta SR. Study on the 5-hydroxytryptamine contents in guinea pig stomach with relation to

phenylbutazone induced gastric ulcers and the effects of curcumin thereon. *Indian J Pharmacol* 1974; 6: 87-96.

99. Sinha R, Anderson DE, Mc Donald SS, Greenwald P. Cancer risk and diet in India. *J Postgrad Med* 2003; 49(3): 222-228.

100. Sivalingam N, Hanumantharaya R, Faith M, Basivireddy J, Balasubramaniam KA Jacob M. Curcumin reduces indomethacin-induced damage in the rat small intestine. *J Appl Toxicol* 2007; (In Press).

101. Skrzypczak-Jankun E, Mc Cabe NP, Selman SH, Jankun J. Curcumin inhibits lipoxygenase by binding to its central cavity: theoretical and X-ray evidence. *Int J Mol Med* 2000; 6: 521-526.

102. Soni KB, Kuttan R. Effect of oral curcumin administration on serum peroxides and cholesterol levels in human volunteers. *Indian J Physiol Pharmacol* 1992; 36: 273-275.

103. Soni KB, Lahiri M, Chackradeo P, Bhide SV, Kuttan R. Protective effect of food additives on aflatoxin-induced mutagenicity and hepatocarcinogenicity. *Cancer Lett* 1997; 121(1): 99-104.

104. Soni KB, Rajan A, Kuttan R. Reversal of aflatoxin induced liver damage by turmeric and curcumin. *Cancer Lett* 1992; 66(2): 115-121.

105. South EH, Exon JH, Hendrix K. Dietary curcumin enhances antibody response in rats. *Immunopharmacol Immunotoxicol* 1997; 19: 105-119.

106. Sreejayan N, Rao MN. Curcuminoids as potent inhibitors of lipid peroxidation. *J Pharm Pharmacol* 1994; 46(12): 1013-1016.

107. Sreejayan N, Rao MN. Nitric oxide scavenging by curcuminoids. *J Pharm Pharmacol* 1997; 49: 105-107.

108. Srihari Rao T, Basu N, Siddqui HH. Antiinflammatory activity of curcumin analogues. *Indian J Med Res* 1982; 75: 574- 578.

109. Srimal RC, Dhawan BN., In. Development of Unani drugs from Herbal Sources and the role of Elements in their Mechanism of Action (ed. Arora, BB), Hamdard National Foundation Monograph, New Delhi, 1985.

110. Srimal RC. Turmeric. a brief review of medicinal properties. *Phytotherapy* 1997; 68: 483–493.

111. Srivastava KC, Bordia A, Verma SK. Curcumin, a major component of food spice turmeric (*Curcuma longa*) inhibits aggregation and alters eicosanoid metbolism in human blood platelets. *Prosataglandins Leukot Essent Fatty Acids* 1995; 52: 223-227.

112. Srivastava R, Dikshit M, Srimal RC, Dhawan BN. Anti-thrombotic effect of curcumin. *Thromb Res* 1985; 40(3): 413-417.

113. Srivastava R. Inhibition of neutrophil response by curcumin. *Agents Actions* 1989; 28: 298-303.

114. Subramaniam M, Sreejayan Rao MNA, Devasagayam TPA, Singh BB. Diminution of singlet oxygen induced DNA damage by curcumin and related antioxidants. *Mutat Res* 1994; 311: 249-255.

115. Sumbilla C, Lewis D, Hammerschmidt T, Inesi G. The slippage of the Ca^{2+} pump and its control by anions and curcumin in skeletal and cardiac sarcoplasmic reticulum. *J Biol Chem* 2002; 277: 13900-13906.

116. Surh YJ, Han SS, Keum YS, Seo HJ, Lee SS. Inhibitory effects of curcumin and capsaicin on phorbol ester-induced activation of eukaryotic transcription factors, NF-kappaB and AP-1. *Biofactors* 2000;12(1-4):107-12.

117. Suryanarayana P, Krishnaswamy K, Reddy GB. Effect of curcumin on galactose-induced cataractogenesis in rats. *Mol Vis* 2003; 9: 223-230.

118. Tantaoui-Elaraki A, Beraoud L. Inhibition of growth and aflatoxin production in *Aspergillus parasiticus* by essential oils of selected plant materials. *J Environ Pathol Toxicol Oncol* 1994; 13: 67-72.

119. Thaloor D, Singh AK, Sidhu GS, Prasad PV, Kleinman HK, Maheshwari RK. Inhibition of angiogenic differentiation of human umbilical vein endothelial cells by curcumin. *Cell Growth Differ* 1998; 9: 305-312.

120. Toda S. Antioxidative components isolated from rhizome of *Curcuma longa* L. *Chem Pharm Bull* 1985; 33: 1725–1728.

121. Unnikrishnan MK, Rao MN. Curcumin inhibits nitrogen dioxide induced oxidation of hemoglobin. *Mol Cell Biochem* 1995; 146(1): 35-37.

122. Vajragupta O, Boonchoong P, Morris GM, Olson AJ. Active site binding modes of curcumin in HIV-1 protese and integrase. *Bioorg Med Chem Lett* 2005; 15: 3364-3368.

123. Wahlstrom B, Blennow G. A study on the fate of curcumin in the rat. *Acta Pharmacol Toxicol* 1978; 43: 86-92.

124. Wallace JM. Nutritional and botanical modulation of the inflammatory cascade-eicosanoids, cyclooxygenases and lipoxygenases-as an adjunct in cancer therapy. *Integr Cancer Ther* 2002; 1: 7-37.

125. Wang YJ, Pan MH, Cheng AL, et. al. Stability of curcumin in buffer solutions and characterization of its degradation products. *J Pharm Biomed Anal* 1997; 15: 1867-1876.

126. Woo JH et. al. Molecular mechanisms of curcumin-induced cytotoxicity: induction of apoptosis through generation of reactive oxygen species, down-regulation of Bcl-XL and IAP, the release of cytochrome *c* and inhibition of Akt. *Carcinogenesis* 2003; 24: 1199-1208.

127. Wuthi-udomlert M, Grisanapan W, Luanrantna O, Caichompoo W. Antifungal activity of *Curcuma longa* grown in Thailand. *Southeast Asian J Trop Med Public Health* 2000; 178-182.

128. Zhang F, Altorki NK, Mestre JR, Subbaramaiah K, Dannenberg AJ. Inhibition of cyclo-oxygenase 2 expression in colon cells by the chemopreventive agent curcumin involves inhibition of NF-kappa B activation via the NIK/IKK signaling complex. *Carcinogenesis* 1999; 20: 445-451.

Some Additional Informations on Turmeric

The curcuminoids and a peptide, turmerine with 40 aminoacids in turmeric have potent antioxidant activities, and they strongly inhibit the free radical damage to biomolecules. The anticarcinogenic, anti-inflammatory, antibiotic and antiatherogenic properties of turmeric are due to the various curcuminoids which make turmeric a wonder drug among the plant kingdom. Turmeric extract in capsule form is available from Pepper India Corporation, K.K, Road, Kottayam, Kerala. Turmerine is water soluble and a methionine rich peptide. It is a more potent antioxidant than the curcuminoids. It is present to the extent of 0.1% in turmeric and active at nanomolar levels. Curcuminoids are present in turmeric to the extent of 3-5%. It was found that the strong nematocidal activity of turmeric is due to a synergistic action of the three curcuminoids referred in the above article (Kiuchi F, Goto Y, Sugimoto N, Akao K, Tsuda Y. Nematocidal activity of turmeric: Synergistic action of curcuminoids. *Chem Pharm Bull (Tokyo)* 1993; 41: 1640-1643., Srinivas, L.,Shalini, V.K and Shylaja, M(1992) Turmerin a water soluble antioxidant peptide from turmeric. Arch. Biochem-Biophy.292, 617).

Editors

4.4 Anti-inflammatory Action of Curcumin

Dr. P. R. Sudhakaran, P.T. Boban and K. Saja
Department of Biochemistry, University of Kerala
Kariavattam campus, Kariavattam 695 581

Introduction

Curcumin, a yellow coloured phenolic pigment is the active component isolated from rhizome of the Indian medicinal plant Curcuma Longa L. Curcuma Longa or turmeric is widely cultivated in southern and southeastern tropical Asia. Turmeric is extensively used as a dietary spice and in traditional medicine for the treatment of various diseases. In traditional Indian medicine, turmeric is used for biliary disorders, anorexia, cough, diabetic wounds, hepatic disorders, rheumatism and sinusitis (Jain & DeFilipps, 1991). Curcumin constitutes about 2-5% of the total spice in turmeric. The crude extract of rhizome of turmeric contains about 77% Curcumin (diferuloylmethane), about 17% curcumin II (demethoxycurcumin) and about 3% curcumin III (bis-demethoxycurcumin). These curcuminoids are responsible for the yellow colour of turmeric. In the pure form curcumin is an orange-yellow crystalline powder and is insoluble in water, but it is soluble in ethanol or dimethylsulfoxide.

(See the figures of Curcuminoids in P. 172 of this book)

Beneficial Effects of Curcumin

Extensive scientific research on curcumin has demonstrated a wide spectrum of beneficial effects (Aggarwal *et. al.* 2005; Joe *et. al.* 2004; Araujo & Leon, 2001). **The different pharmacological activities of curcumin include its anti-inflammatory (Jackson *et. al.* 2006; Chainani-Wu, 2003) and antioxidant (Farombi & Ekor, 2006; Reddy & Lokesh 1994; Joe & Lokesh, 1994; Motterlini *et. al.* 2000) activities. Curcumin has also been reported to have hypolipidemic properties (Olszanecki *et.* al. 2005; Arafa, 2005; Babu & Srinivasan, 1997) and anti-atherogenic activities (Quiles *et. al.* 2002; Ramirez-Tortosa *et. al.* 1999).** *These beneficial effects of curcumin have been attributed to its ability to influence a variety of molecular targets in different cells, which includes transcription factors, enzymes, protein kinases, cell adhesion molecules, gene expression etc. (Aggarwal et. al. 2005).*

Anti-inflammatory Action of Curcumin

Inflammation is a complex set of interactions among soluble factors and cellular components, often accompanied by destruction of connective tissue. Chronic inflammation is a risk factor for a number of diseases. The commonly used anti-inflammatory agents like aspirin and other non-steroidal anti-inflammatory drugs (NSAIDS), act mainly by inhibiting cyclooxygenase, which convert arachidonic acid to prostaglandins that in turn induces inflammatory reactions (Coussens& Werb, 2002) **Curcumin is a potent anti-inflammatory agent that mediates its effects mainly by inhibiting arachidonic acid metabolism (Joe and Lokesh 1997; Srivasthava *et. al.* 1995), cyclooxygenase (Hong *et. al.* 2004; Wallace, 2002), lipooxygenase (Hong *et. al.* 2004; Wallace, 2002), pro-inflammatory cytokines (Abe *et. al.* 1999; Kang *et. al.* 1999) and also by inhibiting the production of reactive oxygen and nitrogen species (Pan *et. al.* 2001; Surh *et. al.* 2001).**

Effect of Curcumin on COX and LOX

Arachidonic acid derived lipid mediators are intimately involved in inflammation. They are synthesised by pathways dependent on cyclooxygenase (COX) and lipooxygenase (LOX) enzymes (Rao CV, 2007). Cox-2 is an inducible form of cyclooxygenase that responds to pro-inflammatory mediators and is responsible for increased production of Prostaglandins (Otto and Smith, 1995) at the site of inflammation. Curcumin has been shown to regulate eicosanoids pathway involving COX and LOX. **Curcumin reduces pro-inflammatory leukotriene synthesis via inhibition of LOX enzyme (Ramsewak, 2000; Skrzypczak-Jankun, 2000; Huang et. al. 1991). A number of evidence indicate that curcumin regulates LOX and COX-2 predominantly at the transcriptional level and to a certain extent at the post- translational level (Rao CV, 2007).**

Effect of Curcumin on Inducible Nitric Oxide Synthase

Inducible nitric oxide synthase (iNOS) is an important enzyme that mediates inflammatory responses. Improper up-regulation of iNOS has been associated with pathophysiology of certain types of human cancers as well as inflammatory disorders. NO released by their constitutive enzymes, produce autocrine and paracrine effects regulating the onset of an inflammatory response. **The actions of all forms of NOS are mediated not only by the free radical oxidant properties of this soluble gas, but also by its activation of guanylate cyclase (GC), leading to the production of cyclic guanosine monophosphate (cGMP) that mediates many of its physiological actions. In addition, NO activates cyclooxygenase and lipoxygenase, leading to the production of physiologically relevant quantities of prostaglandin E2 (PGE2) and leukotrienes (Mc Cann et. al. 1998).**

Recent studies have demonstrated that eukaryotic transcription factor nuclear factor kB (NF-kB) was involved in regulation of iNOS expression. Surh studied the molecular mechanism underlying antiinflammatory activity of curcumin (Surh et. al. 2001). Pan et. al. compared the ability of curcumin and its hydrogenated metabolites to suppress NOS, through down-regulation of I-kB kinase and NF-kB activation in macrophages [Pan et. al. 2001].

Effect of Curcumin on NFκB

NF-κB is a family of transcription factors, which play a pivotal role in chronic inflammatory diseases. In the unstimulated state, NF-κB is found in the cytoplasm and is bound to IκB, which prevents its translocation to the nucleus (Barnes and Karim, 1997). This factor is activated in response to various inflammatory stimuli, resulting in the phosphorylation and degradation of IκB. This leads to the activation of NF-κB and subsequent translocation to nucleus, where it binds to specific sequence in the promoter region of target genes (Karim et. al. 2002). Many laboratories including ours have shown that various stimuli activated NF-κB and that curcumin down-regulates the activation (Singh & Aggarwal, 1995; Saja et. al. 2007). **Curcumin-induced down regulation of NFκβ is shown to be mediated through suppression of Iκβα_1. kinase activation (Jobin et. al. 1999; Plummer et. al. 1999). Down-regulation of COX-2, and iNOS by curcumin is also found to be regulated by NF-κβ as NF-κβ binding element is present in the promoter region of these genes (Plummer et. al. 1999; Pan et. al. 2000).**

Effect of Curcumin on MMPs

Matrix metalloproteinases (MMPs) are a family of structurally related cation-dependent neutral proteinases that degrade almost all the components of the extracellular matrix (ECM). They play a major role in the tissue remodeling and repair in both physiological and pathological conditions. The activity of MMPs is regulated mainly at the level of gene transcription, zymogen activation as well as by tissue inhibitors of metalloproteinases (TIMPs) (Egeblad and Werb, 2002).

Apoptosis and Anti Apoptosis

Abnormal expression of MMPs may contribute to pathological process, especially inflammatory conditions such as tumour metastasis, arthritis, atherosclerosis etc. MMPs including MMP-9, 12 and 14 contribute to the progression of cancer (Fingleton et. al. 2001). MMPs have both apoptotic and anti-apoptotic actions. MMP-3, 7, 9 and 11 regulate apoptosis, MMP-3 induces apoptosis in mammary epithelial cells (Mitsiades et. al. 2001), whereas MMP-7 and MMP-11 inhibit cancer cell apoptosis (Egeblad and Werb, 2002). MMPs also participate in the late event of metastasis process, MMP-9 is required for intravasation and

MMP-14 is found to be necessary for the survival of the cancer cells (Egeblad and Werb, 2002). In rheumatoid arthritis MMP contributes to joint destruction by degrading the cartilage and bone. The major MMPs implicated in this process include MMP-3, MMP-1, MMP-13, MMP-9, MMP-2 and aggrecanases (Jackson et. al. 2001, Nagase and Kashiwagi 2003). A number of studies indicated the localization of MMP-1, 2, 3, 7, 9, 12 and MT1-MMP in atherosclerotic plaque (Uzui et. al. 2002, Katsuda and Kaji 2003), which breaksdown the fibrous caps of atheromas leading to vascular complications of atherosclerosis.

Inflammatory lesions are often associated with significant destruction of extracellular matrix (ECM), with an intense infiltration of inflammatory cells. MMPs produced by these cells play an important role in the migration of these cells to the site of inflammation by degrading the ECM barrier. *Among different MMPs, MMP-9 is an inducible enzyme, which is upregulated in response to various inflammatory signals. Inflammations being a major risk factor for a number of deseases, anti-inflammatory components of natural origin particularly neutraceuticals are potentially useful.* Several studies, including ours have shown that curcumin down-regulates the expression and activity of MMPs, especially MMP-9 in various systems (Lin et. al. 1998; swarnakar et. al. 2005; Saja et. al. 2007). As MMP-9 promoters contain several putative AP-1 and NFκB elements (Eberhardt et. al. 2002; Pan and Hung, 2002; Huhtala et. al. 1991), one of the mechanisms for MMP-9 down-regulation is through these transcription factors. *Curcumin is found to be a potent inhibitor of both AP-1 and NFκB (Biswas et. al. 2005; Prusty et. al. 2005). Reports of Wahl et. al. and ours showed that in inflammatory cells like Mo/Mφ the production of MMP-9 is found to be mediated through inflammatory mediators, mainly prostaglandins (Wahl et. al. 1977; Saja at al 2007). Another possible mechanism for down-regulation of MMP-9 by curcumin is through the inhibition of production of prostaglandins by COX, which in turn is down regulated by curcumin. The anti-inflammatory effect of curcumin involves down regulation of MMP-9.*

Summary

A large number of studies have revealed that curcumin has wide therapeutic actions. Its anti-inflammatory activity is mainly due to inhibition of AA metabolism, COX, LOX, cytokines (ILs and TNF) and NF-kB. In addition to this, down regulation of MMPs by curcumin enhances its therapeutic potential. The most interesting feature of curcumin is lack of gastrointestinal side effects despite being an anti-inflammatory agent. Curcumin appears to be a useful compound for treatment of various inflammatory diseases such as arthritis, cancer, Coronary artery disease, etc.

References

1. **Abe Y,** Hashimoto S, Horie T. Curcumin inhibition of inflammatory cytokine production by human peripheral blood monocytes and alveolar macrophages. Pharmacol Res. 1999; 39: 41-47.
2. **Aggarwal B B**, Kumar A, Aggarwal M S, Shishodia S. Curcumin derived from turmeric (Curcuma Longa): A spice for all seasons. Phytopharmaceuticals in cancer chemoprevention. CRC press LLC. 2005, p. 349.
3. **Arafa HM**. Curcumin attenuates diet-induced hypercholesterolemia in rats. Med Sci Monit. 2005; 11: 228-234.
4. **Araujo CC**, Leon LL. Biological activities of Curcuma longa L. Mem Inst Oswaldo Cruz. 2001; 96: 723-8.
5. **Babu PS**, Srinivasan K. Hypolipidemic action of curcumin, the active principle of turmeric (Curcuma longa) in streptozotocin induced diabetic rats. Mol Cell Biochem. 1997; 166: 169-75.
6. **Barnes PJ**, Karin M. Nuclear factor-kappa B: a pivotal transcription factor in chronic inflammatory diseases. N Engl J Med. 1997; 336: 1066-71.
7. **Biswas SK**, McClure D, Jimenez LA, Megson IL, Rahman I. Curcumin induces glutathione biosynthesis and inhibits NF-kappa B activation and interleukin-8 release in alveolar epithelial cells: mechanism of free radical scavenging activity. Antioxid Redox Signal. 2005; 7: 32-41.
8. **Chainani-Wu N**. Safety and anti-inflammatory activity of curcumin: a component of tumeric (Curcuma longa). J Altern Complement Med. 2003; 9:161-8.
9. **Coussens LM**, Werb Z. Inflammation and cancer. Nature. 2002; 420: 860-7. Egeblad M and Werb Z. New functions for the matrix metalloproteinases in cancer progression. Nat. Rev. Cancer 2002; 2: 163-175.
10. **Eberhardt W**, Schulze M, Engels C, Klasmeier E, Pfeilschifter J. Glucocorticoid-mediated suppression of cytokine-induced matrix metalloproteinase-9 expression in rat mesangial cells: involvement of nuclear factor-kappaB and Ets transcription factors. Mol Endocrinol. 2002 Aug;16(8):1752-66.
11. **Farombi EO**, Ekor M. Curcumin attenuates gentamicin-induced renal oxidative damage in rats. Food Chem Toxicol. 2006; 44: 1443-48.

12. **Fingleton B**, Vargo-Gogola T, Crawford HC, Matrisian LM. Matrilysin (MMP-7) expression selects for cells with reduced sensitivity to apoptosis. Neoplasia. 2001; 3: 459-468.

13. **Hong J**, Bose M, Ju J, Ryu JH, Chen X, Sang S, Lee MJ, Yang CS. Modulation of arachidonic acid metabolism by curcumin and related beta-diketone derivatives: effect of cytosolic phospholipase A(2), cyclooxygenases and 5-lipooxygenase. Carcinogenesis. 2004; 25: 1671-1679.

14. **Huang MT**, Lysz T, Ferraro T, Abidi TF, Laskin JD, Conney AH. Inhibitory effects of curcumin on in vitro lipoxygenase and cyclooxygenase activities in mouse epidermis. Cancer Res. 1991; 51:813-9.

15. **Huhtala P**, Tuuttila A, Chow LT, Lohi J, Keski-Oja J, Tryggvason K. Complete structure of the human gene for 92-KDa Type IV collagenase. Divergent regulation of expression for the 92 and 72 kilodalton enzyme genes in HT-1080 cells. J. Biol. Chem. 1991; 266: 16485-16490.

16. **Jackson C**, Nguyen M, Arkell J, Sambrook P. Selective matrix metalloproteinase (MMP) inhibitor in rheumatoid arthritis – targeting gelatinase A activation. Inflamm. Res. 2001; 50: 183-186.

17. **Jackson JK**, Higo T, Hunter WL, Burt HM. The antioxidants curcumin and quercetin inhibit inflammatory processes associated with arthritis. Inflamm Res.2006; 55: 168-75.

18. **Jain S K**, DeFilipps R A. Medicinal Plants of India, Reference Publications, Algonac, MI, 1991, p. 120.

19. **Jobin C**, Bradham CA, Russo MP,Juma B, Narula AS, Brenner DA,Sator RB.Curcumin blocks cytokine-mediated NF-kappaB activation and proinflammatory gene expession by inhibiting inhibitory factor I-kappaB kinase activity, J.Immunol. 1999;163, 3474-3483.

20. **Joe B**, Lokesh BR. Effect of curcumin and capsaicin on arachidonic acid metabolism and lysosomal enzyme secretion by rat peritoneal macrophage. Lipids. 1997; 32: 1173-1180.

21. **Joe B**, Lokesh BR. Role of capsaicin, curcumin and dietary n-3 fatty acids in lowering the generation of reactive oxygen species in rat peritoneal macrophages. Biochim Biophys Acta. 1994; 1224: 255-63.

22. **Joe B**, Vijaykumar M, Lokesh BR. Biological properties of curcumin-cellular and molecular mechanisms of action. Crit Rev Food Sci Nutr. 2004; 44: 97-111.

23. **Kang BY**, Chung SW, Chung W, Im S, Hwang SY, Kim TS. Inhibition of interleukin-12 production in lipopolysaccharide-activated macrophages by curcumin. Eur J Pharmacol. 1999; 384: 191-195.

24. **Karin M,** Cao Y, Greten FR, Li ZW. NF-kappaB in cancer: from innocent bystander to major culprit. Nat Rev Cancer 2. 2002; 301-310.

25. **Katsuda S** and Kaji T. Atherosclerosis and extracellular matrix. J. Atheroscler. Thromb. 2003; 10: 267-274.

26. **Lin LI,** Ke YF, Ko YC, Lin JK, Curcumin inhibits SK-Hep-1 hepatocellular carcinoma cell invasion in vitro and suppresses matrix metalloproteinase-9 secretion, Oncology, 1998; 55(4) 349-353.

27. **McCann**, S M, Licinio, J, Wong M L, YuW H, Karanth, S, Rettorri V, The nitric oxide hypothesis of aging. Exp-Gerontol. 1998 Nov-Dec; 33(7-8): 813-26.

28. **Mitsiades N**, Poulaki V, Mitsiades CS, Koutras DA, Chrousos GP. Apoptosis induced by FasL and TRAIL/Apo2L in the pathogenesis of thyroid diseases. Trends Endocrinol Metab. 2001; 12(9):384-90.

29. **Motterlini R**, Foresti R, Bassi R, Green CJ. Curcumin, an antioxidant and anti-inflammatory agent, induces heme oxygenase-1 and protects endothelial cells against oxidative stress. Free Radic Biol Med. 2000; 28: 1303-12.

30. **Nagase H**, Kashiwagi M. Aggrecanases and cartilage matrix degradation. Arthritis Res Ther. 2003; 5(2):94-103. Epub 2003 Feb 14.

31. **Olszanecki R**, Jawien J, Gajda M, Mateuszuk L, Gebska A, Korabiowska M, Chlopicki S, Korbut R. Effect of curcumin on atherosclerosis in apoE/LDLR-double knockout mice. J Physiol Pharmacol. 2005; 56: 627-35.

32. **Otto JC**, Smith WL. Prostaglandin endoperoxide synthases-1 and -2. J Lipid Mediat Cell Signal. 1995; 12:139-56.

33. **Pan MR**, Hung WC. Nonsteroidal anti-inflammatory drugs inhibit matrix metalloproteinase-2 via suppression of the ERK/Sp1-mediated transcription. J Biol Chem. 2002 Sep 6; 277(36):32775-80.

34. **Pan MH**, Lin-Shiau SY, Lin JK. Comparative studies on the suppression of nitric oxide synthase by curcumin and its hydrogenated metabolites through down-regulation of IkappaB kinase and NFkappaB activation in macrophages. Biochem Pharmacol. 2001; 60: 1665-1676

35. **Plummer SM**, Holloway KA, Manson MM, Munks RJ, Kaptein A, Farrow S, Howells, L, Inhibitionof cyclo-oxygenase 2 expression in colon cells by the chemopreventive agent curcumin involves inhibition of NF-kappaB activation via the NIK/IKK signaling complex, Oncogene, 1999.;18,6013-6020.

36. **Prusty BK**, Das BC. Constitutive activation of transcription factor AP-1 in cervical cancer and suppression of human papillomavirus (HPV) transcription and AP-1 activity in HeLa cells by curcumin. Int J Cancer. 2005; 113: 951-60.

37. **Quiles JL**, Mesa MD, Ramirez-Tortosa CL, Aguilera CM, Battino M, Gil A, Ramirez-Tortosa MC. Curcuma longa extract supplementation reduces oxidative stress and attenuates aortic fatty streak development in rabbits. Arterioscler Thromb Vasc Biol. 2002; 22: 1225-31.

38. **Ramirez-Tortosa MC**, Mesa MD, Aguilera MC, Quiles JL, Baro L, Ramirez-Tortosa CL, Martinez-Victoria E, Gil A. Oral administration of a turmeric extract inhibits LDL oxidation and has hypocholesterolemic effects in rabbits with experimental atherosclerosis. Atherosclerosis. 1999; 147: 371-8.

39. **Ramsewak RS**, DeWitt DL, Nair MG. Cytotoxicity, antioxidant and anti-inflammatory activities of curcumins I-III from Curcuma longa. Phytomedicine. 2000; 7: 303-8.

40. **Rao CV**. Regulation of COX and LOX by curcumin.Adv Exp Med Biol; 2007:213-26.

41. **Reddy AC**, Lokesh BR. Studies on the inhibitory effects of curcumin and eugenol on the formation of reactive oxygen species and the oxidation of ferrous iron. Mol Cell Biochem. 1994; 137: 1-8.

42. **Saja K**, Babu MS, Karunagaran D, Sudhakaran PR. Anti-inflammatory effect of curcumin involves downregulation of MMP-9 in peripheral bloodmononuclear cells. Int Immunopharmacol, 2007(accepted)

43. **Saja K**, Chatterjee U, Chatterjee BP, Sudhakaran PR. Activation dependent expression of MMPs in peripheral blood mononuclear cells involves protein kinase A. Mol Cell Biochem. 2007 Feb; 296 (1-2):185-92. Epub 2006 Oct 17.

44. **Singh S** and Aggarwal BB, Activation of transcription factor NFκB is suppressed by curcumin, J.Biol.Chem, 1995; 270, 24995-5000.

45. **Skrzypczak-Jankun E**, McCabe NP, Selman SH, Jankun J. Curcumin inhibits lipoxygenase by binding to its central cavity: theoretical and X-ray evidence. Int J Mol Med. 2000; 6: 521-6.

46. **Srivastiva KC**, Bordia A, Verma SK. Curcumin, a major component of food spice turmeric (curcuma longa) inhibits aggregation and alters ecosanoid metabolism in human blood platelets. Prostaglandins Leukot Essent Fatty acids. 1995; 52: 223-227.

47. **Surh YJ**, Chun KS, Cha HH, Han SS, Keum YS, Park KK, Lee SS. Molecular mechanisms underlying chemopreventive activities of anti-inflammatory phytochemicals: down-regulation of COX-2 and iNOS through suppression of NF-kappa B activation. Mutat Res. 2001; 480-481: 243-268.

48. **Swarnakar S**, Ganguly K, Kundu P, Banerjee A, Maity P, Sharma AV. Curcumin regulates expression and activity of matrix metalloproteinases 9 and 2 during prevention and healing of indomethacin-induced gastric ulcer. J Biol Chem. 2005 Mar 11; 280: 9409-15.

49. **Uzui H**, Harpf A, Liu M, Doherty TM, Shukla A, Chai NN, Tripathi PV, Jovinge S, Wilkin DJ, Asotra K, Shah PK, Rajavashisth TB. Increased expression of membrane type 3-matrix metalloproteinase in human atherosclerotic plaque: role of activated macrophages and inflammatory cytokines. Circulation. 2002; 106: 3024-3030.

50. **Wahl LM**, Olsen CE, Sandberg AL, Mergenhagen SE. Prostaglandin regulation of macrophage collagenase production. Proc Natl Acad Sci U S A. 1977; 74:4955-8.

51. **Wallace JM**. Nutritional and botanical modulation of the inflammatory cascade-eicosanoids, cyclooxygenases and lipooxygenases- as an adjunct in cancer therapy. Integr Cancer Ther. 2002; 1: 7-37.

4.5 Curcumin – A Nutraceutical with Potential Chemosensitizing Property

Dr. Ruby John Anto, Smitha V B, Vinesh kumar TP, Sreekanth CN, Vinod BS, Vino T Cherian, Priya R Prabhu and Gayatri LT

Division of Cancer Biology, Rajiv Gandhi Centre for Biotechnology, Thiruvananthapuram 695014

Introduction

Chemosensitization is the enhancement of the action of one chemical by the presence of a second one which may not have direct ability to kill cancer cells. Curcumin (Diferuloyl methane), is the major active component of the food flavor, turmeric (*Curcuma longa*), that has been shown to inhibit the proliferation of a wide variety of cancer cells[1]. But there are several reports that curcumin is unable to inhibit the proliferation of cancer cells in which the anti-apoptotic factors like NF-κB, Bcl-2 etc. are over expressed which is the case in advanced tumors[2, 3]. But it is a well-known chemopreventive agent and the potential of curcumin in sensitizing cancer cells towards other conventional chemotherapeutic drugs is not yet fully explored. Cervical cancer is the second most common cancer among women in the world and the most common type of carcinoma afflicting women in developing countries. Globally, 300,000 women die from cervical cancer every year, and the majority of these deaths occur in poorer countries. Taxol is a widely used clinically effective drug against cervical cancer. But its major disadvantages are high cost and dose limiting toxicity, thus rendering it inaccessible to ordinary people who are most often the real victims of cancer. Hence there is a need for the generation of toxicity-limiting cost effective methods relevant to poorer countries. In view of the known activity of the two agents in several malignancies it would be reasonable to investigate the possible combinations of the two, which can bring about the same therapeutic effect at a lesser toxicity.

Materials and Methods

Maintenance of the Cells

Healthy HeLa cells were seeded into T 25cm^2 tissue culture flask and allowed to become 80% confluent in DMEM containing 10% FBS with antibiotics and antimycotics at 37 ^{0}C in a CO_2 incubator.

Subculturing

When cells were grown to confluency, the medium was removed, and washed once with PBS 0.25% Trypsin-EDTA solution was added, and incubated for 5-10 minutes at 37^{0}C. Fresh medium (with serum) was added and cells were dispersed gently by a pipette. A known number of cells were dispensed into new flasks or microtitre plates for further experiments.

Cytotoxicity Assays

Cytotoxicity assays serves as the means of evaluating the antiproliferating activity and helps to do a preliminary screening of the antitumor activity of the compounds tested. The following techniques were used to evaluate the cytotoxicity of various combinations of taxol and curcumin to different cell lines.

[^{3}H] Thymidine incorporation- Inhibition of DNA synthesis induced by taxol and/or curcumin was assessed by [^{3}H] Thymidine incorporation assay as described previously[2].

Annexin-PI Staining- The membrane flip-flop induced by taxol and/or curcumin was assessed essentially as described previously[3] according to manufacturer's protocol (Annexin V apoptosis detection kit, Santa Cruz Biotechnology).

Detection of caspase 3 cleavage- Western blot analysis was done to detect the active fragments of caspases 3 as described previously[3] and detected by Enhanced Chemi Luminescence (ECL, Amersham Biosciences)

Electrophoretic Mobility Shift Assay (EMSA)- To detect NF-κB activation, EMSA was done and the specificity of the bands was confirmed by super shift[4] and visualized by a Phosphor Imager (Bio-Rad Personal FX).

Results

We examined the effect of taxol and curcumin individually and in combination on DNA synthesis by the method of thymidine **incorporation** assay. We tried various combinations of taxol and curcumin and observed that a combination of 5μM taxol and 5μM curcumin almost brings about the same effect of 10μM taxol when treated alone. When 10 nM and 5 μM taxol induced 53% and 32% cytotoxicity respectively in HeLa cells, a combination of 5μM taxol and 5 μM curcumin induced 48% cytotoxicity (Fig 1). These results indicate that curcumin and taxol when used in combination, induces almost double the amount of cell death than taxol when used alone.

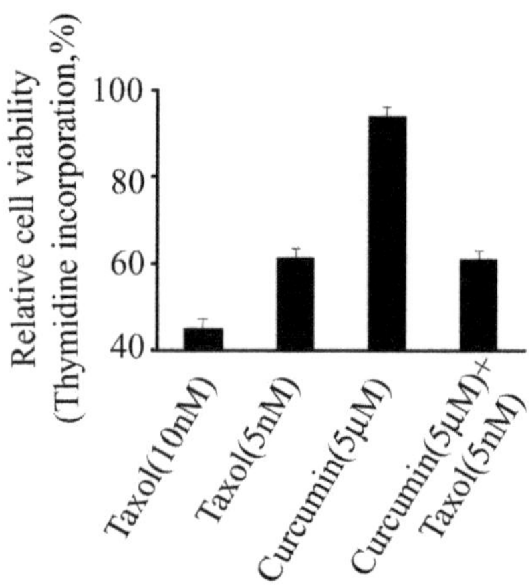

Fig.1 HeLa cells were treated with taxol and/or curcumin as indicated for 24 h and the thymidine incorporation was determined as described in "Materials and Methods".

Taxol induced morphological alterations and cell damage is potentiated by curcumin

When viewed through a phase contrast microscope, the untreated cells looked well spread with flattened morphology, where as some cells in the taxol treated wells and almost all cells in the wells treated with taxol/curcumin combination were showing round off morphology with a lot of apoptotic bodies showing that the extent of apoptosis is much higher in cells treated with the combination.

Annexin staining also gave supporting data for the hypothesis. Bright green annexin was imparted to membranes of the apoptotic cells showing membrane blebbing, one of the early markers of apoptosis. The cells with later stages of apoptosis showed red color of propidium iodide signifying the nuclear damage and condensation and their number is much higher in the wells treated with the combination of curcumin and taxol (Fig. 2).

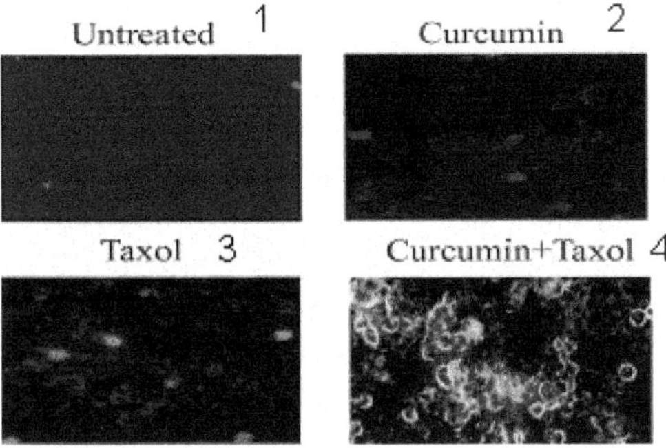

1. Cells have normal and flattened morphology
2. Do
3. Some cells have round off morphology with apoptotic bodies.
4. All cells have round off morphology with a lot of apoptotic bodies.

Fig. 2 HeLa cells were treated with taxol (5 nM) and/or curcumin (5 μM) for 16 h, and stained for annexin-PI positivity as described under "Materials and Methods".

Curcumin Potentiates Taxol Induced Executioner Caspase Activation

Caspases are a family of cysteine proteases that cleave proteins after aspartic acid residues. They are the main effectors of apoptosis or programmed cell death (PCD) and their activation leads to characteristic morphological changes of the cell such as shrinkage, chromatin condensation, DNA fragmentation and plasma membrane blebbing. Initiator caspases are the first to be activated and include caspase-2, 8, 9 and 10. These cleave and activate the effector caspases (3, 6, 7), which cleave, degrade or activate other cellular proteins. We studied the role of the executioner caspase-3, which is a clear indicator of apoptosis by western blot. Taxol-induced cleavage of caspase 3 was also enhanced by curcumin pretreatment (Fig. 3). The above result confirm that a combination of 5nM taxol and 5μM curcumin make HeLa cells much more sensitive to apoptosis than when either of the compounds are used alone as evidenced by higher activation of caspase 3.

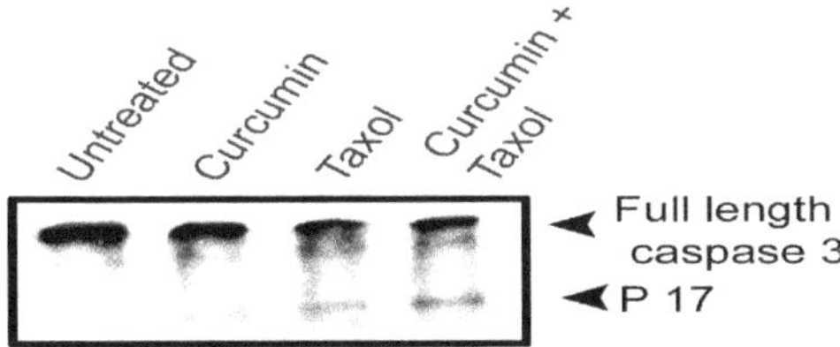

Fig. 3 Western blot-HeLa cells were treated with taxol (5nM) and/or curcumin (5 μM) for 24h, whole cell lysate was resolved on 12% gel, blotted against anti-caspase 3 and detected by ECL.

Taxol induced NF-κB activation and IκBα degradation is inhibited by curcumin

Our next attempt was to find out the possible explanation for this synergistic effect. As taxol has been reported to induce NF-κB activation in certain cell lines[5]. We checked whether taxol is activating NF-κB in HeLa cells. We also checked whether curcumin could inhibit the taxol induced NF-κB activation. Interestingly curcumin pretreatment clearly down regulated the NF-κB activation induced by taxol (Fig. 4). To confirm whether the active complex contains the classical NF-κB partners, p50 and RelA, the nuclear extracts prepared from HeLa cells stimulated with 5nM taxol were incubated with antibodies specific to p50 or RelA and EMSA was carried out. Both antibodies shifted the active NF-κB complex (super shift) where as incubation with excess of an unlabelled oligonucleotide containing the NF-κB binding site completely removed the active complex confirming the specificity of the band (Fig. 4). Nuclear extract of HeLa cells treated with TNF-?, a well-known activator of NF-κB was taken as the positive control. We examined the level of IκB-α in the cytosol of the cells after treatment with taxol and curcumin. Interestingly we found that curcumin is inducing resynthesis or blocking the degradation of IκB-α (Fig. 4). These results confirm that lower concentrations of taxol induces NF-κB in HeLa cells through the degradation of IκB-α and curcumin inhibits NF-κB activation, by blocking degradation or inducing resynthesis of IκB-α.

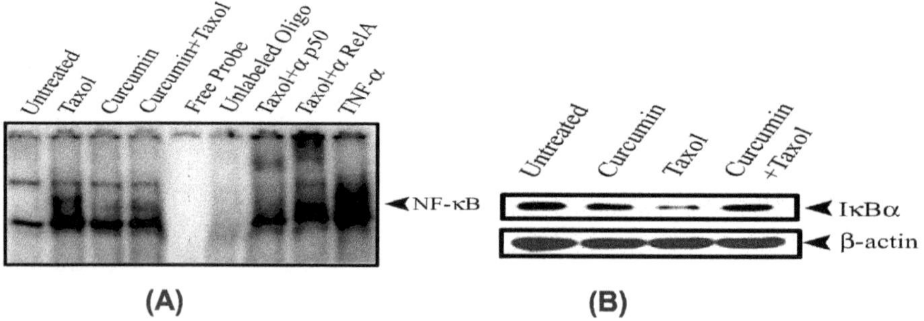

Fig. 4 (A) HeLa cells were treated with taxol (5nM) and/or curcumin (5μM) for 1h. Nuclear extracts were prepared and EMSA was done as described under "Materials and Methods". The nuclear extracts from taxol-stimulated cells were also incubated with either RelA or p50 antibody or unlabeled oligo. Cells treated with 0.1nM TNF was kept as a positive control. The arrowhead shown indicate the positions of the active DNA binding complex of NF-κB. (B) Cytosol of control cells and those treated with taxol and/or curcumin from the above experiment was collected and blotted against anti-IκBα.

Discussion

Many postulates have been suggested to explain the mechanisms by which taxol induces cell death in cancer cells. The primary mechanism of action of taxol is attributed to its ability to bind to microtubules and prevent their assembly. This causes cells to arrest in the G2/M phase of the cell cycle there by blocking cell cycle progression[6]. Although the primary target of paclitaxel is microtubules, its efficacy exceeds that of conventional microtubule-disrupting agents, suggesting that it may have additional cellular effects. Huang et. al.[7] have reported that apoptotic cell death induced by taxol may occur via a pathway independent of mitotic arrest. Our results also leads to the conclusion that apoptosis is a potential mechanism by which taxol exerts its antiproliferative effect.

In HeLa cells we observed a dose dependant cytotoxic effect by taxol, which was potentiated by pretreatment with 5μM curcumin. Curcumin pretreatment also potentiated DNA fragmentation and PARP cleavage induced by taxol. Throughout the present study we did not see a noticeable apoptosis induction by curcumin alone (5μM) at the concentration we studied even though we have noticed induction of the above-mentioned apoptotic parameters by curcumin at a higher concentration (25μM)[3].

Tumor cells often evade apoptosis by over-expressing antiapoptotic proteins such as Bcl-2, NF-κB, Akt etc. which give them survival advantage[8-10]. Lower concentrations of some of the conventional chemotherapeutic drugs also cause up-regulation of these survival signals thereby elevating the effective dose of treatment, which causes damage to the normal cells also. Protective effect of NF-κB against apoptosis has been reported in several cell lines[2]. Taxol activates NF-κB in several cell systems[5]. Several groups have reported that curcumin inhibits NF-κB activation induced by various agents[11,3] in several cell systems. In the present study we observed that taxol-induced NF-κB activation in HeLa cells is down-regulated by curcumin, which may be one of the reasons for the sensitization of taxol-induced apoptosis by curcumin. As we have used a non-toxic concentration of curcumin in this study, we cannot expect an additive effect of both the compounds.

Whether curcumin can regulate taxol induced activation of other antiapoptotic factors is not yet known though curcumin inhibits some of these factors in several cell system. Further studies are in progress to know the role of these proteins in the synergistic effect of taxol and curcumin.

Reference

1. Aggarwal, B.B, Kumar, A, Aggarwal, M.S. and Shihodia, S. Curcumin derived from turmeric: A spice for all seasons. Phytochemicals in cancer prevention.2003.
2. Anto, R. J., Maliekal, T. T., and Karunagaran, D. L-929 cells harboring ectopically expressed RelA resist curcumin-induced apoptosis. J Biol Chem, 275: 15601-15604, 2000.
3. Anto, R. J., Mukhopadhyay, A., Denning, K., and Aggarwal, B. B. Curcumin (diferuloylmethane) induces apoptosis through activation of caspase-8, BID cleavage and cytochrome c release: its suppression by ectopic expression of Bcl-2 and Bcl-xl. Carcinogenesis, 23: 143-150, 2002.
4. Anto, R. J., Mukhopadhyay, A., Shishodia, S., Gairola, C. G., and Aggarwal, B. B. Cigarette smoke condensate activates nuclear transcription factor-kappaB through phosphorylation and degradation of IkappaB(alpha): correlation with induction of cyclooxygenase-2. Carcinogenesis, 23: 1511-1518, 2002.
5. Lee, M. and Jeon, Y. J. Paclitaxel-induced immune suppression is associated with NF-kappaB activation via conventional PKC isotypes in lipopolysaccharide-stimulated 70Z/3 pre-B lymphocyte tumor cells. Mol Pharmacol, 59: 248-253, 2001.
6. Horwitz, S. B. Mechanism of action of taxol. Trends Pharmacol Sci, 13: 134-136, 1992.
7. Huang, Y., Johnson, K. R., Norris, J. S., and Fan, W. Nuclear factor-kappaB/IkappaB signaling pathway may contribute to the mediation of paclitaxel-induced apoptosis in solid tumor cells. Cancer Res, 60: 4426-4432, 2000.
8. Hermine, O., Haioun, C., Lepage, E., d'Agay, M. F., Briere, J., Lavignac, C., Fillet, G., Salles, G., Marolleau, J. P., Diebold, J., Reyas, F., and Gaulard, P. Prognostic significance of bcl-2 protein expression in aggressive non-Hodgkin's lymphoma. Groupe d'Etude des Lymphomes de l'Adulte (GELA). Blood, 87: 265-272, 1996.
9. Wang, W., Abbruzzese, J. L., Evans, D. B., Larry, L., Cleary, K. R., and Chiao, P. J. The nuclear factor-kappa B RelA transcription factor is constitutively activated in human pancreatic adenocarcinoma cells. Clin Cancer Res, 5: 119-127, 1999.
10. Vivanco, I. and Sawyers, C. L. The phosphatidylinositol 3-Kinase AKT pathway in human cancer. Nat Rev Cancer, 2: 489-501, 2002.
11. Singh, S. and Aggarwal, B. B. Activation of transcription factor NF-kappa B is suppressed by curcumin (diferuloylmethane) [corrected]. J Biol Chem, 270: 24995-25000, 1995.

Chapter – 5

Nutraceuticals of Alliums

5.1 Phenolic Acid Composition of Garlic (Allium Sativuml)

Dr. D.P. Singh[1], B.K. Sarma[1], U.P. Singh*, S. Maurya[1] and Mandavi Singh[2].

[1]Department of Mycology and Plant Pathology, Institute of Agril. Sciences

[2]Department of Anatomy, Institute of Medical Sciences, Banaras Hindu University.Varanasi .221005. India

*Corresponding author, e-mail: upneem@sify.com.

(Rtd. Professor of Mycology& Plant Pathology, Institute of Agril. Sciences)

Introduction

The use of traditional plant preparations for curing several diseases entails the realizations for their nutraceutical value for the case of human health (Singh et. al. 2004, Uhl, 2000). Plant based products have been components of phytomedicines throughout human history for treating human and plant diseases. During the last hundred years, plants have become an important source for the discovery of novel pharmaceuticals with many blockbuster drugs being directly or indirectly derived from them. Among various herbals and medicinal plants, garlic (Allium sativum) plays a great role in human disease therapy since time immemorial. It has been an essential component of culinary preparations in India and several other countries of tropical and subtropical zones. Garlic has been used for lowering blood pressure and cholesterol, fighting infections, and also in cancer therapy (Singh et. al. 2001). Antiplatelet aggregation and enhancement of fibrinolytic activity have been found in compounds and crude extracts of garlic. They have also shown antifungal, antibacterial and antiviral activities. Recent researches indicate that phytophenols, being chief secondary metabolites (Runkova and Talieva, 1975, Bravo, 1998) are present in rich amount in several higher plants including garlic.

Keeping this in view, a detailed investigation has been carried out to analyze the presence of phenolic compounds in different parts and different preparations of garlic cloves. The results are presented here.

Materials and Methods

Extractions of Phenolic Acids from raw and various preparations of Allium Sativum

One gram of one and two month old-garlic plant parts, i.e. leaves, sheath, bulb, and roots as well as various preparations of mature garlic bulb along with aerial bulb (syn. Bulbils) was macerated separately in a pestle-mortar. Finely crushed samples were suspended in 5 ml of ethanol-water (80:20 v/v). They were collected in screw-bottles tubes and later suspensions were subjected to ultrasonication (Branson Sonifier, USA) for 15 min at 4°C followed by centrifugations at 7,500 rpm for 15 min. The clear greenish supernatant was subjected to charcoal treatment to remove pigments from each sample and was then transferred to glass tubes. The residue was re-extracted twice and supernatant was pooled prior to evaporation under vacuum (Buchi Rotavapor Re Type). Dried samples were re-suspended in 1.0 ml HPLC grade methanol by vortexing and filtered through membrane filter (pore size 0.45 μm, Millipore) before HPLC analysis (Singh et. al. 2002).

High Performance Liquid Chromatographic (HPLC) Analysis

HPLC **analysis** of the extracted phenolic acids of garlic and their preparations were performed on HPLC system (Shimadzu Corporation, Japan) equipped with two Shimadzu LC-10 ATVP reciprocating pumps, a variable UV-VIS detector (Shimadzu SPD -10 AVP), integrator and Winchrom software for data recording and processing (Winchrom. India). Reversed phase chromatographic analysis was carried out in isocratic conditions using C-18 reversed phase HPLC column {(250×4.6 mm i.d., particle size 5m) Luna 5C-18(2), phenomenex, USA} at 25C. Running conditions included mobile phase methanol-0.4% acetic acid (80:20. v/v, flow rate 1.0 ml/min. injection volume 51 and detection at 290 nm. Tannic (TA), gallic (GA), oxalic (OA), protocatechuic (P-cat-A), caffeic (Caf-A), vanillic (VA), ferulic (FA), o-coumaric (o-Cou-A), chlorogenic (Chl-A), cinnamic acid (CA), gentisic (Gen-A) and salicylic acids (SA) were used as internal and external standards. Phenolic acids present in the sample were identified by comparing retention time (Rt) of standards. e.g. TA (Rt.2.76 min). GA(Rt.2.86 min), OA(3.00 min), P-cat-A(3.05 min), Caf-A(Rt.3.10 min), VA(Rt.3.26 min), FA (Rt.3.42 min), o-Cou-A (Rt.3.58 min), Chl-A (Rt.4.16 min), CA(Rt.4.45 min), Gen-A (4.56 min) and SA (6.36 min). These phenolic acids were identified by co-injection of internal and external standards for their confirmation. Amount of individual compound was calculated by comparing peak areas of reference compounds with those in the samples run under similar elution conditions.

Results and Discussion

HPLC analysis of one and two month-old garlic plants and different preparations of cloves indicated that phenolic acids varied in both types of plant parts and mature cloves. In one-month-old garlic leaves gallic acid (31.31 µg/g) was maximum followed by tannic (2.30 µg/g), cholorogenic and cinnamic acids. Sheath of one-month-old plants had gallic, ferulic and chlorogenic acids. Bulb of one-month-old garlic had four phenolic acids in which gallic (22.2 µg/g) and tannic acids (7.07 µg/g) were maximum followed by ferulic and chlorogenic acids in traces (chart-1). Various phenolic acids were in traces in sheath and scale. However, two-month-old leaves gallic acid (43.54 µg/g) was maximum but caffeic and o-coumaric acids were also detected. Sheath showed three phenolic acids in which protocatechuic acid (23.26 µg/g) was maximum but others were in traces. However, in two-month-old bulb showed only gallic and o-coumaric acids but roots of one-and two months-old plants had five (Tannic, gallic, ferulic, chlorogenic, cinnamic) and four (tannic, gallic, ferulic, chlorogenic) phenolic acids, respectively (chart-2). In mature clove tannic (109 µg/g) and ferulic acids (63.83 µg/g) were in major proportion followed by gallic, cinnamic, chlorogenic, caffeic and o-coumaric acids in traces. Pickles were rich in phenolic acids in which gallic acid (256.04 µg/g) was maximum.

Chart 1: *Order of Phenolic acids in one month old garlic (A sativum) plant parts.* viz; TA = tannic, GA = gallic, FA = ferulic, Chl-A = chlorogenic and CA = cinnamic acid.

Leaves.	GA>TA>FA	Sheath.	GA>FA>Chl.A
Bulb.	GA>TA>FA>chl.A	Roots.	GA>TA>CA

Chart 2: *Order of Phenolic acids in two month old of garlic (A. sativum) plant parts.* viz; TA = tannic, GA = gallic, FA = ferulic, Chl-A = cholorogenic, CA = cinnamic, Caf-A = caffeic, O-Cou-A = O-coumeric and P-Cate-A. Protocatechuice acid.

Leaves.	GA>CA>O.Cou-A	Sheath.	P-Cate-A
Bulb.	GA>O.Cou-A	Root.	TA>FA>GA

The intact and chopped clove of garlic in vinegar had 93.06 µg/g and 46.83 µg/g gallic acid, respectively (Chart.3). Fried garlic in different oils like deshi ghee prepared from cows milk, refined oil and mustard oil indicated that garlic cloves fried in deshi ghee had vanillic, caffeic, gentisic and salisylic acids. However, cloves, fried in refined oil, showed protocatechuic (104.95 µg/g), gallic (67.04 µg/g) and tannic acids (25.79 µg/g) but mustard oil-fried cloves had maximum oxalic acid (1089.6 μg/g) followed by tannic and chlorogenic acids in traces. Bulbils (aerial clove) had four phenolic acids in which gallic acids (10.91 μg/g) was maximum followed by ferulic acid (1.12 μg/g) but cinnamic and salicylic acids were in traces. Dry leaves had gallic, ferulic and salicylic acid in which gallic acids was maximum (67.1 μg/g) (Table 1)

Phenolics constitute an important group of natural products (as antioxidants) contributing significantly to the marked pharmacological value of a number of plants, including fruits, vegetables and spices (Singh et. al. 2001, 2004). They are important components, either in free or conjugated forms, of almost all plants in which they are synthesized via shikimic acid or phenylpropanoid pathways (Agrios.1997). Phenylalanine ammonia lyase (PAL) catalyzing phenylpropanoid pathway, is not found in animals and humans and they neither synthesize phenols nor breakdown phenol ring (Harborne. 1989, 1993). This is why animals solely depend on plants for the accumulation of phenols in their tissues. Presence of various phenolic acids in garlic indicates their therapeutic responsible for human and plant disease therapy. Narbad and Gasson (1998) isolated vanillin (Flavouring Agent) from pseudomonas flourscens, which is found by metabolism of ferulic acid. The present results indicate that vanillic acid was present in rich amount in deshi ghee-fried cloves. Presence of various phenolic acids in different parts of garlic and its preparations indicates their enormous medicinal properties essential for human and plant health.

Chart-3: Order of Phenolic acids in mature garlic (A. sativum) parts and its different preparations.

Pickle –	GA>TA	Scale-	GA>FA
Root-	GA>T.A	Clove in Vinegar	GA>FA
Cloves	TA>FA		

Table 1 Phenolic acid content of fresh aerial bulbills and boiled clove pulp, boiled aqueous extract of clove, fried clove, aerial clove of garlic (bulbil) and dried leaves of garlic.

Short Forms of Phenolic Acids Used

TA = Tannic; GA = Gallic; OA = Oxalic; P-Cat = A Protocatechuic; Caf-A = Caffeic; VA = Vanillic; FA = Ferulic; Chl-A = Chlorogenic; CA = Cinnamic; Gen-A = Gentisic and SA = Salicylic acids, ± Standard error.

Table 1

Preparation of Garlic	Phenolic conc.(μg/g fresh wt)
1. Boiled pulp	GA(11.98±0.98), VA(14.66±1.5), Caf-A(0.01)
2. Boiled clove extract	GA(11.8±0.85), VA(11.2±1.1)
3. Fried clove in ghee	Caf-A(12.5±0.9),VA(60.1±4.5),Gen-A (8.1±1.7) SA(0.18±0.6)
4. Clove in mustard oil	TA(14.6±1.5),OA(1090±14.8),Chl-A(0.26±.0.05)
5. Clove in refined oil	TA(25.8),GA(67.1±6.5)P-Cat(105±4.9)
6. Bulbil	GA (10.9±2.1), FA(1.15±0.15), CA(0.047±0.2) SA(0.143±0.1)
7. Dried leaves	GA(67.1±5.6), SA(0.154±0.2)

Several phytophenols are natural free-radical scavengers because of their structural characteristics and hydrogen-donating properties of the phenol moiety and therefore, their role in protections of both human and plants against oxidative stress have been widely recognized (Bors et. al. 1990, 2001). Presence of gallic acid indicates its possible role as anti-inflammatory and cytotoxic against all cancer cell lines studied in vitro (Inoue, 1995). Its ethyl esters are the most potent scavengers of superoxide radical (Gharzouli et. al. 1999). Gharzouli et. al. (1999) reported that monomeric and polymeric polyphenols in food are multifunctional such as antioxidants, metal chelators and inhibitors as well as strengthening the gastric mucasol barrier and immuno-stimulatory property. Crude extracts and some active principles are also antimicrobial as they have been used in controlling some plant diseases in glasshouse (Singh. et. al. 1990. Prithiviraj et. al. 1998 and Srivastava et. al. 2000). The phenolic acids together with several other compounds are responsible for global gravitation towards garlic consumption and recommendation for its use since time immemorial. The presence of several phenolic acids in bulbils as well as other parts of garlic is being reported for the first time.

Summary

Garlic has plethora of biologically active compounds including phenolic acids. This is the reason that it plays important roles in improving human health. Fresh garlic cloves, other parts and their different preparations contain several phenolic acids such as tannic, gallic, protocatechuic, ferulic, cinnamic, chlorogenic, o-Coumaric, caffeic, vanillic, gentisic, salicylic and oxalic acids. Maximum number and amount of phenolic acids were seen in garlic pickles followed by mature garlic clove, intact clove in vinegar, chopped clove in vinegar, one-and two-month-old leaves, bulb and sheath and minimum in roots and scales of garlic in varying amounts. Some of the phenolic acids are known as antioxidants besides having other therapeutic properties. The results of the present experiments show that clove fried in mustard oil has high amount of oxalic acid as a break down product, which is known for its harmful effects in human beings. Therefore, mustard oil fried garlic cloves should not be taken regularly. Crude extract and some active principles of Garlic are also antifungal and have been successfully used in plant disease control. The presence of several phenolic acids in bulbils and other parts of garlic is being reported for the first time.

NB

Data were collected from Recent Advances in Allium Research Published by Association of Allium Workers in India, Varanasi 2006.

Literature Cited

Agrios, G.N.1997. Plant Pathology, Academic Press, California.

Bors. W, Heller W, Michel C, Saran M. 1990. Flavonoids as antioxidants: Determination of radical-scavenging efficiencies, Meth Enzymol 186:343-355.

Bors W, Michel C, Stettmair K.2001. Structure- activity relationships governing antioxidant capacities of plant polyphenols. Methods Enzymol:335:166-180.

Bravo L 1998. Polyphenols: chemistry, dietary sources, metabolism, and nutritional significance. Nutr Rev 56:317-333.

Gharzouli K.Khennouf S, Amira S & Gharzouli A.1999. Effect of aqueous extracts from Quercus ilex L.root bark, Punica granatum I., fruit peel and Artimisia herba-alba Asso leaves on ethanol induced gastric damage in rats. Phytother.Res.13,42-45.

Harborne J.B.1989. Methods in plant biochemistry, I:Plant phenolics. Academic Press, London, UK

Harborne J.B.1993. The flavanoids: advances in research since 1986. Chapman & Hall, London, UK.

Inoue M.1995. Gallic acid found in Grape Seed Kills Cancer Cells. Biol Pharm Bull;;18:1526-1530.

Narbad, Arjan and Gasson, Michael J.1998. Metabolism of ferulic acid via vanillin using a novel CoA-dependent pathway in a newly isolated strain of Pseudomonas flourescens. Microbiology, 144:13971405 Printed in Great Britain

Prithiviraj. B, Singh, U.P.Singh, K.P.and K.Plank-Schumacher.1998. Field evaluation of ajoene, a constitutent of garlic (Allium sativum) and neemazal, a product of neem (Azadirachta indica) for the control of powdery mildew (Erysiphe pisi) of pea (Pisum sativum). J.PL. Dis.Prot.105:274-278.

Runkova L.V.Talieva M.N.1975.The distribution of phenolic compounds in the leaves of certain Allium spp.Dok.Akad.Nank SSSR.225:232-234.

Singh, U.P, Prithviraj, B,Sarma. B.K., Singh Mandavi and Ray.A.B.2001.Role of garlic (Allium sativum)in human and plant diseases. Indian J.Experimental Biol. 39:310-322.

Singh U.P., Sarma B.K., Singh D.P., Amar Bahadur.2002. Plant growth promoting rhizobacteria mediated induction of phenolics in pea (Pisum sativum) after infection with Erysiphepisi.Curr.Microbiol.44:396-400.

Singh. U.P., Pandey, V.N., Wagner.K.G. and K.P.Singh.1990.Antifungal activity of ajoene, a constitutent of garlic (Allium sativum L.) Can.J.Bot.68:1354-1356

Singh. U.P., Singh, D.P., Singh.M., Maurya.S, Srivastava.J.S., Singh.R.B. and S.P.Singh. 2004. Characterization of phenolic compounds in some Indian mango cultivars. Inter.J.Food Sciences and Nutrition.55(2):163-169.

Srivastava, J.S., Singh, D., Singh.U.P and K.G.Wagner. 2000. Differential sensitivity of rhizobial strains to ajoene, a constituent of garlic (Allium sativum L) New Agriculturist 11:1-4.

Uhl S.2000. Spices:Tools for alternative or complimentary medicine. Food Tech.54:61-65.

N.B. The School of Health Sciences of Kannur University honoured Dr.U.P.Singh with a Life Time Achievement Award for this work on 29th Nov. 2006.

5.2 Evaluation of the Nutritional Constituents of some Onion and Garlic Varieties

Dr. R.P. Gupta, S.R. Bhonde, K.J. Srivastava and D.K. Singh
National Horticultural Research and Development Foundation
Nasik – 422 011 (MS)
e-mail: nhrdf_nsk@sancharnet.in

Introduction

Onion and garlic are the important commercial vegetable and spice crops grown almost all over the country. Both these crops have seasonality in production but are required round the year for domestic as well as export purpose. Onion and garlic are indispensable item of every kitchen. These are the commodity of mass consumption and used by almost all the sections of the society in various ways due to its nutritive value, characteristic flavour, pungent taste and several medicinal properties.

The nutritive value of onion as well as garlic varies from variety to variety. The soil, climate, cultural practices, agro-techniques and nutrient application also have great influence on the chemical composition of the produce. A perusal of the literature reveals that the data on nutritional constituents on onion and garlic are virtually scanty and the parameters studied are limited pertaining to the quality attributes. In view of this, studies were undertaken at National Horticultural Research and Development Foundation (NHRDF), Nasik to assess the nutritional status of different onion and garlic varieties now commonly available and grown in the country by farmers.

Materials and Methods

The onion varieties viz- Agrifound Light Red, Agrifound Dark Red, Agrifound White, Arka Niketan, N-2-4-1, Pusa Red and Pusa Madhavi (Big onions), Arka Bindu and Agrifound Rose (Small onions) and Agrifound Red (Multiplier onion) were included in the study. The bulbs were produced at Regional Research Station, Nasik in a replicated field trial following standard agronomical practices and harvested at crop maturity.

Multiplier onion was obtained from NHRDF, Dindigul. After proper drying, curing and neck cutting, the bulbs were brought to the laboratory for chemical analysis.

The bulbs of garlic varieties viz- Agrifound White (G-41), Yamuna Safed (G-1), Yamuna Safed-2(G-50) and Yamuna Safed-3(G-282) were produced at Regional Research Station, Karnal, however, Agrifound Parvati (G-313) was grown at Karnal (Plain) as well as Kulla (Hill). After harvesting of bulbs, properly dried and cured garlic bulbs of each variety having uniform shape and size were brought to laboratory at Nasik for the analytical studies. The analytical studies were undertaken at 45 days after harvesting in onion while 60 days after harvesting in case of garlic. The bulbs for analytical studies were selected randomly in each variety from each replication in onion as well as garlic. In case of onion, the outer dried skin was removed and the neck and root portions were scooped out, while in garlic, the outer most dry skin (white papery sheath) was removed and all the cloves of the bulbs were separated and peeled out.

For the determination of moisture contents, dry matter and drying ratio, the onion and garlic samples were cut into small pieces, weighed and oven dried at $60 \pm 2^{o}C$ till constant weight, drying ratio was calculated following the method suggested by Creuss (1958). Total Soluble Solids were determined from the onion and garlic juice directly using the hand refractometer. Reducing sugar, non reducing sugar and total sugar contents were estimated as per the standard procedure prescribed by Lane and Eynon (1923). The pyruvic acid contents were measured by adopting the method of Hart and Fisher (1971). The reconstitution (rehydration) ratio was calculated as per the method followed by Anon (1944). Non-enzymatic browning was observed spectrophotometrically. Protein, Sulphur, potassium, Nitrogen, Calcium, Magnesium, Asscorbic acid, Total ash, Crude fat, Sodium, phosphorus, Copper, Iron and Chlorine were determined as per the standard methods described by Ranganna (1986). Each analysis was replicated thrice. The data obtained were scrutinized statistically and are presented in Tables 1 and 2 for onion and garlic, respectively.

Results and Discussion

Onion

The data obtained revealed that all the chemical constituents exhibited significant variation among the varieties studied. Significantly lowest moisture content (78.32%) and highest total soluble (19.50%) and dry matter (21.68%) were recorded in the variety Agrifound Red (multiplier onion) and the moisture content and total soluble solids were found at par in the variety Agrifound Rose (small onion). The moisture contents of a food commodity is a very important factor and determines the shelf life to a large extent. Total soluble solid is an important quality criteria for onions and also contributes towards the flavour (Sharma et. at. 1996). Total soluble solids in onions have been found to form the bulk of dry matter and both these values are correlated (Verma et. al. 2003). About 80% of onion dry matter consists of non-structural carbohydrates (Darbyshise and Henry, 1981). The prominent carbohydrates are glucose, fructose, sucrose and low molecular weight fructons, while starch and raffinose are absent (Benkeblia et. al. 2002). The varieties with higher TSS and dry matter content are considered suitable for dehydration (Verma et. al. 2003; Singh et. al. 2004).

The variety Agrifound Red performed significantly superior in drying ratio (5.75:1) and reconstitution ratio (1:5.76) while the reconstitution ratio was found at par in the variety Agrifound white (big onion, white coloured) and Agrifound Rose (small onion). Drying ratio is commercially an important criterion in onion dehydration as it mainly decides the economics of processing while the rehydration ratio is also an important trait in dehydrated products (Singh and Kumar, 1984) and the values are crucial when the dehydrated product is used for cooking etc. (Singh et. al. 2005).

The sugar contents of onion are major chemical constituents of onion. In browning/discolouration of dehydrated onion, sugar play an important role (Singh and Kumar. 1984). The reducing sugar was found to range from 0.96 to 4.79% (Agrifound Rose and Agrifound White) while non reducing sugar between 5.32 and 11.45% (Pusa Madhvi and Agrifound Rose) and total sugar from 7.64 to 12.61% (Pusa Madhavi and Arka Bindu). This wide variation in constituents among varieties for sugar leaves scope for choosing the variety as per the need and preference. Lowest reducing sugar to non-reducing sugar ratio in onion is considered beneficial to minimize the browning/discolouration (Verma et. al. 2003, Singh et. al. 2004). The ratio between reducing sugars and total sugars is considered as best characters for dehydration in onion (Singh et. al. 2005). The pyruvic acid contents was recorded significantly highest in Arka Bindu (14.93 μ mole/g fresh tissue) followed by Agrifound White (12.00 μ mole/g fresh tissue). According to Singh and Kumar (1984) a high amount of pungency in fresh onion is considered an important criteria for dehydration.

Pyruvic acid content determines the quality of products and highest contents are desirable for high degree of pungency and also essential to retain better flavour in dehydrated products (Singh et. al. 2005). The non-enzymatic browning (NEB) in fresh onion bulbs ranged from 0.027 to 0.150, while in dehydrated product between 0.050 and 0.390. In fresh bulb it was recorded lowest in Agrifound Rose whereas in dehydrated product it was found lowest in Agrifound white and highest in Agrifound Rose.

The lowest in NEB in onion is considered better to minimize the discolouration (Kapur et. al. 1976). The protein content was recorded significantly highest in Agrifound Rose (2.32%) followed by Agrifound Red (2.22%). Significantly highest sulphur (154.65 mg/100g), crude fat (0.17%) and phosphorus (115.66 mg/100 g) were recorded in Agrifound Red. The crude fat was found at par in all the varieties studied.

Significantly highest nitrogen (372.10 mg/100g), ascorbic acid (66.84 mg/100g) and total ash (0.78%) were recorded in Agrifound Rose. The calcium content was recorded significantly highest in Agrifound Light Red (115.33 mg/100g) which was found at par with Pusa Red. The variety Pusa Red recorded significantly highest magnesium (33.60 mg/100g) and was at par with Arka Niketan and Pusa Madhvi.

Significantly highest sodium content was observed in Agrifound White (9.21 mg/100g) while iron (4.29 mg/100g) and chlorine (52.59 mg/100g) were recorded in Arka Niketan where chlorine was found at par in the variety N-2-4-1. The copper content was recorded significantly highest in the onion variety Agrifound Dark Red (2.03 mg/100g). Some aspects of the data are presented in Table 1.

Garlic

The data obtained revealed significant variation in all the parameters and constituents among the varieties studied. Moisture content is an important factor and play crucial role in storage. The total soluble solids is an important quality parameter for garlic and contributes towards flavour. The total soluble solids in garlic have been found to form the bulk of the dry matter and both these values are correlated (Bara et. al. 1994).

According to Pandey et. al. (2003) the higher contents of TSS and dry matter with low moisture are considered beneficial for storage purpose in garlic. Significantly lowest moisture content (56.28%) and highest total soluble solids (42.00%) and dry matter contents (43.72%) were recorded in the variety Yamuna Safed-2 while moisture and dry matter contents were found at par in the variety Yamuna Safed.

The garlic varieties having higher TSS and drymatter are considered best for dehydration purpose. The pyruvic acid content determines the quality of products and are desirable for high degree of pungency and also essential to retain better flavor in dehydrated product (Singh and Gupta, 2002) and it was recorded significantly highest (29.46 μ mole/g) in garlic variety Yamuna Safed. Significantly highest potassium (534.33 mg/100g), calcium (42.64 mg/100g), total ash (1.71%) and iron (4.62 mg/100g) were also recorded in the garlic variety Yamuna Safed.

The garlic variety Agrifound White recorded significantly highest nitrogen (1.45%) and protein (9.06%), whereas highest variety Yamuna Safed-2 recorded the highest value for TSS and Phosphorus and the variety Agrifound Parvati (plain grown) showed least of them. Significantly highest sulphur (85.69 mg/100g), magnesium (22.22 mg/100g), ascorbic acid (10.26 mg/100g), crude fat (10.28%), sodium (138.00 mg/100g) and copper (0.17 m/100g) were recorded in the garlic variety Yamuna Safed-3 while the ascorbic content was at par in variety Agrifound White and copper in variety Agrifound Parvati (plain grown).

Variations in various chemical constituents of different garlic varieties/genotypes were recorded by earlier workers also (Shobahalan and Arunugam, 1991; Brar et. al. 1994; Bhatt et. al. 1998; Chhokar et. al. 2000, Sood et. al. 2000 and Agarwal and Tiwari, 2003). Some aspects of the data are presented in Table 2

Conclusion

The studies on nutritional constituents of onion and garlic revealed that the onion variety agrifound Red (multiplier onion), Agrifound Rose and Arka Bindu (small onion) are better for the nutritional constituents than big onion varieties. Among the garlic varieties, the variety Yamuna Safed, Yamuna Safed-2 and Yamuna Safed-3 were found nutritionally more rich than other varieties studied.

Table 1 Analysis of important Nutritional constituents of different onion varieties. Ascorbic acid and Elements are expressed as mg/100g.

Onion variety	Total soluble solid (TSS)%	Reducing sugar%	Non reducing sugar %	Pyruvic acid (µmol/g)	NEB (Bulbs)	Cu^{2+}	Protein %	Sulfur	Phosph	Potassium	Fe^{2+}	Ca^{2+z}	Mg^{2+}	Ascorbic acid
Agrifound Light Red	13.0	3.52	8.01	12.2	0.07	1.8	1.32	17.9	25.5	114.8	3.3	115.3	17.5	22.7
Agrifound Dark Red	12.0	2.61	9.12	10.07	0.12	2.0*	1.48*	21.2	30.3	124.5	3.2	55.4	22.4	41.7
Agrifound White	13.5	4.79	6.56	12.00	0.04	0.33	1.31	69.5	66.9	115.8	0.9	46.7	16.4	24.3
Agrifound Rose	19.33	0.96	11.45	10.27	0.15	0.73	2.32*	97.6	80.3	208.2	2.7	66.1	18.1	66.8
Agrifound Red	19.50*	1.13	11.00	10.13	0.13	1.8	2.22	154.6*	115.7*	229.9*	1.8	71.7	22.7	56.7
Arka Bindu	15.67	2.21	10.40	14.93*	0.05	0.9	1.17	88.9	26.6	152.8	4.1	108.9	28.8*	14.4
Pusa Red	13.00	2.66	8.17	11.20	0.03+	1.7	1.33	60.9	18.3	101.1	3.3	113.1	33.6	13.2

- These values are quite good and highest also.

+ Non enzymatic browning (NEB) should be lowest to minimize discolouration

Table 1 Analysis of important Nutritional constituents of different onion varieties. Ascorbic acid and Elements are expressed as mg/100g.

Onion variety	Total soluble solid (TSS)%	Reducing sugar%	Non reducing sugar %	Pyruvic acid (µmol/g)	NEB (Bulbs)	Cu^{2+}	Protein %	Sulfur	Phosph	Potassium	Fe^{2+}	Ca^{2+} z	Mg^{2+}	Ascorbic acid
Agrifound Light Red	13.0	3.52	8.01	12.2	0.07	1.8	1.32	17.9	25.5	114.8	3.3	115.3	17.5	22.7
Agrifound Dark Red	12.0	2.61	9.12	10.07	0.12	2.0*	1.48*	21.2	30.3	124.5	3.2	55.4	22.4	41.7
Agrifound White	13.5	4.79	6.56	12.00	0.04	0.33	1.31	69.5	66.9	115.8	0.9	46.7	16.4	24.3
Agrifound Rose	19.33	0.96	11.45	10.27	0.15	0.73	2.32*	97.6	80.3	208.2	2.7	66.1	18.1	66.8
Agrifound Red	19.50*	1.13	11.00	10.13	0.13	1.8	2.22	154.6*	115.7*	229.9*	1.8	71.7	22.7	56.7
Arka Bindu	15.67	2.21	10.40	14.93*	0.05	0.9	1.17	88.9	26.6	152.8	4.1	108.9	28.8*	14.4
Pusa Red	13.00	2.66	8.17	11.20	0.03+	1.7	1.33	60.9	18.3	101.1	3.3	113.1	33.6	13.2

- These values are quite good and highest also.

References

Agarwal, A, and Tiwari.R.S.(2003): Physico chemical characterization of sixteen Germplasm lines of garlic (Allium sativum L.) Approaches for Sustainable Development of Onion and Garlic. Proc. Nat.Symp. on Onion-Garlic: Production and Post Harvest Management-Challenges and Strategies pp.90-94.

Anon (1944): Vegetable and fruit dehydration. U.P. Deptt. Agril., Misc. Publi., 540.

Benkeblia.N; Varoquaux.P., Shiomi N and Sahai.H. (2002): Storage technology of onion blubs C.V. Rouge Amporta: Effects of irradiation, maleic hydrazide carbamate isopropyl, N-phenyl (CIP) on respiration rate and carbohydrates. Int.J.Food Sci Technol. 37:169-175.

Bhat.R.P., Biswas, V.R. and Kumar N.C. (1998): A note on physicochemical characteristics of some genotypes of garlic. Veg.Sci.25: 95-96.

Brar.P.S., Gill, S.P.S. and Sandhu. K.S. (1994): Studies on the physicochemical characteristics of selected varieties of garlic. Haryana J Hort Sci. 23: 173-175.

Chhokar.V: Sood. D.R. and Gupta R.P. (2000): Studies on some biochemical constituents of garlic cloves arranged in different rings. Papers and abstracts – Nat. Sump. On Onion and Garlic – Production and Post Harvest Managements – Challenges and Strategies, Nasic, Nov 19-21 pp .48.

Creuss N.V. (1958): Commercial fruits and vegetables products. M.C.Grow Hill Book Company, Inc. New York.

Darbyshire. B and Henry R.J. (1981): Differences in fructon content and synthesis in some Allium species. New Phytol. 87 : 249-256.

Hart.F.L. and Fisher. H.J.(1971) Modern Food Analysis. Springeruer long Berlin, Neidelberg, New York 432.

Kapur.K.L, Gard. R.C. and Tripathi. M. Preliminary studies on screening of onion varieties for dehydration prog.hort., 7:77.

Lane.J.H. and Eynon, 1. (1923): Determination of sugar. J. Soc.Chem.Ind., 42 and 32T.

Pandey.U.B., Singh, L., Singh.D.K. and Pandey.J.P.N (2003) : Studies on the physico-chemical characteristics of different garlic varieties. NHRDF News Letter, Vol.XXIII(2): 9-12.

Ranganna.S., (1986): Analysis and quality control for fruit and vegetable products. Tata Mc Grow Hill Publishing Company Limited, New Delhi.

Shobhalan and Arumugam.R (1991): Chemical changes in the quality parameter of garlic (Allium sativum L.) during growth and development. South Indian Hort., 39:93.

Singh.D.K., Bhonda.S.R. and Pandey, U.B. (2004): Studies on screening of white onion varieties for dehydration qualities. Proce.of Nat. Seminar on 'New Perspective in Spices, Medicinal and Aromatic Plants' Eds. Korikanthimath et al.pp.181-183.

Singh.D.K., Bhonde.S.R., and Pandey U.B. (2005): Composition of white onion varieties for their qualities for processing by dehydration. Diversification of Agriculture through Horticultural Crops. Pp.291-295.

Singh.D.K, and Gupta.R.P. (2002): Studies on the dehydration qualities of garlic lines. NHRDF News Letter. Vol.XXII(2) : 7-10

Sood.D.R., Chhokar.V. and Singh J(2000): Studies on growth, pungency and flavour characteristics of five varieties of garlic (Allium sativum .L) bulbs during development. Veg.Sci 27(2):180-184.

Verma. L.R. Pandey. U.B. and Srivastava.K.J. (2003): Screening of white onion varieties for processing. Approaches for Sustainable Development of Onion and Garlic-Proc. Nat. Symp. On Onion-Garlic: Production and Post Harvest Management Challenges and Strategies.pp. 122-128.

A Survey on Food Consumption Pattern by people

Conducted by Naufal K.K., Faizal P. Jeena Antony, Sreejith, Priyanka Kavitha, Sumesh and Dr. K.T. Augusti, SHS Kannur University

A survey conducted by the Editors and students among more than thousand people across Kerala showed a pattern of staple diet with vegetables, spices, drinks, fish, and meat consumption as follows:

1. **Various preparations of Rice > Wheat > Cassava (Tapioca).**
2. **Potato > Plantains >Tubers like yams > Amaranthus > Cabbage > Ladies finger > Bringel > Tomato > Carrot > Drum stick > Mango > Bitter gourd > Pumkins > Pappaya > Lime > Amla (goose berries) > Orange and other fruits very rarely.**
3. **Curry leaves > Red pepper > Green pepper > Turmeric > Onion > Garlic > Asafoetida > Ginger> Black pepper > Cardamom > Cumin etc.**
4. **Tea >Coffee > Juices > Alcohol > Milk**
5. **Fish > Eggs > Meat > Mollusk etc.**

5.3 Role of Allium Compounds (Onion and Garlic) in the Prevention of Diseases, recent Findings are Reviewed

Dr. P.K. Joseph*

Former Professor of Medical Biochemistry, St. John's Medical College, Bangalore and

Dr. K.T. Augusti**

Rtd. Professor of Biochemistry, Kerala University, Thiruvananthapuram.

Recent human population studies suggest that regular consumption of Allium plant products lowers the risk of developing heart disease and cancer[1]. More than 2000 scientific papers have been published through the year 2000 itself on scientific research on the chemistry, pharmacology and clinical use of garlic[2]. After 2000 more than 300 papers were published in this field. Each of them describes one or more biological properties of Allium such as antidiabetic, antibiotic, anticoagulant, antiatherogenic, antihyperlipidemic, antihypertensive and anticarcinogenic activities. Many Reviews on these aspects were also written by various people[3-5]. In view of the widespread consumption of Alliums as fresh plants, as well as supplements, the biological activity of these plants is of great current interest.

Chemistry

Onions are rich in two groups of antioxidants viz: the flavonoids, eg. quercetin and the alkyl or alkenyl cysteine sulfoxides e.g. Methyl and Propenyl cysteine sulfoxides. A second type of flavonoids viz: anthocyanins are also present in onions and they give red/purple colors to onions. Quercetin and its derivatives impart yellow and brown colors to the onions. The enzyme alliinase generates the characteristic odour and taste of onion, various allicins type compounds and the unique lachrymatory factor, propane thial S-oxide ($CH_3CH_2CH=S=O$). The various allicins of onion and garlic are represented by the formula R-S-S-(O)-R where R = CH_3 / C_3H_5 / C_3H_7 etc. In onion allicin type compounds are converted to cepaenes (similar to ajoene) and Zwie belanes.

* Presently Prof of Med. Biochemistry. L.F. Inst. Med. Sci. & Research, Angamaly, Kerala and

** Research Prof of Med. Biochemistry, Thalassery Campus of Kannur University.

Alliums and Related Compounds

In the case of garlic, the major sulfoxide aminoacid is alliin or S- allylcysteine sulfoxide (C_3H_5-S(O).CH_2.CH(NH_2)COOH). When garlic is crushed the enzyme alliinase is released and converts alliin to allicin with release of ammonia and pyruvic acid (See reaction in this book P. 243). Allicin in turn is rearranged to other compounds on storage, viz: ajoene[6] as well as diallyl disulfide (DADS), trisulfide (DADT) and tetra sulfide (DATTS) and vinyldithiins[7].

Ajoene is an oligomeric form of allicin i.e. C_3H_5-S(O)-C_3H_4-S-S-C_3H_5. Diallyl polysulfides have the general formula $C_3H_5(S)nC_3H_5$. Vinyldithiins are sulfur containing ringed structures which give flavour to fried preparations of onions and garlic. All of them possess various biological actions such as hypocholesterolemic, antiplatelet aggregration effects etc[3].

Alliums are Rich Sources of the Antioxidant-Se

When allium plants are grown in selenium rich soil, sulphur in cysteine is replaced by Se and thereby Se-methyl Selenocysteine CH_3Se CH_2. CH(NH_2)COOH, its gamma glutamyl derivative and Selenoprotein are produced[8,9]. For details refer Alliums Chemistry by Block[10]. Se and its conjugates have antioxidant and anticancer activity[8].

Major forms of dietary supplements include aged garlic extract, dehydrated preparations, distilled oil and oil macerates. In addition to the small molecular weight sulphur compounds, garlic contains a biologically active protein also. Antifungal[11], hypolipidemic[12] and immunostimulatory[13] effects are ascribed to garlic protein by different workers. There is a recent view that only fresh garlic products such as allicin and its derivatives have a definite biologically significant action such as hypotensive and hypocholesterolemic effect. ***WHO is a promoter of these aspects with relation to garlic and its use. WHO advises people to use 4-5 fresh cloves of garlic daily to prevent essential hypertension***

Garlic is a Panacea for Many Diseases.

Antitumor, antimicrobial, antiplatelet, antithrombotic, hypolipidemic, hypotensive, and antiasthmatic effects as well as immunostimulatory properties are attributed to garlic and other alliums. Consumption of garlic and other alliums along with food in minimal doses (10-15g/day) is said to reduce cancer risk including prostate cancer[14,15].

Anticarcinogenic Activity

Among garlic users an average reduction by 30% in colorectal and by 50% in stomach cancer with a trend towards reduction in prostrate, breast and laryngeal cancers was reported[1].

Laboratory studies on animals show that compounds in garlic inhibit tumor cell metabolism as well as the initiation and promotion of tumor and alter immune responses. For example studies using cell cultures suggest that pure components found in crushed garlic and its oil inhibit cell division and have antimutagenic properties. DADS at a concentration of 263-2630 ppm inhibits the growth of the human breast cancer cells[16]. In another study Selenium enriched garlic given in the diet to female rats at the level of 3 ppm for one and a half months reduced the incidence of carcinogen induced mammary tumors to the extent of 66-70% compared to the control rats. These experiments demonstrate that Se enriched garlic has cancer preventive effects[8,17].

Mechanism of Action of Allium Principles

The anticancer effects of garlic are interpreted by Eric Block[1] as follows: They are likely due to the induction of garlic organosulphur and Se compounds on phase II carcinogen detoxification enzymes, such as *glutathione S-transferase and quinone reductase* in liver and other organs[18-22]. Munday et. al.[20-22] found that onion organosulfur compounds have more or less similar actions to that of garlic. The ability of allicin to react rapidly with free radicals together with its remarkable ability to cross through membranes including those in human red blood cells may also contribute to its antioxidant and anticancer activity[23,24]. Ajoene is reported to possess antiinflammatory activity similar to that of the non-steroidal anti inflammatory drug indomethacin[25]. The anticancer activity of Se enriched garlic can be attributed to the presence of analogs of various garlic sulphur compounds, such as the cysteine derivatives, in which the essential mineral Se replaces sulphur[8,17]. Further allicin induces apoptosis of cancer cells and inhibits the growth of cancer cells of murine and human origin. *Allicin induces the formation of apoptotic bodies, nuclear condensation and a DNA ladder in cancer cells. Activation of caspases-3, -8 and -9 and cleavage of poly (ADP-ribose) polymerase were induced by allicin.* These results provide a mechanistic basis for the antiproliferative effects of allicin and similar compounds in garlic extracts[25]. Antitumor activity of ajoene, particularly the Z-isomer toward human leukemia cells is thought to be associated with its apoptosis inducing effect and activation of caspase – 3 and– 8[26-28]. The anticancer activities of Z-ajoene *in vitro* and *in vivo* were demonstrated against a panel of human tumor cell lines with IC (50) values varying from 5.2 mM to 26.1 mM and at a lower extent in normal marsupial kidney cells.

Garlic oil, DADS & DATS

Garlic oil and its constituents DADS and DATS and bis (1-propenyl) sulfide *are potent inducers of the phase II enzymes quinone reductase and glutathione reductase and S-transferase in rat tissues*[20,29]. DADS and

DATS modulate cytocrome P4501 mediated bio-activation of benzo (a) pyrene in human hepatoma cells, providing a possible explanation for the known protective effect of allyl sulfides on B(a)P-induced carcinogenesis[30]. Diallyl sulfide (DAS), sulfoxide and sulfone reduce the incidence of a multitude of chemically induced tumors in animal models[1]. These compounds are competitive inhibitors of P(450)2E1, diallyl sulfone is also a suicide inhibitor of this cytochrome[31]. It is perhaps significant that allyl methyl sulfone (C_3H_5-$S(O_2)CH_3$) is the ultimate metabolite of DADS, so the possibility exists that the former compound is also an inhibitor of the above cytochrome. It is possible that DADS may be metabolized *in vivo* to its monomethyl analogue and that in turn being converted to allyl methyl sulfone. The impediment of phase 1 activation of various carcinogens due to organosulfur compounds is hypothesized to explain the reduction in tumor incidence.

Balasenthil et. al.[32] carried out several experiments to show the protective effects of garlic extracts and a component in it, viz; S- allyl cysteine[33] against 7,12 – dimethyl benz(a) anthracene (DMBA) – induced hamster buccal pouch carcinoma. After 1½ months DMBA treatment tumor bearing animals showed significantly enhanced level of lipid peroxidation and significantly decreased levels of GSH and vitamins C&E in their plasma and erythrocytes. Administration of aqueous garlic extract, 250mg/kg body weight thrice a week to DMBA treated hamsters ameliorated these conditions, i.e. lipid peroxidation was significantly decreased and the levels of GSH, GPX and vitamins C & E were increased significantly in the plasma and erythrocytes. The incidence of oral neoplasms in the DMBA treated group was 100%, where as in garlic treated group it was only in preneoplastic stage. It was further suggested that the processes of carcinogenesis was inhibited by the garlic principles by apoptosis. In yet another experiment the above team of workers showed that S-allyl cysteine a component of garlic at a dose of 200 mg/kg prevented carcinogenesis in hamsters subjected to DMBA treatment. The mechanism of action of SAC is probably through apoptosis of tumor cells. Work by others also supported the anti-carcinogenic action of SAC/ Ajoene etc in cancer cell line treated animals. These sulphur compounds particularly their sulfoxides are strong antioxidants too[5].

Antibiotic Activity of Garlic Compound

It has been reviewed by Harris et. al.[34] Allicin and similar thiusulfinates, as well as ajoene and related compounds in macerated garlic have a variety of antimicrobial activity[35-37]. In laboratary cell cultures garlic oil and its components diallyl polysulfides show antibacterial activity against multidrug resistant strains of E. Coli and possess antifungal activity against candida albicans with the magnitude of activity of the diallyl polysulfides[38] following the order of DATTS >DATS > DADS > DAS.

Russians used allicin widely when penicillin was on shortage there to cure wounds from various infections. Therefore it earned the name as **"Russian penicillin"**. Allicin has antiparasitic activity against some major human intestinal protozoan parasites including Entamoeba histolytica and giardia[39]. All garlic compounds show substantial activity against the bacteria Helicobacter pylori which causes chronic gastritis and ulcers in the stomach and upper part of the intestine. H. Pylori infection is a major stomach cancer risk factor and garlic has been shown to kill this organism[40]. Allicin may combine with glutathione to form an adduct which itself can function as an antioxidant and protective agent[24]. Allicin is more active than its break down products such as DADS or a mixture of A(S)nA/A(S)nM. in garlic oil, but similar in activity to DATTS a minor component of distilled garlic oil[41]. Oil-macerated garlic constituents are also active against H.Pylori[42]. The mechanism of action of garlic compounds is most likely their binding to -SH groups in enzymes essential to microbial proliferation, thus inhibiting their growth[43]. Allicin and related allyl methyl thiosulfinate inhibit the in vitro growth of E. coli[44] and H. Pylori[45]. Ajoene at concentrations of 82 ppm prevents replication of the immunodeficiency virus (HIV-1)[46].

Garlic is reported to be more effective than penicillin against typhus disease and work well against strep, staph bacteria and the organisms responsible for cholera, dysentery and enteritis. The irritation quality of garlic oil explain its use for respiratory problems by opening up lungs and bronchial tubes (http://www.go – symmetry .com/garlic.htm)

The distilled oils of garlic and onion and their constituent sulfides with three or more sulfur atoms are potent inhibitors of yeast growth. The oils and their constituent sulfides were only very weakly anti bacterial showing minimal inhibitory concentrations (MIC s) of greater than 300 ppm for most of the bacteria tested[47]. Ajoene has an anti proliferative and leishmaniadal effect on various leishmania species and is useful in the treatment of tinea pedis[48,49].

Antiplatelet, Antiatherogenic and Fibrinolytic Actions of Alliums

Allicin and related sulfur containing compounds (thiosulfinates) are implicated as a principal source of the antiplatelet property of garlic juice and are significantly more potent platelet inhibitor than aspirin at nearly equivalent concentrations[50]. They inhibit platelet aggregation and micro particle shedding at a calpin-dependent step[51]. Ajoene also inhibits platelet aggregation in baboon[52] and prevents the development of microangiopathy and thrombotic disorders seen in primates injured with pig cells[53]. Ajoene is thought to prevent blood clotting by selectively blocking the binding of fibrinogen to platelets. This is the crucial step in platelet-platelet interactions leadings to blood clotting[54].

The antiatherogenic actions of garlic may be related to its inhibitory influence on geranyl geranyl transferase I (GGTase I)[55]. DATS a breakdown product of allicin shows antiplatelet activity and inhibits formation of thromboxane[56]. Allyl methyl trisulfide inhibits the arachidonic acid cascade at the reaction site with PGH synthase and specifically inhibits the conversion of PGG2 to PGH2[57]. Onion juice inhibits platelet-mediated thrombosis in dogs[58]. Welsh onion extract inhibits platelet function in vitro while boiled extract activates platelets[59]. With fresh onion extract, induction of an inhibition in platelet aggregation followed by less action was observed in 30 minutes period, while aged extract of onion showed a better platelet inhibition[60]. Augusti et. al.[61] observed an increase in blood fibrinolysis of human volunteers who consumed 125 mg onion oil or cycloallicin. The latter is a cyclic aminoacid formed from propenyl cysteine sulphoxide and isolated from onions. Bordia et. al.[56,62] also observed an enhacement in blood fibrinolysis of human volunteers i.e. normal people as well as CHD patients who consumed garlic oil-equivalent to that in one gram cloves.

Hypolipidemic and Hypotensive Activities of Onion and Garlic

Garlic has the ability to relax vascular smooth muscle[63] and ameliorate hypoxic pulmonary vasoconstriction due to high altitude sickness[64]. *An in vitro experiment using isolated blood vessel demonstrated that aqueous extract of garlic inhibits calcium binding to proteoheparan sulfate receptor, which in turn blocks the interaction of calcium with LDL. This property of garlic prevents calcium dependent generation of atherosclerotic plaque.* It was also observed that the addition of HDL and garlic extract caused freshly, formed nanoplaques to dissolve[65]. Preventive effects of garlic on cardiovascular disease has been reviewed by Gardner et. al.[66] and Banerjee and Maulik[67]. One of the conditions in which garlic treatment brings the fastest and clearly measurable improvements is hypertension. Dr.F.G.Piotrowski of the University of Geneva used garlic on patients with abnormally high blood pressure. *The study revealed that garlic treatment brought "excellent results". Garlic has a dilating effect on blood vessels, thereby it reduces B.P.* (http://www.go-symmetry.com/garlic.htm). Work of Augusti, Joseph and their teams showed the hypolipidemic effects of garlic and onion oils in laboratory animals[5].

Mechanism of Actions

The ability of garlic to reduce blood cholesterol levels is attributed to the effect of allicin on a key enzyme, HMGCoA reductase, involved in cholesterol synthesis in the liver[68,69] Allicin decreases formation of fatty streaks leading to plaque formation in mice fed a cholesterol rich diet[70].

The effect of garlic and allicin to elicit a NO – dependent relaxation in a pulmonary artery isolated from rats, is proposed to be mediated via garlic activation of NO formation rather its stabilization[71,72]. A similar effect is proposed for the antihypertensive effect of onion in spontaneously hypertensive rats[73].

Ajoene and Thiosulfinates

Ajoene inhibits cholesterol biosynthesis by affecting HMGCoA reductase and late enzymatic steps of the mevalonate (MVA) pathway. Mevalonate constitutes the precursor not only of cholesterol, but also of a number of intermediary isoprenoids such as farnesyl and geranyl groups. Covalent attachment of these isoprenoid groups (prenylation) is a required function of several proteins that regulate cell proliferation. Ajoene has been shown to interfere with protein prenylation, an affect that may contribute to its inhibition of smooth muscle cell proliferation[74]. Allicin, methyl allyl and allyl methyl thiosulfinates are more effective inhibitors against geranyl geranyl protein transferase (GGPT) than against farnesyl protein transferase.

Garlic Therapy

Short term garlic therapy in adults with mild hypercholesterolemia was shown to affect neither lipid levels nor various psychopathologic parameters[75]. In one of our studies[76] when aqueous extract of 10 g garlic per day was administered to adults with hypercholesterolemia for two months their cholesterol level was lowered by 28%. In a third study[77], in hypercholesterolemic patients using an enteric coated garlic supplement equivalent to 9.6 mg allicin releasing potential, only a 4-6% cholesterol was lowered during 3 months study. From these experiments it is evident that the effect could be observe only with a higher dose of garlic i.e. equivalent for 25mg allicin /adult/day. WHO recommends to eat 4-5 cloves of fresh garlic daily to reduce hypertension.

Antioxidant and Antidiabetic Actions

Banerjee et. al.[78] has reviewed the antioxidant activity of garlic. Various allium – derived sulfur compounds showed antioxidative activity inhibiting lipid hydroperoxide (LOOH) formation in human LDL[79]. Allicin of garlic is a better antioxidant than corresponding (allicin type) compounds in onion e.g. C_3H_7-S-S(O)-C_3H_7. Unsaturated allyl group in allicin may be responsible for a better activity as against a saturated propyl group in the onion compound. Further di and poly sulfides present in garlic and onion oils are good in capturing electrons and neutralizing free radicals like $OH^{\bullet}$ by a mechanism proposed by Klanns-Dieter[80].

$2RSS(O)R + e^{-}aq \rightarrow RSSR^{\bullet -} + RSS(O_2)R$ 1

$RSSR^{\bullet -} \rightarrow RS^{\bullet} + RS^{-}$ (Free and stable radicals) 2

$RS^{-} + OH^{\bullet} - RS^{\bullet} + OH^{-}$ (Free and stable radicals) 3

$RS^{\bullet} + RS^{\bullet} \rightarrow RSSR$ (Stable radicals) 4

$RSSR + e^{-} \rightarrow RSSR^{\bullet -}$ (Free radicals) 5

And the cycle is repeated and this may account for the antioxidant action of all di and poly sulfide allium compounds. They may also act as insulin secretagogues[81] and release insulin from the pancreas of both normal and alloxan/streptozotocin diabetic animals, which have some functional beta cells. Dava Farva et. al.[82] found that daily administration of garlic oil (100mg/kg/day) to moderate streptozotocin diabetic rats for two months significantly decreased their blood sugar, cholesterol and triacylglycerol in serum and the latter two in liver also. Recently in yet another study Paramesha and Kasinath[83] demonstrated the anti diabetic action of both garlic and onion oils extracted by hexane and fed to alloxan diabetic rats. The former shared far better results in reversing blood sugar level and regenerating the pancreatic beta cells. A synthetic compound diaceto dibutyl disulfide (DADBDS) prepared by Joseph and Kasinath[84] was also tested on the diabetic rats. It was found to be less active than onion oil in the control of blood parameters. It has an advantage that it is free of the obnoxious smell of alliums oils. This compound at a dose of 100mg/kg/day showed significant hypoglycemic and hypercholesterolemic effects in rats fed ethanol (30ml 30%/kg/day) for 45days and it showed no toxicity.

Immune Modulation

The immune stimulatory effect of allicin is mediated by redox-sensitive signaling such as activation of p21(ras). The antitumor effect of allicin is likely related to its immune stimulatory properties[85]. Allicin down regulates T cell functions which explains the beneficial role of it where T cells play an important role. These observations suggest that allicin may be used therapeutically with chronic inflammatory disease[86]. Ajoene shows antiinflammatory activity similar to that of the non-steroidal anti inflammatory drug indomethacin[87]. Work of Girija et. al. given in this volume explains the role of garlic as an immunomodulator.

Hepatic Detoxification Systems

The modulatory effect of garlic oil on hepatic drug metabolizing enzymes can be attributed to the components in the oil viz; DAS, DADS and DATS. They vary in modulatory activity and this variation is related to the number of sulfur atoms in the molecule. The polysulfides also increased glutathione

S-transferase (GST) activity and at the same time lowered N-nitrosodimethylamine.demethylase activity[88]. Allyl sulfides or whole garlic oil and its non polar fraction have been found to protect against liver damage by carbon tetra chloride by Fukas et. al.[89] and Augusti et. al.[90] respectively. According to the work of Hattori et. al.[91] ajoene protects liver from injury by acetaminophen. Work by the authors of this article showed that allium oils or extracts could protect animals from the deleterious effects of sucrose, high fat diet and alcohol[92,93] as well as nicotine[94] and lead toxicity[95]. Garlic flavoured drinks like beer may be suggested as a medicine to prevent obesity and related diseases.

How to Consume Garlic and What Quantity

Ayurvedic physicians suggest that it should not be eaten before breakfast. They as well as Dr. Arun Bordia, a pioneer in garlic research and a Rtd. Cardiologist from Udaipur advice to consume garlic after homogenizing it with very little water and then mixing it with enough boiled milk. As WHO recommends, 3-5 cloves of garlic are enough for any body/day according to each one's choice. Taking garlic with food shall avoid stomach irritation. A homogenate of ginger and garlic in 1:4 by weight along with little black pepper and salt is good and tasty. Everybody may use half a teaspoon daily along with food to drive away all viral fevers. People who are allergic to garlic or anaemic or those who are on the use of anticoagulants may not use garlic. Regular use of garlic, ginger, black pepper preparation (4:1:0.25 ratio) helped a lot of author's students at Kottayam and Kannur to prevent viral fevers that occurred in Kerala during 2006-2007. It cured its after effects like edema and joint pains in many of their viral fever infected countrymen also.

Garlic is five in one

1. Reduces harmful LDL cholesterol and triglycerides that causes CHD.
2. Reduces blood clotting by preventing clumping of blood platelets (better than aspirin)
3. Blocks the ability of chemical carcinogens to transform normal cells into cancer cells.
4. Stimulate various immunological factors that may help combat cancer and infections.
5. Protect cells against damage by oxidizing agents and heavy metals. (http://www.go-symmetry.com/garlic. htm)

How Good are the Spices to Prevent Cancer?

Drs. R.Kuttan and M.C.Unnikrishnan carried out some experiments[96] at Amala cancer Res. Centre Trichur to find out the preventive effects of garlic, ginger, pippali, black pepper, asafoetida, mustard, horsegrame and sesame against cancer. They assessed the tumor reducing activity of these spices in experimentally implanted tumors. There was a significant increase in lifespan of mice treated with the extracts of black pepper, pippali, garlic and asafoetida. Garlic and asafoetida were not only found to increase the lifespan of tumor bearing animals but also was shown to inhibit chemical carcinogenesis. Earlier experiments by others[97,98] proved the efficacy of turmeric/curcumin for the inhibition of tumor promotion brought about by TPA & croton oil.

Antiageing Effect of Garlic

Svendsen, Rattan et. al.[99] demonstrated an age related beneficial change in the morphology of human skin fibroblasts serially passaged in the presence of different amounts of garlic extracts (AS) in the culture medium. A concentration of AS at 250 µg/mL treated culture gave the best growth effect. Therefore A. sativum is useful to prevent ageing.

Dedication

This work is dedicated to the memory of Late Marry Joseph W/o Dr. P.K. Joseph and cousin sister of Dr. Augusti. Both of us mourn the untimely death of her in 1995. Mary and Joseph were instrumental in employing Dr. Augusti as professor in Maiduguri University of Nigeria (1980-85) from where they published several research papers on cabbage and garlic.

Acknowledgement

The authors acknowledge with thanks Dr. Eric Block of State University of New York at Albany and the Secretariat of ISHS Belgium, for sending the necessary literature and the proceedings of the fourth international symposia on Edible Alliacea at Beijing in 2004 to prepare this article.

Reference

1. Eric Block, Biological activity of Alliums compounds; Recent Results in: Proceedings of the fourth International Symposium on Edible Alliacea, Beijing, April 21-26.2004. Editor Lin Guangshu. Published by Chinese Society for Horticultural Science. ISHS Working Group on Edible Alliaceae. Acta Horticulture. pp 41-57.
2. Kiple, K.F and Ornelas, K.C(eds) 2000. The Cambridge World History of Food. Cambridge University Press, Cambridge, U.K.
3. Eric Block. Organo Sulfur Chemistry of the Genus Alliums – Implications for the organic chemistry of sulfur. Angew Chem. Int. Ed. Engl. 31(1992)1135-1178.

4. Barry. S. Kendler. Garlic (Allium sativum) and onion (Allium cepa): A Review of their Relationship to Cardiovascular disease Preventive Medicine 16(1987)670-685.

5. Augusti, K.T. Therapeutic values of onion (Allium cepa L) and garlic (Allium sativum L) Ind. Jour Exp. Biol. 34(1996)634-640 and in: onion and allied crops. Vol. III. Edited by J.L. Brewster and Rabinowitch (CRC Press Inc. Boca Florida) 1990.P83.

6. Block, E; Ahmad, S. et. al. (E-Z)- Ajoene : a potent antithrombotic agent from garlic. J.Am. Chem. Soc. 106 (1984)8295-96.

7. Block, E. The chemistry of garlic and onions. Sci. Am. 252(1985)114-119.

8. Dong, Y; Lisk, D, et. al. Characterization of the biological activity of gammaglutamyl-Se-methyl Seleno cysteine: a novel naturally occurring anti cancer agent from garlic. Cancer Research 61(2001)2923-2928.

9. Yang, W. Studies on the stabilities of bioactive Seleno compounds in Selenium enriched garlic and onion. Wei Sheng Yan Jiu 31(2002)252-255.

10. Block, E. Putman, D and Zhao, S.H. Allium Chemistry GC.MS analysis of thiosulfinates and related compounds from onion, leek, scallion, shallot, chive and Chinese chive. J. Agric. Food Chem. 40(1992)2431-2438.

11. Wang, H.X. and Ng. T.B. Purification of allivin, a novel antifungal protein from bulbs of the round clove garlic. Life Sci. 70(2001) 357-365.

12. Biju C Mathew, Danial R.S. and Augusti K.T. Hypolipidemic effect of garlic protein substituted for casein in diet of rats compared to those of garlic oil. Indian Jour. Exp. Biol. 34(1996)337-340.

13. Hirao, Y; Sumioka, I; Nakagami S, et. al. Activation of immunoresponder cells by the protein fraction from aged garlic extract. Phytother Res. 1(1987)161-164.

14. Grant, W.B.; A multicountry ecologic study of risk and risk reduction factors for prostate cancer mortality. Eur.Urol.45(2004)271-279.

15. Hising, A.W; Chokkalingam, A.P. et. al. Alliums vegetables and risk of prostate cancer: a population based study J. Natl. Cancer Inst. 94(2002)1648-1651.

16. Nakagawa. H ; Tsuta, K. et. al. Growth inhibitory effects of diallyldisulfide on human breast cancer cell lines, carcinogenesis. 22(2001)891-897.

17. Ip, C; Berringer, M; Block, E. et. al. Chemical speciation influences comparative activity of Selenium – enriched garlic and yeast in mammary cancer prevention. J. Agric. Food Chem. 48(2000)2062-70.

18. Guyonnet, D; Belloir, C et. al. Antimutagenic activity of organo sulfur compounds from Allium is associated with phase II enzyme induction, Mutat.Res.495 (2001)135-145.

19. Cohen, L.A; Zhao, Z. et. al. S-allylcysteine, a garlic constituent, fails to inhibit N-methyl nitrosourea – induced rat mammary tumorigenesis. Nutr. Cancer. 35(1999)58-63.

20. Munday, R and Munday, C.M. Relative activities of organo sulfur compounds derived from onions and garlic in increasing tissue activities of quinone reductase and glutathione transferase in rat tissues, Nutr. Cancer, 40(2001)205-21.

21. Munday, R and Munday, J.S Munday, C.M. Comparative effects of mono, di, tri, and tetrasulfides derived from plants of the Allium family: redox cycling in vitro and hemolytic activity and phase 2 enzyme induction in vivo, Free radic. Biol. Med. 34 (2003)1200-01.

22. Munday, R and Munday, C.M Induction of phase II enzymes by aliphatic sulfides derived from garlic and onions: a overview. Methods Enzymol. 382(2004)449-56.

23. Rabinkov, A; Miron, T et. al. The mode of action of allicin: trapping of radicals and interaction with thiol containing proteins. Biochim. Biophys. Acta. 1379(1998)233-244.

24. Rabinkov, A; Miron, T. et. al. S- allylmercapto glutathione: the reaction product of allicin with glutathione possess SH – modifying and antioxidant properties. Biochim. Biophys. Acta 1499(2000)144-153.

25. Oommen, S; Anto, R.J. et. al. Allicin (from garlic) induces caspase – mediated apoptosis in cancer cells. Eur. J. Pharmacol. 485(2004)97-103.

26. Li, M; Ciu, J.R. et. al. Anti tumor activity of Z-ajoene, a natural compound purified from garlic: antimiotic and microtubule – interaction properties. Carcinogenesis 23(2002)573-79.

27. Dirsch, V.M; Antlsperger, D.S et. al. Ajoene, an experimental anti-leukemic drug : mechanism of cell death. Leukemia 16(2002)74-83.

28. Ledezma, E; Apitz-castro, R and Cardier, J. Apoptotic and anti-adhesion effect of ajoene, a garlic derived compound, on the murine melanoma B_{16} F_{10} cells. Possible role of caspose-3 and the alpha (4) beta (1) integrin. Cancer Lett 206(2004)35-41.

29. Wu.C.C. Sheen, L.Y. et. al. Effects of organo sulfur compounds from garlic oil on the antioxidant system in rat liver and red blood cells. Food Chem. Toxicol. 39 (2001)563-69.

30. Chun, H.S; Kim, H.J. and Choi, E.H. Modulation of cytochrome P 4501-mediated bioactivities of benzo(a) pyrene by volatile allyl sulfides in human hepatoma cells. Biosci. Biotech. Biochem 65:2205-2212.

31. Yang. C.S.; Chhabra, S.K. Hong, J.Y and Smith, T.J. Mechanism of inhibition of chemical toxicity and carcinogenesis by diallylsulfide (DAS) and related compounds from garlic. J. Nutr. 131(2001)1041S-1045S.

32. Balasenthil, S.; Arivazhagan, S and Nagini, S. Garlic enhances circulatory antioxidants during 7, 12-dimethyl benz[a]anthracene – induced hamster buccal pouch carcinogenesis. Jour. Ethno pharmacology 72(2000)429-33.

33. Balasenthil, S; Rao, K.S. and Nagini, S. Apoptosis induction by S-allyl cysteine, a garlic constituent, during 7,12-dimethyl benz(a) anthracene – induced hamster buccal pouch carcinogenesis. Cell Biochem Funct 20(2002)263-68.

34. Harris, J.C. and Cottrel, S.L. et. al. Antimicrobial properties of Allium sativum (garlic). Appl.Microbial Biotechnol.57 (2001)282-86.

35. Ankri. S and Mirelman, D. Antimicrobial properties of allicin from garlic. Microbes Infect, 1(1999)125-129.

36. Yoshida, H; Iwata, N et. al. Antimicrobial activity of a compound isolated from an oil-macerated garlic extract. Biosci. Biotech. Biochem. 62 (1998)1014-17.

37. Yoshida, H; Katsuzaki, H et. al. Antimicrobial activity of the thiosulfinates isolated from oil-macerated garlic extract. Biosci. Biotech. Biochem. 63 (1999)591-94.

38. Tsao, S.M. and Yin, M.C. In vitro antimicrobial activity of four diallyl sulfides occurring naturally in garlic and Chinese leek oils. J. Med. Microbial. 50(2001)646-49.

39. Harris, J. C; Plummer, S. et. al. The microaerophilic flagellate Giardia intestinalis; Allium sativum (garlic) is an effective antigiardial. Microbiology. 146pt.14 (2000)3119-27.
40. Ernst, E. Is garlic an effective treatment for helicobacter pylori infection? Arch. Intern. Med. 159 (1999)2484-85
41. O' Gara, E.A. Hill, D.J. and Maslin, D.J. Activities of garlic oil, garlic powder and their diallyl constituents against Helicobacter pylori. Appl. Environ. Microbiol. 66 (2000) 2269-73.
42. Ohta, R; Yamada, N et. al. In vitro inhibition of the growth of Helicobacter pylori by oil-macerated garlic constituents. Antimicrob. Agents. Chemother. 43(1999)1811-12.
43. Ankri, S and Mirelman,d. Antimicrobial properties of allicin from garlic. Microbs Infect, 1(1999)125-29.
44. Seo, K II; Moon, Y.H. et. al. Antibacterial activity of S-methyl methanethiosulfinate and S-methyl 2-propene-1-thiosulfinate from Chinese chive towards Escherichia coli 0157:H7. Biosci. Biotech. Biochem. 65(2001)966-68.
45. Canizares, P; Gracia, I., et. al. Allyl thiosulfinates, the bacteriostatic compounds of garlic against Helicobacter Pylori. Biotechnol. Prog. 20(2004)397-401.
46. Walder, R; Kalvatchev, Z. et. al. In vitro suppression of HIV-1 replication by ajoene (E, Z-4, 5, 9 trithiadodeca-1, 6, 11. triene – 9 oxide) Biomed. Pharmacother.51 (1997)397-403.
47. Kim, J.W; Kim, Y.S. and Kyung, K.H. Inhibitory activity of essential oils of garlic and onion against bacteria and yeasts. J. food. prot. 67 (2004)499-504.
48. Ledezma, E; Marcano, E. et. al. Efficiency of ajoene in the treatment of tinea pedis: a double-blind and comparative study with terbinafine. J. Am. Acad. Dermatol. 43(2000)829-832.
49. Ledezma, E; Jorquera, A et. al. Antiproliferative and leishmanicidal effect of ajoene on various leishmania species: ultra structural study. Parasitol. Res. 88(2002)748-53.
50. Briggs, W.H.; Xiao, H. et. al. Differential inhibition of human platelet aggregation by selected allium thiosulfinates. J. Agric. Food Chem.. 48(2000)5731-35.
51. Rendu, F; Brohard-Bhon, B. et. al. Thiosulfinates inhibit platelet aggregation and micro particle shedding at a calpain dependent step. Thromb. Haemost. 86(2001)1284-91.

52. Teranishi, K; Apitz-Castro, R et. al. Inhibition of baboon platelet aggregation in vitro and in vivo by the garlic derivative ajoene. Xeno transplantation 10(2003)374-79.

53. Benatuil, L. Apitz-castro, R and Romano. Ajoene inhibits the activation of human endothelial cells induced by porcine cells: implications for xeno transplantation. Xeno transplantation 10(2003)368-73.

54. Apitz-Castro, R; Escalante, J. et. al. Ajoene, the antiplatelet principle of garlic, synergistically potentiates the anti aggregatory action of prostacyclin, forskolin, indomethacin and dipiridamole of human platelets. Thromb. Res. 42 (1986)303-11.

55. Golovchenko, I; Yang, C. H. et. al. Garlic extract methyl allyl thiosulfinate blocks insulin potentiation of platelet-derived growth metabolism 52(2003)254-59.

56. Bordia, A. Verma, S.K. and Srivastava, K.C. Effect of garlic (allium sativum) on blood lipids, blood sugar, fibrinogen and fibrinolytic activity Essential Fatty Acids 58(1998)257-63.

57. Ariga, T; Tsuj, K et. al. Anti thrombotic and antineoplastic effects of phyto-organosulfur compounds, Biofactors 13(2000)251-55.

58. Briggs, W.H; Folts, J.D et. al. Administration of raw onion inhibits platelet-mediated thrombosis in dogs. J. Nutr.131 (2001)2619-22.

59. Chen, J.H; Chen, H.I. et. al. Life Sci66(2000)1571-79.

60. Osmont, K.S.; Arnt, C.R. and Goldman, I. L. Temporal aspects of onion induced antiplatelet activity. Plant foods Hum.Nutr.58 (2003)27-40.

61. Augusti, K.T. Benaim, M.E, Dewar, H.A. and Virden, R. Partial identification of the Fibrinolytic activators in onion Atherosclerosis 21(1975)409-416.

62. Bordia, A; Bansal, H.C. et. al. Effect of the essential oils of garlic and onion on alimentary hyperlipidemia. Atherosclerosis 21(1975)15-19.

63. Koch, H.P. and Lawson, L.D. Garlic – The Science and Therapeutic Application of Allium sativum L and Related Species. 2nd edition. 1996. Williams & Wilkins Baltimore.

64. Fallon, M.B. Abrahams, G.A. et. al. Garlic prevents hypoxic pulmonary hypertension in rats. Am. J. Physiol. 275(1998) L283-87.

65. Siegel, G., Malmsten, M et. al. The effect of garlic on arteriosclerosis nanoplaque formation and size. Phytomedicine 11(2004)24-35.

66. Gardner, C.D.; Messina, M et. al. Soy, garlic and ginkobiloba: their potential role in cardiovascular disease prevention and treatment. Curr. Atherosclerosis. Rep. 5 (2003)468-75.

67. Banerjee, S.K. and Maulik, S.K. Effect of garlic on cardiovascular disorders : A Review. Nutr.J.1 (2002)4.

68. Teyssier, C. Guenot, L. Metabolism of diallyl disulfide by human liver microsomal cytochromes. P-450 and flavin – containing mono oxygenases. Drug Metab. Dispos. 27(1999)835-41.

69. Cho, B.H. and Xu, S. Effects of allyl mercaptan and various Allium-derived compounds on cholesterol synthesis and secretion in Hep-G2 cells. Comp. Biochem. Physiol, C. Toxicol. Pharmacol. 126 (2000)195-201.

70. Abramovitz, D; Gavri, S et. al. Allicin induced decrease in formation of fatty streaks (atherosclerosis) in mice fed a cholesterol-rich diet. Coron. Artery. Dis.10 (1999)515-19.

71. Ku, D.D; Abdel-Razek, T.T et. al. Garlic and its active metabolite allicin produce endothelium and nitric oxide dependent relaxation in rat pulmonary arteries. Clin. Exp. Pharmacolol. Physiol. 29(2002)84-91.

72. Schwartz, I.F.; Hershkovitz, R, et. al. Garlic attenuates NO production in rat cardiac myocytes through inhibition of inducible nitric oxide synthase and arginine transporter CAT-2 (Cationic aminoacid transporter-2) Clin. Sci. (London)102(2002)487-93.

73. Sakai, Y; Murakami, T. and Yamamoto, Y. Antihypertensive effects of onion on NO synthase inhibitor – induced hypertensive rats and spontaneously hypertensive rats. Biosci. Biotech. Biochem. 67 (2003)1305-11.

74. Ferri, N.; Yokoyama, K. et. al. Ajoene, a garlic compound, inhibits protein prenylation and arterial smooth muscle cell proliferation. Br. J. Pharmacol. 138 (2003)811-18.

75. Peleg, A; Hersheovici, T. et. al. Effect of garlic on lipid profile and psychopathologic parameters in people with mild to moderate hypercholesterolemia. Isr. Med. Assoc. J.5 (2003)637-40.

76. Augusti, K.T. Hypocholesterolemic effect of garlic Allium sativum Linn. Indian Jour. Exp. Biol, 15 (1977)489-90.

77. Kannar, D; Wattanapenpaiboon, N et. al. Hypocholesterolemic effect of an enteric – coated garlic supplement. J. Am. Coli. Nutr. 20 (2001)225-31.

78. Banerjee, S.K.; Mukherjee, P.K. and Maulik, S.K. Garlic as an antioxidant : the good, the bad and the ugly Phytother. Res. 17(2003)97-106.

79. Higuchi, O. Tateshita, K. and Nishimura, H. Antioxidative activity of sulfur containing compounds in Allium species for human low density lipoprotein (LDL) oxidation in vitro. J.Agric.FoodChem.51 (2003)7208-14.

80. Klanns-Dieter, A. 1983. Sulfur content free radicals. In: Radio protectors and Anticarcinogens, Niggard, O.F. and Simic, M.G. (editors). Academic Press, New York pp.23-42.

81. Hallman, B; Lernmark, A. et. al. On the possible role of thiol groups in the insulin releasing action of mercurials, organic disulfides, alkylating agents and sulfonylureas Endocrinology 99(1976)1398.

82. Farva, D; Goji, I.A.; Joseph, P.K. and Augusti, K.T. Effects of garlic oil on streptozotocin diabetic rats maintained on normal and high fat diets. Indian Jour. Biochem. & Biophys. 23 (1986)24-27.

83. Paramesha, S. and Kasinath, R.T. Antidiabetic and related effects of solvent extracted oils of alliums and a synthetic disulfide in experimental diabetes mellitus. In: Proceeding of the National seminar on the evaluation of nutraceuticals that prevent diseases 29th Nov. to 2nd, Dec.2006. Thalassery Campus of Kannur University – Kerala. Pp.71-75.

84. Joseph, P.K and Kasinath R.T. Hypoglycemic and hypolipidemic effects of diacetodibutyl disulfide. Indian Jour. Clin.Biochem.15 (2) (2000)68-75.

85. Patya, M; Zahalka, M.A. et. al. Allicin stimulates lymphocytes and elicts an anti tumor effect: a possible role of p21ras. Int.Immunol.16 (2004)275-281.

86. Sela, U.; Ganor, S et. al. Allicin inhibits SDF-L alpha – induced T cell interactions with fibronectin and endothelial cells by down – regulating cytoskeleton rearrangement, Pyk,-2 phosphorylation and VLA-4 expression, Immunology III (2004)391-99.

87. Dirsch, V.M. and Vollmar, A.M. Ajoene, a natural product with non-steroidal antiinflammatory drug (NSAID) – like properties? Biochem. Pharmacol. 61 (2001)587-593.

88. Wu, C.C.; Sheen, LY. et. al. Differential effects of garlic oil and its three major organosulfur components on the hepatic detoxification system in rats. J. Agric. Food Chem. 50(2002)378-383.

89. Fukao, T; Hosono, T et. al. The effects of allyl sulfides on the induction of phase II detoxification enzymes and liver injury by carbon tetrachloride. Food.Chem.Toxicol.42 (2004)743-749.

90. Augusti K.T, Anuradha, et. al. Nutraceutical effects of garlic oil, its non polar fraction and Ficus flavonoid as compared to vitamin E. in CCl4 induced liver damage in rats. 43(2005)437-444.

91. Hattori, A; Yamada, N et. al. Protective effect of ajoene on acetaminophen –induced hepatic injury in mice. Biosci. Biotech. Biochem. 65 (2001)2555-57.

92. Ikpeazu, O.V.; Augusti, K.T. and Joseph, P.K. Hypolipidemic Effect of Garlic Extracts Mixed with 3% Ethanol in Rats fed sucrose – high fat diet. Indian Jour. Biochem. Biophys. 24 (1987)252-253.

93. (a) Aminu Bobboi, Augusti, K.T. and Joseph, P.K. Hypolipidemic effects of onion oil and garlic oil in ethanol fed rats. Indian Jour. Biochem. Biophys. 21(1984)211-213.

    (b) Wilcox, B.F.; Joseph, P.K. and Augusti, K.T. Effect of Allyl disulphide isolated from Allium cepa Linn on high – fat fed rats. Indian Jour. Biochem. Biophys. 21(1984)214-216.

94. Helen, A; Rajasree, C.R. et. al. Antioxidant Role of oils isolated from garlic (Allium sativum Linn) and onion (Allium cepa Linn) on Nicotine – induced lipid peroxidation. Vet. Human Toxicol 41(5) (1999)316-319.

95. Augusti, K.T., Andrews, A. et. al. Environmental Hazards from lead salts and the additive effects by alcohol and their amelioration by garlic oil as compared to vitamin E. Extended Abstracts of the 19th Kerala Science Congress. Kannur. 29th to 31st Jan 2007. pp791-93.

96. Unnikrishnan, M.C. and Kuttan, R. Tumor reducing and anticarcinogenesis activity of selected spices. Cancer Letters 51(1990)85-89.

97. Huang, M.T.; Smart, C.R. et. al. Inhibitory effect of curcumin, chlorogenic acid and Ferulic acid on tumor promotion in mouse skin by 12-0-tetradecanoyl phorbol-13-acetate.Cancer Res.48 (1988)5941.

98. Soudamini, K.K. and Kuttan, R. Inhibition of chemical carcinogenesis by curcumin. J. Ethnopharmacol. 27(1989)227.

99. Svendsen, L, Rattan, I.S et. al. Effects of garlic extract on human skin fibroblast growth. J. Ethnopharmacol, 43 (1994) 125-133.

5.4 Some Tips on Garlic, Onions, Cabbage and Broccoli for the Household

Dr. Jasmin Maret

Head of the Dept. of Computer Studies, ST. Kevin College, Omaru. Newzealand.

Let Garlic be the Medicine

Perhaps no vegetable or herb better symbolizes medicinal food than garlic. Fresh garlic has strong immune boosting and antibiotic properties. In order to control hypertension W.H.O recommends to use regularly 4-5 cloves of garlic daily in a raw pulp form. On crushing the cloves the enzyme alliinase is released from the cells of the cloves and it converts S-allylcysteine sulfoxide, (Alliin) the precursor of the oil to allicin, pyruvicacid and ammonia through a process of hydrolysis

$$\underset{\text{Alliin}}{2C_3H_5 - S(O)CH_2\,CH(NH_2)COOH} \xrightarrow[H_2O]{\text{alliinase}} \underset{\text{Allicin}}{C_3H_5 - S - S(O) - C_3H_5} + 2CH_3COCOOH + 2NH_3$$

Chopping up cloves for ten minutes before throwing them into the fry pan allows the allinase enzyme time to produce the cancer fighting allyl sulfur compound (diallyl sulfide and diallyldisulfide). In truth, more than one hundred compounds give garlic its synergistic abilities as a healing herb. Allicin and related compounds reduce the infection stresses imposed upon the body by various diseases[1]. Onion also produces allicin type compounds viz; $CH_3 - S - S(O) - CH_3$ from its precursor amino acids. Ajoen, a polymer of allicin produced on macerating fresh garlic in olive oil helps prevent blood clots and work against certain cancers[2]. Diallyl trisulfide (DATS) is liver friendly and antiviral[3]. These compounds together help reduce blood pressure[4] and blood sugar[5], relieve fatigue[6] and improve blood circulation and heart function[2,7]. Machanism of action of allicin, ajoene, polysulfides etc. may be due to their binding to SH groups in cells or microorganism that in turn inactive each of them and in addition due to their vasodilatory action.

Garlic actually kills infecting bacteria while at the same time boosting the body's immune system to ward off bacterial poisons that are causing an infection[8].

Louis Pasteur's Comments

The forefather of antibiotic medicine Louis Pasteur acknowledged "garlic to be as effective as penicillin" (1858). We call on this herbal antibiotic specifically to thwart a developing sore throat. Dr.K.T. Augusti a pioneer in the field of garlic research experienced that by eating 2-3 cloves of fresh garlic it can dispel cold, sore throat and improve the voice a lot. Tooth ache disappears on sucking a raw garlic clove for a few hours and one can experience its localized effect also. Every day consumption of garlic, both raw and cooked makes for good medicine no matter how deep you go with this amazing plant. However anaemic people may avoid garlic.

The Chinese Practice on Garlic. (Dr. Augusti learnt these things from China in 2004)

In accordance with the recording on the **'Compendium of Materia Medica"** of the Ming dynasty, the following things are noted.

1. *Garlic takes the functions of driving away many diseases*, i.e. of scattering pain and swollen, eliminating wind and evil, killing poisons, getting rid of rheumatism, treating malicious and tinea, doing good for spleen and stomach, stopping cholera and efficiency of solving the pestilence etc. to cure mainly several dozen kinds of diseases. Modern medical sciences proves that the garlic and its products can suppress or kill more than 20 causes of disease fungus such as the golden yellow staphylococcus, pneumonia coccus, green suppuration bacillus, typhoid bacillus, dysentery bacillus, tubercle bacillus, diphtheria bacillus, cold bacillus etc.

2. *The garlic takes health care and treat function to the cardiovascular system*. Chinese take garlic to invigorate blood circulation and eliminate silt, for free movement of the bowels and to prevent and cure the disease with a history of over a thousand years. Modern medical research indicates that the garlic can lower the fat of the blood, lower the blood pressure and expand the blood vessel on function. It can prevent and cure the gruel arteriosclerosis formation. Beijing's China-Japan Friendship Hospital has adopted garlic injection to treat the patients with brain blocking up and coronary heart disease with obvious result. (German Medical Circle considers that the garlic has strange results in preventing and curing the CVD).

3. *There is an anticancer function of the garlic.*

   Garlic can suppress the growth of nitrate reducing fungus in stomach, reducing the content of sub nitrate of gastric juice[9], to block the synthesis of subnitramines, which are carcinogenic. Garlic can promote cancer cell death and prevent colon, bladder, cutaneum, breast, liver and many kinds of cancers. This is in line with the report that the cancer incidence is lower in the main garlic producing region in Shandong province. (sub nitrate is nitrite)

4. *Garlic can strengthen the immune function of organism*: Garlic can activate the function of the human macrophage cell, strengthen the human immunity and immune function of the organism. Experiments by Lau[10] and Girija Kuttan[11a] demonstrated the immunostimulating action of garlic principles.
5. *Garlic as an additive to fish, meat and eggs preparation make them easier to be digested and absorbed.*
6. *The garlic can reduce the blood pressure, platelet aggregation, blood sugar and the content of cholesterol and triglycerides of blood.*
7. *Garlic aminoacids together with thiamine help the human body to control blood sugar leading to a cure of diabetes mellitus.*

Cooking with Garlic

In China, Japan, India, Pakistan, Middle East, Germany, Netherlands and Egypt, garlic is a usual additive to food. Many garlic cook books say that you can make food items with just a touch of garlic here and a bit of garlic there, but that is not enough for your health. If you properly add smashed garlic to your food items (5 g/meal) you need not buy any garlic pill, you get enough daily dose of garlic from your own tasty food prepared as per recipies given in standard cook books as that one prepared by garlic goddess *Pat Report*. Please note to use only macerated garlic.

Ginger Allium Complex

In garlic farms of China a rasayana of ginger and garlic is regularly sold with a claim that it is a good drug to boost one's immunity to all types of infections. According to Dr. Augusti who visited China in 2004 in connection with the Fourth International symposium on alliums, he asked the farm people there about the composition of the rasayana. He was told that fresh garlic and ginger in the ratio of 4:1 were macerated without addition of water and mixed together with little vinegar to preserve it. The rasayana was purchased by many delegates and ever since that Dr. Augusti (75 years) is using the rasayana made at home. He adds enough black pepper and salt to it to make the chutney more palatable. He says it is a tonic for him. It cures all illness of his old age, it keeps him alert and active to carry on his teaching programmes according to schedule. It is an antiaging drug according to Svendsen and Ratan[12]. According to

Dr.Bordia[13a,b] a Cardiologist of Udaipur both garlic and ginger are good to protect the circulation of blood as both of them prevent platelet aggregation. **Therefore ginger allium complex is a drug (nector) that protects our heart.** (Refer Bordia's papers in this book (p. 312).

The Thieves' Decoction

When the City of Basle was infested with the great plague, it is said that the Jewish population who was eating garlic regularly had a much lower fatality rate than others. In the year 1721, the plague raged through Marseille. At that time gangs of thieves passed through the city robbing the sick and dead without infecting themselves. Four thieves confessed to the police that they had regularly consumed a *concoction of garlic with wine* and vinegar. This remedy soon became rather popular and was called vinegar of the four theives[14]. Since then many used the decoction of garlic to prevent all types of infections or even the spread of plague. Many Germans, Jews and others supported the medicinal effects of garlic against all types of infections. This may be one reason that Christians following the customs of Jews make the bread on Maundy Thursday with the addition of little garlic.

How Much Garlic is Usually Taken?

Some people chew one whole clove of raw garlic per day. For those who prefer it, odor-controlled, enteric-coated tablets or capsules with standardized allicin potential can be taken in amounts of 600-900 mg in two or three divided doses (Refer, http: //www.satisfied_mind.com/drugstore/ garlic.htm)

Garlic is mentioned in the Bible and the Talmud as a food additive to promote health. Hippocrates, Galen, Pliny the Elder and Dioscorides all mention the use of garlic for many conditions including parasites, respiratory problems, poor digestion and low energy. Its use in China was mentioned during Ming Dynasty (14th century). Louis Pasteur confirmed the antibacterial action of garlic in 1858 through his own tests.

Cardiovascular Actions of Garlic

Garlic considerably lowers serum cholesterol (LDL) and triglycerides, inhibits platelet stickiness (aggregation) and increases blood fibrinolysis – which results in a slowing of blood coagulation. It is mildly antihypertensive and has antioxidant activity. Three reviews of double blind studies in humans have found that garlic can lower blood cholesterol levels in adults by approximately 10%. However a similar study by Dr. Augusti on giving a decoction of garlic in water equivalent to 10 g garlic daily to adults with hypercholesterolemia for two months lowered their serum cholesterol by 28%[15]. Dr. Bordia did other experiments on blood fibrinolysis and platelet aggregations (PP 312-321) and confirmed the benefits of garlic. Several double blind studies also suggest it can prevent arteriosclerosis. Garlic is also helpful for persons with intermittent claudication (cramping in the lower legs secondary to poor blood flow) according to one controlled study.

Antimicrobial Actions of Garlic

Garlic has antibacterial, antiviral and antifungal activities. It may work against some intestinal parasites. Garlic appears to have roughly 1% the strength of penicillin against certain types of bacteria. This means it is not a substitute for antibiotics but it can be considered as a support against some bacterial infections. Candida albican's growth is inhibited by garlic and it has shown long-term benefit for recurrent yeast infections[2,16,17.] As Russians used garlic extract when penicillin was not available as an antibiotic, it earned the name *Russian penicillin.*

The Kerala Experience

In Kerala when jaundice raged during 2003-04 Dr. Augusti who was a Visiting Professor at M.G. University, Kottayam did a yoe man's work to advocate daily use of garlic juice equevalent to 10 g fresh garlic by every body to protect them from the menace. It worked effectively in those who used it. Similarly when chikunguniya raged Kerala in 2006 and 2007 Dr. Augusti called Press conferences at Kottayam, Trivandrum and Kannur and advocated the use of ginger, allium, black pepper-food complex prepared as a paste with out addition of water in the ratio of 1:4:0.25 by every body to boost up their immuno response against that disease. Many people used this food supplement daily for two weeks or more along with food and escaped from the viral fevers. Those who did not mind to take this preparation got the fevers and they suffered from joint pains and edema. However some 20 of those who suffered from this fever used this preparation daily and slowly they were cured of both edema and joint pains in two weeks time. As Chikungunya disappeared when sanitation improved and rains subsided a follow up of this experiment could not be carried out any longer. This work can be taken up by others. Ayurvedic Physicians used a similar preparation or decoction to prevent viral fevers in Kerala. It was composed of five spices viz; Ginger, Garlic, Black pepper, Long pepper and Cumin. A perusal of literature showed both the peppers contained similar compounds.

A study in India by Vinod and Sadasivan exhibited the supporting action of fresh ethereal oil of garlic for ampicillin. The growth of ampicillin resistant staphylococcus aurues was inhibited significantly by both the garlic preparation (GP) as well as by GP and ampicillin combination. i.e. Inhibitory zones were 8 mm and 14 mm respectively[11(b)]. Onion oil also worked considerably in that manner (See P. 470).

Anticancer Actions of Garlic

Human population studies show that eating garlic regularly reduces the risk of esophageal, stomach and colon cancer. This is partly due to garlic's ability to reduce the formation of carcinogenic compounds, e.g. nitrosamines from nitrate. Nitrates are found as a pollution in our food.

In China residents of the Shandong Province's Cangshan county enjoyed the lowest death rate due to stomach cancer (3 per 100,000), but residents of the county of Qixia had a thirteen-fold higher death rate due to the same cancer. This is because the residents of Cangshan regularly eat 20 g of garlic per day, where as residents of Qixia rarely eat any garlic[9]. Examination of gastric juice of the residents revealed that the former's sample had a lower concentration of nitrites than that found in the latter's sample. In other words garlic protected the stomach against the formation of nitrites from nitrates. The former is a precursor of the carcinogens e.g. nitrosamines. Garlic compound DATS is a potent inhibitor of stomach cancers in a tissue culture according to Pan[18].

Ajoene

Rafael Apitz an investigator of the Venezuelan Institute of Scientific investigations from 1982 began to study alcoholic extracts of garlic for their biological properties. Between many compounds he isolated, only one showed interesting activity like blocking of the action of platelets, which are involved in the formation of thrombus in the blood. The effective compound was a polymer of allicin which he called by the name Ajoene (Spanish name originated from garlic)[19]. This compound does not exist in garlic. It is formed only when the cloves are crushed and kept for some time at low temperature. A methanol extract of garlic kept at 4°C is a good method to produce ajoene. Ajoene inhits plaque formation and also mutation by several carcinogens viz; benzo(a)pyrene and 4 nitro –1, 2-phenylenediamine[20].

Garlic is a Medicine in Homoeopathy Too

According to Dr. Indu Vaid[21] a Research officer of Homoeopathic pharmacopoeia Laboratory, Govt. of India, Ghaziabad, garlic is being prescribed as a medicine by allopaths and homoeopaths alike. She says like ginseng, garlic has come from China and it is widely grown in India too. Pharmacological investigation has resulted in eliciting good values of the drug as hypotensive, antiseptic and cholesterol regulator. Homoeopathic literature speaks highly of garlic because of its action on intestinal mucous membrane increasing peristalsis, vasodilatory properties and arterial hypotension. It used in 3rd and 6th potency and in tuberculosis the use of crude drug has been suggested[22]. Herbal medicine highlights its use in asthma, leprosy and arterioclerosis[23]. Prof. Hans Reuter of Cologne University (Germany) reported that garlic helps breakup cholesterol in blood vessels, thus preventing arterioscleresis, B.P. and heart attacks[24]. Garlic is a tonic for loss of sexual power, impotence and nervous exhaution[25]. Garlic is not known to cause any serious toxic effect acute or chronic.

Selenium Content of Alliums

The selenium content in fresh garlic (0.01-0.6ppm) is very less than that of sulfur, however, because selenium, a nutritionally essential element of the same family as sulfur, can substitute for sulfur (Se can take the place of sulfur in thiols) in the organosulfur compounds of the sulfur rich Allium-species, there has been considerable interest in growing garlic and onion, in Se enriched soils as less toxic vehicles for increasing the dietary levels of this important component of the body's antioxidant enzyme, glutathione peroxidase. Selenium enriched garlic for pharmaceutical purposes has been patented. Se level in garlic can be increased to 0.05 mg/g by cultivating the vegetable in Se enriched soil. *This has improved the anticancer effect of garlic.* Se is present in garlic as Selenoprotein, Se-cysteine and Se-methionine. While garlic oil has been found to contain dimethyl selenide and dimethyl diselenide[26.]

i.e CH_3 – Se-CH_3 and CH_3 – Se-Se-CH_3.

Flavonoid Pigments, Polyphenols and other Nonsulfur Active Principles in Garlic & Onions

Although the coloured flavanoids are quite abundant in onions and other allium species[27], such compounds are shown to be virtually absent in garlic except for trace amounts of quercetin and kaempferol[28]. However the reddish purple color of inner garlic scales has been shown to be due to three anthocyanins: cyanins: cyanidin-3-glucoside and two of their acylated forms on the glucose[29]. Anthocyanins are also present in onions[30]. They are all strong antioxidants and induce pathogen resistance in the plants. **Onion is also a good source of Calcium and its use by women may protect them from osteoperosis.** Small amounts of phenolic acids (total 40 µg/g) have been reported to be present in pure garlic cloves[31], viz; p-hydroxybenzoic acid (13 µg/g), caffeic acid (10 µg/g), ferulic acid (7 µg/g), vanillic acid (6 µg/g), sinapinic acid (2 µg/g) and p-coumaric acid (2 µg/g). Outer scales also contained such compounds except p-hydroxybenzoic acid. *They are all strong antioxidants* and add much value to the medicinal value of garlic.

Tannins (Condensed Phenols)

Tannins, which have antioxidant properties, have been detected in the skin of red onions[32]. Other Allium species also have phenolic compounds, some of which are even more abundant. Lignin, a complex polymer of p-propenol phenols that provide a rigid cell wall structure is found at 1.6% in garlic cloves. These compounds also offer pathogen resistance in the plants. They bind and transport heavy metals in the roots. *Adenosine and guanosine are also present in Alliums.* Adenosine is present in relatively high amounts in garlic and onions viz; 0.2-0.37 mg/g in garlic[33]. Some ascribed to the presence of adenosine[34] for the antithrombotic action of garlic. Both adenosine and guanosine are released only when garlic is crushed or homogenized. The latter is 40% higher in concentration than the former. Some people claim that allicin free non-volatile residue of crushed garlic still retains some antibiotic substance. Machado et. al.[35] named such a nonsulfur yellow compound as garlicina. Residue of steam distilled sample was reported to contain a compound viz; dihydroxycyclohexyl lactone $C_8H_{12}O_4$ with antibiotic activity.

Garlic Protein is with similar composition and Medicinal Properties of Soy Protein

Biju and Augusti[36] isolated a medicinally active protein from garlic. It was found to possess similar amino acid composition and hypolipidemic activity with that of soyprotein[37].

Garlic protein was isolated from an aqueous extract of the vegetable at pH4.5. The yield was around 5.5%. In cholesterol rich diet fed rats incorporation of 16% garlic protein in the diet showed 85% hypolipidemic activity of garlic oil at a dose of 100 mg/kg during a period of 3 months treatment. The hypolipedimic activity of garlic and soy protein is ascribed to a low Lysine/Arginine ratio of each, i.e. 0.77 and 0.84 respectively. Soy protein isolate has a biological value of 74 as compared to egg white protein at 83[38,39]. Hirao et. al.[40] and Lau et. al.[41] reported earlier that garlic protein possesses immunostimulating activity in macrophages. Rajasree et. al.[42] reported on the hypolipidemic action of garlic protein in alchohol induced hyperlipidemia in rats. They identified a low MW protein (11 KD) by electrophoresis which may be responsible for the immunomodulatory effects. More work is warranted in this direction.

Garlic and Onion Oils and Their Precursor Amino Acids

Many scientists reported not only on the antidiabetic and antiatherogenic effects of garlic and onion oils, but also on their precursor amino acids. Viz, S-allyl cysteine sulfoxide (SACS) and S- methyl cysteine sulfoxide (SMCS) respectively. They are significantly active antioxidants and antiatherogenic substances too[43]. **They are the main medicinally active**

compounds in raw form of uncrushed and peeled forms of garlic and onion or in their pickles, but they are less active than the oils produced from each with the action of alliinase. SACS[44] and SMCS[45] are found to be hypocholesterolemic and hypolipidemic in high fat or cholesterol diet fed rats. They are also moderately antidiabetic in action[46]. SACS was also found to ameliorate the deleterious effects of alcohol[47] and nicotine[48] in rats. However onion and garlic oils counteracted the deleterious effects of alcohol[49] and nicotine[50] to a greater extent than their precursors. Garlic[5] and onion oils[1,51] proved to be antidiabetic in action and they are stimulators of blood fibrinolysis[52,53] and hypotensive[2]. Their compounds are immunoboosters, and antiageing agents[11,12]. Diallyl disulfide is an inhibitor of HMGCoA reductase[54]. Juice expressed onion pulp (50 g/adult) improved the tolerance of post prandial blood sugar in diabetic patients[55]. The juice of onion contains only small amount of its oil and the left out residue is rich in oil and its precursors. They are responsible for the antidiabetic action observed in Augusti's experiment. Very recent experiments by Augusti's team, proved that garlic oil feeding to rats can protect them from the damages of lead salt in their drinking water.

Cabbage and Broccoli

They belong to the family of cruciferous vegetables, Itokawa et. al.[56] showed that S-methyl cysteine sulfoxide (SMCS) present in onion and cabbage and S-allyl cysteine sulfoxide (SACS) present in garlic are antihypercholesterolemic in action. They are the precursors of dimethyl disulfide (CH_3-S-S-CH_3) of cabbage and onion oils and diallyl disulfide of garlic oil (C_3H_5-S-S-C_3H_5) respectively. Tarfa et. al.[57] demonstrated the antidiabetic action of cabbage oil in streptozotocin diabetic rats. Ismalia et. al.[58] demonstrated the hypolipidemic action of cabbage oil in ethanol fed red rats. These experiments demonstrated the medicinal value of cabbage oil. Among the cancer fighting vegetables broccoli, cauliflower and cabbage stand out first especially in cancers of bladder. Several studies claim that org. sulfur compounds like isothiocyanates and indol-3-carbinol (1-3C) present in Cabbage are good cancer fighting compounds[59,60] However people with thyroid diseases may not take cabbage regularly.

Broccoli (Brassica Oleracea Italica)

Seventeen phenolic/flavonoid compounds were characterized in this vegetable. They are different glucosides of the following compounds[61a]. Sulforaphane and the indoles have significant anticancer effects[61b]. Quercetin 3-0-Sophoroside, 3-P.coumaroyl quinic acid, Kaempferol 3-0-sophoroside, Kaempferol 3-0 (caffeoyl) – Sophoroside, Sinapic acid, Kaempferol 3-0 (sinapoyl)- sophoroside, Kaempferol 3-0-(feruloyl) Sophoroside, Kaempferol 3-0(p-coumaryol) sophoroside, 4p-Coumaroyl quinic acid, Sinapic acid, Kaempferolo 3-0-Sophoroside, 1,2 disinapic acids, 1-Sinapoyl –2-ferulic Acid, 1,2,2-trisinapic acid, 1,2' disinapoyl –2-ferulic acid. In addition to them, isothiocyanates, sulforaphane, and indol-3-, carbinol(1-3c) are also present in broccoli. They have been identified as anticancer compounds and most of them reduce colorectal or other cancers, although the exact compounds responsible for this benefit have not been identified. Broccoli is also a good source of vitamins, carotenoids, fiber, calcium and folate. Polyphenols and flavonoids act as antioxidants and boost detoxifying enzymes in the body. **Some studies suggest that they may alter body estrogen levels which might reduce breast cancer risk.**

Why an Apple a Day Keeps the Doctor Away?

All types of fruits are rich in antioxidants. However apple has a special place. For the English apple is the most cherished fruit and it is like a medicine for every disease. In Netherland a recent study published in Thorax (2007) says if pregnant women eat four apples per week their new born babies only very rarely get lung diseases and asthma.

Apple is a good source of flavonoids that act as antioxidants. Many of our Indian fruits also contain flavonoids. Fruits juices contain many antioxidants that protect our brain from oxidative stress according to many scientists from U.S. and Japan. Last September issue of the Am. Jour. Med (2006) reports that the risk of Alzheimer's disease was reduced by 76% for those who drank fruit juices more than three times a week compared with others who drank them less than once a week. Cashew fruit is called the Indian apple. Its skin is rich in flavonoids as is the case with those of onions and apple. Pappaya, mangoes, amla and grapes are also good. Let us use all of them at least 3-4 days a week to keep us free from fatal diseases and also from ageing. Just like apple, onion also may keep the doctor away as it is rich in quercetin, org. sulfides and calcium that helps to grow bones stronger.

Dedication

This work is dedicated to the memory of my late father Mr. Philipose Maret, Thiruvananthapuram.

Reference

1. Augusti. K.T., Therapeutic values of onion (Allium Cepa L) and garlic (Allium Sativum L) Indian Jour. Exp. Biol 34(1996)634-640.
2. Block, E. The organosulfur chemistry of the genus Allium; implications for the organic chemistry of sulphur, Angew Chem. Int. Engl, 31 (1992)1135-1178.

3. Wu. C.C, Sheen, L.Y et. al. Differential effects of garlic oil and its three major organosulfur components on the hepatic detoxification system in rats. J. Agric. Food. Chem. 50(2002) 378-383.

4. Mcmahon, FG and Vargas, R. Can garlic lowers blood pressure? A pilot study Pharmacother 13(1993) 106-107.

5. Farva, D; Goji, I A et. al. Effects of garlic oil on streptozotocin diabetic rats maintained on normal and high fat diets. Indian Jour. Biochem & Biophys. 23(1986) 24-27.

6. Hasegawa, Y, Kikuchi N et. al. Clinical effects of kyoleopin against various complaints in the field of internal medicine. Japanese J. New Remedies. 32(1983) 365.

7. Bordia AK, Joshi, HK et. al. Effect of essential oil of garlic on serum fibrinolytic activity in patients with coronary artery disease. Atherosclerosis 28(1977) 155-159.

8. Kandil, OM; Abdullah TH, Elkad, A Garlic and the immune system in humans: its effect on natural killer cells. Federation Proceedings 46(1987) 441.

9. Mei, X; Wang ML et. al. Garlic and gastric cancer. Acta Nutr Sinica 4(1982)53.

10. Lau BHS, Woolley JL et. al. Superiority of intralesional immunotherapy with corynebacterium parvum and Allium Sativum in control of murine transitional cell carcinoma. J.Urol 136(1986)701.

11. (a) Girija Kuttan, Thejass P and Manesh C. Effect of diallylsulphide (DAS) and diallyl disulphide (DADS) two naturally occurring sulphur compounds from garlic on the immune system of normal as well as metastatic turmour bearing animals. Paper presented at the National Seminar on the Evaluation of Nutraceuticals that prevent diseases. Proceedings published by the School of Health Sciences, Thalassery Campus of Kannur University Nov. 29 to 2nd Dec. 2007 pp.39-48

    (b) Vinod, N.V. and Sadasivan C. Seminar paper: Ampicillin Resistant staphylococcus aurues and the synergistic effects with crude extracts of garlic and other plants. Ibid 125-127

12. Svendsen, L et. al. Effects of garlic extracts on Human fibroblasts growth. J. Ethnopharmacol 43(1994)125-133.

13. (a) Bordia. A; Verma, S.K. and Srivastava, K.C. Effect of ginger (Zingiber officnale Rosc) and fenugreek (Trigonella foenugraecum L) on blood lipids, blood sugar and platelet aggregation in patients with coronary artery disease. Prostaglandins, Leukotrienes and Essential Fatty Acids 56(5) (1997)379-384.

(b) Bordia, A; Verma, S.K and Srivastava, K.C. Effect of garlic on platelet aggregation in human: a study in healthy subjects and patients with coronary artery disease. Postaglandins Leukot, Essent Fatty acids, 55(1996)201-205.

14. Gottfried Hain. History, Folk Medicine and Legendary use of garlic. In garlic, The Science and Therapeutic Applicatin of Allium Sativum L and Related Species. 2nd edn. Edited by H.P. Koch and L.D. Lawson 1988.PP 1-24. Williams & Wilkins A Waverly Company. Baltimore, Maryland U.S.A.

15. Augusti. K.T. Hypocholesterolemic effect of garlic, Allium sativum Linn. Indian J. Exp. Biol 15(1977)489-490.

16. Adetumbi, M.A; Javor, GT, Lau, BHS. Allium sativum (garlic) inhibits lipid synthesis by candida albicans. Antimicrob Agents Chemother 30(1986) 499.

17. Adetumbi, M.A, Lau, BHS: Allium sativum (garlic) a natural antibiotic. Med. Hypotheses 12(1983) 227.

18. Pan, XY. Comparison of the cytotoxic effect of fresh garlic, diallyl trisulfide, 5 fluorouracil, mitomycin C and Cis-DDP on two lines of gastric cancer cells. Chung-Hua Chung Liu Tsa Chin 7(1985)103.

19. Apitz-Castro; Cabrera, S et. al. Effects of garlic extract and of three pure components isolated from it on human platelet aggregation, arachidonate metabolism, release reaction and platelet ultrastructure. Thromb. Res. 32(1983)155-169.

20. Ishikawa, K; Naganawa, R et. al. Antimutagenic effects of ajoene an organosulfur compound derived from garlic. Biosci, Biotechnol. Biochem 60(12)(1996)2086-2088.

21. Indu Vaid. Benefits and curative properties of garlic (Allium Sativum) Homoeopathic up-date 2(1994)147-148.

22. William Boericke. Materia Medica with Reportory. B. John publishers, New Delhi, 1991. p.90.

23. Foods that heal. The natural way to good health. H.K. Bokhru. Orient Paper backs 1993.p.115.

24. Koul, M.K. Mirror Monthly Magazine, Bombay June (1986).p40

25. Singh, H.J. Food Remedies, Nature Cure Council of Medical Res. Lucknow. 1982.p.91.

26. Yang. M; Wang. K et. al. Exploration for a natural selenium supplement: Characterization and bioactivities of Se. Containing polysaccharide from garlic. J.Clin. Pharm. Sci. 1(1992)28-32.

27. Omidiji. O. Flavonoid glycosides in the wet scale of the deep purple onion (Allium cepa L) Discovery Innovation 5(1993) 139-141.

28. Leighton, T, Ginther, C et. al. Molecular Charaterization of quercetin and quercetin glucosides in Allium vegetables; their effects on malignant cell transformation. ACS Symp. Ser, 507(1992) 220-238.

29. Borukh, IF and Demkevich, L.I. Pigment substances of some garlic varieties of Western Forest Steppe of the Ukrane. Iz. Vyssh Uchebn. Zaved Pishch. Tekhnol. 1976.47-49.

30. Harborne. J.B. The natural distribution in angiosperms of anthocyanins acylated with aliphatic dicarboxylic acids, Phytochemistry 25(1986)1887-1891.

31. Codignola, A, Verotta, L et. al. Cell Wall bound Phenols in roots of vesicular-arbuscular mycorrhizal plants. New Phytol 112(1989)221-228.

32. Akaranta, O and Odozi. T.O. Antioxidant properties of red onion skin (Allium cepa) tannin extract. Agricultural wastes. 18(1986) 299-303.

33. Lawson, L.D.; Wood, S.G and Hughes, B.G. HPLC analysis of allicin and other thiosulfinates in garlic clove homogenates. Planta Med. 57(1991) 263-270.

34. Koch, H.P. "Hormon Wirkurgen" bei Allium Arten. Historische Berichte und modern wise senschaftliche Erketnntnisse. Z. Phytother 13(1992)177-188.

35. Machado, PA., Duran, M.G. et. al. Garlicina, unknown antibiotic An. Paul. Med. Cir. 55(1948)93-155(Sao Paulo)

36. Biju C, Mathew and Augusti. K.T. Biochemical effects of garlic protein diet and garlic oil on glycosaminoglycan metabolism in cholesterol fed rats. Indian Jour.Exp. Biol, 34(1996)346-350.

37. Hajos, G. et. al. Effects of proteolytic modification and methionine enrichment on the nutritional values of Soya Albumins for rats. Nutri. Biochem. 7(1996)481-487.

38. FAO/WHO/UNU. Expert consultation. Energy and Protein requirements. Technical Report Series 724. World Health Organization, Geneva.

39. Protein, Quality-Report of joint FAO/WHO Expert consultation. Food and Agriculture organization, Rome, FAO, Food and Nutrition paper 51, 1991.

40. Hirao, Y; Sumioka, I et. al. Activation of immunoresponder cells by the protein fraction from aged garlic extract. Phytother Res. 1(1987) 161-164.

41. Lau, BHS; Takeshiyamsaki; and Daila, S. Gridley. Garlic compounds modulate macrophage and T-lymphocyte functions. Mol. Biother 3(1991)103-107.

42. Rajasree. C.R.; Rajmohan, T and Augusti. K.T. Biochemical effects of garlic protein on lipid metabolism in alcohol fed rats. Ind. Jour. Exp. Biol. 37(1999)243-247.

43. Banerjee, S.K., Mukherjee, P.K and Maulik, S.K. Garlic as an antioxidant: the good, the bad and the ugly. Phytother. Res 17(2003)97-106.

44. (a) Augusti. K.T. Onions and allid crops. Brewster, J.L and Rabinowitch(eds) Vol.3 (1990) Biochem. Food Sci & Minor Crops, CRC Press Inc. Boca. Raton Florida pp93-108.

(b) Augusti. K.T. Therapeutic values of onion (Allium Cepa L) and garlic (Allium Sativum L). Indian Jour. Exp. Biol. 34(1996) 634-640.

45. Kumud, K and Augusti, K.T. Lipid lowering effect of S-methyl cysteine sulfoxide from Allium cepa Linn in high Cholesterol diet fed rats Jour. Ethnopharmacology 109 (2007)367-371.

46. Sheela.C.G. Kumari Kumud and Augusti. K.T. Antidiabetic effects of onion and garlic sulfoxide amino acids in rats. Planta Medica 61(1995)72-74 and 356-357.

47. Bindu, M.P., Sreekanth, K.S.; Annamala, P.T and Augusti. K.T. Effect of S-allyl Cystein Sulfoxide on lipid metabolism and free radical scavenger in alcohol fed rats. Current Sci. 82(2002) 628-631.

48. Helen, A; Krishnakumar, K; Vijayammal, P.L and Augusti, K.T. A comparative study of antioxidant S-allyl cystein sulfoxide and vitamin E on the damages induced by nicotine in rats. Pharmacology 67(2003)113-117.

49. Bobboi, A, Augusti, K.T. and Joseph. P.K., Hypolipidemic Effects of onion oil and garlic oil in ethanol-fed rats. Indian Jour. Biochem and Biophys. 21(1984)211-213.

50. Helen, A; Rajasree, C.R; Krishnakumar, K; Augusti, K.T. and Vijayammal, P.L. Antioxidant role of oils isolated from garlic (Allium sativum Linn) and onion (Allium cepa Linn) on Nicotine induced lipid peroxidation. Vet. Human Toxicol 41(5)(1999)316-319.

51. Augusti, K.T. and Benaim, M.E, Effect of Essential oil of onion (Allyl propyl disulphide) on blood glucose, free fatty acid and insulin levels of normal subjects. Clinica Chimica Acta 60(1975)21-123.

52. Bordia, A; Joshi, H.K; Sanadhya, Y.K and Bhu, N. Effect of essential oil of garlic on Serum fibrinolytic activity in patients with coronary artery disease. Atherosclerosis 28(1977)155-159.

53. Augusti, K.T., Benaim, M.E. Dewar, H.A. and Virden.R. Partial identification of the Fibrinolytic activators in onion. Atherosclerosis 21(1975)409-416.

54. Gebhardt, R and Beck, H. Differential inhibitory effects of garlic derived organosulfides on cholesterol biosynthesis in primary rat hepatocyte culture, Lipid 31(1996)1269.

55. Mathew, P.T and Augusti. K.T,. Hypoglycemic effects of onion, Allium cepa Linn, on diabetes mellitus, A Preliminary report. Ind. J. Physiol. Pharmac. 19(4)(1975)213-17

56. Itokawa, Y; Inoue, K et. al. Effect of S-methylcysteine sulfoxide, S-allyl cysteine sulfoxide and related sulfur containing amino acids on lipid metabolism. J. Nutr. 103(1973) 88-92.

57. Tarfa, S.P.; Joseph, P.K and Augusti, K.T., Preliminary studies on the antidiabetic effects of Cabbage (Brassia var capitata L) oil on streptozotocin diabetic rats. Current Sci. 57(1988)32-33.

58. Ismalia Umar, Augusti. K.T. and Joseph, P K, Hypolipidemic Action of Cabbage oil in ethanol fed rats. Indian Jour. Biochem and Biophys. 24(1987)241-43

59. Wattenberg L.W. Inhibitory effects of benzyl isothiocynate administered shortly before diethyl nitrosamine or benzo(a) pyrene on pulmonary and forestomach neoplasia in A/J mice.Carcinogenesis.8(1987)1971-83

60. Block, G; Patterson, B and Subar, A. Fruits, vegetables and cancer prevention: A review of the epidemiological evidence. Nutr.Cancer.17 (1992)1-29

61. (a) Vallejo, F; Tomas-Barteran, F.A; Garcia-Viguera, C, Phenolic compounds content in edible parts of broccoli inflorescences after domestic cooking. J. Sci. Food. Agric, 2003, 83(4).

    (b) Misiewicz, I, Skupinska, K and Kasprzycka-Guttman T. Sulforaphane and 2-oxohexyl isothiocynate induced cell growth arrest and apoptosis in L-1210 leukemia and ME-18 melanoma cells. Oncol Rep.10(6) 2003,2045-50.

5.5 A Review on the Chemistry of Alliums (Onions and Garlic), Peper Nigrum (Black Pepper) and Emblica Officinalis (Amla) with their selected Biological Effects

Sini Jose.T; Devi.S Nadh and Sharlet George,

Dept. of Medical Biochemistry, School of Medical Education, M.G.University, Kottayam-686008

WHO recommends the use of 4-5 cloves of fresh garlic every day to control hypertension. Dr. Banjamin Lau suggests every body to have some garlic cloves daily to drive off viral diseases. Dr. Augusti advocates the use of Allium Ginger Complex (4:1) by every body as is the case with the Chinese to drive away all pestilences as well as heart diseases. Dr. Arun Bordia Rtd. Cardiologist of RNT Medical College, Udaipur proved the efficacy of using both garlic and ginger by the CHD patients to improve their blood functions. At the outset let us learn the chemistry of garlic and onions to know their actual armory.

Both these vegetables contain cysteine sulfoxide derivatives or alliin of the general formula[1,2] $R\text{-}S(O)CH_2\text{-}CH(NH_2)COOH$. Where $R=C_3H_5$ i.e. allyl group $CH_2=CH.\ CH_2$- is present in garlic and propenyl groups CH_3-CH=CH- are present some in garlic and plenty in onions. Besides these R= CH_3 i.e. methyl group is present very little in garlic and in abundance in onions along with $R=C_3H_7$ i.e. propyl group is also present in abundance in the latter. When these vegetables are crushed or chewen the enzyme alliinase breaks these alliins to allicin type compounds $R_1\text{-}S\text{-}S(O)\text{-}R_2$ with groups of methyl, allyl, propenyl and propyl as the case may be with release of ammonia and pyruvic acid as the case may be[3].

$$2R–S(O)\ CH_2CH(NH_2)COOH+H_2O \rightarrow R–S–S(O)–R+ 2NH_3+2CH_3CO\ COOH$$

When R=allylgroup as in garlic and the product is allicin $C_3H_5\text{-}S\text{-}S(O)C_3H_5$ a very potent antibiotic against gram positive bacteria and virus. As the Russians used largely allicin as an antibiotic when there was no supply of penicillin, it earned the nick name "Russian penicillin" Onion produces only allicin type compounds with methyl, propenyl and propyl groups as side chains. As the double bond is towards the outer carbons of allyl group, allicin of garlic is more powerful in reactions with thiol and related groups of bacterial and viral proteins than that of onions which contains any of the methyl and propyl groups with no double bonds or propenyl group with a double bond in the interior carbon chain.

$2RSH + C_3H_5 - S - S(O) - C_3H_5 \rightarrow 2R - S - S - C_3H_5 + H_2O$

Thiol Allicin Mixed disulfide

Thus enzymes and various organisms with thiol groups are inactivated by allicins

Organo Sulfides

When allicin is stored at 4°C it is polymerized into a very active garlic principle called ajoene[4] (C_3H_5-S(O)CH_2-CH = CH-S_2-C_3H_5). This conversion is very fruitful in a medium of methanol. In other conditions of storage very little ajoene and many sulfides of the nature diallylsulfide (DAS), diallyl disulfide (DADS), diallyl trisulfide (DATS), diallyl tetrasulfide (DATTS) and other polysulfides ($C_3H_5(S)_nC_3H_5$) are formed. Out of these DADS is a good anticarcinogenic organosulfur compound[5] and others are more or less with the same property. The corresponding polysulfides of onions[6] are lesser active than those of garlic, again due to the absence or shift in the double bonds in the alkyl group. Allicin type compounds are also called thiosulfinates and their polymers are termed as cepaenes.

The botanical name Alliums for the group of onions, garlic, leeks, chives, scallions, shallot etc. is derived from the celtic word "all" which means pungent, betray the presence of a host of remarkable flavorants and odorants all having in common one sulfur[6]. Many of these flavorful sulfur compounds of garlic contain the allyl group which in turn gets its name from Allium. Onions and other allium products contain any of the alkyl groups like methyl, propenyl, propyl etc. Virtanen et. al.[7] showed that propenyl-L-Cysteine sulfoxide is the precursor of lachrymatory factor (LF) that irritates our eyes when fresh onions are crushed. It's formula is CH_3-CH_2-CH = S=O after a shift of hydrogen. The allinase present in onions converts the propenyl cysteine sulfoxide first to LF which is later rearranged to allicin type dipropenyl disulfide oxide (C_3H_5-S-S(O)C_3H_5). Propenyl-cysteine sulfoxide is present in onion to the extent of 0.2% by weight, while other alkyl derivatives of this nature are present only about 0.02% by weight. The strong flavor of onion is due to the production of a mixture of propenyl, propyl and methyl disulphides. Many glutamyl S-alkyl cysteine derivatives containing peptides are also present in alliums. When the allicin type compounds are subjected to high terperature many cyclic compounds called vinyl dithiin and thiopyran derivatives are formed. Similarly allicins of onions are converted to a group of polysulfides containing sulfoxide group as in ajoene called cepaenes. **At high temperature many sulfur containing heterocyclic compounds are also formed. Each of these allium compounds has one or other physiological property[6], such as antidiabetic, antiatherogenic, antiplatelet aggregation effects etc. (See the diagram for Allium compounds).**

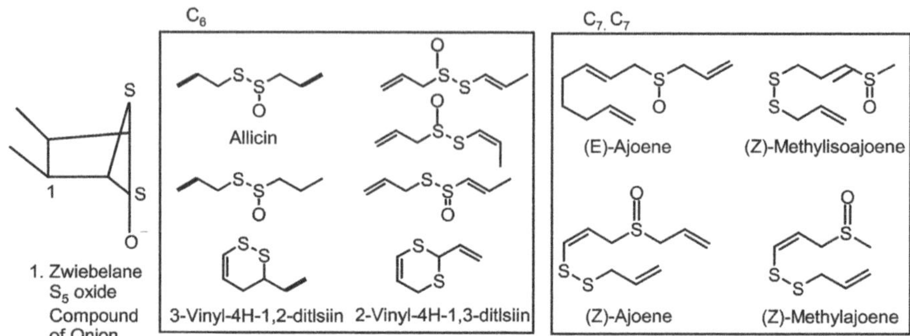

Fig. 1 Allium compounds.

Certain Rare Nutraceuticals Present in Allium Volatile Fractions

(a) Methyl-Se-S-allyl, is a selenium substitute of DADS found in garlic vapours by Cai, Block et. al.[8]. It is a dominant Se compound in this vegetable. Methyl – Se- methyl was also found in garlic volaliles at a concentration of 1% of that of alkyl sulfides. It has a very strong odor.

(b) Two terpenes are also present in garlic. d-limonene and p-cymene are released initially in minute quantities of 1%, but later it increases rapidly in 1-4 hours to levels similar to those of alkyl sulfides according to Ruiz, Hartman et .al.[9].

(c) In the essential oil of other allium species e.g. onion, shallot, leek, chives, rakkyo, scallion and Japanese bunching onion, alkyl furanones and thiophenes have also been found among the volatile flavor compounds according to the work of Galetto and Hoffman [10] and Kameoka, Iida et. al.[11].

Compounds Produced on Cooking Alliums

On heating pure alliin in water (18°C, 1hr) 1% volatiles are formed and they consist mainly of allylalcohol (67%) and acetaldehyde (21%) according to Yu and Wu[12]. As cooking quickly inactivates alliinase only 1% allicin is formed from alliin of garlic in that process. This allicin is quickly converted to DAS, DADS, DATS, DATTS, and to some suphones of the nature C_3H_5-S-S(O_2)-C_3H_5. All of them have one or other biological activity[13].

Heating of aqueous S-allyl cysteine, produces a large variety of volatiles mainly 2-methyl-1, 4 dithiepane (a 7 member ring with two sulfur atoms), allyl thioacetic acid (C_3H_5-S-CH_2COOH), DAS and DADS, but almost no allyl alcohol.

When chopped garlic and a vegetable oil were heated together a novel compound S-allyl thiohexanoate was identified due to the reaction of DADS with an unsaturated oil i.e. dienal according to Hsu, Jeng et. al.[14].

Boiling garlic cloves for 20 min. also causes hydrolysis of 12% of γ-glutamyl cysteine to S-allyl cysteine and S-1-propenyl cysteine and a similar loss of alliin without production of S-allyl cysteine. When garlic is chopped into tiny pieces or is crushed most of cysteine sulfoxides of peptides are transferred into thiosulfinates. Heating the crushed garlic at boiling temperature for 20 min. in a closed container causes complete conversion of the thiosulfinates to DATS and lesser amounts of other diallyl sulfides. However after boiling in an open container for 20 min; 7% of the allicin are retained, but 97% of the sulfides are evaporated off.

Cooking in whole milk in an open vessel causes even more rapid loss of allicin through evaporation and conversion to polysulfides. 70% of the polysulfides are retained by the fat. Baking and microwaving of garlic slices yield maximum volatiles (0.2%) and DADS is the main compound formed. In oil cooked garlic significant amount of allyl methyl disulfide, vinyl dithiins and allylalcohol are formed.

Allithiamine

In the 1950's Japanese workers found that the addition of thiamine (Vitamin B_1) to garlic extracts produced a new form of thiamine that was found to be absorbed much better than thiamine itself and was less toxic than thiamine, yet it had all the physiological effects of thiamine[15]. **This property of allicin type compounds of alliums with thiamine to form allithiamine and enhancement of certain transport mechanism for vitamin B_1 and glucose from the intestine [16] may together explain the efficacy of alliums as a moderator of hyperglycemia.** Satoh in a series of publications[17] demonstrated that garlic fed to animals as well as to humans stimulates thiamine synthesis by intestinal bacteria. **Animal experiments showed that garlic fed mice experienced a weight gain, greater agility and better defense against infections than the controls without garlic in the diet[18].**

Regular consumption of garlic plays an important role in the absorption of vitamin B_1 which is necessary for the function of the nervous system and the coronary vessels, a process that is often disturbed in elderly persons. **Bogin[19] found that garlic extract increases the permeability of certain compounds e.g; ATP through erythrocytes and mitochondrial**

membranes. These mechanisms by allium compounds may explain why they play a role against all types of stress induced problems of the body. Ajoene and similar compounds with or without an alkyl group shift to form the side chain are called cepaenes.

In 1988 Kawakishi and Morimitsu, identified methyl 1-(methyl sulfinyl) propyl disulfide [CH_3-S(O)-CH(CH_2CH_3)-S-S-CH_3]. Which is a cepaene and also obtained as a new platelet aggregation inhibitor from onion extract[20]. During that time Wagner et. al.[21] also reported the isolation of a diastereomeric pairs 1- [(E)-1- Propenyl Sulfinyl] propyl propyl disulfide (CH_3-CH=CH-S(O)-CH(CH_2-CH_3)-S-S-CH_2-CH_2-CH_3) and 1-(E)-1-propenyl sulfide) propyl (E,Z)-1-propenyl disulfide. [CH_3-CH=CH–S(O)–CH(CH_2-CH_3)-S-S-CH=CH.CH_3] with cyclooxygenase and 5-lipoxygenase inhibitory activities from onion extracts[21,22]. Later other cepaenes like 1-(methyl- sulfinyl) propyl (E,Z)-1-propenyl disulfide, [CH_3 –S(O)- CH (CH_2-CH_3)-S-S-CH = CH.CH_3] were also isolated[23]. Individual enantiomers of diastereomeric pairs showed only a two fold to four fold difference in biological activity. **Cepaenes display a variety of biological activites, viz; significant reduction in serum lipids of patients with CHD who consumed capsules containing garlic oil rich in ajoene and dithiins[24-26] for three years. The inhibitory effect of garlic and onions on human platelet aggregation have been attributed mainly to allicine type cepaenes and vinyldithiins[27,28]. Several studies indicate that components of freshly cut garlic[29] and onion[30] inhibit platelet aggregation and smooth muscle contraction through inhibition of cyclooxygenase and related enzymes. The antiasthmatic effects of onion extracts have been demonstrated and attributed to thiosulfinates and cepaenes**. These compounds exert a wide range of pharmacological effects such as inhibition of the cyclooxygenase and lipoxygenase pathways of arachidonic acid metabolism, inhibition of histamine release and leukotriene biosynthesis, prevention of bronchial asthma and platelet activating factor and inhibition of inflammatory cell influx[31]. See Fig. 1. Besides these effects antimicrobial and anticancer effects of allium oils and their compounds like ethyl ethane thiosulfinate ($C_2H_5S(O)SC_2H_5$] have been reported by various workers.

[See the figures and tables of Nutraceuticals given elsewhere]

Makheja, Chow Eng and Bailey determined the antiplatelet activity of onion and garlic extracts *in vitro* system of ADP, arachidonic acid or collagen induced platelet aggregation[34]. The activity of extracts was significant and it was ascribed to the presence of adenosine, allicin type compounds and various paraffinic polysulfides (Cepaenes). The oily fraction of onion and garlic suppressed thromboxane synthesis completely and induced a redistribution in the products of the lipoxygenase pathway.

Adenosine and allicin were present in diethyl ether extract (Polar compounds) and paraffinic polysulfides were present in petroleum ether extract (nonpolar compounds) of alliums. An authentic sample of dimethyl trisulfide duplicated the effects of onion and garlic oil fractions on both aggregation and arachidonic acid metabolism. Black fungus extract contained only adenosine which showed the antiplatelet activity. The activities for onion oil fractions were in the order Nonpolar > adenosine > polar and for garlic oil fractions were in the order Adenosine > Polar > Nonpolar.

Further Block, Iyer et. al.[35] report that garlic thioallyl compounds or related thiols have complementary action to two antioxidants vitamins C and E. Thus Cepaenes have a series of biological activities as nutraceuticals of alliums that prevent diseases.

Black Pepper (Piper Nigrum Linn)

It is called black gold of India as it is in great demand for the foreigners from time immemorial. Black pepper, long pepper, dry ginger, garlic and cumin are used to prepare a decoction to cure viral fevers according to vidhyamadam Cheriya Narayanan Nampoothiri (Mathrubhumi News paper report 3rd June 2007). All the above contain very good nutraceuticals. Black pepper contains a medicinally active alkaloid piperin to the extent of 3-8% and it is the most pungent substance. Other alkaloids are piperanine and piperylin. Pepper volatile compounds are 1-16% α-pinene, 0.2-19% sabinene, 9-30% β caryophyllene, 0- 20 % Δ^3 carene, 16 – 24 % limonene, 5-14% β-pinene etc[36(a)]. Black pepper is used in almost all Ayurvedic preparations. Water and ethanol crude extracts of black pepper were investigated at the department of Chem. Atturk University Faculty of Science & Arts in Turkey, for their antioxidant and radical scavenging activation in six different assays[37] viz: total antioxidant activity, reducing power 1,1-diphenyl-2-pieryl hydrazyl (DPPH) free radical scavenging, super oxide anion radical scavenging, H_2O_2 Scavenging and metal chelating activities. Both water extract and ethanol extract of black pepper exhibited strong total antioxidant activity. Most of the volatiles are mono or sesquiterpenes and they have anticarcinogenic, anti-inflammatory, antiviral and immunostimulatory properties[36(a),38]. **The 75 μg/mL concentration of these extracts showed 95.5 and 93.3% inhibition on peroxidation of linoleic acid emulsion respectively (*in vitro* study). Same concentration of α tocopherol at the same time exhibited only 70.4% inhibition on peroxidation of the above system.**

Total phenolic content in both the above extracts were determined as gallic acid equivalents and values were 54.3 and 42.8 μg gallic equivalent of phenols per mg of water and ethanol extracts in dry form respectively (Folin-ciocuttau procedure). Further work on these antioxidants *in vivo* system is warranted.

In addition to the above black pepper contains the following also[38]

1. **Pinene** which is a monoterpene hydrocarbon with a pleasant aromatic odour.
2. **Myristicin** is a phenyl propaniod ether structurally related to safrol and present in the seeds only in small amounts. It is useful in lower disease, but toxic in high doses according to Hall[39]. Alkamides are also present in black pepper and they are responsible for sharp burning taste. They are long chain unsaturated fatty acid amides.
3. **Piperine** is an alkaloid called 1-piperoyl piperidine. It is present in piper nigrum and piper longum (black and long peppers). Piperine is a stimulant to our system and shown to have hepatoprotective effects though less potent than silmarin[40]. Piperine influences the bioavailability of other compounds, be they herbal or pharmaceutical. This has been related to an interaction of these compounds that leads to alteration in membrane dynamics and permeability in the intestine following ingestion of piperine[41].

Ginger-Allium-Pepper Food Complex

Very recently Dr. Augusti made a preparation of ginger and garlic homogenate in the ratio of 1:4 by weight and added enough black pepper and common salt to improve its taste. This food complex at a dose of 10 g daily with milk or food for 15 days prevented infection of viral fevers and cured the edema and joint pains of many affected by viral fevers in Kerala during 2007. This type of food complex is promoted in china to prevent cancer, CHD and viral infections.

Emblica Officinalis Gaertn (Amla)

Amla or Indian gooseberry is being used against a variety of conditions like liver injury, atherosclerosis[42] and diabetes[43]. It possesses very good hypocholesterolemic effect also[44]. Chavanaprasa and Brahmarasayana contain amla and they are being used for rejuvenating body[45], and also as immunomodulators[46], as paste to lower body temperature, to stop bleeding from nose, head aches and certain psychiatric condition[47]. Amla was also found to enhance interferon production[48]. Maharshi Ayurvedic herbal mixtures M4 and M5 containing amla were reported to have anticarcinogenic property[49]. A very recent finding about amla is its antioxidant action. The antioxidants present in amla are aqueous soluble, extractable with ether and the active fraction contains epigallocatechin gallate (EGCG) and gallic acid derivatives[50]. Apart from the tannins[51], amla contains trigalloylglucose, ellagicacid[52], flavonoids[53] and phyllemblic acid[54]. The antioxidant activity is mainly associated with polyphenols and flavonoids.

1. **An experiment conducted on garlic amla and onions by Dr. Augusti's group[55].**

   We know that animal fats like butter and beef fats are atherogenic in nature as they contain 46% and 57% saturated long chain fatty acids respectively. Moreover butter fat (BUF) contains more cholesterol than beef fat (BF), 727 & 455 mg/100g. In order to study their hypercholesterolemic effects and also to compare the beneficial effects of the three vegetables garlic, amla (Indian goose berry) and onions on hyperlipidemia, they conducted the following experiments on rats. They took nine groups of rats containing five in each. Group I was fed only laboratory rat feed, groups 2 to 5 were fed laboratory diet mixed with 21% of BUF. Besides that homogenized forms of 5% garlic, 5% amla and 5% onions by weight were added to the diets of groups 3, 4, 5 respectively. Groups 6 to 9 were fed laboratory diet mixed with 21%BF. Besides that 5% garlic, 5% amla and 5% onions made as above by weight were added to the diets of groups 7 to 9 respectively. After a period of three months feeding the rats were sacrificed after over night fasting. Their blood, liver, heart and kidneys were collected for various estimations.

   Results

   It was observed that diets containing BUF and BF increased significantly the lipoid profile i.e. total cholesterol, TAG, and VLDL+LDL cholesterol in serum and tissues. Certain marker enzymes i.e. AST and ALT for CHD and liver diseases respectively also increased significantly. Addition of any of the three vegetable separately ameliorated the hyperlipidemic and enzyme raising effects of both BUF & BF. In addition to the above, incorporation of garlic and amla in the diet increased the serum level of HDL cholesterol and thus brought down the atherogenic index i.e. total cholesterol/HDL cholesterol, to the normal level i.e. from 3.7 to 2.5. We also noted that BUF is more harmful than BF in their hyperlipidemic and enzyme altering process.

However the damages brought about by these two saturated fats could not be nullified completely by any of the above three vegetables and the order of their beneficial effects is represented below.

Garlic > Amla > Onion

The better effects demonstrated by garlic and amla than by onions may be because the former two contain biologically more effective unsaturated allyl group or flavonoid type compounds than the last one. i.e. the vegetables on homogenization released the active compounds like allyl and diallyl sulfides, their oxides and ajoene type compounds from garlic and various polyphenols and flavonoids, like ellagic acids, phyllemblic acids etc from amla. Onion compounds are alkyl sulfides, sulfoxides and allicin type compounds with saturated side chains of methyl & propyl groups or an altered form of allyl group such as propenyl group[6]. These last series of compounds are less active than the former two as antioxidants. All these results emphasis the role of functional foods that contain nutraceuticals with various beneficial effects on unwanted dietary compounds such as various saturated lipids and cholesterol.

2. **A Comparative study on the beneficial effects of amla and vitamin C by Dr. Bordia's group[56].**

A comparative study on the effects of amla juice, its pulp and vitamin C (35 mg vitamin C or its equivalent of juice/pulp of amla/kg/day) has been conducted on rabbits fed an atherogenic diet for three months by Bordia's group[56].

Amla juice, its pulp and vitamin significantly prevented the rise in serum cholesterol and TGS and tendency for platelet aggregation due to cholesterol feeding. All three items used above viz; amla juice, its pulp and vitamin C prevented the development of experimental atheroma significantly. However amla juice and pulp were found to be superior to vitamin C as antiatherogenic agents. The researchers attributed these effects of amla primarily to tannins that protect vitamin C as suggested earlier by Brahmachari and Gupta[51] and also to polyphenols such as gallic acid/ellagic acid systems in addition to pectin a soluble fiber present in amla. Tannins and polyphenols are strong antioxidants and their presence in the pulp/juice etc might have been responsible for the antiplatelet aggregation hypocholesterolemic and hypolipidemic effects of amla. [Dr.H.DBrahmachari was the Ph.D. guide of Dr. Augusti at BITS Pilani]

3. **Advantages of mixing equal parts of saturated and unsaturated oils or of feeding of garlic oil along with either of them[57].**

In a previous study Augusti et. al.[58] showed the hypolipidemic effect of garlic oil with coconut oil diet. At present to compare the hypolipidemic effect of garlic oil at a dose of 100 mg/kg in rats fed a diet containing 20% sunflower oil (SFO) and 2% cholesterol with another group whose diet contained 10% each of SFO and CNO along with 2% cholesterol, the following experiment was conducted. Male albino rats of Sprague Dawley Strain were divided into five groups, containing 5 rats in each group. Group 1 was kept as normal control and they were fed on normal laboratory feed. Group 2 was fed 2% cholesterol diet made from normal feed and cholesterol. Group 3 was fed with another diet containing 20% SFO and 2% cholesterol made with the normal feed Group 4 was fed with a diet containing 2% cholesterol, 10% SFO and 10% CNO. Group 5 was fed with the same diet as for group 3, but they were treated by feeding garlic oil (100 mg/kg) for a month. After this period the rats were weighed and after over night fasting they were all sacrificed and the biochemical parameters in blood and tissues were determined. The high cholesterol diet with and without SFO produced certain deleterious effects on serum and tissue lipids and also on certain serum marker enzymes viz; catalase and glutathione reductase. Feeding a diet as for group 4 or on feeding garlic oil to group 5 the deleterious effects of a high cholesterol or high SFO in the diet could be significantly reduced. The advantages of a diet containing equal amounts of saturated CNO and unsaturated SFO for group 4 and the beneficial effects of an antioxidant like garlic oil for group 5 are self evident from the results. These findings high light the beneficial roles of nutraceuticals in our diet and their recent wide range acceptability along with vitamins and minerals as essential modulators for a better health management.

References

1. Virtanen, A.I and Matikkala, E.J. The isolation of S-methyl cysteine sulphoxide and S-n-propylcysteine sulphoxide from onion (Allium cepa) and the antibiotic activity of crushed onion. Acta Chem,. Scand 13(1959)1898-1900

2. Stoll, A and Seebeck, E. Experientia 3(1947)114-115

3. Cavallito, C.J. and Bailey, J.H. Allicin, the antibacterial principle of Allium Sativum-1. Isolation, physical properties and antibacterial action. J. Am. Chem. Soc. 66(1944) 1950-51.
4. Block, E; Ahmad, S; Jain R.W; Cerecely. R and Apitz, Castro M.R. (E.Z.) Ajoene a potent antithrombotic agent from garlic. J. Am. Chem. Soc.106 (1984)8295-96.
5. Maunday, R and Maunday, C.M. Induction of Phase II enzymes by aliphatic sulfides derived from garlic and onions; an overview. Methods Enzymol 382(2004)449-456.
6. Block. E The organosulfur chemistry of the genus Allium. Implications for the organic chemistry of sulfur. Angew Chem. Int. Ed. Engl. 31(1992) 1135-78.
7. Wilkens, W.F. Ph.D Thesis Cornell University, Ithaca, N.Y.(1961).
8. Cai X.J; Block, E et. al. Allium chemistry; identification of Seleno amino acids in ordinary and selenium enriched garlic, onion and broccoli using gas chromatography with atomic detection. J. Agri. Food Chem.. 43(1995) 1754-57.
9. Ruiz.R; Hartman. T.G et. al. Breath analysis of garlic-borne phytochemicals in human subjects: combined absorbent trapping and short path thermal desorption gas chromatography-mass spectrometry. ACS Sympo. Ser. 546(1994) 102-119.
10. (a) Galetto, W.G. and Hoffman,P.G. Synthesis and flavor evaluation of several alkyl furanones found in Allium Species (onion, shallots, leeks) J. Agric Food Chem.. 24 (1976) 854-856.

    (b) Galetto, W.G. and Hoffman, P.G. Synthesis and flavor evaluation of some alkyl thiophenes volatile components of onion. J. Agri. Food. Chem.24(1976)852-854.
11. Kameoka, H; Iida. H et. al. Sulphides and furanones from steam volatile oils of Allium fistulosum and Allium chinense. Phytochemistry 23 (1984)455-58.
12. Yu, T.H; Wu, C.M et. al. Volatile compounds generated from thermal degradation of alliin and deoxy alliin in an aqueous solution. J. Agric. Food chem. 42(1994)146-153.

13. Lawson, L.D. and Wang Z.Y.J. Changes in the organo-sulfur compound released from garlic during aging in water, dilute ethanol, or dilute acid J. toxicology 14 (1995) 214.

14. Hsu, J.P; Jeng. J.G; and Chen. C.C Identification of a novel sulfur compound from the interaction of garlic and heated edible oil. Proc. Int. Conf. Prog. Flavour Precursor Stud 1993. 391-394.

15. Fujiwara, M. Allithiamine and its properties. J. Nutr. Sci. Vitaminol 22(1976)57-62.

16. Kokas, E.V. and Ludany. G.V. die wirkung der Gewurzmittel auf die Bewegungder darmzotten and die glykoseresorption. Arch. Exp. Pathol. Pharmakol 169(1933)140-45.

17. Satoh, Z. Effect of Allium diets on bacterial syntesis of thiamine in the intestinal tract. VII. The invitros synthesis of thiamine from garlic by Escherichia coli. Vitamins[Japan] 5(1952) 585-589.

18. Makowsky, Zur Frage der Beein flussung von Impfgeschewulstender. Mausdurch Gewurzstoffe und Golibakterien. Z Immunitatsforsch. Exp. Ther. 89(1936)123-130.

19. Bogin, E and Abrams, M. The effect of garlic extract on the activity of some enzymes. Food cosmet. Toxicel 14 (1976) 447-49.

20. Kawakishi, S and Morimitsn, Y. Lancet (1988)330.

21. Bayer, T. Wagner, H; Wray, V and Dorch, W. Lancet (1988) 906.

22. Bayer, T. Dissertation, Universitat Munchen. 1988.

23. Morimitsu, Y; Kawakishi, S. Phytochemistry 29(1990) 3435-39

24. Lawson, L.D. Human Medicinal agents from plants (Eds. A.D. Kinghorn and M. Balandarin) American Chemical Society, Washington. D.C 1992.

25. Lawson, L.D; Ranson, D.K. and Hughes, B.G. Thromb. Res 65(1992) 141-156.

26. Makheja, A.N; Vanderhock, J.Y et. al. Adv. Prostaglandin Thromboxane Res.6 (1980) 309-312. and Biochem Pharmacol 29 (1990) -3169-73

27. Ali, M; Thomson, M et. al. Prostaglandin Leukotriene Essential Fatty Acids 41(1990)95-99

28. Boulllin, D.J. Lancet 1981. 776-777.

29. Gaffen, J.D; Tavarer. I.A. and Bennett, A.J. Pharm. Pharmacol. 36(1984)272-274.

30. Morimitsu, Y; Morioka, Y and Kawakishi. S, J. Agric. Food. Chem. 40(1992)368-72

31. Dorseh,W; Schneider, E et. al. Int. Arch. Allergy. Appl. Immunol 92(1992) 39-42. and Wagner, H; Dorseh, W et. al. Prostaglandins, Leukot. Essential Fatty acids. 39(1990) 59-62

32. Weisberger, A.S; Pensky, J. Science Washington. D.C. 126(1957) 1112-1115.

33. Lau, B.H.S; Tadi, P.P; Tosk, J.M. Nutr.Res. (N.Y)10 (1990) 937-48.

34. Makheja. A.N. Chow Eng Low and Bailey, J,M. Biological Nature of platelet inhibitors from A Cepa, A. Sativum and Auricularia Polytrica. Abstract from VIIth International Congress on Thrombosis and Haemostasis. July 1981(See Ref.26)

35. Block, E; Iyer R, et. al. Lipoxygenase inhitors from essential oil of garlic. Morkovnikov addition of the allyldithio radical of olefins. J. Am. Chem. Soc. Soc.110 (1988)7813-7827.

36. (a) Belitz. H.D and Grosch, W. Food Chemistry (1999) p.908. Springer-Verlag. Berlin.

    (b) Dolara, P; Corte, B et. al. Local anaesthetic, antibacterial and antifungal properties from myrrh, planta Medica 66(2000)356-358.

37. Gulcin Ilhami. The antioxidant and radical scavenging activities of black pepper (Peper nigrum) seeds. Int.J. Food. Sci. Nutr.56(7)(2005)491-499.

38. Essential oils and Resin. In: The constituents of medicinal plants Andrew Pengelly (ed) 2nd edn. CABI Publishing, CAB International Walling ford Oxon, U.K. 2004. p.55-90, 96,138.

39. Hall. R. toxicants occurring Naturally in Foods, Ntional Academy of Sciences, Washington, D.C. 1973.

40. Koul, I and Kapil, A. Evaluation of liver protective potential of piperine, an active principle of black and long peppers plant a Media 59(1993)413-417.

41. Khajuria A; thusu, N and Zutshi U; Piperine modulates permedability characteristics of intestine by inducint alterations in membrane dynamics; influences on brush border membrane fluidity, ultrastructure and enzyme kinetics. Phytomedicine 9(2002)224-31.

42. Thakur, C.P Thakur, B et. al. The Ayurvedic Medicines, haritak, amla and bahira reduce cholesterol induced atherosclerosis in rabbits. Indian J. Cardiol 21(1988), 167.

43. Tripathi, S.N; Tiwarim C M. et. al. Screening of hypoglycemic action in certain indigenousdrugs. J Res. Indian Med. Yoga Homoep. 14 (1929)159.

44. Thakur, C.P. Emblica officinalis reduces serum, aestic and hepatic cholesterol in rabbits. Experientia 41 (185) 423.

45. Praveenkumar, V; Kuttttan, R and Kuttan G. Effect of Rasayanas in normal and tuomor bearing mice. J. Exp. Clin. Cancer. Res. 13(1994)67.

46. Ojha, J.K in: Chyavanaprash a scientific study, 1st edn Indeginous drugs of India (VN Dhar & Sons. Published by Tara Books Agency. Varanasi, India) 1985, 506.

47. Balakrishnan, V.V. Fruits and their medicinal properties (DC Books, Kottayam, Kerala, India) 1993, 56.

48. Rao, T.S; kuppuraja, K et. al. Herbal preparations of Emblica officinalis, j. Res Ayur Sidha, 1 94) 1980, 507.

49. Shaema, H.M; Hanna, A.N et. al. Inhibition of uman low density lipoprotein oxidation in vitro by Maharshi ayurveda herbal mixtures, pharma biochem. Behaviour, 43 (1992) 1175.

50. Jeena. K. Jose and Kuttan, R. Antioxidant activity of Emblica officinalis. J.Clin Biochem Nutr19 (1995) 63.

51. Brahmachari, H.D and Gupta, V.S. Studies on Phyllanthus emblica (Amla) part III Role of tannins in stabilizing the ascorbic acid of the fruit. Indian. J. Appl.Chem.21 91958) 173-74.

52. Damodaran, M and Nair, K.R. A tannin from Indian goose berry (Phyllanthus emblica) with protective action on ascorbic acid. Biochem. J. 30 91936) 1014-1020.

53. Khanna, P; taparia, R and Jain, S.C. Flavonoids from Emblica officinalis Gaertn, tissue cultures, Indian J. Bot. 5 91982) 43-44.

54. Pillay, PP and Iyer, M.K. A chemical examination of Emblica officinalis. Curr. Sci.27 91968) 266-267.

55. Augusti, KT; Arahy, S.L et. al. A comparative study on the beneficial effects of garlic, amla and onion on the hyperlipidemia induced by butter fat and beef fat in rats. Ind. Jour. Exp. Biol. 39 92001) 760-66.

56. Bordia, A; Verma, S.K: Mehta, L.K and Andrews, A.M.R Comparative effect of Vitamin C, Amla Juice and amla pulp on blood lipids, platelet aggregation and experimental atheroma in rabbits. Indian heart journal 37 (1985) 179-182.

57. Devi. S. Nadh, Sudheesh M. et. al. Beneficial effects of coconut oil, garlic oil, coconut kernel and ground nuts in cholesterol fed rats. Souvenir, national seminar on coconut oil and coconut production in health and disease 19 – 20 Sept.2003, thiruvananthapuram PP 104-111.

58. Augusti, K.T; Julie chackery, Julie Jacob et. al. Beneficial effects of a polar fraction of garlic (Allium sativum Linn) oil in rats fed with two different high fat diets. Indian Jour. Exp. Biol. 43 (2005) 76-83.

Chapter – 6

Nutraceuticals Vs Diseases

6.1 Role of Dietary Fiber, Functional Foods and Drugs in the Control of Diabetes Mellitus

Dr. K.P. Paulose, Physician,

SUT Hospital, Pattom, Thiruvananthapuram-4

Diabetes Mellitus (DM) is the commonest disease seen in Kerala. It is defined as a syndrome characterized by chronic hyperglycaemia associated with disturbances of carbohydrate, fat and protein metabolism due to absolute or relative deficiency of insulin secretion and/or its action. In this chapter we briefly describe the types of DM and its management by selected forms of insulin and oral drugs with certain adjustments in the diets, particularly with relation to functional foods. As India tops in this disease in the world we should know more about this disease[1]. The new classification of diabetes mellitus is shown below.

New Classification of Diabetes Mellitus

1. **Type 1 Diabetes (Old Iddm)**
   - Auto immune (antibodies present)
   - Idiopathic (no antibodies)
2. **Type 2 Diabetes (Old Niddm)**
3. **Gestational Diabetes**
4. **Other Types**
   (a) Genetic defects
   (b) Endocrinopathies
   (c) Disease of exocrine pancreas including Infection, Calcific pancreatitis
   (d) Drug induced – mainly steroids
   (e) Genetic syndromes

1. **Type-1 Diabetes or Insulin Dependent Diabetes Mellitus (IDDM)**

   These patients depend on insulin for survival. On withdrawal they go into hyperglycemia, ketoacidosis and coma. IDDM has its onset most often in childhood and adolescence although it may occur at any age. Though usually abrupt onset, it can be protracted in its course. The HLA association of autoimmunity and environmental factors are thought to play certain roles in the causation and precipitation of IDDM.

2. **Type-2 Diabetes or Non-Insulin Dependent Diabetes Mellitus**

   NIDDM begins in middle age or after 40 years. The pathophysiological basis is a combination of increased peripheral insulin resistance at receptor/post receptor level, increased hepatic glucose output, hyperinsulinemia and subsequently impaired Beta cell function. Since the incidence of diabetes mellitus is increasing, screening test is essential in all possible cases.

The Major Risk Factors for NIDDM include

1. Family history of diabetes mellitus, 2. obesity, 3. race, 4. age equal or more than 45 years, 5. previously identified glucose intolerance, 6. hypertension and hyperlipidaemias and, 7. women with a bad obstetric history and delivery of big babies. In these patients, screening with fasting blood glucose or in appropriate cases, glucose tolerance test should be performed with oral administration of 75 g of glucose.

As shown by DCCT, UKPDS, and Kumamotto (in Japan) studies; strict control of diabetes mellitus is essential for preventing/retarding hyperglycemia related complications. For striving euglycemia it is mandatory to monitor blood glucose periodically in all cases of diabetes mellitus. In all cases of diabetes mellitus, glycosylated Hb, ECG, microalbuminuria, lipid profile etc should be monitored. Doppler study of peripheral vessels and comprehensive ophthalmic and neurologic examination is mandatory at least on an annual basis. (Full form of DCCT=Diabetes control and complication trials, UKPDS=United Kingdom Prospective Diabetes Study);

Glycosylated Hb has the advantage of assessing glucose control in the preceding 2-3 months and not being influenced by diet, mode of therapy, physical activity, meals and patient's co-operation at the time of blood testing. Glycosylated Hb values may be misleading in conditions where life span of RBCs are altered as in hemolytic anemia or haemoglobinopathies. Glycosylated Hb is not useful for day to day management or in adjusting the dose of insulin or oral hypoglycemic drugs.

Management

Diet is the corner stone in the management of diabetes mellitus. The goals of non-pharmacological therapy in diabetes mellitus are:

1. Improving overall health
2. Achieving euglycemia and eulipidemia (Normal blood sugar and lipids)
3. Providing calories for maintaining weight, growth and development in children and adolescents, to meet the increased metabolic needs during lactation and pregnancy.

The first step in prescribing a diet for diabetes mellitus is calculating the ideal body weight. Simple formula to calculate the ideal body weight of a patient is by subtracting 100 from the patient's height in cm. e.g. Height 170 cm. Ideal wt=170-100=70 kg (Broca's index). The next step is calculation of appropriate calorie for a given patient. For a diabetic patient with ideal body weight, the usual requirement is 30 kcal./kg/day, which may be modified depending upon the weight of the individual. 60% of the calories should be from carbohydrate and proteins should be given to make up to approximately 20% of total calories. The remaining calories should be from fat (20%). The selection of functional foods containing antioxidants as part of the patient's food may be beneficial in the control of DM and that part is separately delt with. Exercise should be individualized for each patient. A comprehensive health check-up is essential before undergoing strenuous exercise. Exercise is relatively contraindicated in patients with severe LV dysfunction and other medical conditions. (LV=Left ventricle).

Pharmacotherapy

Oral hypoglycemic agents (OHAs): Oral hypoglycemic agents are indicated in all cases of diabetes mellitus of mild to moderate severity. The contraindications for oral hypoglycemic agents are: IDDM, pregnancy, severe infections, and allergy to sulphonylurea, liver and kidney diseases and surgery.

OHAs are classified Mainly under 4 Headings

1. Those which stimulate pancreas to produce more insulin – insulin secretogogues.
2. Those which reduce the peripheral insulin resistance – insulin sensitisers
3. Those which suppress appetite as well as hepatic glucose production and
4. Those which reduce the absorption of glucose from the small intestine.

Table 1. Commonly used hypoglycemic agents at present.

Class	Name	Duration of action Hrs.	Daily dose preferable	Type of action*
Sulphonyl-Ureas	Glibenclamide	24	1.25-20 mg	(1)
	Glipizide	24	2.5-20 mg	(1)
	Gliclazide	10-20	80-320 mg	(1)
	Glimiperide	24	4-8 mg	(1)
Nonsulphonyl-Ureas	Nateglenide	8	180-240 mg	(1)
	Repaglinide	8	8-16 mg	(1)
Meglitinides	Rosiglitazone	6-8	8-12 mg	(2)
	Pioglitazone	18-24	45 mg	(2)
Biguanides	Metformin	8	0.5-2 g	(3)
α- Glucosidase Inhibitors	Acarbose	6-8	300 mg	(4)
	Miglitol	6-8	150 mg	(2)

* 1. Insulin secretogogue.
2. Insulin Sensitiser.
3. Enhances peripheral up take of glucose and diminishes hepatic glucose production
4. Inhibits glucosidase

The oral hypoglycemic agents should be started in small dose which may be increased gradually to maximum recommended dose. Complications of oral hypoglycemic agents are few and relatively uncommon. Oral hypoglycemic agents may be combined with insulin and different groups of oral hypoglycemic agents may be combined in appropriate cases. Sulphonylureas act by stimulating beta cells. Biguanides act by many ways viz. inducing anorexia, insulin sensitising, and increased expression of GLUT 4 pathways. Combination of sulphonylurea with Metformin is the standard type of combination therapy. **But, it is not advisable to combine one sulphonyl urea with another sulphonyl urea. More over they are not suitable for obese diabetics.**

Acarbose (A Tetra Saccharide)

It is isolated from fermentation of actinomycetes and it is a nonabsorbable alpha glucosidase inhibitor. It blocks the alpha glucosidase enzyme in the brush border of intestinal enterocyte, thus suppressing the digestion of starch, sucrose and maltose. Additionally acarbose decreases the meal stimulated secretion of gastric inhibitor polypeptide (GIP) and other gastrointestinal hormones. The recommended dose is 50 mg thrice a day – to be increased after 2 weeks to a maximum dose of 600 mg per day. Major side effects of this drug are abdominal fullness and diarrhoea. Hypoglycaemia does not occur when the drug is used alone. This should be taken along with food. Miglitol belongs to the same group, but this is absorbable, however the action is the same. Initial does is 25 mg tds. Side effects are the same.

Meglitinides

This group of drugs e.g.; Rosiglitazone and Pioglitazone are newer oral hypoglycemic agents. They are insulin sensitizing agents and useful in type 2 diabetes. It can be given as monotherapy or in combination with other oral hypoglycemic agents and insulin. Pioglitazone is long acting (maximum dose 45 mg/day) while rosiglitazone is short acting (max.- 12 mg/day). Weight gain is an important side effect, hence contraindicated in patients with heart failure and obesity. Glitazones bind to PPAR receptors (Peroxisome Proliferator activated receptor) and increases insulin sensitity.

Insulin Therapy

The insulin is divided into major categories based on the duration of action: very short acting, intermediate acting and long acting. All types of insulin are available as porcine, bovine, highly purified mono components and human insulin. The important definite indications for insulin therapy are: **Type-I diabetes, gestational diabetes requiring insulin, acute metabolic conditions, sepsis and major stressful situations like surgery.**

Table 2. Insulin Preparations

Insulin Preparations	Onset action	Peak action	Total duration
Short Acting			
Regular	0.5-1 hrs.	2-4 hrs.	4-6 hrs.
Intermediate acting			
NPH	3-4 hrs.	10-16 hrs.	20-24 hrs.
Lente	3-4 hrs.	10-16 hrs.	20-24 hrs.
Long acting			
Ultralente	6-8 hrs.	14-20 hrs.	24-32 hrs.
PZI	6-8 hrs.	14-20 hrs.	24-32 hrs.
Biphasic			
Premix in diff.ratios			
30:70; 50:50	0.5 hrs.	2-10 hrs.	12-18 hrs.
(NPH&Reg)			

Newer Insulins/Insulin Analogues

Lyspro	-	**Short acting**
Insulin Aspart	-	**Short acting, also long acting preparations Combined with protamine.**
Insulin detmir	-	**long acting (not yet available)**
Insulin Glargine	-	**long acting – 24 hr.action, very costly, but effective**

The initial dose required can be calculated as 0.5 units/kg/day for IDDM and 0.2 units/kg/day for NIDDM. If patient is not symptomatic, (osmotic symptoms) 50% of dose calculated by the above formula can be the starting dose and the dose can be gradually increased by 4 units every 4th day. If the patient is symptomatic, the above-calculated dose can be given.

The best time to gauge the effectiveness of morning intermediate acting insulin is to check the fasting blood sugar the next day. If FBS is under control same dose can be continued. If fasting blood glucose is high, in addition to morning dose of insulin, a small dose of intermediate acting insulin (50% of the morning dose) may be given at dinner time. If the patient also has elevated pre lunch blood sugar, regular insulin is usually necessary in the morning to handle post breakfast hyperglycemia.

The above regimen of regular and intermediate insulin in the morning controls hyperglycemia in most cases. If the post dinner blood glucose is high, a small dose of regular insulin is necessary before dinner in addition to morning dose of insulin. Combination of regular and intermediate acting insulin before dinner may be necessary if fasting blood glucose is high. The combination of short and intermediate acting insulin in the morning and evening is known as mixed and split dose insulin regime. Various oral hypoglycemic agents may be combined with insulin preparations. (Example–bed time insulin and day time sulphonylurea (BIDS). *In significant renal and hepatic diseases the only treatment modality for diabetes is insulin when oral hypoglycaemic agents are contraindicated. In gestational diabetes mellitus, human insulin are preferred.* In all insulin requiring patients for major surgery, insulin infusion has to be started on the day of surgery. For minor surgical procedures, in patients on oral hypoglycemic agents and euglycemic no need of starting insulin for a short time. For minor surgery in patients on insulin, the same dose may be continued with slight modifications.

Surveillance for complications of diabetes should be done in all cases of diabetes mellitus. This includes fundus examination, urine examination for albumin, electrocardiogram and echocardiogram for cardiovascular system, Doppler study and biothesiometry, assessment of lipids and if necessary, cases should be referred to concerned specialist in appropriate cases.

Guidelines for Management of Type 2 DM

The corner stone of management of Type 2 Diabetes is non-pharmacological therapy, both diet and exercise. All patients with Type 2 Diabetes Mellitus should be prescribed balanced diet at least for 4-6 weeks before embarking on pharmacotherapy.

For treatment purposes, diabetic patients may be classified into obese and non-obese. After a trial of diet and exercise, if the patient remains uncontrolled with a fasting blood sugar more than 140 mg% or 2 Hr PPBS more than 200 mg%, pharmacotherapy is started.

In obese patients with FBS more than 140 mg% after a month of dietary therapy and exercise, treatment may be started with Metformin, in the usual starting dose of 250-500 mg twice or thrice daily after meals. Depending upon the response, the dose may be increased to a maximum of 2g a day in divided doses. If the blood sugar is not controlled with Metformin alone, Glibenclamide or Glipizide or Gliclazide must be added, starting with 5 mg daily (80 mg gliclazide) and slowly increasing it to 15 mg daily, in divided doses. More patient compliance will be obtained with Glimiperide as a single dose, initially 1mg/day and it can be increased up to 6 mg/day. If the combination OHA therapy fails to achieve adequate control, insulin therapy is necessary. Insulin therapy can be initially started as basal therapy with a night dose of NPH insulin starting with 15 units and increasing it slowly to a maximum of 25 units. If adequate control cannot be achieved with a night dose of 25 units, twice daily use of combination of regular and NPH Insulin to be started.

Non-obese patients with minimal elevation of fasting blood sugar (<140 mg%) require sulphonylurea (glibenclamide, glipizide and glimiperide) for a good control of diabetes, since there is minimal Beta cell reserve of the pancreas. In the second step, metformin may be added to sulphonylurea. In obese patients insulin may be started if glycemic status is not achieved with combination of sulphonylurea and biguanides. Initial therapy with insulin is also advocated by some followed by OHA to increase the β cell reserve.

In both groups of patients with significant elevation of postprandial hyperglycemia, a trial of alpha glycosidase inhibitors like Acarbose or Miglitol may be started before initiating insulin therapy. Acarbose may be started as a single dose of 50 mg with breakfast and addition of second dose may be considered after fifteen days.

Table 3. Proposed criteria for blood sugar and required parameters control in DM patients

Index	Good (mg%)	Fair (mg%)	Poor (mg%)
FBS	<120	120-140	>140
PP(2 hrs)	<160	160-200	>200
S.Lipid TC	200	200-220	>220
TG	180	180-220	>220
HDL chol.	>50	35-45	<35
LDL chol.	130	130-150	>150
Blood pressure	<130/85 mm Hg	<140/90 mm Hg	>140/95 mmHg
HbAIC	<6.5%	6.5%-8%	>8%

All patients should be non smokers

Table 4. Anti-diabetic drugs

Medication	Route & Year of Introduction	Efficacy – HbAIC Reduction
Insulin	S/C (1921)	>2.5
Inhaled Duralin	Pulmonary (2006)	1.5
Sulfonyl Ureas	Oral (1946)	1.5
Biguanides	Oral (1957)	
Metformin	Oral (1995 USA approved)	1.5
α- Glucosidase inhibitors	Oral (1995)	0.5-0.8
Thiozolidinediones[1]	Oral Triglitazone (1997-Withdrawn)	
Rosiglitazone[2]	Oral (1999)	
Pioglitazone[3]	Oral (1999)	
Glinides (Repaglinide, Nateglinide)	Oral (1997)	1-1.5
GLP_1 agonists Exenatides Parenteral	(2005)	0.6
Amylin agonists Parenteral	(2005)	0.6
DPP- IV inhibitors : Sitagliptin	Oral (2006)	0.5-0.9
Vildagliptin	Oral (2006)	0.5-0.9

1, 2, 3 are insulin sensitizers.

Table 5 Main characteristics of currently availableoral blood glucose lowering drugs.

Drug(s)	Reduction in glycated haemo globin (%)	Main mode of action	Benefits	Side effects and limitation
Metformin	1.5	Lowers production of hepatic glucose	No weight gain: cheap	Gastrointestinal complaints; lactic acidosis (very rare)
Sulfonylureas	1.5	Stimulate insulin secretion	Cheap	Hypoglycaemia, sometimes severe and of long duration; weight gain
Thiozolidinediones	0.5-1.5	Improve insulin sensitivity	Improve lipid profile and may reduce risk of cardiovascular disease	Fluid retention, which can cause heart failure (rare); weight gain; expensive
α-Glucosidase inhibitors*	0.5-0.8	Retard intestinal absorption of glucose	No weight gain	Gastrointestinal side effects: multiple daily dosing required; expensive.
Meglitinides*	1-1.5	Stimulate insulin secr etion	Short acting, less risk of hypoglycaemia	Need to be taken at meal time; expensive
Dipeptidylpeptidase 4 inhibitors*	0.5-10	Stimulate insulin secretion	Low risk of hypoglycaemia	Experience limited: expensive

*Not yet licensed for use in the United Kingdom.

Table 6 Main characteristics of parenteral blood glucose lowering agents and inhaled insulin

Drug(s)	Reduction in glycated haemo globin (%)	Main mode of action	Benefits	Side effects and limitation
Pramlintide*	0.5-1.0	Retards gastric emptying and reduces energy intake	Weight loss	Needs to be injected before meals: gastrointestinal side effects; expensive: experience limited.
Exenatide*	0.5-1.0	Stimulates insulin secretion: suppresses glucagons; retards gastric emptying and reduces energy intake	Weight loss	Needs multiple injections; gastrointestinal side effects; expensive: experience limited
Subcutaneous insulin*	>2	Stimulates peripheral glucose uptake and inhibits hepatic glucose output	Reduces severe hyperglycaemia, cheap; much experience	Weight gain; hypoglycaemia; needs to be injected; blood glucose must be monitored
Inhaled insulin*	0.5-1.0	Stimulates peripheral glucose uptake and inhibits hepatic glucose output	No injections needed	Needs multiple daily dosing; blood glucose must be monitored; long term pulmonary effects unknown; expensive and experience limited

*Not yet licensed for use in the United Kingdom.

Obesity is a Pandemic now, although it was an Epidemic in the last Century

There are 110 crores (1100 million) of adults who are overweight/obese in the world, out of which 155 million are children. The prevalence of obesity, has tripled in the developing world and the great threat is in the Middle East Countries, SE Asia, China and Pacific islands, 90% of Type 2 DM is attributable to excess weight. 58 million people die every year from cardiovascular disease for which obesity, diabetes and hypertension are major factors. Overweight also contributes to increased prevalence of hypertension and globally now there are 1000 million of hypertensives which may increase to 1560 million in 2025, obesity increases the insulin resistance and hence the increased prevalence of type 2 DM in obese patients.

In Indian cities the prevalence of overweight/obesity varies from 19% to 30% (Chennai 27%, Bombay 19% in men and 30% in women) and in Kerala it is about 31% in adults (BMI above 25). Obesity is also linked to dyslipidaemia and hypertension, the basic problem is in the adipose tissue which now a days is considered as the largest endocrine gland in the body and in which are produced several cytokines which are responsible for endothelial damage resulting in enhanced atherogenesis resulting in CVD.

Lipids and CVD

It is well known that Low HDL and high LDL are the main causative factors of IHD and hence treatment to maintain normal cholesterol level is absolutely necessary. 1% reduction of LDL can reduce MI by 2%. There are so many drugs which can reduce the LDL and Triglycerides and increase the HDL, including statins, which are inhibitors of HMG-CoA reductase enzyme. Fenofibrates decrease Triglycerides and nicotinic acid increases HDL in the serum.

Diet restriction including restriction of saturated fats and omega 6 fats, increased intake of monounsaturated fats and ω_3 fats and regular exercise are essential to prevent CVD and also dyslipidemia.

Obesity, Cardiovascular Risk and Diabetes

It is Reaven in 1988, while delivering the Banting lecture discussed on a group of patients with certain clinical features and who have a tendency to develop cardiovascular complications like MI, Stroke and Hypertension. The cluster of these clinical features is called Reaven Syndrome/ Metabolic syndrome. Even though obesity was not included earlier, Reavean advocated weight maintenance as an additional treatment. Various definitions of metabolic syndrome are given by WHO, IDF, ATP III, NCEP with minor differences in classification. Obesity is defined as either waist measurement of 102 cm in males and 88 cm in females or waist/hip ratio of 1 in males and 0.9 in females. Asians are more predisposed to this syndrome and in Asians the normal waist measurement is decreased to 90 in males and 80 in females. In WHO definition, FBS above 110 mg/dl is also included as a feature of metabolic syndrome.

IDF=International Diabetic Federation.

ATP III = Adult Treatment Panel III.

NCEP = National Cholesterol eradiation Programme.

Obesity

Driven by the need to survive and influenced by complex genetic emotional and socio cultural factors, the desire to eat is one of the strongest of human instincts. Some time during human evolution the capacity to store fat became a protective mechanism. Obesity which was a feature of affluence is now seen even in underdeveloped countries where poverty is prevalent. Obesity is assessed by the BMI (Body mass index) which is calculated as

$$\text{BMI} = \frac{\text{Wt. in Kg.}}{(\text{Ht in meter})^2}$$

Normal BMI is 25 Kg/m^2 and BMI above 25 is considered as overweight and above 30 is obesity. Obesity due to accumulation of fat in the body is actually due to increased quantity of adipose tissue which is distributed mainly in the subcutaneous tissue, visceral organs and abdomen. Obese people are more prone to Diabetes due to increased insulin resistance, hypertension, IHD, stroke, gall bladder disease, dyslipidaemia, osteoarthritis, restrictive lung disease, sleep apnea, varicose veins, cancer of colon, prostate, breast etc. *Patients with metabolic syndrome have a 4 times risk for myocardial infarction compared to people without metabolic syndrome.*

Control of Diabetes

Diabetes is considered as a 'coronary artery disease equivalent' which means that the frequency of recurrent myocardial infarction is almost the same as in a patient with previous history of MI and in a patient with diabetes mellitus without any history of MI. Control of diabetes (Reduction of HbA_1C) by 1% reduces the incidences of MI by 27%. In view of the high incidence of obesity, diabetes is also increasing (In India it will be 70 million by 2025, a three time rise from 22.5 million of 2000). Diabetic patients usually die of MI (58%) and 40% of the patients who undergo CABG will be diabetics.

(CABG = Coronary Artery Bypass Graft)

Role of Neutraceuticals in the Control of Diabetes

Diet restriction is essential for IHD patients, obese patients, DM patients and patients with hyperlipidaemia.

Nutraceuticals

Viz, Terpenes and terpenoids, carotenoids, phytosterol/Saponins, polyphenols and flavonoids and theols (Alliums sulfur compounds) are strong antioxidants or modulators and many of them are hypoglycemic and hypocholesterolaemic agents too as described in research papers[2-5]. Coloured foods i.e. Pigment containing functional foods e.g. Onion, turmeric, carrot, leaves and many types of fruits e.g. Apple, strawberries, amla, black currant, grapes, pomegranate, tomato, papaya, drumstick, mangoes etc., are good sources of antioxidants and that they are health promoting functional foods. As described elsewhere garlic, as well as onion, amla, turmeric, pomegranate, ginger and fenugreek seeds[4-11] are good sources of nutraceuticals that can comb many toxins and control hypercholesterolaemia and hyperglycemia. In a limited number of studies[12] cumin seeds, ginger, mustard, coriander, and curry leaves also showed reduction on blood sugar. Because of these properties of nutraceuticals they protect our organs especially liver, heart and brain from various ailments. Based on the effective dosages evidenced from experimental data[13], 25-50 g fenugreek seeds, 5-6 nos. of cloves of garlic, 50 g onion and 1g turmeric powder incorporated in the daily diet of diabetics could serve as an effective supportive therapy in the prevention and management of long term complications of diabetes. Their antidiabetic action seems to be mediated through (i) Stimulation of the pancreas to produce and secrete insulin (ii) interference with dietary glucose absorption and (iii) insulin sparing action of the bioactive compounds. Such levels of these spices can be comfortably consumed in regular diet.

As described earlier, central adiposity (accumulation of fat around the waist) is a predisposing factor for CV disease and diabetes. Through diet and exercise one can reduce central adiposity. Chutney made of ginger and garlic (1:4) along with little black pepper and salt, equivalent to ½ a teaspoon being taken with breakfast is useful to reduce weight and for protection from CHD and diabetes. In order to prevent CHD one has to do the following things strictly. Stop smoking (if one has this bad habit), control diabetes, blood pressure, high cholesterol, obesity, alcoholism and stress if one has any of them. Dieting and exercise should be a life style practice in your schedule.

Regular use of functional foods reduces atherogenic index

$$= \frac{\text{Total serum cholesterol}}{\text{HDL cholesterol}}$$

Normal value is around 4.5.

In Conclusion

Insulin resistance is a risk factor for cardiovascular disease and the underlying aetiology for some of the syndrome factors is related to abnormality in adipose tissue. Patient with normal BMI may have abnormal deposition of visceral fat and can have increased waist measures. In fact in S.E. Asians the current abnormal waist measurement is considered as above 90 cm in males and above 80 cm in females. Hence treatment of obesity is very important through dieting and exercise regularly and if required through drug also.

Drugs given for Obesity at the Moment

1. Sibutramine – acts centrally suppresses appetite, to be given for at least 1-2 years
2. Orlistat – Inhibits gastric and pancreatic lipase thus preventing absorption of fat
3. Rimonabant – Blocks cannabinoid B_1 receptor and suppresses appetite, Tgs and increases HDL. It also reduces the weight.

N.B. Honey and garlic in diet also reduce overweight

[Editors]

References

1. Poulose, K.P., Regi Jose, Augusti, K.T. and Joseph, P.K. Diabetes Mellitus and its Management. Ed. Dr. Paul Augustine R.C.C. TVM and published by School of Medical Education, M.G. University, Kottayam. 2001. P.6.
2. (a) Mazza, G. Function Foods. Technomic Publishing Co. 1998

   (b) Bhaskaran, K. Nutraceuticals. Proceeding of the National Seminar on the Evaluation of Nutraceuticals that Prevent Disease. Kannur University, Thalassery. 29th Nov-2nd Dec.2006. PP15-16.
3. Augusti, K.T. Therapeutic values of onion and garlic. Ind. J. Exp. Biol. 34(1996)634-40.

4. Srinivasan, K. Plant Foods in the Management of Diabetes Mellitus: Spices as beneficial antidiabetic food adjuncts. Ind. J. Food. Sci. Nutr. 56(6)2005, 399-414 Quoted in National Product Radiance 5(6) 2006-488-496, with a write up on spices as beneficial antidiabetic food adjuncts.

5. Rajesh Kumar. Cancer chemoprevention by phytochemicals in fruits and vegetables. Amala. Res. Bulletin 18(1998)141-150.

6. (a) Helen, A, Krishnakumar, K et. al. Antioxidant effect of onion oil (A Cepa L) on the damages induced by nicotine in rats as compared to alpha-tocopherol. Toxicology Letters 116 (2000) 61-68.

   (b) Helen, A, Rajasree, C.R. et. al. Antioxidant role of oils isolated from garlic (A. sativum L) and onion (A. cepa. L) on nicotine-induced lipid peroxidation. Vet Human Toxicol 41(5) 1999, 316-319.

7. Tripathi, S.N; Tiwari, C.M; Upadhyay, B.N and Singh, R.S. Screening of hypoglycemic action in certain indigeneous drugs, J. Res. Indian Med. Yoga Homoep. 14 (1979) 159-169.

8. (a) Soni, K.B and Kuttan, R. Effect of oral curcumin administration on serum peroxides and cholesterol levels in human volunteers. Indian J. Physid. Pharmacol. 36(1992) 273 & 293.

   (b) Tank, R, Sharma, N et. al. Antidiabetic activity of C. Longa in alloxan induced diabetic rats, Indian Drugs. 27(11). 1989, 587-589.

9. Aviram, M; Dornfeld, L et. al. Pomegranate juice consumption reduces oxidative stress, atherogenic modification to LDL, and platelet aggregation; Studies in humans and in atherosclerotic apolipoprotein E-deficient mice. Am. Jour. Clin Nutr. 71(2000) 1062-1076.

10. Duke, J.A. and Ayensu, E.S Medicinal plants of China. 1985, 378.

11. Verma, S.K.; Singh, M; Jain, P and Bordia, A. Protective effect of Ginger, Zingiber officinale Rosc on experimental atherosclerosis in rabbits. Indian Jour of Exp. Biol. 42(2004) 736-38.

12. Spices as beneficial antidiabetic food adjuncts. Natural Product Radiance 5(6)2006. pp 488-496.

6.2 Life Style, Dietary Components and Cancer Prevention

Dr. Regi Jose MD, DPH, DNB, Assistant Professor,
Dept. Community Medicine, Dr. SMCSI Medical College Karakonam, Trivandrum, Kerala

Of all the environmental factors, dietary components appear to play an important role in the initiation/progression of the disease according to an article by Krishnaswamy and Polasa[1] from the National Institute of Nutrition, Hyderabad. In the article they say many of the directory factors demonstrate antimutagenic/anticarcinogenic effects also. Spices and vegetables such as turmeric, mustard, green leafy and allium species of vegetables are in the forefront in these aspects. They stress the importance of dietary intervention for cancer prevention, besides avoiding risk factors such as smoking and alcoholism and exposure to genotoxicants. In order to achieve cancer prevention through dietary modulation we need to avoid deep frying, barbecued and fungus infected food items. Lot of green and leafy vegetables, coloured food items such as papaya, carrots, turmeric, onions, garlic and all types of fruits along with complex carbohydrates (fiber rich) with smaller amounts of saturated fats and meat with plenty of fresh water-fish are advisable in a healthy diet. Red meat should be avoided. Fat composition up to 30% containing 10% saturated 10% mono unsaturated and 10% poly unsaturated fat is recommended by various groups of heart and cancer societies for prevention of CHD and cancer.

Chemical Carcinogenesis

It is characterized by three main stages, viz. initiation, promotion and progression. In the initiation process an exogenous or endogenous carcinogen alters the genetic make up of the cell and results in a lesion that confers upon the cell, the potential for neoplastic transformation. A procarcinogen is metabolically converted to carcinogen (step1) and then to reactive electrophiles (mutagens at step 2). Certain dietary factors such as antioxidants/bioantimutagens deactivate the enzymes involved in both the above steps. These types of intervention by antimutagens convert the carcinogenic substances to non toxic products which are easily excreted later. If the dietary factors are not capable of preventing these oxidative steps for the formation of reactive mutagens, they in turn covalently bind to macro molecules such as DNA and proteins and start to do the malfunctions.

Further at the initiation stage1 mutagens form a complex with DNA (DNA adducts). This causes alteration in gene expression. On progression of this at the second stage(II) occurs preneoplasia, this on promotional events proliferate the initiated cells and transform them into cancer cells at the third stage(III). The initiation and promotional stages (I & III) can be effectively inhibited by certain inhibitors and it is believed that certain dietary factors work as bioantimutagens and antipromoters at the initiation (I) and promotional (III) stages.

Procarcinogen $\xrightarrow{I}$ Carcinogen $\xrightarrow{II}$ Reactive electrophilic Mutagens $\rightarrow$ EnterTarget tissues
Air/Food/Water)

Metabolic/Oxidative steps

$\xrightarrow{III}$ Intercalation with DNA $\xrightarrow{IV}$ Preneoplasia $\xrightarrow{V}$ Neoplasia
Initiation ... Progression ... Promotion

Dietary factors (Nutraceuticals) deactivate the transformation of procarcinogens and interaction at steps other than progression. Progression is the expansion of the population of initiated cum promoted cancer cells.

Therefore dietary components play a role as inhibitors both at the bioactivation (oxidative steps) of carcinogens and their interaction with the cell components in the processes of transformation of a normal cell to a cancer cell. An example of procarcinogen is Benzo (a) pyrene formed from protein on deep frying or an direct cooking in fire. This is transformed in our body to hydroxyderivative which form adducts on intercalation with DNA.

Various studies of the National Institute of Nutrition (NIN) Hyderabad on Cancer and related matters can be summarized as follows:

***Alcohol and Tobacco Products*:** They produce mainly cancers of oral cavity and oesophagus, Beta carotene, vitamins (A, B & C) and certain minerals, Zn for the former and iron, zinc and selenium for the latter are preventive factors.

***Low Intake of Lean Meat, Fish, Fruits and Vegetables*:** It may produce cancer of oesophagus and the above mentioned dietary factors may prevent it.

***Nitrates, Nitrites, Pickles, Fried and Smoked Fish*:** It may produce stomach cancer. Complex carbohydrates, proteins, vitamins C and E and Se may prevent this cancer. When nitrate is reduced to nitrite by bacteria, it becomes a precursor of the carcinogen called nitrosamine. Garlic in diet can prevent these reactions.

Low Fiber (Refined Carbohydrates) high fat food: They may produce colon and rectal cancers. Vitamins A and C and low fat food may prevent them.

Tobacco Smoke, Alcohol, Lack of Vegetables etc: They may produce cancer of larynx. Others except alcohol may produce lung cancer. Vitamin A prevents the former and Vitamin A & E prevent the latter. Stopping smoking and alcohol drinks are necessary as early as possible.

***Low in Green and Yellow Vegetables and Obesity*:** The former two conditions in diet may produce prostate cancer and all the three may produce breast cancer. Obesity leads cancer of the colon, cervix, rectum and breast. Beta carotene, Vitamin A and balanced nutrition may prevent them. Increased fat consumption correlates with incidence of breast and colon cancers and a casual relationship may exist between fat intake and carcinogenesis.

***Industrial Chemicals, Artificial Sweeteners and Coffee*:** They produce bladder cancer. Vitamin A may prevent it.

***Low Vegetable Diet*:** It produces cervical cancer. Vitamin A, C and folic acid may prevent it.

***Tobacco Smoke and Coffee*:** They may produce cancer of the Pancreas. Stopping smoking and good nutrition may prevent it. Cigarette smokings increases lung cancer and to certain extend cervical cancer also.

***Aflatoxin*:** It may produce liver cancer. Balanced nutrition is also necessary.

Smoked and Pickled Foods

They increase the incidences of stomach cancer. In costal areas and cold countries smoked fish is a common item for food and it increases stomach cancer. Other works reported elsewhere stated that smoking (even passive) and unhygienic conditions cause cervical cancer. High fat diet may cause colon & rectal cancer; no breast feeding may cause breast cancer and so on. Many claim that regular consumption of allium products, phytoestrogens, curcumin etc. may prevent all types of cancers.

NIN workers report that green vegetables, mustard, onion and garlic are potent inducers of UDP glucutonyl transferase, glutathione S-transferse etc., which prevent cancer production. The NIN workers stress the important role of nutrients such as carotenoids, vitamin A, E and C and the mineral and those of the nutraceuticals such as dithiolthiones, glucosinolates, indols, flavonoids, phenols, isothiocyanates, sterols, diathyl sulfides, limonine etc., that play against the onset of cancer. NIN also confirmed that potent antimutagenic effects of turmeric in *in vitro* studies using rats and carcinogens such as benzo(a) pyrene (B (a) P) and methyl colanthrene[2]. According to them, curcumin the active component in turmeric is antimutagenic to genotoxicants present in tobacco products and carcinogens such as B(a) P and dimethyl benzanthracene (DMBA) *in vitro*[3].

Further *in vitro* studies employing cultured cells such as Chinese hamster ovary cell lines and Dalton's lymphoma ascites tumor cells proved the cytotoxic properties of curcumin and turmeric[4]. NIN workers showed in a human study conducted on smokers that on turmeric administration (1.5 g/d) for 15-30 days decreased the formation and exertion of urinary mutagens[5]. Another group further showed that in addition to curcumin in turmeric it contains a water soluble 5 KDa peptide known as turmerin which has potent antioxidant activity[6].

Some Epidemiological Studies

The nutrition cancer link has been supported by epidemiological studies[7]. Some of the most fascinating comparison has been made between the incidence of cancer in Japan and the United States. Although both countries are civilized, industrialized and developed, the diets of their populations differ dramatically[8] as all the types of cancer developed. In U.S for example, breast cancer, colon cancer and prostate cancer are very common, but they are very rarely seen in Japan. Conversely, stomach cancer is relatively common in Japan and very rare in US. The risk of breast cancer in Japan also differs in rural and urban areas. During 1960-70 period, in rural areas 10%, small cities 15% and in metropolitan areas as high as 21% of the women suffered from breast cancer. Longitudinal studies there in 1950-75 period showed that the average consumption of milk increased by 15 fold, meat, poultry and eggs by 7.5 fold and fat by six fold. However consumption of barley (i.e. Fibre rich carbohydrates) decreased by 97%, of potatoes by 50% and rice by 30%. In Japan consumption of smoked and pickled foods is vary rare and that too prevent cancer. Because of these there were some dramatic changes in the incidence of cancer in Japan.

Breast, colon and lung cancer increased between two and three times where as stomach cancer decreased by 40% and cancer of the uterus decreased by 70%[8]. This means that increased fat consumption increased the incidence of the former three cancers and decreased carbohydrate and smoked food consumption decreased the incidence of stomach and uterus cancers. In Japan increased incidence of lung cancer was probably related to increased smoking of cigarettes.

Colon Cancer

Willett et. al.[9] reported a prospective study of diet and colon cancer in 89000 women during 1980-86 in the west. There was a clinically and statistically significant increase in the incidence of cancer related to ingestion of total fat, saturated fat and red meat. The ingestion of vegetable fat was not significally correlated with that of colon cancer. Finally, there was a negative correlation between the amount of chicken and fish ingested and the incidence of colon cancer in women.

Their work further showed that in countries whose population consumed > 120 g of fat per day e.g. Austria, Sweden, Switzerland, Australia, France, the United States, New Zealand and Canada have very high death rates from colon cancer. In countries such as Thailand, El Salvador and Columbia where fat consumption is quite minimal i.e. $\leq$ 50 g per day, the incidence of deaths from colon cancer is extremely low. The American Cancer Society recommends a diet containing, 30% of calories from fat. [10] However Bernard E Statland of National Reference Laboratory at Nashville and author of an article “Nutrition and Cancer” believes that the consumption of 30% calorie equivalent of fat is quite high and it should be reduced to half of that value per day[11]. Many claim that high fat intake may lead to an increased secretion of bile acids and their conversion to secondary bile acids by altering the bacterial population in the large bowel. On the contrary with a low fat diet, the bacterial population is primarily aerobic and they will not convert the primary bile acids to secondary ones. In the presence of high fat in the bowel the bacteria becomes anaerobic with consequent production of secondary bile acids viz. deoxycholic and lithocholic acids which are thought to be promoters of lesions in the large bowel[12].

This hypothesis may also explain why fat rich meat in the diet is an inducer of colon cancer. Antibiotic components in the diet for e.g. onions and garlic may inhibit the growth of certain bacteria like Helicobacter pylori[13,14]. The incidence of stomach cancer is strongly correlated with H.pylori infection and epidemiological studies show an inverse relationship between stomach cancer incidence and the consumption of Allium vegetables[15,16]. Some others showed that garlic oil (G.O) as well as garlic powder (G.P) has considerable antibacterial effects when tested against a wide range of enteric bacteria also[17]. All the garlic material tested revealed substantial anti-H. Pylori effects against all strains and isolates[18]. These findings suggest that dietary garlic may reduce the infections by H. Pylori and related cancers.

Fiber and Colon Cancer

Fiber intake is inversely related to the incidence of colon cancer as per the original work of Burkitt[19] on the people of Africa. The Africans consumed high fiber diet Viz.Tubers, leaves, whole wheat preparations and unskinned fruits e.g. Mangoes, Gua etc, the English consume refined food free of fiber. In an African village school he studied the transit time of fecal material in the pupils there and compared the same with those in a neighbouring English School. In African children the average transit time from ingestion to evacuation was 45 hrs, and the daily weight of stool was 200 g. In the African English School Children, the transit time was 80hrs and the daily weight of stool was 100 g. In the African adults the corresponding time was 35 hrs and weight was 400 g. He found an inverse relationship between fiber ingestion and colon cancer in the African and English population. Dietary fiber is defined as components of cell wall origin of the food materials that are not degraded during digestion and thus dilute the intestinal and colonic contents and absorb many toxic materials and fat as some fiber forms gels with water.

This is due to the hydroxyls present in the fiber which is mostly cellulose. These processes limit contact between any carcinogen that may be present in the diet and subsequently in the stool and the colonic mucosa. Thus due to the presence of fiber concentrations of carcinogens and promotes such as secondary bile acids are reduced in the lower part of intestines and above in the colon. Fiber also decreases fecal pH which tends to have of an inhibitory effect on various potential carcinogens. In short the amount of fecal mutagens will be reduced[20].

Foods high in fiber include various berries, brussal sprouts, oat flakes, pumpkin, carrots, brown rice, whole wheat, lettuce, cucumber, mangoes, and apple[21].

Breast Cancer, Role of Diet, life Style and Heredity

Breast Cancer is the most common cancer among women and it is second to lung cancer in terms of mortality. About 11% women will develop breast cancer and about 35% of them may die as a result of this disease. Risk factors are being a women, high fat diet, being post menopausal, family history of breast cancer (mostly from mother's side) being nulliparous, having first child after the age of 30, and obesity.

Note that a high fat diet with less vegetable[1] is implicated in the promotion of this disease[22,23]. Relationship of breast cancer Vs fat consumption is as strong as that of colon cancer verses the above. In western countries and Australia where the fat consumption is > 120 g per day the incidence of breast cancer death is very high. In those countries in which fat consumption is < 50 g. per day and vegetable diet is high i.e. Thailand, Japan, Elsalvador, Sri Lanka and Taiwan the incidence of breast cancer is much lower. India and Pakistan are sandwiched between these two groups of countries with modern fast food culture and the women there are increasingly at a greater risk of breast cancer than those in S.E Asia.

Suggested Role of High Fat in the Body

It is known that high fat diets lead to an increased secretion of prolactin and biosynthesis of prostaglandins. Further fat cells increase the biosynthesis of estrogen also[24a]. Heber et. al.[24b] observed that on decreasing the fat consumption to ≤ 10% of the required energy values with a diet of complex carbohydrate in post menopausal women for 22 days their estradiol value dropped from 18.1 to 94 ng/L. Barbosa et. al.[25] also observed significantly lower levels of body fat and serum estradiol in vegetarian women than in non vegetarian women. Vegetarians consumed a diet rich in fiber and low in cholesterol and saturated fats. It appears that a high fat diet is associated with an early menarche as well as a later menopause. This long period of estrogen production in women predisposes them likely to an incidence of breast cancer.

Prostate Cancer

As seen earlier for breast and colon cancers there is a strong relationship between prostate cancer deaths and fat consumption. In countries with highest fat consumption i.e., Denmark, Holland, the United States, Canada and U.K statistically significant rise in prostate cancer deaths are observed[26]. The countries with the lowest fat consumption i.e. the Philippines, Elsalvador and Japan are correlated with an extremely low prostate cancer death rate. Further it was observed that in men put on low fat and complex carbohydrate diets for 26 days there was a profound decrease in serum estradoil from 47.2 ng/L to 23.8 ng/L[27]. In this group their serum cholesterol, triglycerides and body weight also decreased. The speculation is that estradoil acts as a promoter of prostate cancer as it apparently does for breast cancer.

The Role of Micronutrients, Carcinogens and Antioxidants/ Nutraceuticals

Salting, pickling and smoking foods may result in an increased incidence of cancer, especially cancer of the stomach. Smoked fish in Japan and Java beans in Columbia are considered potential carcinogens. These food tend to support conversion of nitrates to nitrites. Nitrites in turn react to form the strong carcinogens Viz, nitrosamines and nitrosamides. It has been suggested that antioxidants in garlic [28] and ascorbic acid actually block the conversion of nitrates to nitrites and they might act as antipromoters of cancer. Deep frying or high temperature cooking produce many potential carcinogens Viz.; polycyclic hydrocarbons, hetrocyclic amines, nitrosamines and nitroaromatics. Fried coffee seeds contain carcinogens like caffeine acid, catechol, furfural, hydroquinone and hydrogen peroxide. Many chemicals like ethylene dibromide, ethylene dichloride, 1, 3 butadiene, tetra chloro ethylene, propylene oxide, chloroform, formaldehyde, Methylene chloride, dioxane and benzene are potential carcinogens in our working environment[29]. Various carcinogens cause oxidative damage to the DNA in cells. Lipid peroxidation, methylation, deamination etc., can also cause damages to DNA and that in turn produces mutation and cancer.

Many antioxidants in the form of micronutrients or nutraceutials in the diet have been termed as antipromoters of cancer. They include vitamins C and E., β carotene, selenium[11,30], polyphenols, indoles, aromatic thiocyanates, coumarins, phytosterols, etc. Anticarcinogenic mechanism of actions of various nutraceuticals have been described[31] e.g. inhitions at initiation and promotional stages. As mentioned earlier, smoked, pickled and cured foods contain nitrites and various antioxidants present in our diet inhibit their conversion to nitrosamines[32] the potential carcinogens in our stomach.

The American Cancer Society and Health Association recommend a proper maintenance of body weight and consumption of a diet that includes a variety of both vegetables and fruits daily, eating more high fiber foods and limiting consumption of alcoholic beverages, high fats and salt cured, smoked and nitrite preserved foods[10, 33] to prevent cancer and CHD.

References

1. Kamala Krishnaswamy and Kalpagam Polasa. Diet, Nutrition and Cancer- the Indian Scenario. Indian. J. Med. Res., 102(1995)200-209.
2. Polasa, K; Sesikeran, B; Krishna, T.P and Krishnaswamy, K, Turmeric (Curcuma longa) induced reduction in urinary mutagens Food Chem., Toxicol 29(1991)699-706.
3. Nagabhushan, M; Amonkar, AJ, Bhide, S.V. In vitro antimutagencity of curcumin against environmental mutagens. Food Chem. Toxicol 25(1987)545-547.
4. Soudamini, K.K; Kuttan, R. Cytotoxic and Tumor reducing properties of curcumin. Indian J Pharmacol 20(1998)95-101.
5. Polasa, K, Raghuram, T.C et. al. Effect of turmeric on urinary mutagens in smokers. Mutagenesis. 1(1972)107-109.
6. Srinivas, L; Shalini, V.K and Shylaja, M. Turmerin, A water soluble antioxidant peptide from turmeric (curcuma longa) Arch. Biochem. Biophys 292(1992)617-623.
7. Cohen, I.A. Diet and Cancer. Sci. Am 5(1987)42-48.

8. Kagawa, Y. Nutrition of Japanese; its biochemical back ground. Kagaku (Science) 45(1975)740-749.

9. Willet, W.C, Stampfer, M.J. et. al. Relationship of meat, fat and fiber intake to the risk of colon cancer in a prospective study among women. N. Engl. J. Med 323(1990) 1664-1672.

10. Weinhouse S, Bal, D.G, Adamson R, et. al. American Cancer Society Guidelines on diet, nutrition, and cancer. CA Cancer. J. Clin 41(1991) 334-338.

11. Bernard E. Statland, Nutrition and Cancer Clin. Chem. 38(8) (1992) 1587-1594.

12. Reddy, B.S. Diet and excretion of bile acids. Cancer Res. 41(1981) 3766-3768.

13. Jonkers, D; Vanden Broek E, et. al. Antibacterial effect of garlic and omeprazole on Helicobacter pylori. J. Antimicrob. Chemoth, 43(1999) 837-839.

14. Ohta, R. In vitro inhibition of the growth of Helicobacter pylori by oil-macerated garlic constituents. Antimicrobe agents Ch.43(1999) 1811-1812.

15. You, W.C; Blot, W.J et. al. Diet and high risk of stomach Cancer in Shandong. China. Cancer Res. 48(1988)3518-3523.

16. Buiatti, E; Palli, D et. al. A case control study of gastric cancer and diet in Italy. 44(1989)611-616.

17. Ross, Z.M ; O' Gara, E.A et. al. The antimicrobial properties of garlic oil against Human Enteric Bacteria- Evaluation of Methodologies and Comparisons with garlic oil sulphides and garlic powder. Cited by David J.Maslin of the University of Wolver Hampton, U.K under publication (2000).

18. 'O' Gara, E.A. Hill, D.J and Maslin, D.J. The antibacterial activity of garlic oil, garlic powder and their diallyl constituents against Helicobacter pylori, J App and Env. Microbiology. 66(2000)2269-73

19. Burkitt, D.P. Epidemiology of Cancer of the colon and rectum cancer 28 (1971)3-13

20. Reddy, B.S; Sharma C, Simi, B, et. al. Metabolic epidemiology of colon cancer: effect of dietary fiber on fecal mutagens and bile acids in healthy subjects. Cancer Res.47(1987)644-48.

21. Krishnan, JD. Fiber content In: Nutritional Research Inc. Nutritional almanac, Newyork. McGraw Hill. 1979.257

22. Carroll, K.K Experimental evidence of dietary factors and hormone dependent Cancers.Cancer Res. 35(1975)3374-83

23. Rao, B.S.N. Bioactive phytochemicals in Indian foods. Bull NFI. 16(1)1995:1-5

24. (a) Sehindler, A.E, Ebert, A and Friedrich, E Conversion of androstene doine to estrone by human fat tissue. J. Clin. Endocrinol Metab. 35(1972)627-30.

(b) Heber D; Ashley J M; Leaf D.A, Barnard RJ. Reduction of serum estradiol in post menoposal women given free access to low-fat high carbohydrate diet. Nutrition 7 (1991) 137-140.

25. Barbosa, J.C, Schultz, T.D et. al. The relationship among adiposity, diet and hormone concentrations in vegetarian and non vegetarian postmenopausal women. An. J.Clin. Nutr. 51(1990)798-803.

26. Reddy, B.S, Nutrition and its relationship to cancer. Ad. Cancer Res. 32(1980) 237-246

27. Rosenthal, M.B; Barnard, R.J et. al. Effects of a high complex carbohydrate, low fat, low cholesterol diet on levels of serum lipids and estradiol. Am. J. Med.78(1985) 23-27.

28. Mei, X; Wang, M.C et. al. Garlic and gastric cancer- the effect of garlic on nitrite and nitrate in garlic juice. Acta Nutr Sinica 4(1982)53-58.

29. Gold, L.S; Backman, G.M. et. al. Ranking the potential carcinogenic hazards to workers from exposure to chemicals that are tumorigenic in rodents. Environ Health Perspect. 76(1987)211-219.

30. Watten Berg, L.W. Inhibition of neoplasia by minor dietary constituents. Cancer Res. 43(1983)2248S-53S

31. Weisburger, J.H. Nutritional approach to cancer prevention with emphasis on Vitamins, antioxidants and carotenoids. Am .J. Clin. Nutr. 53(1991) 226S-37S.

32. Comstock, G.W et. al. Prediagnostic Serum levels of carotenoids and Vitamin E as related to subsequent cancer in Washington County, Maryland. Am. J. Clin. Nutr. 53(1991) 298S-304S.

33. Garewal, H.S. potential role of β-carotene in prevention of oral cancer. Am. J.Clin. Nutr. 53(1991)294S-97S.

6.3 Diet and Cancer – An Indian Perspective

Dr. Kalpagam Polasa, Ph.D., MBA
Deputy Director and Head of the Department
and

Dr. P. Rajendra Prasad, MBBS, M.Sc., Ph.D.
Assistant Director
Food and Drug Toxicology Research Centre, National Institute of Nutrition (Indian Council of Medical Research)
Hyderabad – 500 007

Diet and Cancer – An Indian Perspective

Cancer is one of the major cause of mortality. This is largely due to the fact that people tend to live longer, with fewer people dying from other causes such as infectious diseases. In 2000, over 6 million people died from cancer and there were an estimated 10 million new cases. Between 2000 and 2020, the total number of cases of cancer is predicted to increase by 73% in the developing world and by 29% in the developed world, largely as a result of demographic shift in geriatric population[1]. A report on the incidence of common cancers in India in 2004 showed it as around 154 thousands and 267 thousands in males and females respectively [2]

During the past two decades, data on diet and cancer have greatly increased and this reinforces the belief that a substantial proportion of cancer is potentially preventable by nutritional means. Quantitative estimates of the preventable proportion in Western countries remain approximately 30% to 40%[2]. Presently there is abundant information on specific aspects of nutrition.

The relationships between specific dietary components and cancers are less well established than that of diet and cardiovascular disease. This is due to the fact that the role of diet in the causation of cancer has always been difficult to study and quantify partly because the diet encompasses a wide variety of foods, dietary traditions, habits and is a complex mixture of nutrients and non nutrients.

In theory, there are several possible ways that diet can influence human cancers[3] **(Fig.1)**

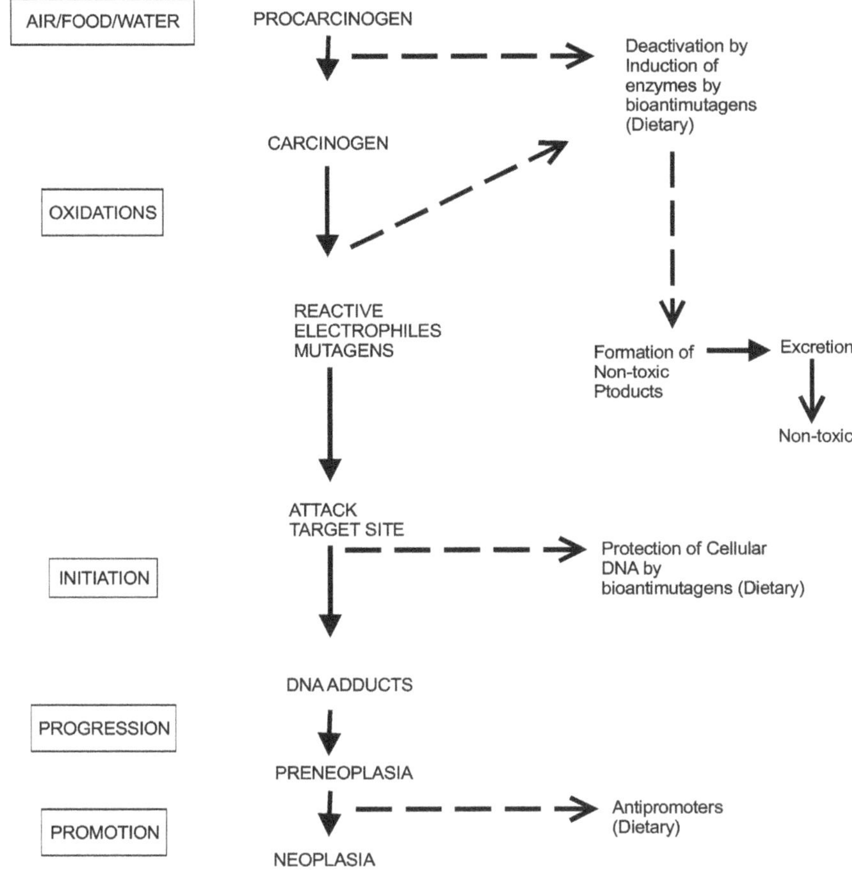

Fig. 1 Role of dietary factors in carcinogenic process.

Diet is composed of macronutrients like protein, carbohydrate and fats and micronutrients namely vitamins and minerals. Diet can be a source of agents that promote carcinogenesis as well as inhibitors of the process.

Dietary Mutagens/Carcinogens

These may occur endogenously in the diet or may be of exogenous in origin. Toxicants present in foods may be mycotoxins, or may be formed in the food during cooking, processing and storage or they may originate from extraneous sources like pesticides, fungicides and food preservatives.

Of the well known food derived mutagens are the heterocyclic amines formed during cooking. Foods like fish and beef are known to form mutagenic substances during smoking and frying[4]. Other food

items like alcoholic beverages are known to contain substances that have been reported to induce mutations in bacteria[5].

Evidences from literature have strongly implicated nitrates, nitrites and nitrosomines in the development of tumors in humans. Nitrates are ubiquitously present in water and food. Though nitrates are not harmful it can be reduced to nitrite under certain conditions both in food and in the body which combines with amines in food to form nitroso compounds. Many food items such as meat, meat products, fish and fish products, smoked grilled foods, sea foods, sausages and spices, pickled vegetables and beverages such as alcoholic drinks are major sources of preformed nitroso compounds. Several of the nitroso compounds have been related to gastro intestinal cancers. Studies initiated in this direction show that alcoholic beverages particularly beers contain nitroso compounds which are relatively higher in Indian beer, as compared to beer manufactured in other Western countries[6]. In alcoholic beverages like beer, the source of nitrosamines is the malt which is used at around 10% in such products (Prasad MPR, 1994). As malt is prepared by roasting germinating cereals like wheat, at temperatures of 1200°C or more, the amines get nitrosated by the action of nitrites in the atmosphere. This usually happens if open-harth method is adopted for preparing malt. As it is usually added at low concentrations beer contains a small percentage of the nitrosamines present in malt.

High nitrate containing foods with high salt intakes may increase the risk of gastric cancer.

Epidemiological evidence in India from places such as Kashmir, have identified salted and fried fish and red chilies as risk factors for esophageal and stomach cancer[7]. Nitrosodimethyl amine has been consistently found in such foods which though not identified as an esophageal carcinogen, is known to be an etiologic factor for gastric cancers.

Similarly flesh foods especially sea fish and salted dry fish have been found to contain nitrosamines. Moreover fish is either fried in oil or boiled with different spices including red chillies, which also add to the load of nitrosamines which humans get exposed when consumed.

The prevalence of esophageal cancers is also high in Kashmir[8] and the salted tea and chilies consumed in Kashmir are sources of nitrosocompounds. Certain spices, which are sun dried like black pepper, dry coriander seeds, cumin, red chilies have all shown to contain nitrosamines.

Pickles having spices and salt have also been a regular source of nitrosamines. The acidic medium is conducive for the formation of nitrosamines and hence people with regular use of such foods are potentially at risk of getting exposed to carcinogens. **The levels of these carcinogens and *in vivo* nitrosations can be reduced by consuming vitamin C rich antioxidants in foods like fruits and vegetables. Certain spices like turmeric*, antioxidants such as vitamin C, can inhibit nitrosation under *in vitro* conditions. Vitamin C is also a potent inhibitor of *in vivo* nitrosation[9].**

(*Chinese workers like Mei reported that garlic sulfides can also prevent nitrosation reactions – (editor)

Chemopreventers in Diet

Several epidemiological studies highlighted the role of vegetables and fruits in reducing the risk of cancer in a variety of organs and tissues[10]. Nutrients that demonstrate modulatory effects in experimental cancers include macronutrients such as fats, carbohydrates, proteins, fibers and micronutrients such as vitamins – folic acid, riboflavin, ß-carotene, retinol, α-tocopherol, vitamin B_{12} and minerals such as selenium, zinc, magnesium and calcium. *Presently, focus has shifted to non-nutritional components in our diet, which have antimutagenic and anticarcinogenic properties[11]. These are known as bioactive compounds or chemopreventers[11]. These are found in all food categories although fruits and vegetables are rich sources. They belong to over 25 classes of chemicals and include some vitamins, food polyphenols and other regular food ingredients[12]. They are also known as phytochemicals (or nutraceuticals). They are safe and have low or no toxicity.*

Mechanism of Action of Chemopreventers

Mechanism of action of chemopreventer is complex. It can be categorized according to the site of action or by specific type of action. The activity could be the result of simultaneous action of several factors on the same event. It appears that most chemopreventers act primarily as antioxidants. Broadly the mechanism of action of chemopreventers can be categorized, depending on whether they act extracellularly or intracellularly[13] (Table 1).

Table 1

Chemopreventers	Mechanism of action
Category	**Mechanism**
Inhibitors of carcinogen formation Ascorbic acid, caffeic acid, ferulic acid	Inhibit insitu formation of carcinogen eg. Nitrosomines formation
Blocking agents Isothiocyanates, diallylsulphide, ellagic acid, ferulic acid and dithiocarbonates	Inhibit the activity of cytochrome p450 and block conversion of procarcinogens to carcinogens
Inducing agents Isothiocyanates, sulforaphane d-limonene, terpenoids	Stimulate enzymatic system which are involved in detoxification of carcinogens
Trapping agents Ellagic acid, N-acetylcysteine, vitamin E, Flavonoids	Physically react with carcinogens and conjugate them and eliminating them as potential carcinogens
Suppressing agents Isoflavones, phytoestrogens, epigallocatechin gallate (EGCG), selenium, soy products source (1).	Suppress different steps in metabolic pathways required for tumor development.

The chemopreventers may act through detoxification mechanism or by antimutagenic processes at initiation, promotion or both the steps.

Detoxificants

The phytochemicals induce drug metabolizing enzymes in the body and act by detoxifying the harmful substances capable of producing deleterious effects. The antineoplastic effects of inducing and inhibiting agents in foods focus on specific monooxygenases like arylhydrocarbon hydroxylase (AHH), uridine diphosphate glucuronyl transferase (UDPGT), glutathione-s-transferases (GST), quionone reductase (DR) and antioxidant enzymes[14].

Antimutagens

Carcinogens bind to the cell macro molecules namely, DNA, RNA and proteins and result in mutagenic events leading to cell transformation and neoplastic changes. Some phytochemicals prevent these changes from occurring either by directly binding to the carcinogens / their metabolites or by metabolizing and eliminating toxic xenobiotics[14]. These are known as antimutagens/anticarcinogens.

Spices as Antimutagens/Anticarcinogens

Turmeric

Turmeric is used extensively in Indian culinary practice for its colour, taste and flavour. It is also added to food as a preservative. In traditional medicine it is used as potent anti-inflammatory agent, carminative and antiseptic agent. Curcumin, the active principle in turmeric, has strong antioxidant and anti-inflammatory potential. Its potent antimutagenic effects were demonstrated against well known carcinogens in *in vivo* rat model[15]. In rats turmeric intake was observed to elevate levels of tissue xenobiotic enzymes that are protective in nature against carcinogen metabolism (16). There was decreased binding of liver DNA to the carcinogen benzo(a)pyrene as quantitated by ^{32}P post label assay.

In oral cancer model turmeric/curcumin painting of Syrian Golden Hamster cheeck pouch resulted in retardation of tumors induced by exposure of cheek pouch to carcinogen dimethyl benzanthracene (DMBA)[17].

In mice forestomach tumors were induced by benzo(a)pyrene and efficacy of turmeric and curcumin as antiinitiator and antipromoter was tested. While turmeric inhibits both the phases, curcumin could only inhibit post initiation process[18].

DNA repair is one of the important mechanisms of protecting the system from the toxicity of environmental toxicants. Protective effect of curcumin against induction of single strand breaks in DNA was observed in yeast cells treated with UV radiation, 8 methoxypsoralen and BP[19].

Antimutagenicity of turmeric was demonstrated in human smokers who are known to excrete mutagens. The excretion of urinary mutagens was reduced at the end of 15 days of turmeric ingestion (1.5 g/day orally for 30 days) and further by 30 days time[20].

Alliums

Among the vegetables, those belonging to the allium family have received increased attention in recent times. Onion and garlic are commonly consumed through the diet. Their homogenates contain sulphur compounds like diallyl sulphide, diallyl disulphide, alliin, allicin, ajoene etc. Prior feeding of onion at 1 and 5 % levels and garlic at 0.1, 0.5, 1 % levels through diet showed decreased excretion of urinary mutagens by rats exposed to mutagens[21]. **Stimulation of the activity of liver cytosolic glutathione-S-transferase, increase in activity of the antioxidant enzyme quinone reductase in liver and lung microsomes was observed in garlic fed rats. In onion fed rats also stimulation in detoxification**

enzymes were reported[22]. These findings suggest that toxicity due to exposure of endogenous or exogenous carcinogens can be averted by consuming alliums regularly.

Ginger

Ginger is a condiment, which is used in various forms throughout the world. In traditional medicine ginger in the form of dried powder, raw form and juice have been prescribed to ameliorate conditions like rheumatic disorders, inflammation and gastrointestinal discomforts.

Cytogenetic damage to tissue is considered as one of the biomarker of genotoxicity[23]. Human blood lymphocytes of male smokers, male non smokers and female non smokers were exposed to trans stillbene oxide in the presence and absence of ginger. **The cytogenetic damage in terms of micronuclei was significantly reduced due to the presence of ginger[24]. Ginger was also observed to counteract induced DNA damage in human peripheral blood lymphocytes. The excretion of urinary mutagens by benzo(a)pyrene exposed rats that were fed ginger was reduced significantly[25]. Ginger feeding also stimulated the levels of detoxification enzymes and antioxidant enzymes proving that ginger can be an effective antimutagenic and anticancer agent[26,27].**

Effect of Cooking on Antimutagens in Spices

The studies on antimutagenic potentials are conducted using raw form or powder. But most of the spices are subjected to boiling or frying while cooking food and may undergo thermal denaturation. Turmeric, curcumin, alliums and ginger were tested for their antimutagenic potential after subjecting them to heat treatment to simulate cooking conditions. The spices and their active principles did not show alteration in their antimutagenic properties suggesting that they can liberally be incorporated during cooking and consumed[28].

Process of Chemical Carcinogenesis

In order to understand the diet and cancer relationship, it is essential to understand cancer process itself, which is broadly characterized by three main stages viz., initiation, promotion and progression. It consists of a distinct initiating process where an exogenous or an endogenous carcinogen alters the genetic makeup of the cell and results in a lesion that confers upon the cell the potential for neoplastic transformation.

Procarcinogens after entry into the host system are converted through the sequential enzymatic process into electrophilic reactive substances which covalently bind to cell macromolecules such as DNA, protein and RNA. Unless these lesions are repaired effectively, these are propogated.

The second major step in carcinogenesis involves, alterations in gene expression and cell proliferation that transforms the initiated cell into a cancer cell. The promotional events can be inhibited by inhibitors, which suppress neoplasia. Inhibitors/antipromoters act by removing initiators or promoting agents, through detoxification or by regulating cellular receptors/differentiation or by inducing repair mechanisms. **Progression is the expansion of the initiated cum promoted cancer cells. The process of neoplastic transformation can be influenced by dietary factors at several stages. Diet associated carcinogens; mutagens and inhibitors of the carcinogenic process play a vital role. The various dietary and nutritional factors implicated in cancer, by site, are summarized in Table 2.**

Table 2 Dietary / nutritional factors in cancer

CANCERS	DIETARY FACTORS CAUSING CANCER	NUTRIENTS FOR PREVENTION
Oral Cavity	Alcohol, Tobacco as snuff or through chewing	Beta-carotene, Vitamins A, C & Riboflavin & Zn.
Oesophagus	Low intake of meat, fish, fruits and vegetables, corn as the staple, alcohol, tobacco, bracken fern aflatoxins	Poor nutritional status, Beta-carotene, vit. A, Iron, Riboflavin, Zn, Se
Stomach	Nitrates, nitrites and nitrosamines; Pickled vegetables, salted substances; Fried foods, Smoked fish Undernutrition	Vitamin C, Vitamin E, Protein Complex carbohydrates, Selenium
Colon and rectal	Low fibre, Refined carbohydrates	High fat and protein Vitamin A, C
Larynx	Tobacco smoke, Alcohol	Vitamin A
Lung	Cigarettes, Low in green Vegetables	Vitamin A, E
Bladder	Industrial chemicals, Artificial sweetners, Coffee consumption	Vitamin A
Prostate	Low in green and yellow vegetables	Higher Vitamin A, Overnutrition, High fat and protein
Breast	Obesity, Low in vegetables	Beta-carotene, Vitamin A, High fat and protein
Cervical cancer	Low in vegetables	Vitamin A, C Folic acid Poor nutrition, Over nutrition
Pancreas	Tobacco smoke, Coffee	Over nutrition
Liver	Aflatoxin	Poor nutrition

There are several aspects of diet-cancer interrelationships, such as the metabolic susceptibility, case-control studies to identify risk factors, intervention studies to determine the role of nutrients and non-nutrient components of the diet which have a positive impact on carcinogenesis and diet associated carcinogens (Table 3).

Table 3 Food sources of non-nutrients

Non-nutrients	Food Source
Carotenoids	Yellow / orange vegetables, fruits and dark green leafy vegetables
Allium compounds	Onion, garlic, chives, leeks
Dithiolthiones / glucosinolates	Cruciferous
Isothiocyanates	Cruciferous
Terpenoids	Oil of citrus fruit peel
Phytoestrogens	Cereals, pulses, sorghum
Protease inhibitors	Cereals, barley, wheat, oats, rye, soyabeans, kidney beans and chick peas
Phytic acid	Cereals, nuts, seeds, sesame seeds, lime beans, peanuts and soyabeans.
Flavonoids	Fruits and vegetables
Phenolic compounds	Fruits, vegetables and tea
Plant sterols	Vegetables
Saponins	Soyabeans, yam and colacasia

Metabolic Susceptibility

Most of the efforts on human subjects with regards to genetic and metabolic susceptibility are focused around identifying the high risk subjects. This involves studying xenobiotic metabolizing enzymes which activate and deactivate carcinogens. Metabolism by these enzymes appear to be an expression of the interplay of genetic, environmental, physiological and pathological factors. The metabolic oxidation plays a central role in the activation processes and mediates mutagenesis and carcinogenesis through formation of active electrophilic molecules which attach the nucleophilic centres in DNA. **The phase-II drug metabolizing enzymes, are mainly conjugating group of enzymes moping the electrophilic substances and detoxifying them to nontoxic products.** The relative activities of these enzymes in the body appear to determine the dose of carcinogen which can reach the critical macromolecules and control the adverse biological effects. Nutritionstatus influences the biotransformation of drugs and foreign chemicals[29,30].

Undernutrition itself influences the hepatic microsomal enzymes in humans. Enzymes such as arylhydrocarbon hydroxylase (AHH), UDP glucuronyl transferase (UDPGT) and glutathione-s-transferase (GST). There is an induction of phase I enzymes and impairment of conjugating enzymes resulting in formation of highly electrophilic substances. There appears to be greater susceptibility to toxicity due to exposure to xenobiotics[31]. **An experiment in animals revealed that chronic undernutrition decreased the protective conjugation enzymes with concomitant increase in activating enzymes which resulted in susceptibility to damage induced by carcinogens such as acetominofluorene, mycotoxins[32,33].**

Though restriction of calorie intake is known to reduce spontaneous and induced tumours, the process of initiation or damage to critical molecules can be higher in diet restriction[34]. Micronutrient deficiencies such as vitamin A[35], riboflavin[36], zinc[37], and Iron deficiency[38] in animals indicated that formation of electrophilic substances, detoxification and antioxidant mechanisms are adversely affected and increase the risk of cancer.

Case Control Studies

One of the ten most important cancers in the world is cancer of oral cavity and pharynx. In India, the oral and pharyngeal cancers are the most common forms of cancers in males and the third most common in females[39]. In South East Asia, including India, the habit of chewing betel leaves, tobacco with other ingredients is one of the main risk factor in the causation of oral cancer[40]. Use of tobacco in other forms like smoking is also implicated in oral cancers.

There is marked variation in the incidence of cancers of the oesophagus and stomach around the world[1]. A case control study was conducted to understand the role of dietary factors in the incidence of oropharyngeal and oesophageal cancers. Detailed personal and dietary history were obtained and dietary nutritional correlates of cancers were evaluated[41,42]. The studies revealed that intakes of green vegetables and fruits were significantly low in cases as compared to controls. The food frequency questionnaire showed higher risk association with less frequently intake of vegetables and higher consumption of fried foods. The odds ratios calculated revealed high risk estimates with low intakes of beta carotene, thiamin, riboflavin, folic acid, iron, magnesium and copper. The odds estimates were also higher for low levels of hemoglobin, albumin, folate, zinc and vitamins A and E and selenium in plasma. Similar observations were made for oesophageal cancers [41,42].

Epidemiological evidences indicate an inverse relationship between vegetables and fruits consumption and human cancers at several sites[1]. This association is significant for epithelial cancers particularly those involving alimentary and respiratory tracts. Anticarcinogenic agents present in the diet as nutrient and non-nutrient components appear to possess inhibitory effects. Other studies in India have documented low vegetable intakes and vitamin A and B complex deficiencies in oral cancer[42].

Another important epithelial cancer that has been associated with diet is cervical cancer[43]. Cancer of the cervix in women is one of the world's most commonly causing cancers and its incidence in women of India is very high. Presently in developed countries the overall incidence rates of cervical cancer are now on a decline while in developing countries its incidence is high. Even though viral etiology may be a major causative factor in the incidence of cervical cancers, lifestyle factors like cigarette smoking, unhygienic sexual practices may have a contributing role. Deficiencies of antioxidant micronutrients such as vitamin A, folate and vitamin C present in plant foods may be other important risk factors.

Intervention Trials

Studies conducted in high-risk individuals of reverse smokers in Srikakulam District of Andhra Pradesh revealed that the micronutrient supplements given as cocktail of nutrients in prescriptive approach resulted in regression of preneoplastic lesions[44].

In this study in reverse smokers 298 subjects were chosen out of whom 150 received vitamin A, riboflavin, zinc and selenium supplements. The 148 control received placebo, one capsule twice a week for one year. The complete regression was 57% in supplemented group whereas 8 percent in control. The micronuclei and DNA adducts in buccal cells, which were significantly elevated in subjects with lesions showed 95% decrease in DNA adducts with all categories of lesions and 72% in subjects without lesion. The micronuclei decreased significantly, with or without lesions[45].

Cancer Prevention through Dietary Intervention

Dietary intervention is based on the knowledge acquired so far that could help in effective decrease in cancer incidence. Broadly, the interventions are of two types.

(i) First approach is through supplements with vitamins, antioxidants and minor dietary factors.

(ii) Second approach is by dietary modification in which target levels are established for consumption of meat, fat, fiber or fruits and vegetables[31]

Conclusions

Results from experiments in animals and epidemiological studies in humans provide unequivocal evidence that chemopreventers, in the levels found in human diet are sage. Diet rich in chemopreventers will have beneficial health effects, cost of treatment of cancer are higher than cost of providing diets rich in phytochemical and modifying eating habits. While there is a need to identify these substances, tendency to take artificial supplements must be avoided as against a back drop of poor diet, no nutrient can produce desired outcome.

A more appropriate approach is one in which the importance of foods in the diet is stressed. Nutrition education will promote public awareness of the dietary guidelines for promotion of healthy life.

References

1. World Cancer Research Fund, American Institute for Cancer Research, Foods Nutrition and the prevention of cancer: a global perspective. Washington DC: American Institute for Cancer Research, 1997.
2. National Commission on Macroeconomic and Health Background papers – Burden of Disease in India, 2005.
3. Krishnaswamy K. and Polasa P. Diet, nutrition and cancer – the Indian scenario. IJMR. 1995; 102: 200-9.
4. Sugimora T, Wakaboyashi K, Nakagama H, Nagao M. Heterocyclic amines: Mutagens / carcinogens produced during cooking of meat and fish. Cancer Sci. 2004; 95: 290-99.
5. Yahagi T, Nagao M, Takahashi Y, Wakabuyashi K, Sugimura T. Mutagenecity of alcoholic beverages. Mutant Res. 1981; 88: 147-54.
6. Prasad MPR, Krishnaswamy K. N-nitrosomines in Indian beer. Ind. J. Med. Res. 1994; 100: 299-301.
7. Siddiqui M, Tricker AR, Preussmann R. The occurrence of preformed N-nitrosocompounds in food samples from a high risk area of oesophageal cancers in Kashmir, India. Cancer Lett, 1988; 39: 37-43.
8. Siddiqui M, Preussmann R. Esophageal cancer in Kashmir – an assessment. Cancer Res. Clin Oncol. 1989; 115: 111-7.
9. Prasad MPR. N-nitrosamines: Potential carcinogens in Indian diet. Amala.Res. Bull. 2000; 20: 54-57.

10. Block G, Patterson B, Subar A. Fruits, vegetables and cancer prevention. A review of the epidemiologic evidence. Nutr. Cancer. 1992; 18: 1-29.

11. Stavric B. Role of chemopreventors in human diet. Clin. Biochem. 1994; 27: 319-332.

12. Wattenberg LW. Inhibition of carcinogenesis by minor dietary constituents. Cancer Res. 1992; 52: 2248S-2253S.

13. Lee KW, Lee HJ, Lee CY. Vitamins, Phytochemicals, Diets and their implementation in Cancer Chemoprevention. Crit. Reviews in Fd. Sci. and Nutr. 2004; 44: 437-452.

14. Polasa K. Nonnutrients and cancer prevention. ICMR Bulletin, 2001, 31: 1-9.

15. Polasa K, Sesikeran B, Krishna T.P. and Krishnaswamy K. Turmeric (curcuma longa) induced reduction in urinary mutagens. Food. Chem. Toxicol. 1991; 29: 699-706.

16. Goud, VK, Polasa K. and Krishnaswamy K. Effect of turmeric on xenobiotic metabolizing enzymes. Plant Foods for Human Nutrition, 1992; 47: 87-92.

17. Krishnaswamy K, Goud V.K., Sesikeran B, Mukundan MA, Krishna TP. Retardation of experimental tumorigenesis and reduction in DNA adducts by turmeric and curcumin. Nutr. Cancer, 1998; 30(2): 163-166.

18. Mukundan, MA, Chacko, MC, Annapurna V.V., Krishnaswamy, K. Effect of turmeric and curcumin on BP-DNA adducts. Carcinogenesis, 1993; 14(3), 493-496.

19. Polasa K, Averbeck D and Krishnaswamy K. Studies on the influence of curcumin on the induction and repair of DNA single strand breaks (ssb) produced by genotoxic agents. Amala Research Bull. 2002; 32: 178-190.

20. Polasa K, Raghuram TC, Krishna TP and Krishnaswamy K. Effect of turmeric on urinary mutagens in smokers. Mutagenesis. 1992; 7: 107-109.

21. Polasa K. and Krishnaswamy K. Reduction of urinary mutagen excretion in rats fed garlic. Cancer Letters. 1997; 114: 185-186.

22. Soni, M.G., Polasa K. and Krishnaswamy K. Alterations in rat tissue glutathione-s-transferase and its isozyme (class Mu) during onion feeding. Indian Journal of Pharmacology, 1999; 31(3): 239-240.

23. Nirmala K, Krishna TP. and Polasa K. Inhibition of induced micronuclei formation in human lymphocytes by ginger (under publication).

24. Nirmala K, Krishna TP and Polasa K. Protective effect of ginger against Benzo(a)pyrene induced DNA damage. International Journal of Cancer Research, 2007; 3(1): 13-24.

25. Nirmala K. Krishna TP. And Polasa K. *In vivo* antimutagenic potential of ginger on formation and excretion of urinary mutagens. International Journal of Cancer Research (In press).

26. Nirmala K, Krishna TP. And Polasa K. Elevation in the levels of detoxifying Phase II enzymes in rats fed with ginger, 2007 (under publication).

27. Nirmala K, Krishna TP. and Polasa K. Alternations in antioxidant status of rats following intake of ginger through diet, 2007 (under publication).

28. Polasa K, Annapurna VV, Krishna TP. and Krishnaswamy K. Inhibitory effect of unprocessed / processed Alliums under *in vitro / in vivo* conditions on carcinogen induced mutagenesis using different assay. International Journal of Cancer Research. 2006'; (3): 199-211.

29. Kato R. Drug metabolism under pathological and abnormal physiological status in animals and man. Xenobiotics. 1977; 7: 25-92.

30. Anderson KE. Influences of diet and nutrition on clinical pharmacokinetics. W Clin Pharmacokin 1988; 14 : 325-346.

31. Kirshnaswamy K. Drug metabolism and pharmacokinetics in malnutrition. Clin Pharmacokin 1978; 13: 216-240.

32. Ramesh RP, Krishnaswamy K. Effect of chronic undernutrition on glucuronide and glutathione conjugation in rat liver. Drug Nutr Interact 1985; 3 : 121-128.

33. Ramesh RP, Krishnaswamy K. Differences in response of glucuronide and glutathione conjugating enzymes of aflatoxin B1 and N-acetyl-aminofluorene in underfed rats. J Toxicol Environ Health 1988; 26 : 103-109.

34. Newberne PM, Schrager TF. Conner, M.W. Experimental evidence on the nutritional prevention of cancer. In : Moon TE, Micozzi MS. Editors. Nutrition and cancer prevention : Investigating the role of micronutrients. New York, Marcel Dekkar Inc. 1989; 32-82.

35. Kalamegham R, Krishnaswamy K. Benzo(a)pyrene metabolism in vitamin A deficient rats. Life Sci. 1980; 27 : 33-38.

36. Pangrekar J, Krishnaswamy K, Jagadeesan V. Effects of riboflavin deficiency and riboflavin administration on carcinogen – DNA binding. Food Chem Toxicol 1993; 31 : 745-750.

37. Jagadeesan V, Oesch F. Effect of dietary zinc deficiency on the activity of enzymes associated with Phase I and Phase II of drug metabolism in Fischer 344 rats. Drug Nutr Interact 1988; 5 : 403-413.

38. Jagadeesan V, Jayanthi Rao, Sesikeran B. Effects of iron deficiency on the incidence of dimethyl hydrazine induced tumors in fisher rats. Nutr Cancer 1994; 22 : 285-291.

39. Consolidated Report of the Population Based Cancer Registries. National Cancer Registry, ICMR, New Delhi, 1990-1996.

40. Gupta PC, Mehta FS, Daftry DK. Incidence rate of oral cancers and natural history of oral precancerous lesions in a 10 year follow up study of Indian villagers. Commun Dent Oral Epidemiol 1980; 81 : 287-333.

41. Prasad MPR, Krishna TP, Pasricha S, Quereshi MA, Krishnaswamy K. Diet and oral cancer – A case control study. Asia Pacific J Clin Nutrition. 1995; 4 :259-264.

42. Prasad MPR, Krishna TP, Pasricha S, Krishnaswamy K, Qureshi MA. Oesophageal cancer and diet – A case control study. Nutr Cancer 1992; 17: 85-93.

43. Willet WC, Trichopoulos D. Nutrition and Cancer: a summary of evidence. Cancer Causes Control. 1996; 7: 178-180.

44. Krishnaswamy K, Prasad MPR, Krishna TP, Annapurna VV, Reddy GA. A case study of nutrient intervention of oral precancerous lesions in India. Eur J Cancer 1995; 318 : 41-48.

45. Prasad MPR, Mukundan MA, Krishnaswamy K. Micronuclei and carcinogenic DNA adducts as intermediate end points in nutrient intervention trial of precancerous lesions in the oral cancer. Eur J. Cancer. 1995; 31B, 155-159.

6.4 Studies on the Beneficial Effects of Functional Foods like Garlic, Ginger, Fenugreek and Amla with special reference to Ischemic Heart Disease

Drs. Arun Bordia*, S.K. Verma* & Vartika Jain**

*Indigenous Drug Research Center, Department of Medicine, RNT Medical College, Udaipur, Rajasthan, INDIA. E-mail: drskverma@prontomail.com

**Department of Botany, M.L. Sukhadia University, Udaipur, Rajasthan, INDIA.

Introduction

It is widely accepted that efforts directed towards the prevention of chronic diseases like atherosclerosis, coronary artery disease (CAD), cancer and arthritis by means of dietary modifications, herb supplementation and physical activity would be sounder and economically viable than treatment and hospitalizations which involve enormous costs. From this point of view, disease prevention and cause modification by the use of 'non-nutritive' secondary plant metabolites i.e. phytochemicals in human diet is gaining much significance. Various dietary components from vegetables, herbs and spices which possess disease preventive properties are being pursued. Phytochemicals from spices by virtue of their anti-platelet activity, arachidonic acid metabolism modulating activities, antioxidant properties, hypolipidaemic effect and fibrinolysis enhancing capabilities along with anti-inflammatory, antibacterial, antihyperglycemic and anti-carcinogenic properties could be of significance in disease prevention. The present paper deals with beneficial effect of some of the phytochemicals (functional foods) from Garlic, Ginger, Fenugreek and Amla for disease prevention with special reference to athero-thrombotic diseases.

Garlic- "The Spice of Life"

According to our studies garlic, juice and its oil gave several health benefiting effects such as control of blood lipids, platelet aggregation, and improvement in fibrinolytic activity, exercise tolerance, protection from radiation and atherosclerosis. In the initial studies, garlic juice or its essential oil was employed. However, in most of the human studies, garlic oil extracted in ethyl acetate and mixed with soya oil was used in capsule form. The dose varies in different studies.

(A) Clinical Studies

Hypolipidemic Effect

Prospective, placebo controlled studies of the effect of garlic oil administration to the CAD patients with mild and moderate hyperlipidaemia were conducted. The dosage and duration of administration was different. Sixty CAD patients, with mild hyperlipidaemia were divided in two groups of 30 each. In the treated group, consumption of 4 capsules of garlic oil per day in two divided doses for 3 months reduced serum cholesterol by 12.8% and serum triglycerides by 15.2% ($p < 0.01$). The placebo group ($N = 30$), however, did not show any significant alteration in the lipid levels[1]. Each capsule contained garlic oil obtained from one gram garlic, i.e.; 3 to 4 mg of garlic oil.

In the second group, garlic oil was administered (essential oil 0.25 mg/kg in two divided doses) to 33, CAD patients with moderate hyperlipidaemia for 10 months, while, 29 similar patients served as control (placebo group). In the treated group, serum cholesterol level decreased by 18% and serum triglycerides by 19.7% while HDL cholesterol increased significantly ($p < 0.001$)[2].

Hypolipidaemic and Fibrinolysis Enhancing Activity

75 g butter feeding in 40 healthy individuals caused significant increase in triglycerides level and decrease in fibrinolytic activity at the end of 3 weeks. This was prevented when garlic was added to it[3]. Garlic administration (essential oil extract from 1 g of raw garlic/kg in two divided doses) in 20 patients with acute myocardial infarction, increased fibrinolytic activity by 95.5% at the end of 20 days ($p < 0.001$) while in control group of 20 patients, the increase was only 24%. When garlic administration was stopped, such effects disappeared in the test group[4]. Other single-dose studies, involving healthy individuals as well as patients with CHD and increased serum cholesterol values have revealed equally good results[1,5].

The effect of garlic on enhancement of fibrinolysis is unequivocal as most of the studies throughout the world, with oil preparation of garlic, have documented this beneficial effect.

Effect of Garlic on Platelet Aggregation

Garlic oil prepared by extraction of macerated garlic with ethyl acetate was used for this study. Acute effect of garlic oil on *in vitro* platelet aggregation was dose related in man[6]. Long term administration of garlic (6 capsules /day) for one month in 10 healthy individuals reduced platelet aggregation induced by both ADP and epinephrine. However, in patients with CAD, the effect of garlic was observed only in epinephrine induced aggregation ($p<0.05$)[6].

Acute physical stress in healthy individuals resulted in a significant decrease in platelet aggregation, while it produced increased aggregation and cortisol production in patients with CAD. Garlic oil administration (1 to 3 capsules/day) for 6 months favorably modified the stress induced changes in platelet aggregation and cortisol levels. After garlic administration the rise in platelet aggregation and cortisol levels was not as significant as before[7].

Beneficial Effect of Garlic Oil on Cardiac Performance and Exercise Tolerance (Treadmill Stress) in Patients with CAD

Six week administration of garlic oil (4 capsules, twice a day) to 30 CAD patients for two months reduced their heart rat at peak exercise, and an index called double product i.e. maximum heart rate × maximum systolic. BP during stress induced by treadmill exercise and increased the duration of exercise tolerance significantly. Garlic oil was prepared by extracting macerated garlic by ethyl acetate. The solvent free oil was dissolved in soy oil and encapsulated. Each capsule contained garlic oil equivalent to one gram raw garlic and 260 mg soy oil. No side effects were observed[8]. Similar effects were observed in animal experiments also by others. Garlic oil administration in stress affected mice prevented decrease in physical strength and promoted recovery from the affected condition along with lower cortisone level[9]. In another study the degree of myocardial damage, produced by isoprenaline was reduced significantly by garlic oil feeding[10].

Effect on Blood Cholesterol in Butter Fed Subjects

Both freshly pressed juice from 50 g garlic and an ether extract from the same amount juice caused significant decrease in cholesterol levels ($p<0.001$) i.e. 7% decrease for juice and 9% decrease for garlic oil compared to a 7% increase in control group, at 3 hours in normal subjects whose serum cholesterol levels were elevated by consumption of 100 g butter[11].

In a nutshell, consumption of garlic oil dissolved in vegetable oil, lowered serum lipids in patients. Three of these studies used an ether extract at a dose of 0.25 mg sulfur compounds/kg body weight[2,12]. In the same studies Bordia and associates also used an oil macerate of garlic at 0.03 mg sulfur compound /kg and the serum cholesterol of the patients decreased significantly and they attributed the activity to allicin and its derivatives in garlic oil.

In patients suffering from arteriosclerosis, Bordia et. al.[13,14] observed that administration of garlic extract as well as garlic oil ameliorated the disease with an improved blood fibrinolysis. Some studies objectively showed that activities of endogenous fibrinolysis by small doses of garlic is real and occurs rapidly i.e. when garlic is taken regularly for several months an increase in fibrinolysis occurs without fail[15].

In vitro Effects of Garlic oil on Arachidonic acid Metabolism in Platelets

The effects of garlic oil on the production of eicosanoids (prostaglandins and thromboxane) from labeled (1-^{14}C) arachidonic acid (AA) platelets were studied[6]. Garlic oil (200 µg/ml) did not show any *in vitro* effect on the deacylation of platelet phospholipids. However, it inhibited the enzymes of AA cascade resulting in reduced formation of thromboxane B_2, hydroxyl heptadecatrienoic acid (HHT) and 12-hydroxy eicosatetraenoic acid (12-HETE) with concomitant increase in AA. Garlic oil administration reduced lipid peroxidation also. Both Diallyl disulphide (DADS) and Diallyl trisulphide (DATS) showed inhibitory effects on TxB_2 formation from platelets *in vitro*[1].

Mechanism of Action

The mechanism of action of garlic principles may be related to suppression of the stress induced activities of the peripheral sympathetic system without affecting adrenal medulla and pituitary adrenocortical system[7]. The corticoids are thereby spared which are known to enhance adaptability. A study on hospital patients also showed the values of garlic in psychological stress in human beings and animals[16,17].

Previous studies showed that the therapeutic effects of garlic were dose dependent[6]. Therefore, Bordia *et. al.*[5] recommend a minimum dose of garlic oil equivalent for 8 g garlic for a person to get some benefits. Bordia group published many papers showing the medicinal properties of garlic in human beings which have been reviewed[18].

(B) Animal Studies

Protective Effect of Garlic on Irradiated Rats

A group of 40 rats were subjected to 400 rads irradiation. 20 rats were kept as control and 20 others were treated with garlic for 5 weeks. While the entire untreated control group died in that period, the treated rats survived[19].

Reversibility of Experimental Atherosclerosis

Rabbits fed with cholesterol rich diet for 3 months were treated with garlic (essential oil extract equivalent to 2 grams raw garlic/kg) for 9 months. Their plasma cholesterol, aorta lipid deposit and atheroma lipid grading etc., reduced significnaly[20]. Similar effects of garlic were observed in other experimental studies also[21,22].

Human Health Benefits

The health benefits of garlic and its products may be due to their antioxidant, anti-inflammatory, antiplatelet aggregation and vasodilatory action as reported by various workers. In addition to these properties of garlic products, they may increase blood flow also as observed by Harenberg et.al.[23]. Administration of single doses of 600-1200 mg dry garlic powder produced pronounced changes in plasma viscosity, tissue plasminogen activator (TPA) activity and hematocrit level. The maximal decrease in hematocrit level was in the range of 5-10%. This is interpreted as a rheoregulatory effect due to an internal hemodilution from garlic's peripheral vasodilatative effect[24]. Similar results were also reported by Kiesewetter also using a daily dose of 800 mg dry garlic powder given for 4 weeks in a double blind study in patients with stage II peripheral arterial occlusive diseae[25]. The anti-platelet aggregation effect of garlic products may be due to their inhibitory effects on cyclooxygenase catalyzed formation of endoperoxides from AA, by inhibiting the release of platelet constituents and by increasing cAMP level as reported by Kawakishi and Morimitsu[26]. All these findings support the health benefits which our team already observed with garlic products.

Ginger (*Zingiber Officinale*) – The Universal Medicine

Antioxidant Activity of Ginger

It contains components with strong antiplatelet and prostanoid synthesis inhibitory activity which prompted us to study its antioxidant effect in healthy subjects and patients with CAD[27]. For this 20 healthy individuals (Group A) and 20 patients with coronary artery disease (Group B) were selected. Both groups were randomly assigned either 5 g dry ginger powder or matched placebo (Lactose powder) for 4 weeks. Blood lipids and lipoprotein oxidation susceptibility (LOS) were estimated initially and at the end of the study and the results were analyzed using paired t-test.

Ginger administration significantly ($p < 0.001$) decreased lipoprotein oxidation susceptibility in healthy subjects as well as in patients with CAD without any effect on blood lipids. No adverse effects were observed. It is well known that essential oil of ginger contains various terpenes and sesquiterepenes (e.g.: Zingiberene). The oxy methyl phenols like shogaol, zingerone and gingerol are responsible for ginger's antioxidant property[28]. Other studies[29,30] also documented the antioxidant properties of ginger essential oil.

Anti-Platelet Aggregation Effect

An ethanolic ginger extract found to contain 40 mg/g active compounds like gingerol, shogaol and zingerone and 90 mg/g total phenols which have been reported by Fuhrman to inhibit LDL oxidation and to reduce the development of atherosclerosis in mice as compared to control group[28]. Ginger has been a popular food spice possessing many medicinal properties[31,32]. Gingerol and Shogaol were found to be potent inhibitors of platelet aggregation both *ex vivo*[33,34] and *in vitro*[35] for healthy as well as CAD groups. Ginger has also shown to ameliorate pain and inflammation in patients with rheumatism, musculo-skeletal disorders and migraine[36].

Effect of Ginger on Platelet Aggregation in Man

Dietary supplementation of 100 g butter in 20 healthy male volunteers for 7 days was found to enhance platelet aggregation significantly ($p < 0.001$). Addition of 5 g of dry ginger in two divided dose with the fatty meal in 10 volunteers significantly inhibited ($p < 0.001$) the platelet aggregation induced by ADP and epinephrine; while in the placebo control group (10 volunteers) there was no significant alteration in platelet aggregation[34]. Serum lipids remained unchanged in both groups. Ginger has also been reported to contain antihistamine and antioxidant[37] as well as antirheumatic and antigout factors[38]. It is used traditionally to relieve colds and flu for its warming properties and to improve circulation[37, 38].

Ginger has been reported to inhibit prostaglandins synthesis *in vitro*[39,40]. It has been suggested that dietary fat content and composition affect platelet aggregation by modulating prostaglandin metabolism[41]. Administration of ginger along with fatty diet might inhibit the conversion of arachidonic acid to thromboxane and decrease the sensitivity of platelets to various aggregating agents. As the serum lipids profile was not significantly changed either by fat or ginger administration, the effect on platelet is possibly not through alteration of lipid levels but by its direct effect on prosta-glandin metabolism. Recent *in vitro* studies have further demonstrated that ginger is a dual inhibitor i.e. it inhibits the cyclooxygenase and lipooxygenase pathways, thus producing reduced amounts of prosta-glandins and leukotrienes respectively[42]. As there is sufficient evidence supporting the involvement of platelets in the genesis of atherosclerosis, administration of natural products like ginger may prove beneficial in thrombo-atherosclerosis.

Effect of Ginger Pearls in Patients with Musculo-Skeletal Disorders

As ginger has been reported to contain antihistaminic and antioxidant factors[37,43] and inhibitors of eicosanoid synthesis[35], a study was conducted on 30 patients of musculo-skeletal disorders i.e. 10 patients in each group with rheumatoid arthritis, osteoarthritis and soft tissue rheumatism respectively in order to assess the effects of ginger on these patients[44].

Ginger pearls were supplied by Seven Seas Ltd., England. Each gelatin capsule contained 100 mg of standardized ginger extract equivalent to approximately 12 g of fresh ginger root. After careful clinical evaluation, the initial blood samples were collected and one ginger pearl was administered twice a day after meals for a period of three months. Patients were evaluated for their symptoms of joint pain, swelling, stiffness, muscle pain and general feeling of well being, along with any side effect every month. The improvement in their symptoms were graded on an arbitrary scale ranging from no improvement (Grade 0) to marked improvement (Grades as follows). Percentage is given in parenthesis. Grade I (<10%); II (>10%); III (>20%); IV (>50%); V (>75%). After 3 months treatment, ginger pearls were stopped and matched placebo was administered for one month to all patients in each group. Blood samples were taken at the completion of treatment i.e. 3 months and again after the placebo at the end of 4th month. ESR, rheumatoid factor, L.E. cell phenomenon and uric acid were estimated.

The symptoms of joint pain, swelling, stiffness, muscle pain and feeling of well being were improved in 20-50% of the patients with arthritis. In patients with rheumatoid arthritis there was only minimal improvement (Grade II) in joint pain and stiffness, while very minimal improvement (Grade I) was observed in swelling and feeling of well being. In patients with osteoarthritis, 30% showed minimal improvement (Grade II) in joint pains, while very minimal effect was (Grade I) on joint stiffness. The patients with soft tissue rheumatism demonstrated moderate improvement in feeling of well being in 50 % of the patients and at the end of 3 months. Ginger pearls were tolerated well by all patients without any side effects. After three months of ginger treatment ESR decreased by 90% in patients of rheumatoid arthritis and by 43% in patients of soft tissue rheumatism. Uric acid level was within normal range for all the patients. Rheumatoid factor was positive in two patients. In patients with osteoarthritis, all laboratory investigations were normal. These levels remained more or less same at the end of placebo therapy.

The dual inhibitor property of ginger on cyclo-oxygenase and lipo-oxygenase enzymes is responsible for its ameliorative effect in musculoskeletal diseases. Some of the active principles isolated from ginger have been found to be even more active inhibitors in prosta-glandin synthesis than indomethacin[45]. When we administered whole ginger in place of ginger pearls the amelioration of the symptoms for the diseases in some patients were more satisfactory than the cases reported above. This may be because the pearl contains only extractable principles and that may be lacking some of the very active principles of ginger[44].

Effect of Ginger and Fenugreek on Blood Lipids, Blood Sugar and Platelet Aggregation in Patients of CAD

In a placebo controlled study, the effects of ginger and fenugreek was examined on blood lipids, blood sugar, platelet aggregation, fibrinogen and fibrinolytic activity[33]. The subjects included in this study were healthy individuals, patients with CAD and patients with NIDDM (Type 2 diabetes mellitus) who either had CAD or were without CAD. In 30 patients with CAD, powdered ginger was administered in a dose of 4 g daily for 3 months did not affect ADP and epinephrine induced platelet aggregation. Also no change in the fibrinolytic activity and fibrinogen level was observed. However a single dose of 10 g powdered ginger administered to CAD patients produced a significant reduction in platelet aggregation induced by the two agonists. Ginger did not affect the blood lipids and blood sugar. Fenugreek given in a dose of 2.5 g twice daily for 3 months to healthy individuals did not affect the blood lipids and blood sugar (fasting and post prandial). However, administered in the same daily dose for the same duration to 30 CAD patients with NIDDM, fenugreek decreased significantly the blood lipids (total cholesterol and triglycerides) without affecting HDL-C. When administered in the same daily dose to 20 mild NIDDM (non-CAD) patients, fenugreek reduced both fasting and post-prandial blood sugar significantly ($p < 0.001$). In severe NIDDM cases, fasting and post-prandial blood sugar levels were reduced but the changes were not significant. Fenugreek administration did not affect platelet aggregation, fibrinolytic activity and fibrinogen[33].

In Vitro Studies

Ginger powder was extracted in n-hexane and the solvent evaporated completely. The residue was dissolved in HPLC grade ethanol and appropriate dilutions were made. Platelet aggregation was performed using sodium arachidonate (AA) and adrenaline as agonist. A dose dependant inhibition of aggregation was observed with ginger extract. The extract was found to be more effective in AA induced aggregation. A dose dependant inhibition of thromboxane formation was observed on challenging washed platelets with ^{14}C labeled AA in the presence of ginger extract. 12-HHT formation was reduced with a concomitant increase in 12-HETE. 125 µg/ml of the extract inhibited the incorporation of labeled AA into platelet phospholipids only by 9% which was statistically not significant[42].

n-hexane extract of fenugreek however did not affect the AA induced aggregation or alter the AA metabolism. Aqueous extract did not inhibit the platelet aggregation induced by AA and adrenaline.

In the case of ginger, its inhibitory effect on platelet aggregation with the blood of healthy subjects who consumed 5 g ginger daily for 7 days was reported earlier[34]. In the present study, on CAD patients, daily consumption of 4 g, ginger for 3 months did not produce any effect on platelet aggregation. However a single dose of 10g produced a significant reduction of ADP and epinephrine induced aggregation[33]. In the former study, enhanced platelet aggregation was caused by fat ingestion and it was neutralized by ginger. In the latter case the elevation was due to CAD and hence a greater dose of ginger was required to show a significant effect. As fenugreek did not show an effect on the AA metabolism, its benefit against CAD could be considered only in the light of its effects on blood lipids and blood sugar.

Protective Effect of Ginger on Experimental Atherosclerosis in Rabbits

Our group studied the effects of air dried ginger powder (0.1 g/kg body weight PO, for 75 days) on experimentally induced atherosclerosis (feeding cholesterol 0.3 g/kg body weight) in rabbits[46]. Cholesterol feeding for 75 days led to distinct development of atheroma in the aorta and coronary arteries of the rabbits and this was significantly inhibited by about 50 % following ginger administration. There was distinct decrease in lipid peroxidation and enhancement of fibrinolytic activity in ginger treated animals. However, ginger did not lower blood lipids to any significant extent. This protection from the development of atherosclerosis by ginger is probably because of its free radical scavenging, prosta-glandin inhibitory and fibrinolysis enhancing properties as reported earlier by us. As LDL oxidation is an initiative process for atherosclerosis[47] its inhibition by ginger's strong antioxidant property may be the major factor in prevention of atherosclerosis in spite of its insignificant effect on blood lipids.

The two active principles present in ginger viz; shogaol and zingerone have been ascribed with strong antioxidant properties[37]. Ginger not only inhibits thromboxane synthetase but also raises levels of prostacyclin without a concomitant rise in PGE_2 or PGF_2[48]. The phenol content of ginger is high due to the presence of the above two along with gingerol (550 ± 44 mg/100g). The total flavonoid content (such as quercetin, kaempferol, luteolin and pelargonidin) is however low (38 ± 3 mg/100g)[49]. The clinical potential of such a dietary condiment against atherosclerosis warrants further study.

Comparative Effects of Vitamin C and Amla (*Embilica officinalis*) on Blood Lipids, Platelet Aggregation and Experimental Atheroma in Rabbits

In yet another study, our team assessed the comparative effects of vitamin C (35 mg/kg/day) and Amla juice and pulp that contain approximately an equivalent dose of Vitamin C per day, on cholesterol fed rabbits for a period of three months[50]. Vitamin C and both the Amla products significantly prevented the rise in serum cholesterol and triglycerides and also reduced the tendency of platelet aggregation as compared to untreated cholesterol fed rabbits. All the three prevented the development of experimental atheroma significantly. In these respects amla products were found to be more effective than Vitamin C. Further amla pulp was found to be superior to Amla juice in reducing the development of atheroma both in aorta and coronary arteries. This may be due to the presence of fiber pectin, ellegic and gallic acids and PUFA present in the former in addition to Vitamin C for their antiatherogenic actions. Some workers[51,52] reported on the absence of hypocholesterolemic action by Vitamin C in humans. However it has significant cholesterol lowering action in experimental animals according to many[53,54]. As the effects of Chyavanprash[55] is largely due to amla with respect to improvement in enhancing fibrinolysis and in reducing platelet aggregation and blood lipids in humans, the therapeutic value of this vegetable in man cannot be ignored. However further studies are warranted to make use of amla as a functional food.

Conclusion

During the last 30 years, we have been working on various health beneficial effect of functional food from spices, herbs and condiments and reached to the conclusion that garlic, ginger, fenugreek and other spices have definite role in modifying the risk parameters of athero-thrombotic cardiovascular diseases. In this regards, hypolipidaemic effect, platelet aggregation inhibition, fibrinolysis enhancement and antioxidant properties are some of the noteworthy effects that warrant further attention and exploration.

References

1. Bordia, A; Verma, S.K. and Srivastava K.C. Effect of garlic (*Allium sativum*) on blood lipids, blood sugar, fibrinogen and fibrinolytic activity in patients with coronary artery disease. Prost Leuk. Essent. Fatty Acids 58(1998) 257.
2. Bordia, A. Effect of garlic on blood lipids in patients with coronary heart disease. Am. J. Clin. Nutr. 34(1981) 2100-2103.

3. Bordia, A; Bansal, H.C. et.al. Effect of the essential oil (active principle) of garlic on serum cholesterol, plasma fibrinogen, whole blood coagulation time and fibrinolytic activity in alimentary lipaemia. J. Assoc. Physicians. India. 22(1974) 267-270.

4. Bordia, A; Joshi, H.K. et. al. Effect of essential oil of garlic on serum fibrinolytic activity in patients with coronary artery disease. Atherosclerosis. 28(1977) 155-159.

5. Bordia, A and Bansal, H.C. Essential oil of garlic on prevention of atherosclerosis. Lancet. 2(1973) 1491-92.

6. Bordia, A; Verma, S.K. and Srivastava K.C. Effect of garlic on platelet aggregation in human: a study in healthy subjects and patients with coronary artery disease. Prost Leuk. Essent. Fatty Acids. 55(1996) 201-205.

7. Verma, S.K; Bordia, A and Srivastava K.C. Garlic in physical stress induced platelet aggregation and stress tolerance: A study in patients with coronary artery disease. South Asian J Preventive Cardiology. 7(2003) 128.

8. Verma, S.K; Rajeevan, V; Jain, P and Bordia, A. Effect of garlic (Allium sativum) oil on exercise tolerance in patients with coronary artery disease. Indian J Physiol. Pharmacol. 49(2005) 115-118.

9. Takasugi, N; Kotoo, K; Fuwa, A and Saito, H. Effects of garlic on mice exposed to various stresses. Oyo Tukurl Pharmacometrics. 28(1984) 991-1002.

10. Saxena K.K; Gupta,B. et.al. Effect of garlic pretreatment on isoprenaline induced myocardial necrosis in albino rats. Indian J Physiol Pharmacol. 24(1980) 233-236.

11. Bordia, A; Bansal, H.C. et. al. Effect of the essential oils of garlic and onion on alimentary hyperlipemia. Atherosclerosis. 21(1975) 15-19.

12. Bordia, A; Sharma, K.D. et. al. Protective effect of garlic oil on the changes produced by 3 weeks of fatty diet on serum cholesterol, serum triglycerides and platelet adhesiveness in man. Indian Heart J. 34(1982) 86-88.

13. Bordia, A and Joshi, H.K. Garlic on fibrinolytic activity in cases of acute myocardial infarction. J. Assoc. Physicians. India. 26(1978) 324-326.

14. Bordia, A and Joshi, H.K. et.al. Effect of essential oil of garlic on serum fibrinolytic activity in patients with coronary artery disease. Atherosclerosis. 28(1978) 155-159.

15. Chutani, S.K. and Bordia, A. The effect of fried versus raw garlic on fibrinolytic activity in man. Atherosclerosis. 38(1981) 417-421.

16. Kajiyama, J. Clinical studies of Kyoleopin. Jap. J. Clin. Rep. 16(1982) 1515-1518.

17. Kventnansky, R; Takasagi, N. et.al. Neuroendocrinological effects of aged garlic extract in control and stress rats. Abst. 25. First world congress of the Health significance of garlic and garlic constituents (1990) Washingtorn DC. (USA).

18. Srivastava K.C; Bordia, A. and Verma, S.K; Garlic (*Allium sativum*) for disease prevention. South African J Science. 91(1995) 68-77.

19. Jaiswal, S.K. and Bordia, A. Radio-protective effect of garlic (*Allium sativum* Linn.) in albino rats. Ind. J. Med. Sci. 50(1996) 231-234.

20. Bordia, A and Verma, S.K. Garlic on the reversibility of experimental atherosclerosis. Indian Heart J. 30(1978) 47-80.

21. Bordia, A; Verma, S.K. et.al. Effect of essential oil of onion and garlic on experimental atherosclerosis in rabbits. Atherosclerosis. 26(1977) 379-386.

22. Bordia, A and Verma, S.K. Effect of garlic feeding on regression of experimental atherosclerosis in rabbits. Artery. 7(1980) 428-437.

23. Harenberg, J; Giese, C. and Zimmermann R. Effect of dried garlic on blood coagulation, fibrinolysis, platelet aggregation and serum cholesterol levels in patients with hyperlipoprotinemia. Atherosclerosis. 74(1988) 247-249.

24. Kiesewetter, H. and Jung, E. Beeinflubt Knoblauch die Atherosklerose? Med. Welt. 12(1991) 21-23.

25. Kiesewetter, H; Jung, E; et.al. Effects of garlic on blood fluidity and fibrinolytic activity: a randomized placebo-controlled, double blind study. Brit. J. Clin. Pract. 44(1990) 24-29.

26. Kawakishi, S. and Morimitsu, Y. Sulfur chemistry of onions and inhibitory factors of the arachidonic acid cascade. ACS Symp. Ser. I. Food Phytochemicals for cancer prevention. 546(1994) 120-127.

27. Verma, S.K; Bordia, A; Jain, P. and Srivastava, K.C. Antioxidant property of ginger in patients with coronary artery disease. South Asian J Preventive Cardiology. 8(4)(2004) 199-204.

28. Fuhrman, B. Ginger extracts consumption decreases plasma cholesterol, inhibits LDL oxidation and attenuates development of atherosclerosis in atherosclerotic, apolipoprotein E- deficient mice. J. Nutr. 130(2000) 1124-1131.

29. Reddy, A.C. and Lokesh, B.R. Studies of spice principle as antioxidants in the inhibition of lipid peroxidation of rat liver microsomes. Mol. Cell. Biochem. 111(1992) 117-124.

30. Krishnakanth, T.P. and Lokesh, B.R. Scavenging of superoxide anions by spice principles. Indian J Biochem Biophys. 30(1993) 133-134.

31. Schulick, P. Ginger- common spice and wonder drug- 2nd Ed. (1994) pp 111-125. Herbal Free Press Ltd. Brattle boro Vermont, USA.

32. James, J; Anderson, L.A. and Phillipson, J.D. Herbal Medicines. 2nd Ed. (2002) pp 243-249. Pharmaceutical Press, London.

33. Bordia, A; Verma, S.K. and Srivastava K.C. Effect of ginger (*Zingiber officinale*) and fenugreek (*Trigonella foenum-graecum*) on blood lipids, blood sugar and platelet aggregation in patients with coronary artery disease. Prost Leuk. Essent. Fatty Acids 56(1997) 379-384.

34. Verma, S.K; Singh, J. et.al. Effect of ginger on platelet aggregation in man. Indian J. Med. Res. 98(1993) 240-242.

35. Srivastava, K.C. Isolation and effect of some ginger components on platelet aggregation and eicosanoid biosynthesis. Prost Leukotr. Med. 25(1986) 187-98.

36. Srivastava K.C.; Verma, S.K; Bordia, A. Spices; A source of phytochemicals protective in human health with special reference to cardiovascular disease. South Asian J Preventive Cardiology. 3(1999) 95-102.

37. The Wealth of India. Vol XI (1976) p. 102. Publications and Information Directorate, New Delhi.

38. Chopra, R.N. Indigenous drugs of India. 2nd ed. 1958. p. 255. G.N. Dhar and Sons Pvt. Ltd. Calcutta.

39. Dorso, C.R, Levin, R.I. et.al. Chinese food and platelets (Letter) N. Engl. J. Med. 303(1980) 756.

40. Kiuchi, F; Shibuya, M and Sankara, U. Inhibition of prostaglandin biosynthesis from ginger. Chem Pharm Bull. 30(1982) 747-754.

41. Editorial. Lipid, platelets and atherosclerosis. Lancet. 1(1980) 464.

42. Srivastava, K.C. Effect of onion and ginger consumption on platelet thromboxane production in humans. Prost Leukot. Essent. Fatty Acids. 35(1989) 183.

43. Duke, J.A and Ayensu, E.S: Medicinal plants of China. Reference Publications. Inc. Michigan, 1985, p. 657.

44. Verma, S.K; Jain, P and Bordia, A. Effect of ginger pearls in patients with musculoskeletal disorders. The Antiseptic. 101(4) 2004, 133-135.

45. Srivastava, K.C. and Mustafa, T. Ginger (*Zingiber officinale*) in rheumatism and musculoskeletal disorders. Med. Hypotheses. 39(1992) 342-348.

46. Verma, S.K; Singh, M; Jain, P and Bordia, A. Protective effect of ginger, *Zingiber officinale* Roxb. On experimental atherosclerosis in rabbits. India J Exp.Biol. 42(2004) 736-738.

47. Diaz, M.N; Frei, B; Vita, J.A. and Keaney, J.F. Jr. Antioxidant and atherosclerotic heart disease, N. Engl. J. Med. 337(1997) 408.

48. Backon, J. Ginger: Inhibition of thromboxane synthetase and stimulation of prostacycline. Relevance for medicine and Psychiatry. Med. Hypotheses, 20(1986) 271.

49. Gupta, R and Nair, S. Antioxidant flavonoids in Indian diet. South Asian J Prev Cardiol. 3(1999) 83-86.

50. Bordia, A; Verma, S.K; Mehta, L.K. and Andrews AMR. Comparative effect of Vitamin C, Amla Juice and Amla pulp on blood lipids, platelet aggregation and experimental atheroma in rabbits. Indian Heart Journal. 37(1985) 179-182.

51. Crawford, GPM; Warloro, CP et. al. The effect of Vitamin C supplements on serum cholesterol, coagulation, fibrinolysis and platelet adhesiveness. Atherosclerosis. 21(1975) 451.

52. Peterson, V.E; Phyllis, BP. et. al. Quantification of plasma cholesterol and triglycerides level in hypercholesterolemic subjects receiving ascorbic acid supplements. Am. J. Clin. Nutr. 28(1975) 584.

53. Ginter, E: Atherosclerosis and Vitamin C. Lancet. 1(1972) 1233.

54. Nambisan, B and Kurup, P.A. Ascorbic acid and glycosoaminoglycan and lipid metabolism in guinea pigs fed normal and atherogenic diet. Atherogenesis. 22(1975) 447.

55. Bordia, A; Verma, S.K. et. al. The effect of Chyavanprash on blood lipids, fibrinolysis, platelet adhesiveness and Vitamin C levels in man. Nagarjun. 25(1981) 44-48.

6.5 Role of Certain Nutraceuticals as Radioprotectors

Drs. Venugopal P. Menon* and Marimuthu Srinivasan
Department of Biochemistry and Biotechnology, Faculty of Science, Annamalai University, Annamalainagar 608 002, Tamil Nadu, India

Introduction

Radiation Induced Damages

Among the physical agents, ionizing radiations are the major ones which cause damage to living organism[1]. Ionizing radiation inflicts deleterious effects on living cells through the generation of reactive oxygen species (ROS) and reactive nitrogen species (RNS) that damage vital cellular targets such as DNA, proteins and lipids. The radiation induced lesions in the cellular DNA are mainly strand breaks, damage to sugar moiety, alteration and elimination of bases, cross links of the intra and inner strand type and cross links to proteins, while peroxidation of the lipids and oxidation of proteins constitute the major lesions in the membranes[2]. Humans are exposed to ionizing radiations for diagnostic or therapeutic purposes and in occupational settings. Apart from these man made exposures, humans are also exposed to cosmic radiations that arise from solar flares and other cosmic interactions during air and space travel[3].

Role of Radioprotectors

Radioprotectors might offer a tactical advantage on the battlefield in the event of a nuclear warfare of radiation leakage from an atomic power station. Radioprotectors are essential to reduce the cancer risk to populations exposed to radiations directly or indirectly through industrial and military applications. They are also required to reduce the normal tissue injury during radiotherapy of cancer. The earlier work were centered around on thiols, amino thiols and their derivatives and found the "gold standard" radioprotective drug amifostin or ethyol or WR2127. Free radical

Address for Correspondence
*Dr. Venugopal P. Menon Professor and Head Dean, Faculty of Science
Department of Biochemistry and Biotechnology
Annamalai University, Annamalainagar-608 002 Tamil Nadu, India.
FAX: (91) 4144-239141, OFF: (91) 4144-238343
E.Mail: **biocmr@sify.com**; cmrana@sify.com

scavengers like chlorogenic acid, β-carotene, vitamins C and E (which are present in many vegetables like alliums, carrot, germinated seeds and citrus fruits) have been shown to have radioprotective effect against micronuclei induction and dicentric aberrations in γ-irradiated mice[4]. Lau et. al.[5] studied the protective effects of cysteine and a garlic preparation against UV-radiation damages of lymphocytes. Both cysteine and garlic compounds protected the cells from radiation through the free radical scavenging reactions of thiols. During radiation, water is spilt into hydrogen atom; OH°, H_3O^+ etc and thiols (RSH) counteract the free radicals formed.

The development of radioprotective agent is important, as it can protect normal cells, from the toxicity and damage associated with chemotherapy and radiotherapy of cancer. A wide variety of compounds have been tested for radioprotective activity including thiols, ginseng extract, interleukin-1, different vitamins, amino acids and antioxidants[6]. Of all the compounds studied as potential radioprotective agents, amino thiols (e.g. cystine) and their derivatives like cystine, methionine, GSH, RSH, R-S-(O)-S- etc are still considered as the best, unfortunately, available radioprotective substances possess unacceptable toxicity limiting its clinical usefulness. Therefore it is necessary to develop protectors that will minimize toxicity while maintaining efficacy[7]. Most of the thiols protect cellular membranes and biomolecules such as DNA and proteins *in vitro*. However most of them are only of limited human applications and the synthetic compounds have toxic effects. Recent studies have shown that a number of phytochemicals, medicinal plants and nutraceuticals possess radioprotective property and they also have less side effects. These have also been found to possess good antioxidant or free radical scavenging and radioprotective property[8].

Radiotherapy

1. Garlic Extracts of Various Nature

Benjamin Lau et. al.[5] conducted an experiment to determine whether garlic powder could provide protection against radiation. They incubated human lymphocytes for two hours with and with out a Japanese preparation of garlic called kyolic (2.5 mg/ml) or fresh garlic extract. They compared with their standard compounds like L-cysteine (1 mg/ml), a thiol known to protect against radiation damage. They then irradiated all the set of cultures with 2000 rads from a Therac-20 linear accelerator; unirradiated culture served as control. They then tested the viability of the cells with tryphan blue dye at 3, 24, 48 and 72 hours following irradiation. The unirradiated lymphocytes remained viable during the three days period (72 hours) of observation. Irradiated control cultures not infused with any of the protective agents steadily declined to 60%, 40% and 25% survival rates of the unirradiated samples on 1st, 2nd and 3rd day respectively. On the other hand cells incubated with Kyolic or L-cysteine was significantly protected from radiation. About 90% to 85% of the cells survived respectively from 1st day onwards at a steady level. However fresh garlic extract proved extremely toxic to the lymphocytes. About 50% of the cells died within 3 hours and none survived beyond 24 hrs. The reason for the toxicity of fresh garlic extract may be due to the very aggressive thiol disulfide interactions of allicin on the thiol groups of lymphocytes.

$$\text{R-S-S (O)-R} + 2\ \text{R}_1\text{SH} \rightarrow \text{R-S-S-R} + \text{R}_1\text{-S-S--R}_1 + \text{H}_2\text{O}$$

This is not the case with aged form of garlic i.e. Kyolic, which may contain only ajoene type compounds that may protect the cells by their free radical scavenging action. Benjamin Lau et. al.[5,9] also showed the immuno stimulation by garlic[6]. Nakagawa et. al.[10] reported that prolonged feeding of raw garlic to rats caused anemia, weight loss and failure to grow. They recommended the use of garlic only when allicine type compounds are transformed on standing to less active compounds like ajoene, diallyl poly sulfides or sulfones i.e. compounds containing-$S(O_2)$-groups. Kyolic is such a suitable preparation due to the ageing of garlic extract that contains enough ajoene and related compounds.

2. Sesamol

Sesamol (Fig.1) is a potent antioxidant present in processed sesame oil[11]. It is a phenolic derivative with a methylene dioxy group and like vitamin E known to be an antioxidant[12]. Recent studies have shown that sesamol is a strong antioxidant[13] and that it possesses chemopreventive, antimutagenic and antihepatoxic properties[14-16]. From time immemorial South Indians use sesame oil for cooking and it has earned the name "Idayam Nallanna" meaning an oil very good for heart in Tamil Nadu. Now we know the sesamol oil contains a suitable proportion of saturated, monosaturated and polyunsaturated fatty acids in the form of triglycerides. More over this oil is rich in an antioxidant called sesamol. Very little work has been carried out on the role of sesamol in protecting the tissues from environmental hazards like chemicals and radiation. Rajendra Prasad et. al.[17] have shown the radioprotective effect of this antioxidant in cultured lymphocytes subjected to γ-radiation.

Cultured human lymphocytes were pretreated with three different concentrations of sesamol *viz.,* 1, 5 and 10 μg/ml. When cultured lymphocytes were exposed to γ-radiation at 1, 2 and 4 Gy in the absence of sesamol it resulted in a significant increase in the frequencies of dicentric aberrations (DC). Maximum numbers of DC (63 ± 1.5) was observed at 4 Gy. Pretreatment of lymphocytes with 1, 5 and 10 μg/ml of sesamol significantly decreased the DC frequencies when the lymphocytes were exposed to 1 Gy. At 2 Gy irradiation, 5 and 10 μg/ml of sesamol brought the DC to near normal. Only 10 μg/ml of sesamol brings down the DC frequency to near normal level when the lymphocytes were exposed to 4 Gy irradiation.

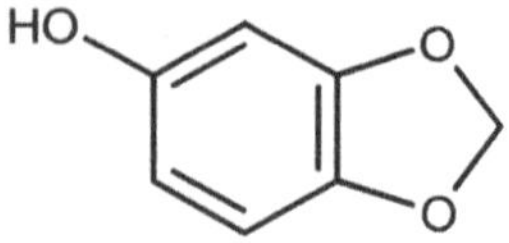

HO, O, O

Fig. 1 Structure of sesamol.

Pretreatment of lymphocytes with sesamol significantly decreased the number of micro nuclei (MN) even at 1 μg/ml concentration at lower dose of irradiation (1 Gy). At 2 Gy irradiation 5 and 10 μg/ml of sesamol brought MN to near normal level. At 4 Gy irradiation 10 μg/ml of sesamol brought the MN to near normal level (24 ± 1.5). Hiramoto *et. al.*[18] showed sesamol protects hydroxyl radical induced DNA damage. The concentrations of TBARS increased and that of GSH decreased significantly in γ-irradiated lymphocytes. Similarly the activities of the antioxidant enzymes SOD, CAT and GPx decreased in γ-irradiated lymphocytes. Pretreatment of lymphocytes with 1, 5 and 10 μg/ml concentrations of sesamol progressively reversed the level of the above parameters.

Sato *et. al.*[19] showed that radiation protective mechanism of sesamol is by protecting DNA and antioxidant enzymes in X-ray induced skin injury. This information high lights the necessity of using vegetables and oils rich in antioxidants that protect our body from various types of radiations.

3. Emblica Officinalis (Amla)

According to the studies of Chandhur[20] Emblica (goose berries) helps in protecting the skin from damaging effect of UV-radiation. Emblica extract was also found to inhibit nitrosation reaction in stomach, which might be helpful in reducing stomach cancers[21]. It was also found to inhibit mutagenesis induced by certain chemicals in *salmonella typhymurium*[22] and the clastogenicity induced by various metals[23]. Emblica was also found to be hepatoprotective[24] and an anti-diabetic agent[25]. It inhibited N-Nitrisodiethylamine induced hepato carcinogenesis and 20-methyl chloranthrene induced sarcoma in experimental animals[26]. Emblica has been reported to contain many polyphenols, ellagitannins such as phyllemblin, ellagic acid, trigalloyl glucose, phyllantidin, mucic acid, emblicannin, and furosin[27], and some of them have been reported to have antioxidant and anticarcinogenic activity. Rajesh Kumar *et. al.*[28] have identified epigallocatchin gallate as one of the major polyphenol present in the ethyl acetate fraction of fresh Emblica. Harikumar *et. al.*[29] at Amala Cancer Research Centre, Trichur, Kerala, evaluated the possible role of Emblica as a radioprotective agent against sub lethal dose of γ-radiation in mice.

They found that radiation caused a reduction in the body weight of all the exposed animals but the reduction was not significant. However radiation significantly lowered the total leukocyte count in the irradiated animals (group I) but on pretreatment with Emblica extract (group II), the leukocyte counts was found to be enhanced when compared with irradiation control (group I) and group III animals also showed significantly higher leukocytes counts after 10 days pretreatment and 15 days post treatment with Emblica extracts when compared with group I and II. This indicated the Emblica extract feeding stimulated the hemopoietic system in a concentration dependent manner. Bone marrow cellularity and Hb levels significantly decreased on the 15th day after γ-irradiation for group I and II. Beneficial effect of Emblica extract was further supported by the enhanced bone narrow cellularity and increased Hb levels in group III. However differential event did not show any significant variation.

In a second series of experiments, four groups of mice with nine in each group were taken and first three groups were subjected to γ-radiation and the fourth group was kept as normal control with out any treatment. On days 5, 10 and 15 after γ-radiation exposure of 7 Gy, three animals from each group were sacrificed and their blood was collected. The activities of enzymic antioxidants like GPx, GST, SOD, CAT and the levels of non-enzymic antioxidants like GSH were estimated. The antioxidant enzymes and GSH levels were decreased significantly in γ-irradiated group. In the Emblica extract treated groups there was a significant increase in the activities of these antioxidant enzymes and GSH levels when compared with irradiation control.

Radiation increased the levels of lipid peroxidation in γ-radiation exposed animal. However by treatment with Emblica extract production of MDA was decreased progressively from the 5th to 15th day in both the treated groups with a better effect in the post irradiation treated group.

4. *Glycyrrhiza Glabra* L. (Yashtimadhu)

Glycyrrhiza glabra L. is also called yashtimadhu in Hindi. Erattimadhuram in Malayalam. It is an ingredient of Ayurvedic decoctions also. It is a rich source of antioxidants. Jisha Joy and C.K.K. Nair[30] studied the radioprotective effects of the ethanolic extracts of *Glycyrrhiza glabra* L. and Holarrhena Antidysenterica wall at Amala Cancer Research Centre, Trichur. The latter is a medicinal plant whose bark is used to prepare decoction to treat dysentery.

DPPH (2,2 diphenyl –I-pieryl-hydrazyl) is a stable free radical and has been used as a model free radical compound to evaluate the effectiveness of antioxidants. The extracts of the above two plants contained sufficient antioxidant as per the experiments showed on DPPH. Damages to membranes in cells and tissues, by γ-radiation can be assessed in terms of peroxidation of membrane lipids. Swiss albino mice were exposed to 4 Gy of whole body γ-radiation at a dose rate of 1.88 Gy/min. The animals were sacrificed by cervical dislocation after 1 hr of γ-irradiation and the liver was removed for *in vitro* experiments.

The membrane damage was estimated using lipid peroxidative indices like thiobarbituric acid reactive substances (TBARS). Exposure of mice to whole body γ-radiation (4 Gy) resulted in elevated levels of TBARS in liver. This may be due to radiation induced peroxidative damage to membrane lipids. Administration of lyophilized residues of the 70% ethanol extracts of both the above plant materials (100 mg/kg b. wt) to the two groups prior to radiation exposure inhibited the peroxidative damage to the liver. Similarly when the liver cells were exposed to γ-irradiation at 25 Gy with the presence of *Glycyrrhiza glabra* L extracts it inhibited the lipid peroxidation of the liver cells. The extracts also protected super coiled DNA of the plasmid PBR-322 from γ-radiation induced strand breaks. The radioprotective property of the extracts has been attributed to the free radical scavenging and antioxidant activities. Studies have shown that *Glycyrrhiza glabra* L protects DNA against γ-radiation induced $OH^{\bullet}$ radical meditated damage. The mechanism of radioprotection is mediated by scavenging of free radicals. The major compounds reported in the extract of *G. glabra* L. are glycyrrhizic acid, glycyrrhitinic acid, glabridin and some flavonosides (glycosides of flavonoids) e.g. 5, 8-dihydroxy flavone, 7-O-beta-D-glucuronide, glychionide A and 5-hydroxy-8-methoxyl flavone-7-O-beta-D-glucuronide-glychionide B.[31] *Glycyrrhiza glabra* L extracts does not possess any cytotoxicity and have been used in medicine for ages. They may be useful for developing effective radioprotectors for human use.

5. Ferulic Acid

Ferulic acid (Fig.2) is a phenolic compound, formed during the metabolism of phenylalanine and tyrosine. It occurs primarily in rice, wheat, barely, oat, roasted coffee, tomatoes, vegetables and citrus fruits[32].

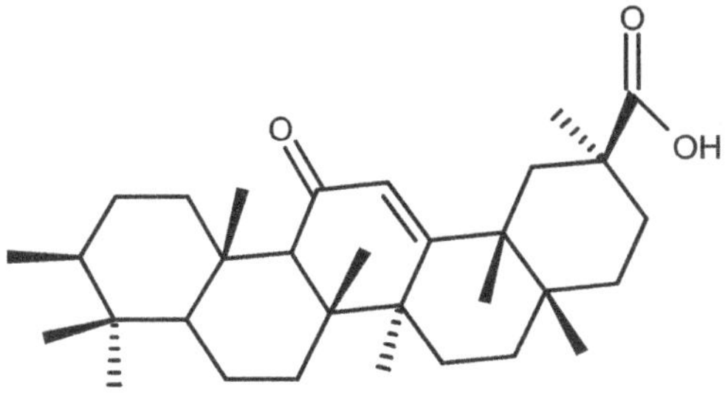

Glycyrrhetinic acid

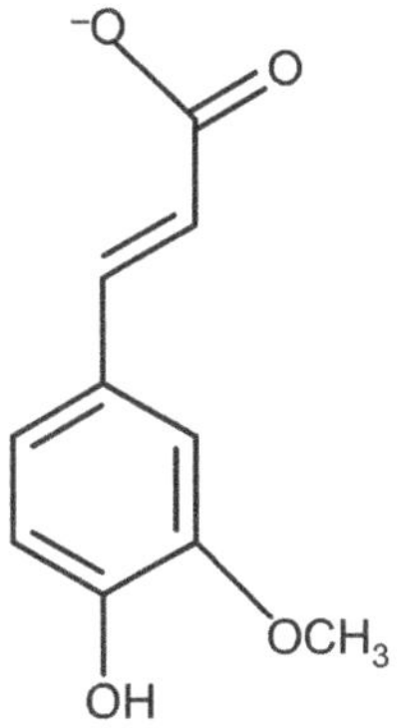

Ferrulic acid

Glycyrrhizin	
Chemical name	(3-β,20-β)-20-Carboxy-11-oxo-30-norolean-12-en-3-yl 2-O-β-D-glucopyranuronosyl-α-D-glucopyranosiduronic acid
Other names	Glycyrrhizin Glycyrrhizinic acid Glycyrrhizic acid
Chemical formula	$C_{42}H_{62}O_{16}$

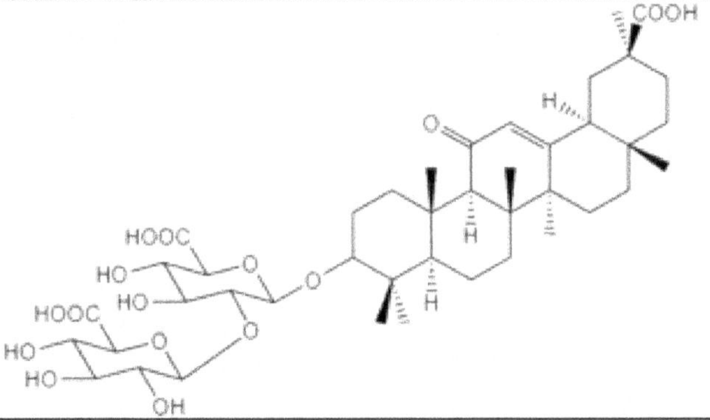

Fig 2 Chemical structures of glycyrrhetinic acid and Ferulic acid. The former is effective in the treatment of peptic ulcer and as an expectorant and the latter is a strong antioxidant.

Ferulic acid acts as a strong membrane antioxidant in humans and is known to be effective against skin disorders, skin cancer, ageing, fatigue, muscle wasting, cold, flu and influenza[33]. Ferulic acid has a high antioxidant potential due to its resonance-stabilized phenoxy radical structure. It is an effective scavenger of free radicals and has been approved in certain countries as food additive to prevent LPO[34]. Studies have shown that ferulic acid is an effective scavenger of free radicals and it inhibits the lipid peroxidation in γ-irradiated rat hepatocytes *in vitro*. The levels of GSH, vitamins A, E, C, ceruloplasmin and uric acid were increased significantly on pretreatment with ferulic acid. It also enhances the activities of SOD, CAT and GPx in γ-irradiated hepatocytes[35]. As seen in Fig-2, Ferulic acid possesses distinct structural motifs that can possibly contribute to the free radical scavenging capability of this compound. The presence of electron donating groups on the benzene ring [3-methoxy and more importantly 4-hydroxyl] of ferulic acid gives additional property for terminating free radical chain reaction. The next functionality – the carboxylic acid group in ferulic acid with adjacent unsaturated C-C double bond can provide additional attack sites for free radicals and thus prevent them from attacking the membrane. In addition, the carboxylic acid group acts as an anchor of ferulic acid by which it binds to the lipid bilayer providing some protection against LPO. Clearly, the presence of electron donating substitutents enhances the antioxidant properties of ferulic acid[36]. The dose dependent study of ferulic acid in γ-irradiated human lymphocytes has been reported to reduce the frequencies of dicentric aberration and micronuclei. The levels of TBARS were decreased and those of GSH and activities of antioxidant enzymes like SOD, CAT and GPx were increased on ferulic acid pretreatment. This might be because of ferulic acid that scavenges superoxide anion radical and inhibits lipid peroxidation induced by superoxide and the effect of ferulic acid is similar to that of SOD[37].

6. Curcumin

Curcumin (Fig. 3) is a dietary antioxidant derived from turmeric (*Curcuma longa*, Zingiberaceae) and has been known since ancient times to possess therapeutic properties. The health benefits of curcumin include many pharmacological activities such as hypocholesteremia, anti-inflammatory, anti-platelet, anticancer, antimutagenic, anti-HIV etc[38]. It has been reported to scavenge oxygen free radicals and to inhibit lipid peroxidation and protect the cellular macromolecules, including DNA from oxidative damage[39, 40].

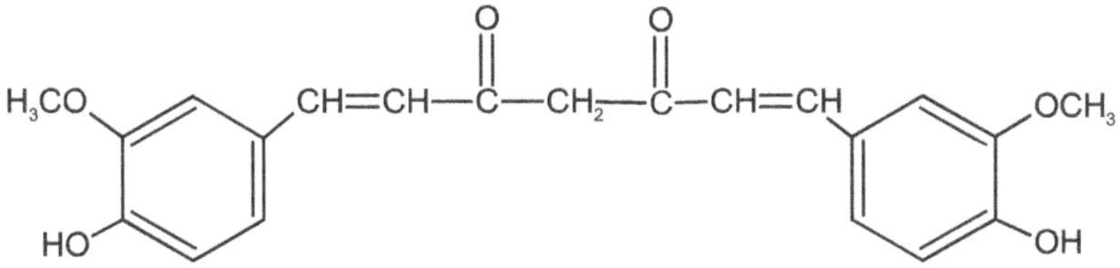

Fig. 3 Structure of curcumin.

Including previous reports have shown that curcumin possesses strong antioxidant and anticancer properties by regulating the expression of genes that require the activation of activator protein (AP-1) and Nuclear factor KB (NF-KB)[41]. Pretreatment of mice with a single dose of curcumin 100 mg/kg body weight before exposure to different doses (2, 4, 6 or 8 Gy) of whole body irradiation resulted in an enhancement of wound healing, as evidenced by increased wound contraction and reduced wound healing time[42]. The oral administration of curcumin to rats before and/ or after irradiation significantly inhibits the tumorigenesis of mammary and pituitary glands[43].

Studies have also shown that curcumin significantly enhance the synthesis of antioxidant enzymes such as SOD, CAT and GPx. Dinkova-Kostova et. al.[44] have also reported that curcumin and several other structurally related polyphenolic compounds induce the activities of phase II detoxification enzymes, which appear to be crucial in the protection against carcinogenesis and oxidative stress. Pretreatment of curcumin to γ-irradiated lymphocytes resulted in decreased lipid peroxidation and improved antioxidant status preventing the damage to the lymphocytes. The presence of π conjugation in curcumin makes it more hydrophobic. As a result curcumin get localized in the lipid bilayer membrane. Curcumin, being lipid soluble, reacts with the lipid peroxyl radicals and acts as a chain terminating antioxidant. It has also been known to inhibit radiation induced lipid peroxidation in rat liver microsomes[45]. Curcumin possesses distinct structural motifs that are responsible for its antioxidant activity. The presence of electron donating groups like phenolic hydroxyl groups and a β-diketone structure are responsible for the free radical scavenging activity and inhibiting lipid peroxidation[46].

Curcumin has the ability to protect cells from DNA damage. Curcumin, being a hydrophobic molecule, passes easily through the plasma membrane into the cytosol[47,48]. The presence of curcumin in the cytosol directly scavenges the free radicals like superoxide anion, hydroxyl radical and lipid peroxyl radicals etc and results in the formation of phenoxyl radicals[49] produced by the electron transfer followed by the proton loss at the phenolic-OH site. The phenoxyl radicals of curcumin thus produced are stabilized over the extended conjugation[45]. Studies have shown that curcumin and related compounds have the potential to protect DNA against oxidative damage induced by singlet oxygen[50]. It was also reported that curcumin significantly protect the B (a) P induced single strand breaks in human peripheral blood lymphocytes[40]. Antunes et. al.[51] have reported that curcumin reduces the chromosomal aberrations in rodent bone marrow cells exposed to γ-radiation or treated with the antitumour drug, cisplatin. Administration of curcumin to mice was found to inhibit radiation-induced chromosomal damage in micronucleated polychromatic erythrocytes. **Curcumin acts as a radiosensitizing agent on squamous carcinoma cells and selectively protects the normal cells against radiation damage during cancer treatment. Curcumin, a polyphenol confers radiosensitizing effects in prostate cancer cell line by inhibiting the growth of human prostate PC-3 cancer cells and down regulating radiation induced prosurvival factors[52].** Moreover curcumin has also been shown to inhibit human myeloid leukemia cells, epidermoid carcinoma cells, HT29 colon cancer cells and human colon epithelial cells[53,54]. Thus curcumin acts as a radioprotector during radiotherapy[53]. The pharmacological safety of curcumin is demonstrated by its consumption for centuries at levels of up to 100 mg/day by people in certain countries[55].

7. Lycopene

Lycopene is a dietary carotenoid synthesized by plants and microorganisms (see structures in P. 51 under nutraceuticals). It occurs primarily in red fruits, vegetables, tomatoes, watermelon, pink grape fruit, apricots, pink guava and papaya[56]. Recent epidemiological studies have shown that supplementation of diets rich in lycopene is associated with reduced risk of many chronic diseases, such as cancer and heart diseases[57]. The antioxidant activity of lycopene has been extensively evaluated based on its ability to scavenge free radicals in cell culture and in animal models.[58] Experimental evidence also suggests that lycopene can quench singlet oxygen ($^1O_2$), scavenge free nitrogen dioxide ($NO_2^\bullet$), thiyl ($RS^\bullet$) and sulphonyl ($RSO_2^\bullet$) radicals[59]. It has been reported that increased DNA damage and elevated levels of lipid peroxidation in γ-irradiated hepatocytes are accompanied by a decrease in the free radical scavenging properties as related to SOD, CAT, GPx, GSH, vitamins A, E, C, ceruloplasmin and uric acid[60]. Pretreatment with lycopene resulted in increased levels of these antioxidants. These may be attributed to lycopene's ability to acts as an antioxidant and singlet oxygen quencher, thereby inhibiting the destructive effects of ROS[61]. In addition to its antioxidant activity; lycopene has been shown to modulate phase II enzymes like GST, GR and GPx, as well as GSH levels in experimental models[62]. These antioxidant enzymes are regulated at the transcriptional level by consensus sequences for the antioxidant response element (ARE) found in their promotor regions[63]. Although it is not clear how lycopene induces phase II enzymes, an antioxidant mechanism is conceivable[64]. Matos et. al.[65] have reported that lycopene supplementation has decreased 77 % of 8-oxodguanosine levels in Fe-NTA/ascorbate treated cells. These results indicate that lycopene provided strong protection against DNA-based oxidation. Furthermore, consumption of tomato products was reported to reduce the susceptibility of lymphocyte DNA to oxidative damage[66]. Silva et. al.[67] also suggested that pretreatment with carotenoid reduced the total number of chromosomal aberrations in cisplatin treated rats.

8. Mangiferin

Mangifera indica (Mango tree), is widely used in India and Southeast Asia as a food supplement in the form of pickle, and the fruit is eaten as such or its juice is drunk. Mango has been widely used as an anti-inflammatory, antipyretic, diuretic, antidiarrheal, antiviral, antibacterial and hypoglycemic in the traditional system of medicine in India[68, 69]. It has also been found to inibit α-glucosidase and α-amylase activities *in vitro*. The flavonoids from M. indica have been found to be antihypolipidemic in rats[70,71]. Mangiferin, a C-glucosylxanthone (1,3,6,7-tetra-hydroxyxanthone-c2-β-D-glucoside) (see P. 49) purified from *M indica* and *Anemarrhena asphodeloides* has been found to inhibit proliferation of neoplastic cells *in vitro* and *in vivo* and antagonize the cytopathic effect of HIV[72]. Pretreatment with mangiferin has been found to reduce the radiation-induced micronuclei formation in human peripheral blood lymphocytes and increase the survival of animals exposed to different doses of γ-radiation[73]. It has also been reported that in human peripheral blood lymphocytes exposed to 3 Gy irradiation, there is nic, double strand breaks as studied by fluorescence analysis of DNA unwinding assay. The lymphocytes when exposed to 3 Gy γ-irradiation caused a drastic reduction in the undamaged DNA double strand Pretreatment of lymphocytes with different concentrations of mangiferin (50 and 100 μg/ml) resulted in a progressive repair of DNA strand breaks when compared with irradiation control group. The highest amount of undamaged DNA double strand was observed in 50 μg/ml of mangiferin pretreatment. The protection afforded by mangiferin to radiation-induced DNA damage could be attributed to scavenging of free radicals by mangiferin and may have played an important role in protecting the DNA from the radiation-induced damage[74]. (phenolic hydroxyl groups of mangiferin are responsible for its antioxidant action).

Conclusion

The interaction of ionizing radiation with biological system results in the generation of many highly reactive short lived ROS mainly due to hydrolysis of water. They include mainly $H^{\bullet}$, $OH^{\bullet}$, $ROO^{\bullet}$ H_3O^+ etc. In addition to them several RNS are also formed. These ROS and RNS attack cellular macromolecules like, DNA, RNA, proteins, membrane and lipids and cause its dysfunction and damage. ROS increase the membrane lipid peroxidation, which results in the alteration of the integrity of membrane structure leading to inactivation of membrane bound enzymes, loss of permeability of the membrane and decrease in membrane fluidity[75]. Radiation also produce a change in antioxidant status in the body as mentioned in various studies conducted in the field. These altered parameters are more or less repaired by the administration of various dietary agents which possess antioxidant property as observed with curcumin, ferulic acid, lycopene, mangiferin, sesamol of sesame oil, sulfoxides and polysulfides of alliums, polyphenols of amla and the flavonosides of the sweetener *G. glabra* L. These dietary nutraceuticals also work as immuno modulators and stimulates the hepatopoietic system as observed in most of the result. Therefore regular consumption of selected vegetables that may contain nutraceuticals with radioprotective action and antioxidant properties is highly beneficial. Use of nutraceuticals may reduce the radiation-induced toxic effects under going radiotherapy as well as during occupational exposures, space and air flights, accidental exposures, and nuclear terror attacks.

References

1. Sulton, D. Text book of radiology and imaging, International Students Edition. 1 (1965) 675-1024.
2. Nair, C.K.K., Parida, D.K and Namura, T. Radio protectors in radiotherapy. J. Radiat. Res. 42 (2001) 21-37.
3. Jagetia, G.C and Venkatesha V.A. Mangiferin protects human peripheral blood lymphocytes against γ-radiation-induced DNA strand breaks: a fluorescence analysis of DNA unwinding assay. Nutrition Res. 26 (1988) 303-311.
4. Abraham, S.K., Sarma, L and Kesavan, P.C. Protective effects of chlorogenic acid, curcumin and β-carotene against γ-radiation induced *in vivo* chromosomal damage. Mutat. Res., 303 (1993) 109-112.
5. Lau, B.H.S. Garlic for Health. Lotus Light Publications. P.O. Box. 2 Wilmot Wl. 53192 (1988) pp 33-35.

6. Durakovic, A. Radioprotective agent in medicine. Arh. Hig. Rada. Toksikol. 44 (1993) 331-354.

7. Weiss, J.F., Kumar, K.S et. al. Advances in radioprotection through use of combined agent legions. Int. J. Radiat. Biol. 57 (1990) 709-718.

8. Maurya, D.K., Devasagayam, T.P.A and Nair, C.K.K. Some novel approaches for radioprotection and the beneficial effects of natural products. Ind. J. Exp. Biol., 44 (2006) 93-114.

9. Lau, B.H.S and Woolley, J.L. Superiority of intralesional immunotherapy with *Corynebacterium parvum* and *Allium sativum* in control of Murine transitional cell Carcinoma. J. Urol., 136 (1986) 701.

10. Nakagawa, S., Masamoto, K et. al. Effect of raw and extracted aged garlic juice on growth of young rats and their organs after per oral administration. J. Toxicol. Sci. 5 (1980) 91.

11. Ando, K; Sako, K.I et. al. Increased band 3 protein aggregation and anti-band 3 binding of erythrocyte membrane on treatment with sesamol. Biol. Pharm. Bull., 23(2) (2000) 159-164.

12. Uchida, M., Nakajin, S. and Toyoshima, M. Antioxidative effect of sesamol and related compounds on lipid peroxidation. Biol. Pharm. Bull., 19(4): (1996) 623-626.

13. Suja, K.P., Jayalakshmy, A. and Arumugham, C. Free radical scavenging behaviour of antioxidant compounds of sesame. (*Sesamum indicum*) in DPPH system. J. Agric. Food Chem., 25 52(4) (2004) 912-15.

14. Kaur, I.P and Saini, A. Sesamol exhibits antimutagenic activity against oxygen species medicated mutagenicity. Mutat. Res., 470(1) (2000) 71-76.

15. Ohta, S., Suzuki, M et. al. Protective effects of sesamol and its related compounds on carbon tetrachloride induced liver injury in rats. Yakuge- ku. Zasshi. 114(11) (1994) 901-910.

16. Kapadia, G.J; Azuine, M.A et. al. Chemopreventive effect of resveratrol, sesamol, sesame oil and sunflower oil in the Epstein Barr Virus early antigen activation assay and the mouse skin two state carcinogenesis. Pharmcol. Res. 45(6) (2002) 499-505.

17. Rajendra Prasad, N., Venugopal, P. Menon., Vasudev, V and Pugalendi, K.V. Radioprotective effect of sesamol on γ-radiation induced DNA damage, lipid peroxidation and antioxidants levels in cultured human lymphocytes. Toxicology 209 (2005) 225-235.

18. Hiramoto, K,. Ojima, N et. al. Effect of plant phenolics on the formation of the spin-adduct of hydroxyl radical and the DNA strand breaking by hydroxyl radical. Biol. Pharm. Bull. 19(4) (1996) 558-563.

19. Sato, Y., Kumazawa, N et. al. Studies on chemical protectors against radiation XXX III. Protective mechanisms of various compounds against skin injury induced by radiation. Yakugaku Zasshi III (1) 1991) 51-58.

20. Chaudhuri, R.K. Emblica cascading antioxidants. A novel natural skin care ingredient. Skin pharmacology and applied skin physiology, 15 (2002) 374-380.

21. Xu, G.P., Song, P.J and Reed, P.I. Hypothesis on the relationship between intragastric nitrosation: N-nitrosamine in gastric juice of subjects from high risk area for gastric cancer and inhibition of N-nitrosamine formation by fruit juices. European Jour of Cancer Prevention, 2 (1993) 25-36.

22. Jeena, K.J., Josely, G and Kuttan, R. Antimutagenic and anticarcinogenic activity of Emblica officinalis Gaertn. Jour. Clin. Biochem. Nutrition, 22 (1997) 171-176.

23. Dhir, H; Agarwal, K et. al. Modifying the role of phyllanthus emblica and ascorbic acid against nickel induced clastogenicity in mice. *Cancer Lettters,* 59 (1991) 9-12.

24. Jeena, K. and Kuttan, R. Hepatoprotective effect of Emblica officinalis and Chyvnaprash. Jour. Ethno. Pharmacology, 72 (2000) 135-140.

25. Sabu, M.C and Kuttan, R. Antidiabetic activity of medicinal plants and its relationship with antioxidant property. Jour. Ethnopharmacologty, 81 (2002) 155-160.

26. Jeena, K.J., Kuttan, R. and Bhattacharya, R.K. Effect of Emblica officinalis extract on hepatocarcinogenesis and carcinogen metabolism. Jour. Clin. Biochem. Nutrition, 25 (1998) 31-39.

27. Zhang, Y., Abe, T., Yang, C. and Kouno, I. Phyllanemblinins A-F, New ellagitannins from phyllanthus emblica. Jour. Natural Products, 64 (2001) 1527-1532.

28. Rajesh Kumar, N.V., Pillai, M.R. and Kuttan, R. Induction of apoptosis in mouse and human carcinoma cell lines by Emblica officinalis polyphenols and its effect on chemical carcinogenesis, Jour Exp. Clin. Cancer Res., 22 (2003) 201-212.

29. Harikumar, K.B., Sabu, M.C., Lima, P.S. and Kuttan, R. Radio protective effect of an extract of Emblica officinalis fruit pulp in mice. Amala Res. Bulletin. 24 (2004) 250-260.

30. Jisha Joy and C.K.K. Nair Radio Protection by *Glycyrrhiza glabra* L. Amala Res. Bulletin, 26 (2006) 159-167.

31. Li, J.R., Wang, Y.Q. and Deng, Z.Z. Two new compounds from *Glycyrrhiza glabra.* J. Asian Nat. Prod. Res., 7(4) (2005) 677-80.

32. Graf, E. Antioxidant potential of ferulic acid. Free Radic. Biol. Med. 13(4) (2000) 435-448.

33. Rukkumani, R., Aruna, K., Suresh Varma, P and Menon, V.P. Hepatoprotective role of ferulic acid: A dose dependent study. J. Med. Food 7(4) (2004.), 456-461.

34. Adam, A., Crespy, V., Levrat Verny, M.A., Leenhardt, F., Leuillet, M., Demigne, C and Remesy, C. The bioavailability of ferulic acid is governed primarily by the food matrix rather than its metabolism in intestine and liver in rats. J. Nutr. 132 (2002) 1962-1968.

35. Srinivasan, M., Ram Sudheer, A., Raveendran Pillai, K., Raghu Kumar, P., Sudhakaran, P.R and Menon, V.P. Influence of ferulic acid on γ-radiation induced DNA damage, lipid peroxidation and antioxidant status in primary culture of isolated rat hepatocytes. Toxicology 228 (2006) 249-258.

36. Kanski, J., Aksenova, M., Stoyanova, A., Butter Field, D.A. Ferulic acid antioxidant protection against hydroxyl and peroxyl radical oxidation in synaptosomal and neuronal cell culture systems in vitro: structure activity studies. J. Nutr. Biochem. 13 (2002) 273-281.

37. Rajendra Prasad, N., Srinivasan, M., Pugalendi, K.V., and Venugopal P. Menon. Protective effect of ferulic acid on γ-radiation induced micronuclei, dicentric aberration and lipid peroxidation in human cultured human lymphocytes. Mutat. Res. 603 (2006) 129-134

38. Sharma, R.A., Gescher, A.J and Steward, W.P. Curcumin: The story so far; Eur. J. Cancer 41 (2005)1955-1968.

39. Kalpana, C and Menon, V.P. Curcumin ameliorates oxidative stress during Nicotine induced lung toxicity in Wistar rats, Ital. J. Biochem. 53(2) (2004) 82-86.

40. Polasa, K, Naidu, N.A., Ravindranath, I and Krishanaswamy, K; Inhibition of B(a)P induced strand breaks in presence of curcumin, Mutation Res.557 (2004) 203-213.

41. Sarkar, F.M and Li, Y. Cell signalling pathways altered by natural chemopreventive agents. Mutation. Res. 555 (2004) 53-64.

42. Jagetia, G.C and Rajanikant, G.K. Role of curcumin, a naturally occurring phenolic compound of turmeric in accelerating the repair of excision wound, in mice whole body exposed to various doses of γ-radiation, J. Surg. Res. 120 (2004) 127-138.

43. Inano, H and Onoda, M. Radioprotective action of curcumin extracted from *Curcuma longa* Linn. Inhibitory effect on formation of urinary 8-hydroxy-2′-deoxyguanosine, tumorigenesis, but not mortality, induced by γ-ray irradiation, Int. J. Radiat. Oncol. Biol. Phys. 53 (2002) 735-743.

44. Dinkova-Kostava, A.T., Masiah, M.A., Bozak, R.E., Hicks, R.J and Talalay, P. Potency of Michael reaction acceptors as inducers of enzyme that protect against carcinogenesis depends on their reactivity with sulfhydryl groups, Proc. Natl. Acad. Sci. USA. 98, 3404-3409.

45. Khopde, S.M., Priyadarsini, K.I., Guha, S.N., Satav, J.G., Venkatesan, P and Rao, M.N. Inhibition of radiation-induced lipid peroxidation by tetrahydro curcumin: Possible mechanism by pulse radiolysis, Biosci. Biotechnol. Biochem. 64(3) (2000) 503-509.

46. Osawa, T., Sugiyama, Y., Inayoshi, M and Kawakishi, S. Antioxidant activity of tetrahydrocurcuminoids, Biosci. Biotechnol. Biochem. 59 (1995)1609-1612.

47. Ashok Khar, A., Mubarak Ali, B.V.V., Zareena Begum, P and Anjum, R. Antitumor activity of curcumin is mediated through the induction of apoptosis in AK-5 tumor cell, FEBS Lett. 445 (1999) 165-168.

48. Oetari, S., Sudibyo, M., Commandur, J.N.M., Samhoedi, R and Vermeulen, N.P.E. Effects of curcumin on cytochrome P450 and glutathione S-transferase activities in rat liver, Biochem. Pharmacol. 51 (1996) 39-45.

49. Priyadarsini, K.I. Free radical reactions of curcumin in membrane models, Free Rad. Biol. Med. 23 (1997) 838-843.

50. Subramanian, M., Sreejayam, M.N.A. Rao, Devasagayam, T.P.A and Singh, B.B. Diminution of singlet oxygen-induced DNA damage by curcumin and related antioxidants, Mutation Res. 311 (1997) 249-255.

51. Antunes, L.M.G., Araujo, M.C.P., Dias, P.D.L and Takahashi, C.S. Effects of H_2O_2, Fe^{2+} and Fe^{3+} on curcumin-induced chromosomal aberrations in CHO cells, Genetics Mol. Biol. 28 (2005) 161-164.

52. Chendil, D., Ranga, R.S., Meigooni, D., Sathish Kumar, S and Ahmed, M.M. Curcumin confers radiosensitizing effect in prostate cancer cell line PC-3, Oncogene 23 (2004) 1599-1607.

53. Khafif, A.V.I., Hurst, R., Kyker, K., Fliss, D.M., Gil, Z and Medina, J.E. Curcumin: A new radio-sensitizer of squamous cell carcinoma cells, Otolaryngol. Head. Neck. Surg. 132 (2005) 317-321.

54. Shimizu, M and Weinstein, B. Modulation of signal transduction by tea catechins and related phytochemicals, Mutation Res. 591(2005) 147-160.

55. Mahesh, T., Balasubashini, M and Menon, V.P. Photo-irradiated curcumin supplementation in streptozotocin-induced diabetic rats: Effect on lipid peroxidation, Therapie 59 (2004) 639-644.

56. Edward, G. Tomato, tomato-based products, lycopene, and cancer: Review of the epidemiologic literature, J. National Canc. Inst. 91 (1999) 317-331.

57. Rao, A.V and Agarwal, S. Role of lycopene as antioxidant carotenoid in the prevention of chronic diseases: A review, Nutrit. Res. 19 (1999) 305-323.

58. Di Mascio, P., Kaiser, S., and Sies, H. Lycopene as the most efficient biological carotenoid singlet oxygen quencher, Arch. Biochem. Biophys. 1 (1989) 532-538.

59. Yaping, Z., Suping, Q., Weni, Y., Zheng, X., Hong, S., Side, Y and Dapu, W. Antioxidant activity of lycopene extracted from paste towards trichloromethyl peroxyl radical CCl_3O_2, Food Chem. 77 (2002) 209-212.

60. Srinivasan, M., Ram Sudheer, A., Raveendran Pillai, K., Raghu Kumar, P., Sudhakaran, P.R and Menon, V.P. Lycopene as a natural protector against γ-radiation induced DNA damage, lipid peroxidation and antioxidant status in primary culture of isolated rat hepatocytes in vitro. Biochim. Biophysic. Acta 1770 (2007) 659-665.

61. Rao, A.V and Agarwal S. Bioavailability and in vivo antioxidant properties of lycopene from tomato products and their possible role in the prevention of cancer, Nutr. Cancer 31 (3) (1998) 199-203.

62. Breinholt, V., Lauridsen, S.T., Daneshvar, B and Jakabesen, J. Dose-response effect of lycopene on selected drug-metabolizing and antioxidant enzymes in the rat, Cancer Lett. 154 (2000) 201-210.

63. Nguyen, T., Yang, C.S and Pickett, C.B. The pathways and molecular mechanisms regulating Nrf2 activation in response to chemical stress, Free Radic. Biol. Med. 37 (2004) 433-441.

64. Cantelli-Forti, G., Hrelia, P and Paolin, M. The pitfall of detoxifying enzymes, Mutat. Res. 402 (1998) 179-183.

65. Matos, H.R., Capelozzi, V.L., Gomes, O.F., Mascio, P.D and Medeiros, M.H.G. Lycopene inhibits DNA damage and liver necrosis in rats treated with ferric nitrilotriacetate, Arch. Biochem. Biophys. 396 (2001) 171-177.

66. Riso, P., Pinder, A., Santangelo, A and Porini, M. Does tomato consumption effectively increase the resistance of lymphocyte DNA to oxidative damage? Am. J. Clin. Nutr. 69 (1999) 712-718.

67. Silva, C.R., Antunes, L.M and Bianchi, M.D.P. Antioxidant action of bixin against cisplatin-induced chromosome aberrations and lipid peroxidation in rats, Pharmacol. Res. 43 (2001) 561-566.

68. Markare, N., Bodhankar, S., and Rangari, V. Immunomodulatory activity of alcoholic extract of *Mangifera indica L.* in mice. J. Ethanopharmacol. 78 (2001) 133-137.

69. Sairam, K., Hemalatha, S., Kumar, A., Srinivasan, T., Ganesh, J., Shankar, M. Evaluation of anti-diarrhoeal activity in seed extracts of *Mangifera indica.* J. Ethanopharmacol. 84 (2003) 11-15.

70. Prashanth, D., Padmaja, R., and Samiulla, D.S. Effect of certain plant extracts on alpha-amylase activity. Fitoterapia 72 (2001) 179-181.

71. Anila, L., and Vijayalakshmi, N.R. Flavonoids from Emblica officinals and *Mangifera indica* effectiveness for dyslipidemia. J. Ethanopharmacol 79 (2002) 81-87.

72. Aritomi, M., and Kawasaki, T. A new xanthone C-glucoside position isomer of mangiferin, from Anemarrhena asphodeloides. Bunge. Tetrahedron Lett. 12 (1969) 941-944.

73. Jagetia, G.C., and Baliga, M.S. Radioprotection by mangiferin in DBAxc57BL mice: a preliminary study. Phytomedicine 12(3) (2005) 209-215.

74. Gracy, R.W. Talent, J.M. Reactive oxygen species the unavoidable environmental insults. Mutation Research. 428 (1999) 17-22.

75. Agarwal, A and Kale, R.K. Radiation induced feroxidative damage. Mechanism and significance. Indian Jour. Exp. Biol., 39 (2001) 291-309.

Chapter – 7

Role of Allium Principles as Anticancer Agents

7.1 Effect of Diallyl Sulphide (Das) and Diallyl Disulphide (Dads), Two naturally occurring Sulphur compounds from Garlic, on the Immune System of Normal as well as Metastatic Tumour bearing Animals

Dr. Girija Kuttan*, P. Thejass and C. Manesh

Amala Cancer Research Centre, Amala Nagar, Thrissur 680 555

Abstract

The immunomodulatory activity of two garlic constituents, Diallyl sulphide (DAS) and Diallyl disulphide (DADS), was studied in normal BALB/c mice as well as metastatic tumour bearing C57BL/6 mice. Administration of 5 doses of both these compounds, DADS in particular, significantly enhanced the total white blood cell (WBC) count. Bone marrow cellularity and number of α-esterase positive cells were also increased by the administration of DAS and DADS. Treatment with these sulphur compounds along with the antigen, sheep red blood cells (SRBC), produced an enhancement in the circulating antibody titre and the number of plaque forming cells (PFC) in the spleen. The weight of vital organs such as spleen and thymus was also significantly enhanced by the treatment with DAS and DADS. Administration of DAS and DADS significantly enhanced natural killer (NK) cell activity in metastatic tumour bearing animals and the activity was observed earlier than metastatic tumour bearing control animals. Antibody dependent cellular cytotoxicity (ADCC) was also enhanced significantly in metastatic tumour bearing animals after DAS and DADS administration compared to untreated control metastatic tumour bearing animals. An early antibody dependent complement mediated cytotoxicity (ACC) was also observed in DAS and DADS treated metastatic tumour bearing animals. These compounds, especially DADS, significantly down regulated the production of proinflammatory cytokines such as IL-1β, IL-6, GM-CSF and TNF-α during metastasis and up regulated the production of IL-2, which is an activator of NK cells. These results clearly demonstrate the immunomodulatory activity of these two garlic constituents

---

Address for Correspondence

Dr. Girija Kuttan, Ph.D, Professor, Winner of Dr. H.D. Brahmachari Award,

Dept. Immunology, Amala Cancer Research Centre, Amala Nagar, Thrissur, Kerala State, India 680555, Ph: 91 487 2307950, Fax: 91 487 2307868,

E-Mail: amalaresearch@rediffmail.com

Introduction

Metastasis remains to be the major cause of death in cancer patients. Although several drugs have been recommended for cancer therapy there are no drugs presently available which can specifically arrest the metastatic process. The ability to interfere with the process of metastasis is, therefore, of critical importance to cancer therapy. All standard combinations for metastatic therapy have low efficiency and low response rate and it also produced a number of side effects[1] Immuno suppression is one of the major side effects of chemotherapy as well as radiation therapy. Side effects produced by both of these conventional therapies of cancer are nausea, vomiting, mucosal ulceration, interstitial pulmonary fibrosis, lymphocytopenia, hepatic and cardiac toxicity etc. Therefore, standard chemotherapy and radiotherapy might negate or reduce the therapeutic benefits obtained by the increased tumour killing of the treatment. Thus combination of chemotherapy or radiotherapy with immunomodulating agents may provide a strategy for overcoming the immunosuppressive effects of chemotherapy or radiotherapy.

Use of plant products as immunomodulators is getting more and more importance in the field of cancer research. Some of the plants with known immunomodulatory activities are V*isum album*[2], *Panax ginseng*[3], *Tinospora cordifolia*[4] etc.

Garlic and its organosulphur compounds have shown to be effective in altering the bioactivation of diverse carcinogens such as nitrosamines and polycyclic hydrocarbons[5,6]. The protection of tumour incidence by garlic organosulphur compounds such as Diallyl sulphide (DAS), Diallyl disulphide (DADS), Allyl methyl sulphide (AMS) etc. may arise from several mechanisms, including the blockage of N-nitroso compound formation, suppression of the bioactivation of several carcinogens, enhanced DNA repair, reduced cell proliferation and induction of apoptosis. DAS have been reported to have anti-oxidant, anti-tumorigenic, anti-biotic, detoxifying and other properties[7]. The detoxifying effects of garlic and its organosulphur compounds are thought to be related to their ability to inhibit phase I enzymes, induce phase-II enzymes, or bind to exogenous toxins through sulfhydryl groups[8]. Another lipid-soluble sulphur compound, DADS has been found to markedly inhibit the growth of both canine and human tumour cells in culture[9].

In this report, the Immunomodulatory activity of DAS and DADS in normal BALB/c mice as well as metastatic tumour bearing C57BL/6 mice have been analyzed.

Materials and Methods

Animals

BALB/c mice (4-6 weeks old) were taken from small animal breeding station of Amala Cancer Research Centre. C57BL/6 mice (4-6 weeks) weighing 20-25 g were purchased from National Institute of Nutrition, Hyderabad, India. All animal experiments were performed according to the rules and regulations of the Animal Ethical Committee, Govt. of India.

Cell lines

B16F-10 melanoma cells and K562 human leukemic cells were used for this study. Sheep red blood cells (SRBC) were collected from local slaughter house in Alsever's solution.

Administration of Test Compounds

Diallyl sulfide (DAS) and Diallyl disulfide (DADS) were purchased from Sigma, St. Louis, USA. DAS and DADS were suspended in liquid paraffin oil and administered intraperitoneally (i.p) at a dosage of 250 μg/dose/animal.

Determination of the effect of DAS and DADS on the Immune system of normal BALB/c mice

BALB/c mice (6 Nos /group) were divided into three groups. Group I animals were kept as untreated control. Group II and III animals were treated with DAS and DADS respectively at a concentration of 250 μg/ dose/ animal (i.p)/day for 5 consecutive days. Various haematological parameters such as total WBC count (Hemocytometer), differential count (Leishman's stain) and hemoglobin (Hb) content (Cyanmethemoglobin method) were determined. The change in body weight was also recorded. Weight of the vital organs such as liver, spleen, thymus, lungs and kidneys were recorded and expressed as relative organ weights. Bone marrow cellularity was determined by the method of Sredni et. al.[10]. The number of α-esterase positive cells was determined by the azodye coupling method[11]. Antibody titre was conducted by Haemagglutination assay using SRBC as antigen[3]. Jerne's plaque assay[12] was also conducted to determine the effect of these sulphur compounds on the number of antibody producing cells.

Determination of the effect of DAS and DADS on cell m*ediated immune response in metastatic tumour bearing animals*

C_{57}BL/6 mice were divided into 3 groups (n=12/group). All the animals were injected with B16F-10 cells (106 cells/animals) intravenously. Group I animals were kept as untreated tumour bearing controls. Group II and III animals were treated with 5 consecutive doses of DAS and DADS (250 μg/dose/animal) respectively. The animals were sacrificed at different time points after 24 h of tumour induction and spleen and blood were collected.

Spleen cells were processed to single cell suspension and used as effector cells for NK and ADCC. Serum was separated from the blood and used for the estimation of ACC[13]. Natural killer cell activity was determined by 4 h chromium release assay[14] using K-562 cells as the target. Antibody dependent cell mediated cytotoxicity was determined by 4 h chromium release assay[14] using SRBC as the target. The level of proinflammatory cytokines such as IL1β, IL-2, IL-6, GM-CSF and TNF-α during metastasis were estimated using respective Elisa kits, according to manufacturer's protocol[15] at two time points – 7th and 21st day.

Statistical Analysis

Results were expressed as Mean ± SD. The statistical analysis was done by using one-way ANOVA followed by Dunnett's test.

Results

Effect of DAS and DADS on the Immune System of Normal BALB/c Mice

Administration of both these garlic constituents, especially DADS increased the total WBC counts in normal BALB/c mice (Figure.1). The maximum WBC count obtained for DADS was 17800 cells/mm^3 on the 6th day while DAS showed the maximum of 13,600 cells/mm^3 on the 9th day. However, administration of these compounds produced no effect on lymphocyte-neutrophil ratio as well as haemoglobin content (Data not shown).

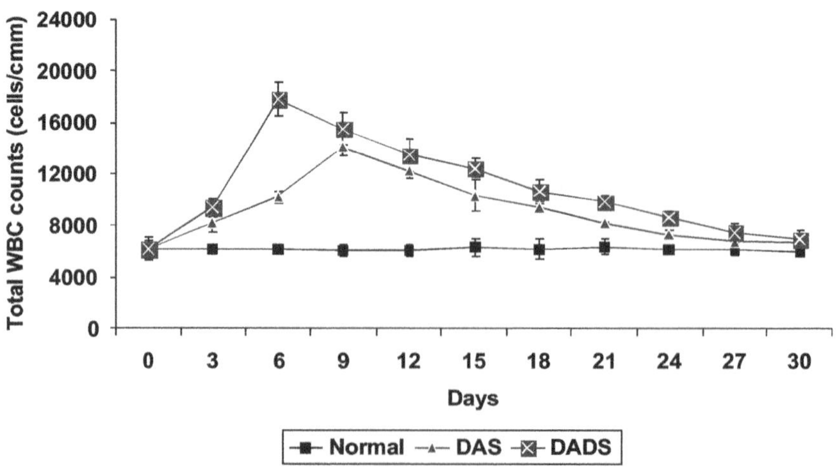

Fig. 1 Effect of DAS & DADS on total WBC count.

There was significant enhancement in the weight of thymus on treatment with DAS (0.14 ± 0.04 g/100 g body wt) and DADS (0.17 ± 0.03 g/100 g body wt) compared to normal (0.08 ±. 0.04 g/100g body wt). The size and weight of spleen was also enhanced significantly by the administration of DAS (0.51 ± 0.03 g/100 body wt.) and DADS (0.59 ± 0.05 g/100/g body wt) compared to normal (0.33 g/100 g body wt.) (Table 1).

Table 1 Effect of sulphur compounds on relative organ weights

Treatment	Relative organ weights (g/100g body. Wt.)				
	Spleen	Thymus	Liver	Kidney	Lungs
Normal	0.33 ± 0.22	0.08±0.04	4.47±0.96	1.15±0.06	0.60±0.19
DAS	0.51±0.03*	0.14±0.04	5.67±0.18*	1.66±0.03*	0.61±0.12
DADS	0.59±0.05*	0.17±0.03	5.43±0.11*	1.66±0.04*	0.59±0.14

Animals were treated with five doses of AITC and PITC (25 mg/dose/animal) *P < 0.001

Administration of DADS significantly enhanced the bone marrow cellularity to 24.7×10^6 cells/ femur compared to normal (18.6×10^6 cells/ femur). Bone marrow cell number in the case of DAS treated animals was only 19.6×10^6 cells/femur. There was a significant increase in the number of α-esterase positive cells in DADS (1748/4000 cells) and DAS (1315/4000 cells) treated animals compared to normal (911 cells/4000 cells) (Table 2).

Table 2 Effect of sulphur compounds on bone marrow cellularity and α-esterase activity

Treatment	Bone marrow Cellularity (cells/femur × 10^6)	a-esterase activity (No.of α-esterase positive cells/4000 cells)
Normal	18.2 ± 0.2	911.0 ± 39.4
DAS	19.6 ± 0.4	1315.0 ± 9.1*
DADS	24.7 ± 1.4*	1748.0 ± 47.7*

Treated animals received five doses of DAS and DADS (250 mg/dose/animal) *P < 0.001

The maximum antibody titre value of 1024 was observed on 15th day in DADS treated animals whereas the control animals showed the maximum titre value of only 128 on the same day. Treatment with DAS was also found to enhance the production of specific antibody with a maximum titre value of 512 on day 12 (Fig. 2).

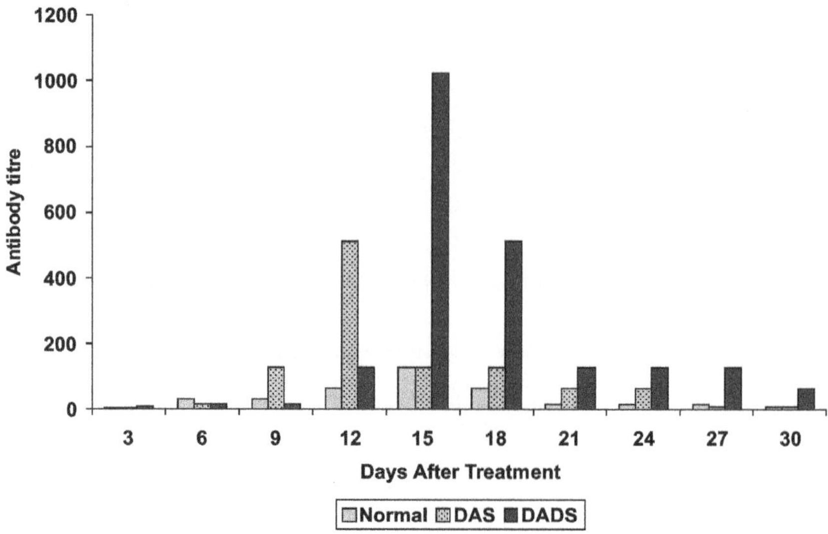

Fig. 2 Effect of DAS & DADS on circulating antibody titre.

DADS administration produced the maximum number of antibody producing cells (1409PFC/10^6 spleen cells) on the 6th day after antigen administration. The maximum number of antibody producing cells in DAS (641PFC/10^6 cells) treated group was observed on the 5th day while control animals had a maximum of 268 plaque forming cells/10^6 spleen cells on the 5th day (Fig. 3).

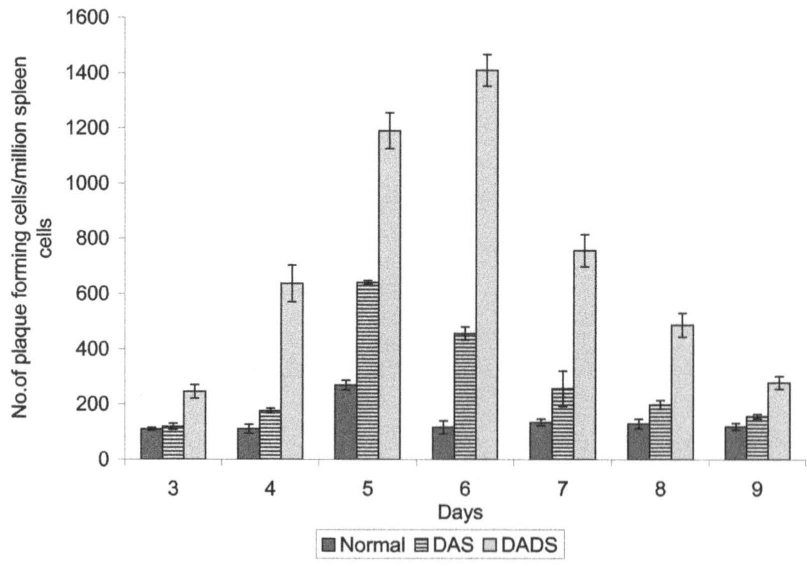

Fig. 3 Effect of DAS & DADS on antibody producing cells.

Effect of DAS and DADS on Cell Mediated Immune Response in Metastatic Tumour Bearing Animals

Administration of DAS and DADS significantly enhanced the NK cell activity in metastatic tumour bearing animals and this occurred much earlier when compared to untreated metastatic tumour bearing animals. Maximum NK cell mediated cell lysis was observed on 5th day for all the animals treated with the compounds at an effector-target ratio of 100% and it was 65.4% and 47% for DADS and DAS respectively. Metastatic tumour bearing control animals showed lowered levels of NK activity and maximum lysis was observed on 17th day and it was only 27.6% (Figure 4).

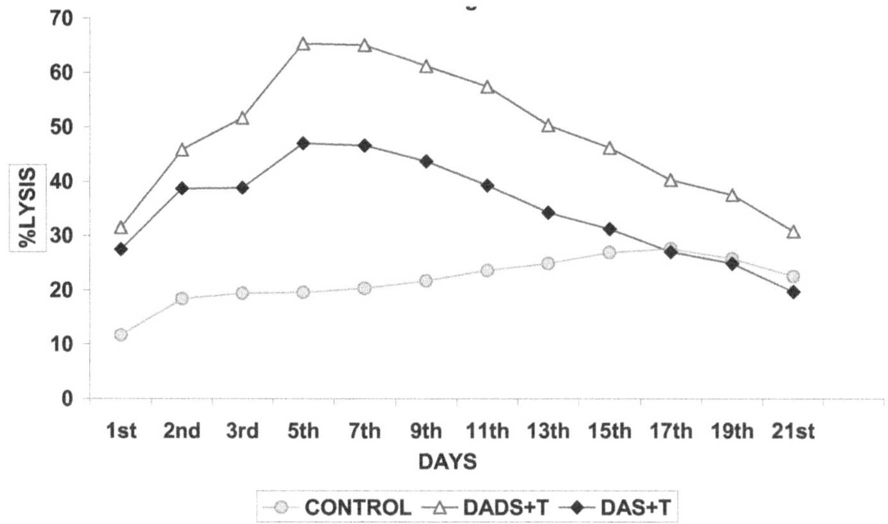

Fig. 4 Effect of DAS & DADS on NK cell activity in metastatic tumour bearing animals, on treatment (T).

ADCC activity was also elevated by the treatment with DAS and DADS compared to metastatic tumour bearing control animals (21% on 17th day). For all the compounds, maximum ADCC activity was observed on 13th day at an effector : target ratio of 100%. For DADS maximum ADCC activity was observed on 13th day (50.3%) and for DAS, the maximum was 34.2% on the same day (see Fig. 5).

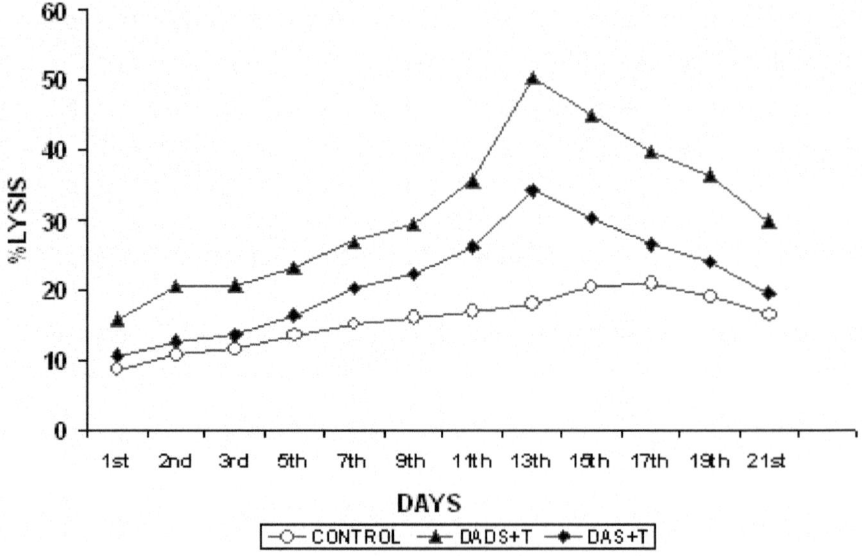

Fig. 5 Effect of DAS & DADS on ADCC in metastatic tumour bearing animals, on treatment (T).

ACC was also enhanced by the treatment with DAS and DADS. Maximum cell lysis was observed on 17th day for both these compounds. For DADS, maximum cell lysis was 31.3% and for DAS it was 23.3%. But for metastatic tumour bearing control animals, the maximum cell lysis was observed on 19th day and it was only 13.3% (Fig. 6).

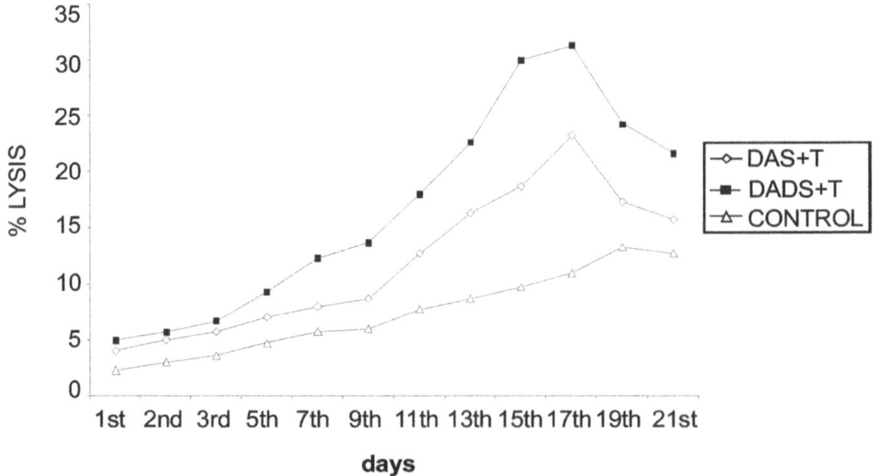

Fig. 6 Effect of DAS & DADS on ACC in metastatic tumour bearing animals, on treatment (T).

As shown in Table 3, 7th day after tumour inoculation, the level of TNF-α (38.5 ± 1.6 pg/ml), GM-CSF (23.8 ± 0.8 pg/ml) and IL-6 (37.6 ± 1.6 pg/ml) was significantly reduced by DADS treatment compared to the metastatic tumour bearing control animals. There was no effect on the level of IL-1β by the treatment of DADS. The level of IL-2 was significantly enhanced by the treatment with DADS (46.8 ± 0.5 pg/ml) compared to untreated control animals (24.9 ± 0.6 pg/ml). DAS treatment has no profound effect on the cytokine levels in metastatic tumour bearing animals on day 7.

On 21st day after tumour inoculation also, the enhanced level of TNF-α, GM-CSF and IL-6 in metastatic tumour bearing animals was significantly reduced by the treatment of DADS. DAS was also found to be effective. The enhanced level of IL-1β was also effectively reduced by the treatment of DADS (28.7 ± 0.4 pg/ml) and DAS (42.5± 1.4 pg/ml) compared to control animals (60.3 ± 1.3 pg/ml). Reduced level of IL-2 in control animals (7.4 ± 0.9 pg/ml) was significantly enhanced by the treatment of DADS (38.3 ± 1.3 pg/ml).

Discussion

Modulation of the immune system by cytostatic agents is emerging as a major area in pharmacology, especially in cases where undesired immunosuppression is the result of therapy. Immunomodulatory agents can enhance or inhibit the immunological responsiveness of an organism by interfering with its regulatory mechanisms. They may selectively activate either cell mediated or humoral immunity by stimulating either TH_1 or TH_2 type cell response respectively. Immunomodulatory agents that are free from side effects and which can be administered for long duration to obtain a continuous immune activation are highly desirable for the prevention of diseases. The modulation of immune response using medicinal plant products as a possible therapeutic measure has become a subject of active scientific investigations[16]. Our laboratory has reported earlier that an extract from plants such as Withania somnifera[17], Piper longum[18] etc could stimulate the immunity in normal mice. The present study demonstrates that unlike other chemically defined compounds, DAS and DADS modulate the immune system without undesired side effects.

Table 3 Effect of DADS, AITC and DAS on serum cytokine levels in Metastatic tumour bearinganimals

Treatment	**Serum cytokine level (pg/ml)**		**7th day**			**21st day**				
	IL-Ib	IL-2	TNF-a	IL-6	GM-CSF	IL-Ib	IL-2	TNF-a	IL-6	GM-CSF
Normal	16.0±2.1	27.4±1.8	20.0±3.5	35.0±3.5	7.8±1.1					
Control	44.8±0.6	24.9±0.6	24.1±3.5	370.1±7.4	37.9±1.1	60.3±1.3	7.4±0.9	334.9±27.5	559.8±46.9	21.8±4.4
DADS+T	36.3±1.6	46.8±0.5	38.5±1.6	37.6±1.3	23.8±0.8	28.7±0.4	38.3±1.3	69.6±6.6	370.7±20.9	7.9±0.8
DAS+T	38.0±2.3	29.4±1.2	198.4±19.2	176±16.4	30.8±2.4	42.5±1.4	20.8±1.9	278±29.3	491±35.4	17.6±1.9

Animals were injected with B16F-10 cells (10^6) intravenously. Animals were treated with 5 consecutive doses of DAS and DADS (250 µg/dose.animal). Blood was collected by tail bleeding on 7th and 21st day after tumour inoculation. Serum separated and used for assays.

Note: The cytokine IL-2 increased significantly on treatment with DADS both in the 1st and 3rd weeks. Most of others decreased. IL-2 is a mediation of T and NK cells activity to destroy cancer cells. This is a mechanism of action of many nutraceuticals.

The effect of these compounds on total WBC count and bone marrow cells indicate that these compounds significantly stimulated hematopoiesis, especially the cell mediated immune system. Both innate and adaptive immunity depends upon the activities of WBCs. The mononuclear phagocyte system is composed of bone marrow monocyte precursors, circulating monocytes and macrophages in all tissues including lung, liver, spleen, adrenal glands, intestine and bone marrow. These cells are highly phagocytic and play an active role in antigen processing. Like proliferating bone marrow cells, bone marrow monocytes show non-specific esterase activity. Administration of DAS and DADS stimulated stem cell proliferation and differentiation as there was significant enhancement in the number of α-esterase positive bone marrow cells.

These compounds stimulated the humoral immune response. DADS showed the highest stimulatory effect, which was observed both in an enhanced antibody titre and increased number of plaque forming cells. The increased titre remained for several days indicating that there is a sustained immunological activity even after the treatment. The enhancement of spleen and thymus after DAS and DADS administration also support their stimulatory effect on the immune system.

We also analyzed the immunostimulatory effects of DAS and DADS in C_{57}BL/6 mice bearing the highly invasive B16F-10 melanoma cells and found that both these compounds significantly enhanced the cell mediated immune response. The fate of the host tumour interactions is considered to depend on the balance between the inherent metastatic potential of the tumour and the strength of the host immune response. Cytotoxic Tlymphocyte and NK activity play an important role in immunological surveillance in neoplasia and metastasis[19]. In contrast to CTL, which are triggered by class I MHC molecules, NK cells mediate lysis of target cells which fail to express MHC class I molecules[20]. NK cells are large granular lymphocytes capable of lysing many types of tumour and virus infected cells without prior sensitization. The enhanced cell mediated immune responses and increased productions of NK cells are the major protective measures of the immune system during metastasis. Here DAS and DADS treatment resulted in much earlier and enhanced activation of NK cell mediated tumour cell lysis compared to untreated metastatic tumour bearing control animals.

Although the presence of a humoral immunity is not consistently correlated with increased tumour resistance in the host, the antibodies can mediate cell destruction either via binding with complement or by acting as an opsonin to fascilitate phagocytosis by macrophages or other phagocytic cell bearing Fc receptors. Natural killer cells also have Fc receptors CD_{16} on their surface which allow them to kill antibody coated target cells

(ADCC), thus providing another form of immune response[21,22]. The elevated NK cell activity by DAS and DADS administration resulted in significant enhancement of ADCC in metastatic tumour bearing animals where as untreated metastatic tumour bearing animals with low NK cell activity showed decreased ADCC activity. Complement mediated cytolysis was also enhanced by the treatment with these sulphur compounds. **The treatment with these compounds has stimulated host defence response, as demonstrated by the enhanced level of IL-2, which is an important mediator of NK cell activity.**

The levels of proinflammatory cytokines, such as IL-1β, IL-6, TNF-α and GM-CSF, evaluated in this study is also important in the process of metastasis because of their significant pro-metastatic effects and it was found that these sulphur compounds, DADS in particular, significantly down regulated the production of these proinflammatory cytokines. Increased TNF-α has been thought to contribute to cancer cachexia that is manifested by body weight loss, chronic nausea, fatigue, insomnia and profuse sweating. Drugs that down regulate TNF-α can result in improvements of cancer cachexia. Both these sulphur compounds, especially DADS, effectively reduced the level of TNF-α in metastatic animals. In malignancy elevated GM-CSF may promote metastasis by activating macrophages to produce TNF-α and IL-1.

In conclusion, our study clearly demonstrated the immunostimulatory activity of two allium constituents–DAS and DADS–in normal as well as metastatic tumour bearing animals. Thus, the results obtained herein may provide two potential agents for cancer therapy in the future.

Acknowledgment

The present study was financially aided by the department of Biotechnology, New Delhi, India. We sincerely thank Dr. Ramadasan Kuttan, Research Director, Amala Cancer Research Centre, for his valuable suggestions and support throughout this study.

References

1. Hersh EM., Freirich EJ. In: Bush H, (ed). Methods in cancer research, vol.4. New York: Academic press. 1986, P.335.
2. Kuttan G., Kuttan R. Immunomodulatory activity of a peptide isolated from Viscum album extract. Immunol.Invest. 1992, 21, 285-296.

3. Singh V.K., Aggarval S. Immunomodulatory activity of Panax ginseng extract. Planta Med. 1984, 50, 462-465.

4. Sonel M., Kuttan G. Immunomodulatory and antitumour activities of Tinospora cordifolia. Fitoterapia 1999, 70, 35-43.

5. Mignard D.H., Suschetet M., Berges R. Inhibition of aflatoxin B1 and N- nitrosodiethylamine induced liver preneoplastic foci in rats fed naturally occurring allyl sulfides. Nutrition and Cancer 1996, 25, 61-70.

6. Reddy B.S., Rao C.V., Rivenson A., Kelloff G. Chemoprevention of colon carcinogenesis by organosulfur compounds. Cancer Research 1993, 53, 3493-3498.

7. Wargovich M.J., Imada O., Stephens L.C. Initiation and post-initiation chemopreventive effects of di allyl sulfide in esophageal carcinogenesis. Cancer Lett 1992, 64, 39-42.

8. Dausch G., Nixon D.W. Garlic: a review of its relationship to its malignant disease. Preventive Medicine 1990, 19, 346-361.

9. Sundaram S.G., Milner J.A. Impact of Organosulphur compounds in garlic on canine mammary tumour cells in culture. cancer Lett, 1993, 74,85-90.

10. Sredni B., Albeck M., Kazimirsky G., Shalet F. Immunomodulator AS101 administered orally as a chemoprotective and radioprotective agent. Int. J.Immunopharmacol. 1992, 14, 613-619.

11. Bancroft J.D., Cook H.F. Manual of Histologic Techniques. Churchill Livingston, London. 1992, pp-171-174.

12. Jerne N.K., Nordin A.A. Plaque formation in agar by single antibody producing cells. Science 1963, 140, 405-408.

13. Gupta S.K., Bhattacharya, B. Cytotoxicity assays. In : A hand book of practical immunolog; Talwar, G.P., Ed., Vikas publishing house, New Delhi, 1983, 328-333.

14. Kim Y.B., Huh N.D., Koren H.S., Amos D.B. Natural killing (NK) and antibody dependent cellular cytotoxicity (ADCC) in specific pathogen free (SPF) miniature swine and germ free piglets. 1. comparison of NK and ADCC. J. Immunol. 1980, 125, 755-762.

15. Leyon P.V., Kuttan G. Effect of Tinospora cordifolia on the cytokine profile of angiogenesis induced animals. International Immunopharmacol 2004, 4, 1569-1575.

16. Bhat B.A., Dhar K.L., Puri S. C., Quirishi M.A., Khajuria A., Gupta A., Quazi G.N. Isolation, characterization and biological evaluation of Datura lactones as potential immunomodulators. Bio Org. Med. Chemistry 2005, 13, 6672-6677.

17. Davis L., Kuttan G. Effect of Withania somnifera in the cell mediated immune response. J. Expt. Clin. Cancer Res. 2002, 21, 585-590.

18. Sunila E.S., Kuttan, G. Immunomodulatory and antitumour activity of Piper longum Linn. and Piperine. J. Ethnopharmacol. 2004, 90, 339-346.

19. Cooper M.A.; Fehniger T.A.; Caligiuri M.A. The biology of human natural killer cell subsets. Trend Immunol. 2001, 22, 633-640.

20. Moretta L., Bottino C., Pende D., Mingari M.C., Biassoni R., Moretta A. Human Natural Killer cells: their origin, receptors and function. Eur. J. Immunol. 2002, 32, 1205-1211.

21. Henney C.S., Kuribayashi K., Kern D.E., Gillis S. Interleukin-2 augments natural killer activity. Nature 1981, 291, 335-338.

22. Mandelboim O., Malik P., Davis M.D., Jo C.H., Boyson J.E., Strominger J.L. Human CD16 as a lysis receptor mediating direct natural killer cytotoxicity. Proc. Natl. Acad. Sci. USA 1999, 96, 5640-5644.

7.2 Approaches to contain Oxidative Stress in Human Tumors and protection by Plant products

Dr. B. Nagarajan,
Senior Scientist, Cancer Institute, Chennai, India

The tumor registry data at the Madras Cancer Institute has shown high incidence of cancer stomach in South Indian males and cancer cervix in females. Almost 80-90 percent of human cancers are associated and promoted by environmental risk factors. Cancer is a disease that hallmarks self-sufficiency in growth signal, insensitivity to anti growth signal, evasion of apoptosis, limitless replicative potential, sustained angiogenesis and metastasis. The prognosis depends on both clinical stage and molecular status. The progressive changes are reflected with pathology-normal epithelium, hyperplasia, carcinoma and invasive carcinoma. Chromosomal abnormalities and clonal proliferation of malignancies have been well documented by molecular profile that also helps assess the efficacy of treatment and monitor remission. Metastasis involves interplay between extracellular matrix degradation, proteolysis, cell adhesion, cell migration, angiogenesis and tissue homing. At the new site, tumor growth resumes disrupting normal growth and function that is again modulated by regulation by primary tumor.

Epidemiological surveys showed several risk factors for gastric cancer mainly environment-oriented and food related[1]. Gastric carcinoma develops by intermediate cells of abnormal cell differentiation metaplasia and dysplasia that line up the gastric mucosa directly contacting contents of the stomach. Several molecular events are involved in stomach carcinogenesis that comprise of alterations in the p^{53} and c-met genes, CD44 variant transcripts, genetic instability and telomerase activity. Further amplification of cyclin D, inactivation of APC and mutated K-ras and loss of heterozygosity and apoptotic rate are implicated in the genesis.

Cytokines in Cervical Cancer

Different abnormalities in the level of cytokine production have been found in invasive cervical carcinomas such as an increase of IL6 production and a deficit in IFNγ mRNA expression in cancer patients. By means of new biotechnologies such as quantitative Polymerase Chain Reaction (PCR) or *in situ* PCR, we aim to determine their concentration and distribution directly at the tumor site. A comparison of these molecular diagnosis approaches with reference techniques such as ELISA or immunocytochemistry are performed.

We have identified the potential of a new cytokine, IL-17 as clinical prognosis marker in cervical tumors[2]. More than 200 biopsies derived from cervical cancer patient were collected. They mostly include stage II and III tumors in order to have an homogenous group of cancer patients. mRNA extraction was performed in all these biopsies and quantitative measurement of cytokine mRNA carried out. Tissues were also processed for immunohistochemical analysis such as CD3, CD4, CD8, CD68, IL-6, IL-8, IFN-γ and IL-2Rα. For all patients, clinical parameters were recorded as available from the Tumor Registry. We attempt to demonstrate tangible correlation between biological and clinical parameters.

Studies in Cancer Cervix Patients through Radiation Therapy

We address the issue of residual tumors in human cervical cancer patients post radiation therapy. After successful external radiation/intracavitary and interstitial radiation therapy some patients presented with recurrent tumors on 6-12 months follow up period. These patients had high level of IL-6 on first reporting. This augurs well with the thesis that up regulation of pro-inflammatory protein IL-6 might be involved in tumor progression. Moreover T cells recruited to the tumor site were not sufficient and possibly developed anergy. Further, over expression of IL-6 stromal cells reflected a favorable factor for tumor growth. Biopsies derived from cervical cancer patients were analyzed by RT-PCR method to quantify cytokine mRNA[3]. Different cytokines such as IL-6, IFN-γ and TNF-∝ were successfully analyzed and also antigen presenting dendritic cells as well. CD4 helper cells are involved in MHC II mediated antigen presentation and divided into Th-1 cells that secrete IL-2, IFN-γ, TNF-β while Th-2 cells release IL-4, IL-5, IL-6, IL-10 and IL-13. To address whether this down regulation of Th-1 cytokines is associated with Th-2 polarization of immune response or deactivation of intra tumoral T cells, we have identified and characterized a group of cervical carcinoma patients with undetectable intratumoral T-cell derived cytokine mRNA such as IFN-γ, IL-4 and IL-17. Absence of IFN-γ seems to be more frequent in advanced stage II and III tumors than in localized stage I tumors. Significant correlations between the stromal positivity of IL-6 and IL-8 with macrophages infiltration tend to confirm the macrophages as chief sources of this cytokine. In addition, differential staining for dendritic cells (DC) showed that most tumors contained mature DC located around the tumor, whereas immature DC appeared inside the tumor suggesting a maturation block of dendritic cells and impaired cytokine activity.

DNA Adduct Assay

DNA adduct formation caused by genotoxicants is implicated in tumorigenesis. These adducts are dose dependent and show different mutation efficiencies. For dosimetry of DNA adducts, ^{32}p-post labeling technique has been one of the most sensitive methods for detection. Individuals exposed to genotoxicants show adduct spots by ^{32}p-post labeling and there is good correlation with documented human exposure. DNA damage mediated through reactive oxygen species is implicated in several degenerative disorders such as cancer, reproductive cell death and ageing. The most significant one is the formation of 8-oxodeoxyguanosine.

DNA Instability in Stomach Cancer

We switch to another common cancer and address semi quantitative dosimetry of aberrant DNA in stomach cancer. We hypothesize both acquired and inherited host factors predispose to cancer as a result of oxidative and other damage events in DNA. An attempt was made to critically look at carcinogen-molecular adducts, mutations and DNA alterations in the target epithelial and surrogate blood cells as well.

Single Cell Gel Electrophoresis

The clinical specimens, both biopsy and surgical samples from cancer stomach patients were collected for single cell gel electrophoresis. Gastric tumor tissues and corresponding distal mucosa were collected from patients undergoing gastrectomy and endoscopy. The samples were immediately placed on ice, minced in phosphate buffered saline, filtered and suspension was centrifuged at 1000 rpm for 10 minutes. The isolated cells were resuspended in 50 μl buffer and electrophoresed. A clearly significant increase in the mean comet length was observed in the tumor cell population that correlated with histological grading. Gastritis a putative precancerous condition showed definitive changes as mixture of normal and damaged cells as comets. To correlate this finding, we showed increased levels of N^7-methylguanine both in tumor and distal mucosa. Although these findings do not categorically prove that nitrosating or alkylating agents are responsible for the DNA modification detected, alkylating agents like nitrosamines are ubiquitous contaminants of different industrial and agricultural activities and so also high levels of nitrate from drinking water. Furthermore, this underscores the role of inflammation in putative carcinogenesis. Human DNA adduct is a promising marker for cancer epidemiology and risk assessment, in addition to the above toxic biological end points.

Chemoprevention with Naturally occurring Compounds

Since it is well established that oxidative damage plays a key role in carcinogeneic process both synthetic and natural antioxidants such as flavanoids, terpenes, allium and polyphenolic compounds are the potential candidates in ameliorating approaches. We have shown the antitumor potential of quercetin and luteolin in experimental animal tumors. We have also shown the beneficial effect of ursolic acid and oleolic acid in protecting cardiotoxicity induced by adriamycin.

The cumulative cardiotoxicity of adriamycin (ADR) is a constraint on therapeutic use. Generation of drug induced oxygen radicals lead to cardiac lipid membrane peroxidation. We studied the free radical scavenging potential of two compounds olearolic acid (OA) from *Eugenia Jumbolana* and ursolic acid (UA) damage from *Ocimum Sactum* against ADR induced lipid peroxidation and showed a strong protective action of OA and mild one with UA. It would be of interest to study the combined effect of OA and UA to augment protection in chemotherapeutic management.

Salted sun dried and deep-fried fish and mutton were screened for their mutagenicity by the AMES test, single gel electrophoresis assay, chromosomal aberrations, and micronucleus test. Fish and mutton given at 20% in the diet to the rats daily for two months resulted in cytogenetic damage, which could not be repaired on withdrawal. However the temporary damage was reversed at a10% dose upon withdrawal after the same period. The maximum chromatid damage found as breaks and gaps was in agreement with the increased number of strand breaks. Treated rats also showed DNA strand breaks in hepatocytes and lymphocytes, more so in hepatocytes. Lime and onion extracts inhibited the nitrosation of fish and mutton, and were antitoxic

Studies from our laboratory have shown the clastogenic effects of long-term feeding on deep-fried fish and mutton in rat bone marrow cells. We report the chemopreventive action of two flavanoids, quercetin (Qn) and luteolin (Ln) against the induced mutagenicity by fish and mutton extract.

Groups of rats were treated with flavanoids through presimultaneous and post- treatment regimens and killed at the end of treatment. The bone morrow was removed and analyzed for the presence of micronuclei (MN) and chromosome aberrations (CA). Pre-treatment showed most effectively a good inhibition of mutagenicity at every dose tested. Luteolin was a better protective agent than quercetin. It protected the cells against genetic damage to 93% in the micronucleus assay and to 95% in the chromosome aberrations induced by fish extract ($p<0.001$ in both the groups). Mutton extract-induced micronuclei and chromosome aberrations were protected 85% and 90%, respectively, by luteolin and 79% and 76%, respectively, by quercetin. Our results tend to suggest that quercetin and luteolin are potential chemopreventive compounds.

Molecular immunology is an emerging area of current research with potential to develop prophylactic and therapeutic vaccines. Some of the second-generation chemotherapeutic drugs developed have passed clinical trials and are in vogue.

References

1. Xu, G.P; Song, P.J. and Reed, P.I. (1993) Hypothesis on the relationship between intragastric nitrosation, N-nitrosamine in gastric juice of subjects from high risk area for gastric cancer and inhibition of N-nitrosamine formation by fruit juices. European Jour. of Cancer Prevention, 2, 25-36.
2. B. Nagarajan (2005), Molecular Markers in Human Epithelial Tumors: excerpts from Dr. V. R. Khanolkar Oration, Annals National Academy Med. Sciences, India, 39, 61-65.
3. Radha Munagala, and B. Nagarajan (2007), Isolation of RNA From Cell Scrapings and blood samples from cervical cancer Patients Current Science, 93 (No. 2)138-139.

7.3 Medicinal Importance of Garlic (Allium Sativum Linn) Ancient and Modern View

Dr. K.P. Sathia Gopal B.A.M.S.

Senior Medical Officer, Cholayil Sanjeevanam, Holloway Road (Opp. Josegiri Hospital), Thalassery 670 101.

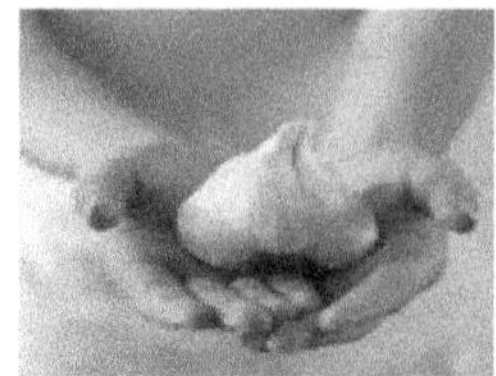

Abstract

Actions and uses: According to ayurvedic concepts Garlic is hot, stimulant, carminative, anti rheumatic and anthelmintic, oil from the seed is stimulant. Garlic acts as vermifuge expelling round worms- oil is a powerful antiseptic[1]. The essential oil of garlic is absorbed into the circulation and is excreted through the lungs and bronchial mucosa acting as a good antiseptic and antispasmodic. When there is much gastro intestinal catarrh, garlic in the form of an ointment is rubbed on the abdomen, a binder being applied after wards (milk or egg white). It is said to be very effective in bronchial and asthmatic complaints. It also acts as a prophylactic for typhus, typhoid, diphtheria and many other infectious diseases. There are several garlic preparations in the market which contains either garlic juice or its constituents.

Nutritional Profile

- Garlic is rich in a variety of powerful sulfur containing Compounds including Thiosulfinates (allicin). Sulfoxides (alliin) and dithiins, ajoene etc[2].
- These compounds are responsible for garlic's characteristically pungent odor.
- Garlic is an excellent source of manganese, a very good source of vitamin B6 and vitamin C and a good source of selenium.
- Nutritional value per 100 gm(edible part) is 150 Kcal

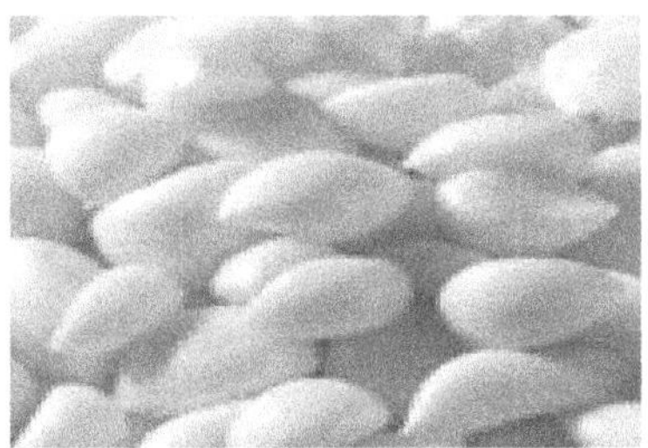

Garlic cloves

Action & Medicinal Uses

- Garlic is hot, stimulants carminative, anti rheumatic & anti helminthic. Oil from the seed is stimulant.

  Garlic act as vermifuge expelling round worms. Oil is a powerful antiseptic.
- The essential oil of garlic is absorbed in to the circulation and is excreted through the lungs and bronchial mucosa acting as a good antiseptic and antispasmodic.
- When there is much gastro intestinal catarrh, garlic in the form of an ointment is rubbed on the abdomen, a binder being applied afterwards (milk or egg white). It is said to show very effective in Bronchial and Asthmatics complaints. Also it acts as a Prophylactic for Typhus, Typhoid, Diphtheria and Viral fevers.
- There are several proprietary preparations on the market at the present moment which contain either the juices of Garlic or its constituents
- Garlic and ginger paste in butter milk is good to be consumed daily to prevent viral diseases like jaundice and chikungunia.

Benefits of Garlic

- The Garlic renew the blood, cleanse it of all impurities, regulate the digestion and remove all parasites in the intestines which might be injurious to health and are recommended for discards of the lungs, antennae – sclerosis, high blood pressure, gout, rheumatism, asthma, instestinal complaints, loss of appetite, constipates and worms. Used extensively as a spice in India for chutneys and curries for flavoring pickles.
- Externally the oil is used in paralytic and rheumatic affections.
- The oil from seeds is prescribed internally as a febrifuge to prevent recurrence of the cold, fits of intermittent fever.
- As resolvent the garlic is applied to indolent tumors. Internally it is given with common salt in afflictions of the nervous system, headache, flatulence, hysteria, coughs etc.

- Externally the juice used as a rubefacient liniment acts very beneficially in infantile convulsions, other nervous and spasmodic affections, relaxed sore throat, in asthma, general paralysis, facial paralysis, gout, sciatica, and in skin.
- Diseases including leprosy.
- When eaten in cold season it is said to ward of attacks of rheumatism and neuralgia.
- Mustard or coconut oil in which garlic has been fried is an excellent antiseptic application for scabies and maggots infesting ulcers, ulcerated surfaces and wounds.
- Its juice mixed with salt is applied to bruises and sprains and also to relieve neuralgia and earache.
- Garlic is applied externally for ear pain. Garlic juice mixed with 4 parts of distilled water has been used as a lotion for washing wounds and ulcers. Garlic produces copious diuresis
- It's applied like onions to the nose in case of fainting in the form of confection it is given in RHEUMATISM.
- Cures irregular menstrual problems.
- Maintains BP level & Cholesterol Level.

Garlic Vs Diseases. Garlic oil and its precursors are found to be very effective in ameliorating diabetes, CVD, and in preventing platelet aggregation and for enhancing blood fibrinolysis[2,3] and also for blocking liver injuries by chemicals[3,4].

Garlic is found very effective in:

- Swasam, Kasam, Arsas, Kushtam, Krimi, Agnimadyam, Paralysis, Forgetfulness,
- Tremor, Colicky pain of the intestine, internal ulcers of the lungs
- Secretes Serum, Chronic fevers.

Garlic in Ayurvedic Preparations

- Astavargam Kasayam., Lasunerandathi Kasayam, Lasunathi Grutham
- **Ulli-vedukathi Kasyam, Vajalasunathi Thailam**
- Garlic is an ingredient for a decoction along with dry ginger, black pepper, long pepper and cumin to treat viral fevers[5].

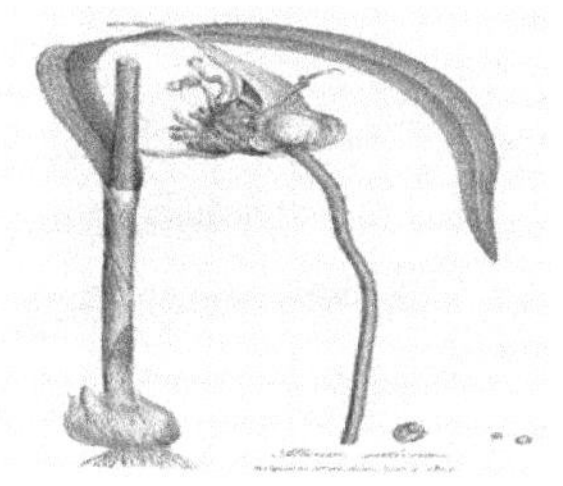
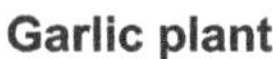

Garlic plant

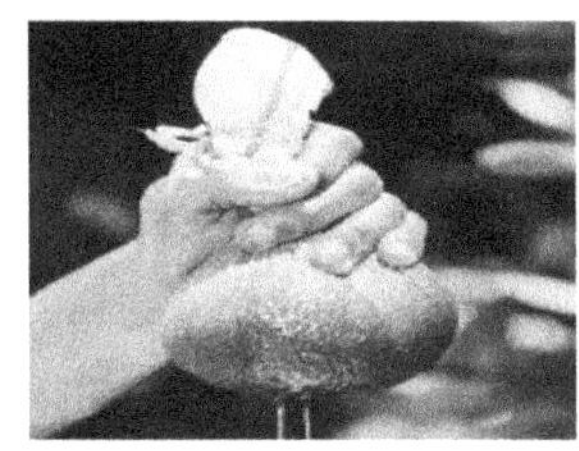

Garlic paste bag for massage

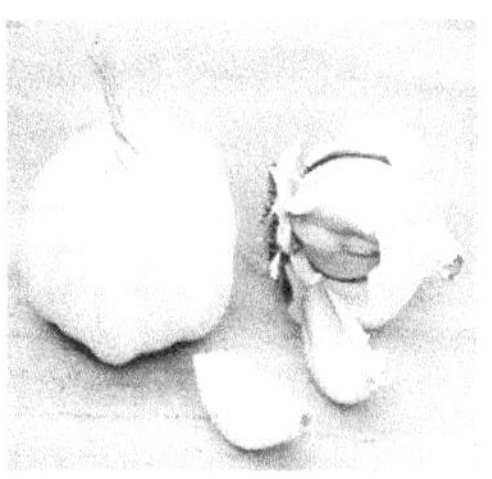

Garlic pearls

References

1. Nadkarni, KM. Indian Materia Medica. 3 rd edn.1954.Vol.1. 66-71.
2. Bordia, A; Joshi, HK et. al. Effect of essential oil of garlic on serum fibrinolytic activity in patients with coronary artery diseases. Atherosclerosis 28 (1978)155-59.
3. Mukerji, B; J. Sci. Ind. Res (India), 1957. 16 a, No, 10; Suppl.1-18.
4. Hikino H, Tohkin, M et. al. Antihepatotoxic actions of Allium sativum bulbs. Planta Medica. 53(1986)163.
5. Vydyamadom Cheriya Narayanan Nampoothiri. Mathrubhoomy daily. June 3rd 2007.

7.4 Cells of the Immune System and their Mechanism of Action

Miss. M.S. Resmy. & Arunkumar, S.
Lecturers, Department of Medical Laboratory Technology, SHS, Thalassery campus of Kannur University
Email-arunkumars123@yahoo.co.in

A wide variety of leucocytes (white blood cells) participate in an immune response. However, only the lymphocytes possess the attributes of diversity, specificity, memory, and self/nonself recognition. All of the other cells have only an accessory function: viz; activation of lymphocytes, phagocytosis/antigen clearance, secretion of cytokines.

Monocytes and Macrophages

(also called mononuclear cells)

- Monocytes circulate in the blood and lymph (represent 5-8% of WBCs in the blood)
- From monocytes macrophages are formed.
- This transition occurs as the monocytes enter the tissues.
- Changes which occur during this transition:
    - Cells enlarge [5-10x].
    - Intracellular organelles increase in number and complexity.
    - Cells acquire increased phagocytic ability.
    - Secretion of many soluble factors.

Macrophages play the following important roles:

1. Phagocytosis
2. Antimicrobial activity
3. Antigen presentation
4. Secretion of soluble factors

Macrophages are activated by a variety of stimuli in the course of an immune response. Phagocyotosis itself is an initial activating stimulus. Macrophages are further activated by cytokines secreted by

T helper cells [IFN-gamma], by mediators of the inflammatory response and by various microbial products.

Phagocytosis

The process of Phagocytosis involves:

- Chemotaxis
- Extension of pseudopodia
- Formation of a phagosome
- Fusion with lysosome to form phagolysosome
  [Lysosome contains hydrogen peroxide, oxygen free radicals, peroxidase, lysozyme, and hydrolytic enzymes]
- Elimination of digested components via exocytosis

Antimicrobial Activity

Following Phagocytosis, microorganisms are killed by both oxygen dependent and oxygen independent mechanisms.

Oxygen Dependent

Respiratory burst involves the activation of a membrane-bound oxidase that catalyzes the reduction of oxygen to superoxide anion (O_2^{-}) which is extremely toxic.

The O_2^{-} also generates other powerful oxidizing agents:

- Hydroxyl radicals ($OH^{\cdot}$)
- Singlet oxygen ($^1O_2$)
- Hydrogen peroxide (H_2O_2)

Macrophages activated with LPS or other microbial products together with **IFN-gamma** also express high levels of enzyme **nitric oxide synthestase**

This enzyme oxidizes L-arginine to yield citrulline and **nitric oxide (NO).** NO is a very potent toxic agent. When it combines with the superoxide anion O_2^{-} it is even more toxic. Nitric Oxide-mediated killing may be more important than respiratory burst in the destruction of intracellular pathogens.

Oxygen Independent

- Lysozyme.
- Other Hydrolytic enzymes.
- Defensins [cysteine-rich cationic peptides - circularize due to the presence of 3 intramolecular disulfide bonds-] Form ion-permeable channels in bacterial and mammalian cell membranes
- Tumor necrosis factor alpha

  (Produced by activated macrophages - cytotoxic effect on some cell types)

Secretion of Cytokines

- **IL-1** - multiple effects (activation of TH cells, affects vascular endothelial cells thus influencing inflammatory response, affects the thermoregulatory center in the hypothalamus leading to fever.
- **Tumor necrosis factor alpha** (kills a variety of cells)
- **IL-12 (enhances INFγ production and destroys cancer cells)**

plus a large number of cytokines which play a role in hematopoiesis [**IL-6, GM-CSF, G-CSF, M-CSF**]

Other Soluble Factors

- Several of the complement proteins
- Various hydrolytic enzymes

Macrophages possess in their membrane, receptors for certain classes of antibody (**Fc receptors**), receptors for complement components (**CRs**), allowing for opsonization.

Granulocytic Cells

(Large leucocytes which contain cytoplasmic granules) Neutrophils, Eosinophils, Basophils (Mast Cells)

Neutrophil - 50-70% of circulating WBC

- If higher numbers, a good sign of bacterial infection.
- Sometimes called PMN (Polymorphonuclear) cell because of multi-lobed nucleus.

- The fine granules stain poorly with acidic and basic dyes, thus the name- neutrophil.
- These granules fuse with phagosome to destroy internalized bacteria.

Primary Granules: electron dense and contain bactericidal enzymes such as lysozyme and myeloperoxidase; neutral proteases (i.e. elastase); and acid hydrolases (B-glucoronidase and cathepsin B)

Secondary Granules: not electron dense. Contain lysozyme, collagenase and lactoferrin.

Oxygen dependent and **Oxygen independent mechanisms** are used to kill internalized microorganisms.

Neutrophils are more likely than macrophages to kill ingested microorganisms. Neutrophils also exhibit a larger respiratory burst than macrophages and consequently are able to generate more reactive oxygen intermediates. In addition, neutrophils express higher levels of defensins.

The neutrophil is a phagocytic cell, particularly important in the phagocytosis of bacteria. However, these cells DO NOT function as Antigen Presenting Cs.

A number of substances produced during an inflammatory response recruit neutrophils to a site of inflammation. Neutrophils are the 1st cells to arrive.

Eosinophil (represent 1-3% of circulating WBCs)

- Possess a bi-lobed nucleus and a heavily granulated cytoplasm.
- Granules stain orange/red with the acidic dye Eosin Y.
- Phagocytic but DO NOT act as APCs.

The major role of the eosinophil is believed to be against parasites, particularly parasitic worms.

Eosinophils kill by ADCC [antibody dependent cell-mediated cytotoxicity] by binding to parasite - specific **Ig E** via cell surface **FcRs**.

When eosinophils bind to IgE on the surface of a worm, the cell is triggered to degranulate. The contents of the granules cause damage to the worm's tegument.

Basophil - <1% of circulaing WBC

Lobed nucleus--more variable, large coarse granules stain blue with basic dye **methylene blue**.

Basophils are **not** phagocytic.

They play a major role in the allergic response when they release their granules (containing **histamine, serotonin, prostan glandin, etc**).

Basophils also bear Fc receptors for IgE. When an individual is exposed to an allergen, allergen specific IgE is produced. This IgE binds to the surface of basophils [in the **sensitization phase** of the allergic response]. Upon re-exposure to the allergen, the allergen binds to IgE on the surface of basophils resulting in degranulation.

Mast Cells

Mast cells are released from the bone marrow as undifferentiated precursor cells and do not differentiate until they enter the tissues (skin, connective tissue, mucosal epithelium, etc.)

Morphology and function similar to circulating basophils.

Mast cells bear Fc receptors for IgE and contain large numbers of cytoplasmic granules which also play a very important role in the allergic response.

Dendritic Cells

Cells which are covered with a maze of long membrane processes resembling dendrites of nerve cells. These cells function as antigen presenting cells. They have high levels of **Class II MHC** molecules and the co-stimulatory molecule known as **B7**. They capture antigen in the tissues and migrate to various lymphoid organs where they present the antigen to **T helper lymphocytes.**

They are termed:

Langerhan cells in skin

Veiled cells in lymph

Interdigitating dendritic cells in T cell areas of secondary lymphoid tissue and thymic medulla.

Interstitial dendritic cells populate most organs (e.g. heart, lungs, liver, kidney, GI tract)

Follicular Dendritic Cells: do not express MHC class II and do not present antigen to Th cells. Exclusive location in **lymphoid follicles**, B cell rich areas of lymph node. Express high levels of membrane receptors for antibody and complement. Binding of immune complexes to these cells is thought to facilitate B cell activation. Complexes are retained for very long periods of time.

Lymphocytes

Leucocytes which are responsible for the specific immune response. Represent 20-40% of circulating WBC in blood - 99% of cells in lymph.

Lymphocytes circulate in the blood and lymph but can also enter the tissues. Broadly divided into T lymphocytes and B lymphocytes and null cells. All three are small, motile, nonphagocytic cells which cannot be distinguished from each other morphologically.

B and T lymphocytes which have not interacted with antigen are said to be resting [virgin or naive] lymphocytes. These cells have little visible cytoplasm around their nucleus. Once stimulated with antigen (and appropriate cytokine/cellular signals) the cell progresses through the cell cycle and enlarges into a blast cell. Lymphoblasts further differentiate into effector cells or memory cells. [Plasma cells, Th cells, T cytotoxic cells]. The memory cells are long-lived cells that reside in the Go phase of the cell cycle until activated by a secondary encounter with antigen.

Different lineages or different maturational stages of lymphocytes can be distinguished by their expression of membrane molecules recognized by particular monoclonal antibodies. Molecules recognized are referred to as **CD molecules** (now well over 100) **Cluster of Differentiation** (CD)

Null Cells

Small group of peripheral blood lymphocytes. They fail to express membrane molecules, Ig or TcR or typical CD molecules. One functional population of these cells are the **NK cells** (Natural Killer cells).

These cells are large, granular, and represent 5-10% of the peripheral blood lymphocytes. NK cells kill tumor cells or virally-infected cells by direct membrane contact or through antibody-dependent cell-mediated cytotoxicity. A type of lymphocyte found in secondary lymph organs.

They are activated by substances called interleukins and interferons.

Recognise infected cells especially those attacked by viral agencies.

Destroy body's own cells if invaded.

Also have the ability to attack aberrant cells that could cause tumours.

Megakaryocyte

Giant polyploid cells. Nucleus undergoes multiple mitotic divisions with no cytoplasmic divisions. Megakaryocytes give rise to platelets when fragments or pieces of cytoplasm break or "bleb" off of the cell body. Platelets are involved in the blood clotting process.

Mature B lymphocytes bear ~150,000 immunoglobulin molecules on their surface. Each of these 150,000 immunoglobulins (**Ig**) possesses an identical binding site for antigen. In other words, a particular B lymphocyte is specific for only one antigen.

In addition to surface Ig, B lymphocytes possess other characteristic surface proteins:

Class II MHC proteins (MHC stands for Major Histocompatability Complex)

The presence of Class II MHC proteins permits B lymphocytes to act as Antigen Presenting Cells (**APCs**) to T helper lymphocytes.

When a mature, but naive (or virgin) B lymphocyte encounters antigen and receives the proper signals from an antigen-specific T helper lymphocyte, the B lymphocyte will be activated to proliferate and to differentiate into immunoglobulin-secreting **plasma cells**. A certain sub-population of cells will differentiate into **memory B lymphocytes**. These cells are long-lived and are responsible for the memory component of the acquired immune response.

Mature **T lymphocytes**

The T lymphocytes (so-called because they complete their maturation in the thymus), bear T cell receptors (**TcRs**) on their surface. As with Ig on B lymphocytes, the TcRs on a single T lymphocyte have identical binding sites .

TcRs **only function** as cell surface receptors for antigen + MHC and the TcRs are not secreted.

In addition to surface TcRs, T lymphocytes possess other characteristic surface proteins:

Thy-1: This protein is the earliest marker of the T cell lineage and is expressed on the surface of all T lymphocytes.

CD_3: The term CD3 refers to a protein complex which is **always** associated with the TcR.

CD_{28}: The receptor for B7 [which is found on the surface of APCs]

CD_{45}: A signal transduction protein which binds to CD_{45L} (CD_{45} ligand) on the surface of antigen presenting cells.

In addition, T helper lymphocytes express **CD_4** on their surface, while T cytotoxic lymphocytes express **CD_8**.

Garlic Vs Stress and /Immune System

Our immune system employs at least four major branches viz;

1. **The B lymphocytes.**
2. **The T lymphocytes,**
3. **The Phagocytes (Macrophages) and**
4. **The Natural killer cells** (See Fig 1). The B lymphocytes respond to various stimuli by producing antibodies, which help fight off many common infections. The other four types of immune cells directly attack foreign invaders, such as cancer cells, bacteria, viruses or fungi. Some carry out their attack by secreting powerful chemicals called cytokines; examples are interferons and interleukins.

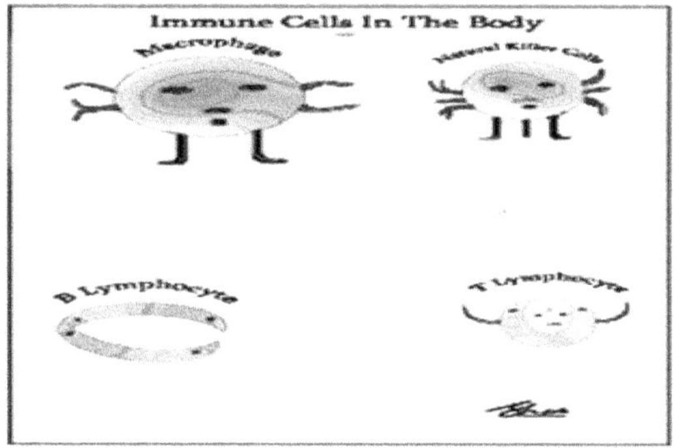

1. Macrophages 2. NK cells
3. T Lymphocytes 4. B Lymphocytes

Fig. 1 Immune Cells are given in clockwise direction.

In our body we have B lymphocytes, T lymphocytes, Macrophages and Natural Killer cells.

Garlic attracts immune cells to the site of injury. Various Nutraceuticals function in a similar way and boost up the immune system. Apart from garlic, onions, ginger, turmeric, apple, pomegranate, mushrooms and various vegetables also contain such nutraceuticals and therefore these are called functional foods.

One paper published by Lau et. al. in 1986 on immunotherapy with corynebacterium parvum and allium sativum for the control of murine transitional cell carcinoma[1,] explained that lymphocytes and macrophages were attracted to the site where garlic was injected. Other researchers have also noticed that garlic extract attracted immune cells.

Garlic Stimulates the Immune Cells

In a second series of experiments Lau's team used three groups of mice. To the first group, they injected 0.1 ml of a 1:2 dilution of kyolic liquid garlic extract subcutaneously in to the inguinal (groin) area. Kyolic is a Japanese preparation of odorless garlic. The second group received 0.1 ml of diluted kyolic liquid garlic extract systemically in to the peritoneal cavity. The third group which served as control did not receive any treatment. Four days after the injection they examined the leukocytes from the peritoneal cavity, spleens and lymphnodes as to how well the leukocytes could engulf and destroy foreign particles by a method of chemiluminescence assay. Compared with the controls the mice which received subcutaneous injection of kyolic showed only slight increase of phagocytic activity with their leukocytes from the peritonial cavity and spleen. However significantly higher activity was obtained with leukocytes from the inguinal lymphnodes.

Again compared with the control the mice which received kyolic intraperitoneally showed increased activity of leukocytes from all three sites; particularly higher with cells from peritonial cavity and spleen. These effects were more than in the inguinal lymphnodes. Obviously if the disease is localized, a localized treatment should be given, where as systemic disease should be treated systemically. In other words systemic therapy shouldn't always be the automatic choice of treatment.

Similar findings have been confirmed in other studies also. One study in Japan showed that certain fractions of kyolic, i.e. odorless garlic extract stimulated macrophages to kill tumor cells and to clear carbon particles from animal's bodies. The same researchers showed

that garlic fractions stimulated B Lymphocytes, the type of cells that produce antibodies[2].

A Florida pathologist Dr. Tarig Abdullah et. al.[3] showed the effect of raw garlic on the action of natural killer cells of human volunteers. He divided the volunteers in to three groups randomly. The first group took 0.5 g/kg body weight of raw garlic everyday for three weeks. The second group took 1.8 g Kyolic (6 capsules) everyday for three weeks. The third group used no garlic and served as controls.

After three weeks the researchers took blood samples from each volunteer and used the blood on tumor cells in a laboratory culture; they wanted to know how active each volunteer's Natural Killer cells were against the tumor cells. The NK cells of those who ate raw garlic killed 139% more tumour cells than those of the control group. The NK cells of those who took Kyolic capsules killed 1.59% more tumour cells than those of the control. Kyolic is an aged form of unheated garlic and it may contain polymerized forms of allyl sulfides like Diallyl Tetrasulfide (DATTS), Ajoene etc. These components may have a better immunostimulating effect than that with raw garlic.

Garlic Vs Stress and Immune System

Through various experiments Lau's team showed the antibiotic[4], antiatherogenic[5], anticarcinogenic[6], heavy metal and toxin detoxification and antiradiation[7] effects of garlic *in vivo* and *in vitro* systems and these findings were reviewed by others elsewhere in this book. Therefore I review only the effects of garlic with relation to stress and immune system of the body.

There are many papers now documenting that stress impairs our immune system, making it difficult for us to fight infection and even cancer[8-10]. Dr Tohru Fuwa and associates[11-13] conducted three studies to unveal the beneficial effects of garlic against stress. Two of them are described below. In the first study the researchers randomly divided mice in to three groups. The first group was subjected to cold temperature (environmental stress); the second group was put in a box that was mounted on an oscillator that shook the box at 129 cycles per minute for 4 hours (Physical Stress). Researchers noted that the stresses caused the mice to behave abnormally, all suffered loss of motor co-ordination, extreme fatigue and loss of appetite. Half of the mice were then given garlic (Kyolic liquid extract) and the experiment was repeated. Those who ate the Kyolic was able to maintain motor co-ordination, recover rapidly from fatigue and function more efficiently than those who did not eat garlic. In another experiment, the researchers restrained a group of mice for 12 hours a day for four consecutive days – an experiment designed to mimic the effects of psychological stress. **At the end of the four days, the mice showed markedly reduced weight of spleen and thymus and markedly fewer B lymphocytes with which to fight infection. In other words, Researchers found that stress can impair the function of the immune system. When part of the mice was supplemented with garlic extract no weight loss occurred and the optimum number of B lymphocytes was restored, boosting the immune system.**

One of the main symptoms of stress, regardless of its source, is lack of energy supply; the victim of stress tires easily, becomes depressed, lacks motivation and is filled with dread. Two groups of Indian scientists tested the effects of garlic on stress induced physical endurance to determine whether garlic could boost endurance. Saxena, Gupta et. al.[14] measured the endurance of rats in terms of their capacity as to how long they can swim in a pond of water before becoming too fatigued to continue. He took one control group and two test groups for garlic juice and its oil respectively.

The control rats who received only saline swarm for an average of 480 Seconds. They were then injected with isoproterenol, a drug that damages the heart muscle and their swimming endurance was again measured and it was an average of 78 seconds only. But the rats that had been fed garlic oil (! mg/day) for seven days swarm for an average of 840 seconds before and 560 seconds !!! after IP injection. The group that was fed with garlic juice (1ml/day) for seven days could swim for 516 seconds and 352 seconds before and after IP injection respectively. **This study proved two things: Garlic principles boosted normal endurance of rats for swimming and again they protected the rats somehow from complete damages of the heart muscles due to IP injection and enabled them to maintain their endurance for swimming to around 65-68%. Dr. Lau repeated this experiment in his laboratory for the benefit of the students and obtained the same results.**

In another set of experiments conducted by Dr. Bordia (Rtd. Cardiologist)[15] and others in RNT Medical College at Udaipur, India, they observed a positive effect of garlic oil on the physical endurance and adaptability in patient's with coronary artery diseases. The effect of six week garlic oil administration was observed on cardiac performance and exercise tolerance in 30 patients of coronary disease. After initial treadmill stress, they were administered garlic oil in the dose of four capsules (around 6 mg) twice a day for six weeks and treadmill test was repeated. Garlic oil significantly ($p < 0.01$) reduced the heart rate at peak exercise and also significantly reduced the workload upon the heart, resulting in better exercise tolerance ($p < 0.05$) as compared to the initial test. Garlic appeared to be a good adaptogen to be utilized in patient's with C.V.D.

Experiment with a Stress Machine

In an effort to measure garlic's effect on stress, Lau's team tested mice with Moloney Sarcoma Virus (MSV) induced tumors[16]. They used a stress machine to test the mice that has MSV tumors. The mice was placed on top of the machine that rotated at 45 rpms for 10 minutes, every hour. Control group of mice was fed a regular diet. Test group's diet was supplemented with 25 mg/day/mouse of a special garlic preparation (SGP powder from Wakunga Pharmaceuticals). At the end of a week they estimated the levels of blood corticoid, the stress hormone that is secreted by the body under stress. The control group's blood showed a corticoid level of 500 ng /ml as against a lowered level of the same at 100 ng/ml for the garlic supplemented group. After the third week the tumor size in each group was measured. Those on a regular diet showed progressive increase in the size of tumors, while those who ate garlic had growth of tumors until the third week, thereafter the size of them decreased steadily.

Further three clinical studies conducted by Japanese workers[17] showed some impact of garlic on stress. In the 1st more than a thousand patients in seven University teaching hospitals were given individually 2 ml Kyolic everyday for four weeks. At the end of four weeks test period 50 to 80% of the patients on Kyolic test suffered less fatigue, depression and anxiety.

A second group involved patients[18] with gynecological malignancies who underwent radiotherapy and or even chemotherapy. Those who took two capsules of Kyolic a day for one to nine months enjoyed significantly fewer side effects from radiotherapy and chemotherapy and 67% of them had absolutely, no side effects.

A third group at Sakitama Hospital[19] involved two groups of hospitalized patients. One group of twenty patients took four capsules of kyolic a day for 50 days, the control group took a placebo only for the same period. At the end of the experiment the kyolic group showed more rapid recovery from exhaustion, had fewer complaints of fatigue after manual labour, and reported less feeling of cold in the extremities than did the placebo group. Interestingly those over fifty years of age benefited more from the Kyolic in terms of endurance possibly because their age group control had a lower level of endurance than that corresponding of the younger group. It is told that the Pharaohs of Egypt used to give Garlic diet to labourers of Pyramid to boost up their stamina. It is assumed that garlic somehow makes more ATP available in the muscle for a continuous work. (or it increases the permeability of ATP into muscle)

Editors' note: When ever I do not get tea at time as my wife is away or busy I grind a single clove of garlic and eat it with a glass of water. It worked wonders within minutes, all my fatigues disappear. Readers can test this claim. This is a 2008-march discovery. For this I thank my wife Alice].

Infection vs Immunity

The three factors influencing infection are, the Etiology (The assignment of a cause or reason), the Susceptible host due to impaired immunity, and Predisposing factors as remarked by Dr.Lau

Mechanisms of Actions of Immune Cells against Infections

It is stated that in a healthy body NK cells are inhibited from killing normal cells because all nucleated normal cells express self class I MHC (Major Histo Compatability Complex) molecules for their protection. But when normal cells becomes infected their class I molecule expression get reduced and inhibitory signals delivered to NK cells are interrupted (i.e. Activation Signal Triggers) and lysis of the infected cell occurs.

Natural Killer cells consist of 10-15 % of Peripheral blood lymphocytes.

It can be considered under the category of Large Granular Lymphocytes.

When a normal cell is infected with virus or undergone malignant transformation the NK cell activating receptors will be expressed more and they will bind with their corresponding elevated ligands (stress induced proteins, viral proteins etc., on the surface of infected cells.

The receptors expressed on the surface of the NK cells include members from NKG_2D and Immunoglobulin supergene families. There on the surface of infected cells ligands include, stress induced proteins, viral proteins, and other protein molecules produced in neoplasm.

NK cells have receptors to bind with ligands of normal cells which are infected.

NK cell is the one of the major cells that is having a defence mechanism against viral infections.

This explains why the NK cells do not cause any damage to normal cells.

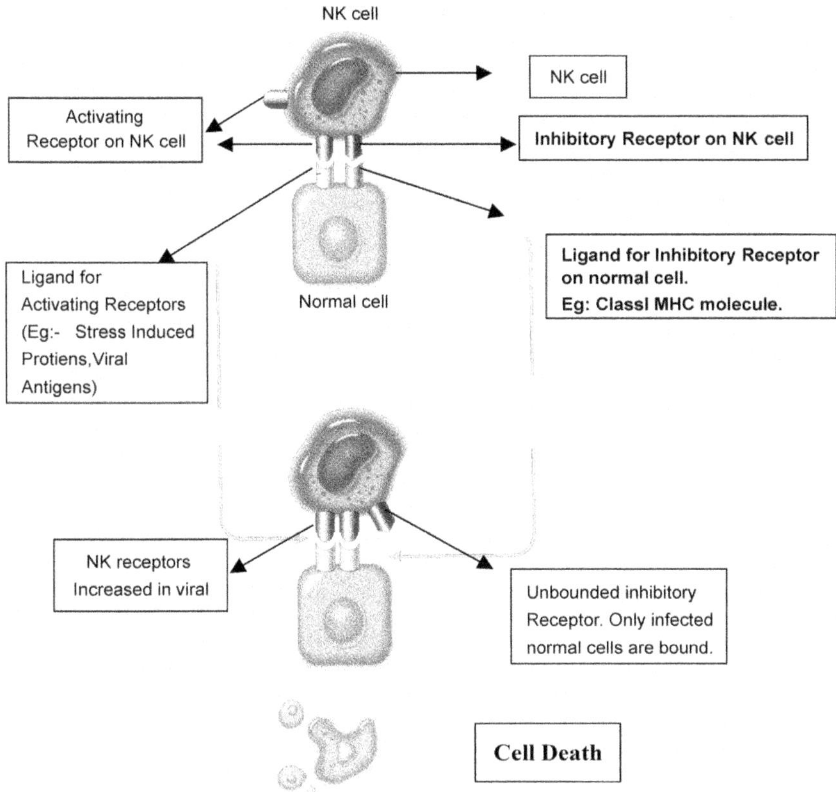

Fig. 2 By killing the viral infected cells, infection is stopped.

Macrophages

Incase of macrophages cytokines control/Modulate the phenotype of macrophages. Immunologically activated macrophages express the capacity to produce antimicrobial products including lyzozyme reactive oxygen and nitrogen species. e.g. NO.

IFNγ (Interferon) characteristically enhances proinflammatory and antimicrobial effects. Interleukin-4 and Interleukin-13 produced by the Macrophages can actvate other immune cells which can kill the infected cells.

Alternative activation of Macrophages promotes humoral immunity and repair process.

Eosinophils mediate cytotoxicity by a process called exocytosis.

The intermediates produced by the eosinophils during the activation damage the virus infected cells.

T and B Lymphocytes

T lymphocytes (both cytotoxic T cells & Helper T cells) and B lymphocyte can mediate damage functions against infectious agents which may be mediated through their cytotoxic effect or antibody dependent mechanisms. There are reports that various nutraceuticals can boost up the functions of immune cells and such nutraceuticals are present in functional foods and mushrooms.

Looking at the mode of infection it does not succeed in infecting a host unless he or she is susceptible. Even if the host is susceptible, the process of infection need to be triggered by certain predisposing factors such as trauma, poor nutrition etc., as suggested by Dr. Lau elsewhere. For this reason, in the prevention or treatment of an infectious disease, we need to look at all three factors rather than just one of them. Merely killing the microbes may not be the best solution. Indeed often carried with it is the price of unwanted side effects. Typical examples are yeast infections such as Candida oral thrush and Candida Vaginitis following the use of a broad spectrum antibiotic.

With respect to the infections from mosquitoes, flies etc., in the tropical countries along with the vector control, good clothing, nutritious and nutraceutical rich food, and pretreatment of underlying diseases are required to contain the infections. Clothing protects the body from insect bites, nutritious food helps the body to build up immunity through synthesis of various immunoglobulins, nutraceuticals through functional foods help the cells to scavenge free radicals, boost up immunity through stimulation of B and T lymphocytes and associated groups such as macrophages, and natural killer cells.

How to Stop Infections like Chikunguniya?

When we plan to stop infections of any nature we have to take into account all the three factors mentioned earlier with equal importance. Not only the government, but also the press, Nongovernmental organizations (NGOS), local authorities and youth organizations should jump in to action and conduct awareness programmes among all the people to control the vectors of the germs, to treat the underlying diseases and to supply to the needy food supplements containing the nutraceuticals mentioned above, clothing and a square meal if needed free or at a reasonable price.

In order to boost up the immunoresponse a Chinese made food supplement is very good. For this ginger-garlic food supplement should be made as a paste without addition of any water in the ratio of 1:4 by weight. Keep it in vinegar or add little black pepper powder and salt to improve its taste and action. According to the Senior editor Dr. Augusti daily intake of half a tea spoon of it (for two weeks) along with food protected many from the infection of jaundice and viral fever raged Kerala during 2006 and 2007. This food supplement also cured the inflammation and pains of many viral infected patients in Kerala as claimed by Dr. Augusti.

Garlic is rated as the best functional food against all the above diseases as it can inhibit the growth of microbes, enhance the function of phagocytes, and natural killer cells. In addition to that garlic nullifies some of the toxins that impair the immune system. In order to protect the heart garlic[21] and ginger[22] lower the serum lipids, platelet aggregation, hardening of blood vessel, and inflammations of various types. In China a garlic ginger food supplement is used widely to fight viral infections[23] from the time of Ming dynasty (14th Century).

Functional Foods

Further garlic enhances weight reduction, vasodilation, blood fibrinolysis and thinning of blood[6,24,25]. Ginger, turmeric, onions, garlic and black pepper, the major food adjuncts of the East contain many antioxidants. Antioxidants play a big role in containing infections, radiations and lipid peroxidations. Further Garlic is a proved medicine to prevent cancer generating compounds like nitrates, DMBA, benzopyrene etc[24]. Ginger and black peper, two important ingredients in the ayurvedic preparations of India, warrant further study for their actions against viruses, CHD, cancer etc. However all these functional foods should be tested separately as well as in combined form to stop infections of the diseases like jaundice, chikunguniya, dengue fever and related viral fevers occassionaly raging the tropical areas like India.

According to the work of Drs Lau, Augusti and others garlic detoxifies the system of heavy metal (like lead) poisoning, protects against irradiation and even kills microbes[25]. Have you had your garlic today? Dr. Augusti, our teacher, takes it everyday from 2000. It keeps him energetic and free of infections at his old age. It is advisable for everybody above the age of 50 to use one functional food a day atleast.

References

1. Lau, BHS; Woolley. JT. et. al. Superiority of intralesional immunotherapy with Corynebacterium parvum and Allium sativum in control of murine transitional cell carcinoma. J.Urol, 136(1986)701.

2. Hirao, Y; Sumioka, I, et. al. Activation of immunoresponder cells by the protein fraction from aged garlic extract. Phytotherapy Res, 1(1987)161.

3. Kandil, OM; Abdullah, TH;Elkadi, A; Garlic and the immune system in humans: Its effect on natural killer cells.Federation Proceedings 46(1987)441.

4. Adetumbi, MA; Javor, GT; Lau BHS. Alliium sativum (garlic) inhibits lipid synthesis by Candida albicans. Antimicrob Agents.Chemother 30(1986)499.

5. (a) Lau, BHS; Lam F; Wang-Cheng, R. Efeect of an odor modified garlic preparation on blood lipids. Nutr Res. 7(1987)139.

   (b) Lau, BHS; Lam F. Lipid lowering action of garlic oil on lipid fed rats.Nutr Res.5(1986)223.

6. Lau, BHS; Marsh, CL. et. al. Effects of biological response modifies on marine bladder tumour.Nat Immune Cell Growth Regul4(1985)260

7. Lau, BHS. Detoxifying, radioprotective and phagocyte-enhancing effects of garlic.Intern Clin. Nutr Rev9(1987)27.

8. Ader, R. Psychoneuroimmunology. Academic Press. 1981.

9. Riley. V. Psychoneuroendocrine influence on immunocompetence and neoplasia. Science212(1981)1100.

10. Max, JL. The immune system 'Belongs in the body'. Science 227(1985)1190.

11. Taka Sugi, N; Kotook et. al. Effect of garlic on mice exposed to various stresses. Oyo Yakuri-Pharmacometrics 28 (1984)991.

12. Taka Sugi N, Kira, K and Fuwa, T. Effects of garlic extract preparation containing vitamin B1 on mice exposed to stresses. Oyo Yakuri-Pharmacometrics, 31 (1986)967.

13. Yokoyma, K; Uda, N et. al. Antistress effects of garlic extract preparation containing vitamins and ginsung-garlic preparation containing vitamin B_1 in mice. Oyo-Yakuri-Pharmacometrics31(1986)977.

14. Saxena, KK; Gupta, B et. al. Effects of garlic pretreatment on isoprenaline-induced myocardial necrosis in albino rats. Indian J Physiol Pharmac 24(1980)233.

15. Verma, SK; Rajeevan, V; Jain P and Bordia A. Effects of garlic (Allium sativum) oil on exercise tolerance in patients with coronary artery disease. Indian J Physiol Pharmacol 49 (1) 2005,115.

16. Lau BHS. in garlic for health. Stress- the hidden cause of disease. 1988.pp.51,59. Lotus Light Publications. P.O. Box 2, Wilmot, w1. 53192.

17. Hiroshima University group (G. Kajiama), Clinical studies of Kyoleopin.Japanese J Clin Rep 16(1982)1515.

18. Tanaka, M; Clinical studies of kyleopin on complaints following treatment of gynecological malignancies. Japanese J. New Remedies 31(1982)1349.

19. Hasegawa, Y; Kikuchi N, et. al. Clinical effects of *kyoleopin a*gainst various complaints in the field of intestinal medicine.Japanese J New Remedies. 32(1983)365.

20. Lau, BHS. Garlic Research Update. 1991.P.24. Published by Odyssey Publishing Inc.2135.West 45th AvenueVancouver, B.C., CanadaV_2 M_2T_2.

21. Bordia A; Joshi, H.K et. al. Effect of essential oil of garlic on serum fibrinolytic activity in patients with coronary artery disease. Atherosclerosis 28(1977)155.

22. Verma, SK; Bordia, A; Jain, P and Srivastava, KC. Antioxidant property of ginger in patients with coronary artery disease. South Asian Jour Preventive Cardiology 8(4)2004.199.

23. Compendium Of Materia Medica Of the Ming dynasty, Palmlet supplied by Beijing Sanbao New Technology Dev. Centre Of Chinese Acad. Sci. at the 4th International Symposium on edible Alliaceac in Nov.2004 which was attended by Dr.K.T.Agusti.

24. Block, E. The organo sulfur chemistry of the Genus Allium – Implications for the organic chemistry of sulfur. Angew Chem Insta. Ed. Engl.31(1992)1135.

25. Proceedings of the National seminar on the Evaluation of Nutraceuticals that prevent diseases. Nov 29th to 2nd December, 2006. Thalassery campus of Kannur University. PP 27-170.

Reference Books

Books Referred : Immunology (Ivan.P.Roitt)- 7th Edition- page no .249

Immunology (Kuby) Richard Goldsby et. al. (editors) 6th edition – page no. 464

Pathologic basis of diseases (Robbins) – Kumar and Abbas (Editors) – 7th edition – page 201 - 202

Chapter – 8

Cancer and Ageing – Causation and Prevention

8.1 Three decades of Garlic Research

Dr. Benjamin H.S. Lau, M.D., Ph.D. (Emeritus Professor)
School of Medicine, Loma Linda University,
Loma Linda, California 92350, U.S.A.
E-mail: blau2005@sbcglobal.net

Garlic is a common plant used as a food item in many different cultures of the world. For thousands of years it has been used as a folk remedy for a variety of ailments. However, only in the past several decades has it been subjected to scientific scrutiny. A recent computer search reveals more than 2,000 references published in the last three decades on various aspects of garlic research. In this paper, I would like to summarize the research conducted by my colleagues, students, postdoctoral fellows, and myself over a period of three decades in four major areas: 1. Antimicrobial effects, 2. Cancer control, 3. Cardiovascular health, and 4. Anti-aging and life-extension potentials.

Antimicrobial Effects

My associates and I at Loma Linda University have been involved in immunology research with special interest in finding means for preventing diseases. This is how I was introduced to garlic research.

As I was visiting a physician friend in his home, he told me that he had used garlic in his practice and that his patients had enjoyed relief from a variety of complaints. In the course of our conversation, he mentioned that garlic is a potent antibiotic and inhibitor of many germs. As a professor of microbiology, I began devising in my mind a test to find out if my friend was right. At the time, my students and I were doing experiments testing the activity of several new antibiotics on bacteria and fungi. **Upon returning to my laboratory, I prepared diluted garlic extract, introduced a small quantity into several bacterial cultures and let them incubate overnight. The next day I was astounded to find that the diluted garlic extract did indeed stop the growth of those bacteria — more effectively, in fact, than some of the potent antibiotics we were testing at that time.**

I shared the finding with my doctoral student, Moses Adetumbi, who immediately went to the library to check out the literature. He found that a number of papers had already been published by microbiologists and other researchers, showing garlic to be a potent broad-spectrum antibiotic. We wrote a paper, "*Allium sativum* (garlic) – a natural antibiotic"[1] and were gratified to receive many requests for that paper.

Dr. Adetumbi, now a professor at Johns Hopkins University, performed several studies demonstrating that garlic can efficiently stop the growth of *Candida albicans*[2], an important yeast organism, and *Coccidioides immitis*, a mold which causes "Valley Fever" in the western United States[3]. He also found out that garlic stops the growth of microorganisms by preventing their synthesis of lipids, important constituents of the cell membrane, which is vital for these organisms[2].

Cancer Control

My associates and I have studied bladder cancer in animals, with the interest of building up the animals' immunity to fight cancer. We studied BCG (a live bacterial vaccine) and *Corynebacterium parvum* (a killed bacterial vaccine), and decided to include garlic extract in our testing. In the articles we published in the *Journal of Urology*[4,5], we showed that treatment with a garlic extract prevented bladder cancer more effectively than the vaccines did. **Garlic apparently stimulates the immune system, particularly enhancing the lymphocytes and macrophages[6], the body's anti-cancer militia, to destroy cancer cells. Our studies also showed that the best results were obtained when garlic was exposed directly to the tumor site. In another experiment, we gave animals five treatments of garlic extract instead of one and were surprised to find these treatments actually cured the cancer[4].**

Another aspect of garlic that has intrigued researchers pertains to its potential effects against carcinogenesis or cancer development. One of my doctoral students, Padma Tadi, now a professor at Loma Linda University School of Public Health, pursued the study of anticarcinogenic activity using two *in vitro* assays: a "mutagenesis assay" which determines if a chemical can cause a change in chromosomes in the direction of cancer formation, and a "DNA-binding assay" which determines if a chemical can attach itself to the DNA of chromosomes leading to cancer development. **Dr. Tadi has identified compounds in garlic that inhibit mutagenesis induced by the carcinogen benzo[a]pyrene, found in charcoal-broiled**

meat, cigarette smoke, and air pollutants[7,8] and aflatoxin B_1[9], a fungal toxin which is also a liver carcinogen. She also found garlic compounds prevent these chemical carcinogens from binding to DNA and thus nullifying their effects in causing cancer[10].

Dr. Takeshi Yamasaki, a postdoctoral fellow from Japan, has been interested in a phenolic compound allixin, a phytoalexin produced by garlic. Plants do not have immune system. They produce bioactive chemicals to protect themselves from pathogens and insect pests. These chemicals are called "phytoalexins" (phyto = plant, alexin = to ward off) and they are major weapons for plant defense. Dr. Yamasaki showed that allixin inhibited mutagenesis induced by aflatoxin B_1 and also prevented its binding to calf thymus DNA[11]. **The effect of allixin on aflatoxin B_1-induced mutagenesis and DNA binding was shown to be mediated through an inhibition of microsomal P-450 enzymes, suggesting that allixin may be useful in the chemoprevention of cancer.**

It is now recognized that a great majority of human cancers, perhaps as many as 80-90%, are attributable to environmental factors[12-14]. A number of these factors have been identified, such as the association between smoking and lung cancer, and high fat intake with breast, colon, and several other malignancies[15-17]. More recently, high intake of dairy products has been linked to increased incidence of ovarian cancer in females and prostate cancer in males[18, 19].

While modern surgery has significantly reduced cancer mortality, the use of additional treatment modalities such as radiotherapy and chemotherapy have resulted in no more than a 5% reduction in the number of death[20]. It is apparent, then, that the most economical means of cancer control lies in prevention. Thus, dietary modification has been considered a powerful and cost-effective method for reducing cancer risks. **Dietary factors which may lower cancer risks have been identified. Examples include dietary fiber, cruciferous vegetables and antioxidant vitamins and minerals[21-23].**

In our review of world literature on the role of garlic in cancer prevention[24], we noted, from epidemiological studies, an inverse relationship between garlic consumption and death rate for gastrointestinal cancers, suggesting a role for garlic in the prevention of human cancer. In animal studies, garlic has been shown to inhibit the growth of transplantable tumors and to reduce the incidence of certain spontaneously-occurring tumors. Garlic compounds have also been found to inhibit the activity of diverse chemical carcinogens during both the initiation and promotion phases of carcinogenesis. There is also evidence that components of garlic modulate specific and nonspecific anti-cancer immunity.

It appears that garlic may be a candidate as a dietary anticarcinogen for cancer prevention. Garlic may exert its protective effects in three ways: 1. A direct inhibition of tumor cell metabolism – this is useful when the tumor size or number of tumor cells is small; 2. Inhibition of the initiation and/or promotion phases of carcinogenesis – this may well turn out to be the most promising aspect of garlic; and 3. Modulating host immune response – this effect, of course, is useful in all phases of cancer control[24].

Cardiovascular Health

Among the various medicinal properties of garlic, the effects on blood lipids and blood coagulation have received the most interest. My associates and I published a paper "*Allium sativum* (garlic) and atherosclerosis: a review"[25], and were indeed very much surprised to receive more than 1,000 requests from nearly every university in the world for that paper! In this paper we reviewed world literature published in English showing that garlic consumption lowers cholesterol and triglycerides in the blood, prevents blood clotting and thus prevents heart attacks and strokes.

Since then, more reports confirming these findings have appeared in the literature. We have come across only a few studies that reported an absence of effect of garlic on lipids or blood coagulation. These studies showing "no effects" used commercially prepared garlic tablets or capsules which probably lacked active components. **By and large, the majority of the research reports beneficial effects of garlic on prevention of diseases of the heart and blood vessels, and several studies also report lowering of blood pressure as I have summarized these findings in a book chapter[26].**

One of the problems of using garlic is the odor, which is not universally welcomed by everyone, so my associates and I decided to conduct a research experiment using an odor-modified garlic extract (Kyolic) prepared by a Japanese pharmaceutical company. The results were published in *Nutrition Research*[27]. **Lowering of cholesterol, triglycerides, low density and very low density lipoproteins (LDL and VLDL) with rise of high density lipoprotein (HDL) was observed in the majority of subjects who took garlic extract; the effect was clearly more significant than with subjects taking placebo.** Garlic extract did not significantly influence the levels of cholesterol and triglycerides in subjects whose initial cholesterol levels were relatively low. Of special interest was the initial rise of cholesterol and triglycerides with garlic supplementation, suggesting possible mobilization of tissue lipids into the circulation during this phase of garlic ingestion. This study shows that odor-modified garlic preparation "Kyolic" may be used in conjunction with dietary modification for control of hyperlipidemia.

Cardiovascular diseases (heart attacks and strokes) are the major cause of death in all affluent societies. Three main groups of risk factors have been recognized: diet related, lifestyle related, and uncontrollable factors[28-30]. Lifestyle-related risk factors include smoking, inactivity, and stress. The uncontrollable factors include heredity, gender, and age. Cardiovascular risk is greater for men than for premenopausal women. As a person ages, there is a greater risk of cardiovascular disease. Studies have now suggested that even these so-called uncontrollable factors can actually be controlled or modified[31,32]. **S-allyl cysteine (a garlic compound), for example, has been shown to regulate transcriptional factors that are required for gene expression[33, 34]. Hence, dietary modification may help keep undesirable genes suppressed.**

The most prominent cardiovascular disease risk factors are diet related. Hyperlipidemia has long been considered a major risk factor for atherosclerosis[35], and lowering cholesterol can significantly reduce the risk for cardiovascular diseases. Oxidation of LDL has recently been recognized as playing an important role in the initiation and progression of atherosclerosis[36, 37]. Oxidized LDL, but not native LDL, promotes vascular dysfunction by exerting direct cytotoxicity to endothelial cells, by increasing chemotactic properties of monocytes, by transforming macrophages to foam cells, and enhancing the proliferation of endothelial cells, monocytes, and muscle cells[38]; all of these events contribute to the vascular dysfunction leading to atherogenesis[39]. **In a series of studies, we demonstrated that several garlic compounds can minimize LDL oxidation *in vitro*[40-43]. Short-term supplementation of garlic in human subjects has demonstrated an increased resistance of LDL to oxidation[44]. Our data thus suggest that suppressed LDL oxidation may be one possible mechanism that contributes to the beneficial effects of garlic in cardiovascular health.**

Anti-Oxidant and Anti-Aging Potentials

In this most recent past decade, my associates and I have been actively engaged in investigating the antioxidant properties of garlic. We found a number of garlic compounds are potent antioxidants. Using bovine pulmonary artery endothelial cells as a model, we demonstrated that aged garlic extract (Kyolic), S-allyl cysteine, fructosyl arginine, and several other minor garlic compounds can protect endothelial cells from oxidant-induced injury[45,46]. Aged garlic extract (Kyolic) was shown to modulate glutathione redox cycle and superoxide dismutase activity in vascular endothelial cells[47]. It was further shown to inhibit the generation of free radicals (hydrogen peroxide and superoxide anion), and at the same time, to increase the levels and activity of endogenous antioxidant enzymes[48]. Allicin, an unstable garlic compound, was however, shown to be an oxidant rather than an antioxidant[39, 40, 44].

The antioxidant properties of garlic compounds prompted us to look into the anti-aging potentials of garlic. Using PC12 cells as a model for studying Alzheimer's disease, aged garlic extract and S-allyl cysteine were shown to protect neuronal cells from amyloid-β peptide-induced apoptosis, suggesting the neuroprotective role of garlic[49].

Our colleagues in China and Japan have already reported that aged garlic extract improved declined immune function, learning behavior, memory, and life span in senescence-accelerated mice – genetically established mice used for studying aging and spontaneous senescence[50-52]. *Among theories attempting to explain aging process, the free radical theory[53] and the neuroendocrine theory[54] appear to be most promising. The first theory maintains that aging is the result of accumulation of free radical oxidants and thus antioxidants such as garlic compounds can delay the aging process. In the neuroendocrine theory, it is believed that the decline of thymic hormone and growth hormone accelerates the aging process.* **Using genetically-engineered human keratinocytes, we showed that Kyolic garlic extract and S-allyl cysteine isolated from garlic significantly increased the secretion of human growth hormone *in vitro*[55]. It will be interesting to determine if garlic supplementation can actually increase the level of growth hormone in humans.**

Conclusion – The Triangle of Disease

To conclude this paper, I would like to share with the readers an important concept that I have used in my teaching of immunology and medical microbiology. This concept is called "The Triangle of Disease" (see Fig.1).

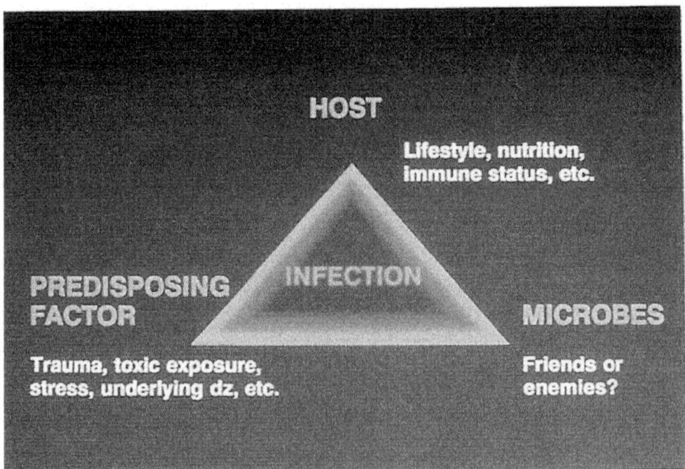

Fig.1 Top Corner (1) Life style, nutrition, immune status, etc. (2) Bottom right. Microbes, Friends or enemies. (3) Bottom left. Predisposing factors, Trauma, toxic exposure, stress, underlying diseases, etc.

The disease process can be illustrated using a triangle. The three angles are: the etiology (Webster defines it as "the assignment of a cause or reason"), the susceptible host, and predisposing factors. If we use infection as an example, the three angles are: (1) microbes as the etiological agent; (2) a susceptible host or a person who is susceptible because of impaired immunity, poor nutrition and/or a risky lifestyle determining the susceptibility; and (3) certain factors such as trauma, toxic exposure, stress and underlying disease which predispose a person to infection.

Looking at the triangle, one needs to recognize that microorganisms alone do not usually cause infection unless there is a susceptible host, even though we give the textbook definition of infection as an invasion of the body by microorganisms. The concept that I want to emphasize is that microorganisms alone do not usually cause infection unless there is a susceptible human being or animal. Having said that, let me hasten to add that even with a susceptible host and the presence of microbes, there still may not be an infection unless the process is triggered by certain predisposing factors. For this reason, in the prevention or treatment of an infectious disease, we need to look at all these three angles rather than just one of these angles. Conventional "wisdom" is to take antibiotics if you have an infection. This practice may lead to undesirable consequences. Merely killing the microbes may not be the best solution. Indeed often carried with it is the price of unwanted side effects. Typical examples are yeast infections such as *Candida* oral thrush and *Candida* vaginitis following the use of a broad spectrum antibiotic.

In the case of infection we obviously need to consider the microbes as the primary factor, and the host and predisposing factors as secondary factors. However, it is equally important to bear in mind when considering a disease that all three angles have equal weight or significance. An example of a clinical entity I often use with my medical students is diarrhea. It has been estimated that in the world each day there are 20 million people suffering from diarrhea. We all know that often our diarrhea is simply due to eating the wrong kind of food. In other words, it may not have anything to do with the microbes. In the figure under microbes, I have "friends or enemies". The point is that it may not be easy to know which microbe is the enemy and which is the friend. For example, a person eats the wrong kind of food and has diarrhea. If he consults a physician and gets a course of antibiotic, he will be killing friendly bacteria without touching the enemy at all, since there may not be any enemy to begin with.

Looking at the third angle, the predisposing factors, it is my practice to constantly remind my students that this angle is a very important one. It too may be the primary cause of a complaint, rather than secondary. Again, take the complaint of diarrhea. It is true that we do not want to miss those germs like *Salmonella*, *Shigella*, *Campylobacter*, and *Vibrio* that are famous intestinal pathogens. What I want to remind my students is that before they write a prescription for a potent drug, find out and *study* what drugs the patient has been taking. In my own experience, I have seen case after case of patients complaining of diarrhea or other gastrointestinal discomfort due to one or more drugs received from a doctor. Many drugs have gastrointestinal side effects. So the emphasis is: each of the three angles can have equal importance.

It is important to point out that the triangle and its basic principle applies not only to infection but also to most, if not all, major diseases inflicting the human race. For example, we can change the entity from infection to cancer and all we need to modify is just one of the angles – adding chemical carcinogens and radiation to the microbes (the three best known causes of cancer are carcinogens, radiation, and viruses). With that in mind, the prevention and treatment of cancer should thus encompass all three angles. Merely killing the viruses is not the solution. For that matter, current methods of focusing only at killing cancer cells is neither adequate nor desirable. One needs to strengthen the host and to remove the predisposing factors in order to obtain a satisfactory and lasting results[56].

In a book entitled ***The Ministry of Healing*** written by Ellen G. White a century ago[57], there is this statement: "In case of sickness, the cause should be ascertained. Unhealthful condition should be changed, wrong habits corrected. Then nature is to be assisted in her effort to expel impurities and to re-establish right conditions in the system." Let us apply this statement to our triangle. In case of sickness (again, let's say in this case we are dealing with infection), we are to do five things:

1. Cause should be ascertained (not just the microbes but the whole triangle).
2. Unhealthful conditions should be changed (this means maybe we need to change our lifestyle).
3. Wrong habits should be corrected (including dietary habits).
4. Assist nature to expel impurities (such as toxic exposure).
5. Re-establish right conditions in the system (we need to cooperate with nature and allow our body to heal itself).

Now, some may ask: "What does garlic have to do with all these?" Please note point number four again. Garlic can help our bodies expel impurities – garlic has been shown to detoxify the system of heavy metal poisoning[58], protect against irradiation[58], and of course, kill microbes[1]. Looking at the triangle again, we see that components of

garlic actually encompass all these three angles. It is amazing that nature has provided us with such an "all around" product that is useful for one's health.

Recently, I made a presentation of our garlic research to a large group of physicians and pharmacists visiting California. At the end of my presentation, I used the word "GARLIC" as an acronym to summarize its major health benefits:

G – Good for many things

A – Antioxidant and anti-aging effects

R – Restoration of memory

L – Life extension

I – Immune modulation

C – Cancer control/prevention

Garlic, especially when used in conjunction with a healthful lifestyle, can indeed enhance our health and well being. Satisfy all the needs of the points mised by the corners of the triangle.

(Editors)

References

1. Adetumbi MA, Lau BHS. 1983. *Allium sativum* (garlic) – a natural antibiotic. Medical Hypothesis 12:227-237.
2. Adetumbi MA, Javor GT, Lau BHS. 1986. *Allium sativum* (garlic) inhibits lipid synthesis by *Candida albicans*. Antimicrob Agents Chemother 30:499-501.
3. Adetumbi MA, Lau BHS. 1986. Inhibition of *in vitro* germination and spherulation of *Coccidioides immitis* by *Allium sativum*. Current Microbiol 13:73-76.
4. Lau BHS, Woolley JL, Marsh CL, Barker GR, Koobs DH, Torrey RR. 1986. Superiority of intralesional immunotherapy with *Corynebacterium parvum* and *Allium sativu*m in control of murine transitional cell carcinoma. J Urol 136:701-705.
5. Marsh CL, Torrey RR, Woolley JL, Barker GR, Lau BHS. 1987. Superiority of intravesical immunotherapy with *Corynebacterium parvum* and *Allium sativum* in control of murine bladder cancer. J Urol 137:359-362.
6. Lau BHS, Yamasaki T, Gridley, DS. 1991. Garlic compounds modulate macrophage and T-lymphocyte function. Mol Biother 3:103-107.

7. Tadi PP, Teel RW, Lau BHS. 1990. Anticandidal and anticarcinogenic potentials of garlic. Int Clin Nutr Rev 10:423-429.
8. Lau BHS. 1991. Garlic Research Update. Odyssey Publishing Inc., Canada.
9. Tadi PP, Teel RW, Lau BHS. 1991. Organosulfur compounds of garlic modulate mutagenesis, metabolism, and DNA binding of aflatoxin B_1. Nutr Cancer 15:87-95.
10. Tadi PP, Lau BHS, Teel RW, Herrmann CE. 1991. Binding of aflatoxin B_1 to DNA inhibited by ajoene and diallyl sulfide. Anticancer Res 11:450-454.
11. Yamasaki T, Teel RW, Lau BHS. 1991. Effect of allixin, a phytoalexin produced by garlic, on mutagenesis, DNA-binding and metabolism of aflatoxin B_1. Cancer Lett 59:89-94.
12. Doll R. 1977. Strategy for detection of cancer hazards to man. Nature 265:589-596.
13. Doll R, Peto R. 1981. The causes of cancer: quantitative estimates of avoidable risks of cancer in the United States today. J Natl Cancer Inst 66:1193-1308.
14. Epstein S. 1974. Environmental determinants of human cancer. Cancer Res 34:2425-2435.
15. Loeb LA, Ernster VL, Warner KE, Abbots J, Laszo J. 1984. Cancer Res 44:5940-5958.
16. Wynder EL. 1976. Nutrition and cancer. Fed Proc 35:1309-1315.
17. Willett WC, MacMahon B. 1984. Diet and cancer – an overview. New Eng J Med 310:633-638, 697-703.
18. Larsson SC, Orsini N, Wolk A. 2006. Milk, milk products and lactose intake and ovarian cancer risk: a meta-analysis of epidemiological studies. Int J Cancer 118:431-441.
19. Chan JM, Giovannucci EL. 2001. Dairy products, calcium, and vitamin D and risk of prostate cancer. Epidemiol Rev 23: 87-92.
20. Cairns J. 1985. The treatment of disease and the war against cancer. Sci Am 253:31-39.
21. Fiala ES, Reddy BS, Weisburger JH. 1985. Naturally occurring anticarcinogenic substances in foodstuffs. Ann Rev Nutr 5:295-321.
22. Wattenberg LW. 1985. Chemoprevention of cancer, Cancer Res 45:1-8.

23. Ames BN. 1983. Dietary carcinogens and anticarcinogens. Science 221:1256-1264.

24. Lau BHS, Tadi PP, Tosk JM. 1990. *Allium sativum* (garlic) and cancer prevention. Nutr Res 10:937-948.

25. Lau BHS, Adetumbi MA, Sanchez A. 1983. *Allium sativum* (garlic) and atherosclerosis: a review. Nutr Res 3:119-128.

26. Lau BHS. 1989. Anticoagulant and lipid regulating effects of garlic (*Allium sativum*). In: New Protective Roles of Selected Nutrients in Human Nutrition. Gene A. Spiller and James Scala, editors, Alan R. Liss, Publishers, p. 295-325.

27. Lau BHS, Lam F, Wang-Cheng R. 1987. Effect of an odor-modified garlic preparation on blood lipids. Nutr Res7:139-149.

28. Howard G, Wagenknecht LE, Burke GL, Diez-Roux A, Evans GW, McGovem P, Nieto FJ, Tell GS. 1998. Cigarette smoking and progression of atherosclerosis: the atherosclerosis risk in communities (ARIC) study, JAMA 279:119-124.

29. Steyn K, Steyn M, Swanepoel AS, Jordaan PC, Jooste PL, Fourie JM, Rossouw JE. 1997. Twelve-year results of the coronary risk factor study (CORIS). Int J Epidemiol 26:964-971.

30. Villeneuve PJ, Morrison HI, Craig CL, Schaubel DE. 1998. Physical activity, physical fitness, and risk of dying. Epidemiology 9:626-631.

31. Gomez del Arco P, Martinez-Martinez S, Calvo V, Armessilla AL, Redondo JM. 1997. Antioxidants and AP-1 activation: a brief overview. Immunobiology198:273-278.

32. Waleh NS, Calaoagan J, Murphy BJ, Knapp AM, Sutherland RM, Laderoute KR. 1998. The redox-sensitive human antioxidant responsive element induces gene expression under low oxygen conditions. Carcinogenesis 19:1333-1337.

33. Geng Z, Rong Y, Lau BHS. 1997. S-allyl cysteine inhibits activation of nuclear factor kappa B in human T cells. Free Radic Biol Med 23:345-350.

34. Ide N, Lau BHS. 2001. Garlic compounds minimize intracellular oxidative stress and inhibit nuclear factor κB activation. J Nutr 131:1020S-1026S.

35. Kannel WB, Castelli WP, Gordon T, McNamara PM. 1971. Serum cholesterol, lipoproteins, and the risk of coronary heart disease. The Framingham study. Ann Intern Med 74:1-12.

36. Steinberg D, Parthasarathy S, Carew TE, Khoo JC, Witztum JL. 1989. Beyond cholesterol, modifications of low-density lipoprotein that increase its atherogenicity. New Engl J Med 320:915-924.

37. Steinberg D.1997. Low density lipoprotein oxidation and its pathobiological significance. J Biol Chem 272:20963-20966.

38. Chan AC. 1998. Vitamin E and atherosclerosis. J Nutr 128:1593-1596.

39. Lau BHS. 2001. Suppression of LDL oxidation by garlic. J Nutr 131:985S-988S.

40. Ide N, Nelson AB, Lau BHS. 1997. Aged garlic extract and its constituents inhibit Cu^{2+}-induced oxidative modification of low density lipoprotein. Planta Medica 63:263-264.

41. Ide N, Lau BHS. 1997. Garlic compounds protect vascular endothelial cells from oxidized low density lipoprotein-induced injury. J Pharm Pharmacol 49:908-911.

42. Ide N, Lau BHS. 1999. Aged garlic extract attenuates intracellular oxidative stress. Phytomedicine 6:125-131.

43. Ho SE, Ide N, Lau BHS. 2001. S-allyl cysteine reduces oxidant load in cells involved in the atherogenic process. Phytomedicine 8:39-46.

44. Lau BHS. 2006. Suppression of LDL oxidation by garlic compounds is a possible mechanism of cardiovascular health benefit. J Nutr 136:765S-768S.

45. Yamasaki T, Li L, Lau BHS. 1994. Garlic compounds protect vascular endothelial cells from hydrogen peroxide-induced oxidant injury. Phytotherapy Res 8:408-412.

46. Ide N, Lau BHS, Ryu K, Matsuura H, Itakura Y. 1999. Antioxidant effects of fructosyl arginine, a Maillard reaction product in aged garlic extract. J Nutr Biochem 10:372-376.

47. Geng Z, Lau BHS. 1997. Aged garlic extract modulates glutathione redox cycle and superoxide dismutase activity in vascular endothelial cells. Phytotherapy Res 11:54-56.

48. Wei ZH, Lau BHS. 1998. Garlic inhibits free radical generation and augments antioxidant enzyme activity in vascular endothelial cells. Nutr Res 18:61-70.

49. Peng Q, Buz'Zard AR, Lau BHS. 2002. Neuroprotective effect of garlic compounds in amyloid-β peptide-induced apoptosis *in vitro*. Med Sci Monit 8:328-337.

50. Zhang YX, Saito H, Nishiyama N. 1994. Ameliorating effect of aged garlic extract (AGE) on learning behaviors in thymectomized senescence accelerated mice. Proceedings of the First International Conference on Senescence, p. 451-453.

51. Moriguchi T, Takashina K, Chu PJ, Saito H, Nishiyama N. 1994. Prolongation of life span and improved learning in the senescence accelerated mouse produced by aged garlic extract. Biol Pharm Bull 17:1589-1594.

52. Nishiyama N, Moriguchi T, Saito H. 1997. Beneficial effects of aged garlic extract on learning and memory impairment in senescence-accelerated mouse. Exp Gerontol 32:149-160.

53. Harman D. 2006. Free radicals: aging and disease. Ann N Y Acad Sci 1067:10-21.

54. Cuneo RC, Salomon F, McGauley GA, Sonksen PH. 1992. The growth hormone deficiency syndrome in adults, Clin Endocrinol (Oxford) 37:387-397.

55. Buz'Zard AR, Peng Q, Lau BHS. 2002. Kyolic and Pycnogenol increase human growth hormone secretion in genetically-engineered keratinocytes. Growth Hormone IGF Res 12:34-40.

56. Lau BHS. 1998. Garlic and You – The Modern Medicine. Apple Publishing Co., Canada.

57. White EG. 1905. The Ministry of Healing. Pacific Press, Mountain View, California, p. 127.

58. Lau, BHS. 1989. Detoxifying, radioprotective and phagocyte-enhancing effects of garlic. Int Clin Nutr Rev 9:27-31.

N.B Recently Dr. Ritu Singh, of the Dept. of Lady Harding Medical College, Delhi narrated to the chief editor as to what way her maternal grand father cured his T.B in the early 1940s when there was no proper drug available or effective against T.B. On some body's advice he started consuming more than 30 g of fresh garlic syrup daily for a year or so and look !!! the patches on his lungs slowly disappeared and he looked very healthy. However he continued this practice throughout his life and he lived as a T.B. free man to the surprise of many. This claim by Ritu Singh came when the editor quoted the works of Dr. Lau and himself at a Seminar at Tirupati on detoxification of lead and other heavy metals by garlic oil (22-23 Dec.2007).

8.2 Role of Food components in the Causation and Prevention of Cancer – A Review

Dr. M. Iqbal Ahammed,
Director, Malabar Cancer Centre, Thalassery,

Dr. K.T. Augusti & P. Faizal,
SHS of Kannur University, Thalassery Campus, Kerala

Traditionally the causative factors for the incidence of cancer are radiation, chemical carcinogens and viruses. These factors one way or other bring about mutation in genes and induce cancer. i.e. uncontrolled multiplication of cells in the animal body. It is known that in everybody's body there are hundreds of thousands of genes and many of them find expression only when the conditions are ripe for its action. Oncogenes or tumour producing genes belong to a particular category that is triggered only by agents like radiation, carcinogens and viruses. The oncogenes are segments of DNA, like any other gene and mutation i.e. knocking out of certain bases in the DNA that changes the order of bases and thus the code in the genetic material, alters the expression pattern of the genes. This situation may lead to deficiency of certain enzymes and over production of some other enzymes thus changing the character of the cells.

Virus can direct the synthesis of new DNAs as copies of its genetic material (DNA or RNA)and incorporate them into the host's cellular DNA. All these processes change the position of oncogenes in the host's cellular DNA and trigger them into action i.e. to synthesize proteins including enzymes which can stimulate the cells to multiply uncontrollably. This type of situation in the body leads to the growth of tumours which in due course become cancer. Therefore we have to avoid the agents that may trigger the oncogenes and we have to assimilate certain other agents that may protect our body from the harmful agents. The protective agents include fiber, vitamins, certain minerals and non-nutrients which shall be discussed at the end of this article.

Carcinogenic effects of high fat and high Protein Diets

Recently dietary components have also been ascribed with certain role in the development or prevention of cancer. It is found that 35% of cancer deaths are due to excessive use of dietary components. It may be surprising to know that the type of protein or fat may determine whether it is a causative factor for cancer or not. Seidman[1] in 1970, Haenszel[2] in 1971 and Cunningham[3] in 1976 found that over nourishment with animal proteins, fat and excess calories have a strong correlation with the incidence of cancer in humans.

Bovine protein was found to be the main culprit in inducing lymphoma according to the epidemiological studies conducted in 15 countries by Cunningham. A detailed study in Italy by Franceschi and team[4] showed that diet containing animal products like liver, milk, butter and and unsaturated oils have a strong correlation with the incidence of Non-Hodgkin's Lymphoma (a hetergenous group of tumors) in humans. Consumption of whole grain bread or pasta reduced this risk greatly and use of green vegetables and carrots showed slight reduction in the risk. However optimum consumption of protein is necessary otherwise a deficiency of it in the diet may reduce the immune response in our body. A 11.5 year follow up study on 15,914 individuals in Norway by Ursin[5] and his team showed that even high consumption of milk (Two glasses or more/day) significantly increases the risk of cancer in the lymphatic system. The increase in risk was strongest for lymphosarcoma. The possible culprits in milk are "protein and fat". The mechanism of action of animal protein is that it may release antigenic peptides, pass them through the mucosal endothelium and elicit an immune response.

Such processes result in active secretion of specific antibodies into the gut and it has been thought that prolonged stimulation of immune system may be casually related to the development of lymphoma[6]. Alternatively it has been suggested that chronic lympboid stimulation of this type may serve as a cofactor or act in predisposing to cancer with other factors such as oncogenic viruses or genetic susceptibility to increase the risk of cancer. Another thing to be noted is that in barbecued or burnt meat, proteins may be converted to benzopyrene like carcinogens and such meat should not be eaten as far as possible.

Drasar[7] and Miller[8] and their team found that high fat intake and cancer are intimately associated. Later many others including Goodwin[9], Prentice[10], Kelsely[11] and Howe[12] and their team also found that increase in dietary fat is a risk factor for breast cancer in woman. As alcohol is lipogenic (fat producing) even moderate daily drinking of alcohol also increases breast cancer in many woman[13]. According to the studies of Allexopoulose and others[14] serum cholesterol and triglycerides (fat) are increased in patients with breast cancer. Lately Willett and his team[15] reported that high fat or high meat intake increases colon cancer in humans and that fiber counteracts such effects. Ames[16] suggested that fatty acid peroxides, endoperoxides and epoxides (which may be produced from unsaturated oils) are strong mutagens and that may be the reason for the deleterious effects of high fat diets in women. According to Tornberg and team[17] serum cholesterol and β-lipoprotein (LDL) together have a strong correlation to the incidence of rectal and colon cancer in man. The possible mechanisms of their actions are that polyunsaturated fatty acids with an immunosuppressive effect[18] and the metabolic products of cholesterol, mainly the secondary bile acids (viz, Deoxy cholic and lithocholic acids) with a tumor promoting action on the mucosa may induce cancer in the colon[19]. Thus one has to avoid high fat and meat intake to escape from cancer of varied nature.

Anticarcinogenic Effects of Vitamins

The vitamins particularly nicotinic acid of the B complex is good to lower the serum cholesterol level in our body[20], generally the B complex vitamins and vitamins A and C have beneficial effects on the control of serum cholesterol[21-23]. As we have seen above a control of serum cholesterol shall definitely decrease the chances of not only atherosclerosis but also cancer, the anticarcinogenic effects of β carotene is mainly due to its vitamin A production, The retinoids form epoxides and dislocate many epoxides of carcinogens from adduct formation with DNA. They also inhibit ornithine decarboxylase enzyme that promote tumours[24]. Vitamin A can reduce the damages from radiation also[25] and β carotene is a scavenger for free radicals[26]. Free radicals promote cancer production in tissues. Many chemicals and alcohol that stimulate free radical formation are therefore strong promoters of cancer[16, 27].

Many non-nutrients (Nutraceuticals) in our diet and Vitamin E are also scavengers of free radicals and hence they are able to prevent induction of cancer[28]. Vitamin D is also ascribed with an anticarcinogenic effect[29] due to an inhibitory effect on ornithine decarboxylase enzyme that promotes cancer. Further nitrosocomponds are potent carcinogens and their formation is inhibited by vitamin C[30]. Moreover this vitamin inactivates singlet oxygen also which is harmful to the body[28]. These findings stress the role of vitamins in the prevention of cancer.

Anticarcinogenic Effects of Fiber and Non-Nutrients/ Nutraceuticals in Food

Fiber is ascribed with an hypocholesteremic action. It is mainly because it prevents the absorption of cholesterol from intestines and facilitates its metabolism and excretion. Further it also prevents the absorption of carcinogens from the intestines and facilitates their metabolism and excretion along with feces[31]. Fiber is present in crude forms of cereals, pulses and tubers and diets rich in these ingredients are the best for the prevention of colon cancer [32].

Refined flour and bread made out of it are poor in fiber content. In affluent countries like America, heart diseases and cancer are common and this is partly due to their high intake of fat, proteins and sweets (60% of the diet). Now the scientists recommend to reduce them to 40% in total and to contain less than 30% fats in it with a sufficient increase in fiber to 5% or more and starch to 50% and mineral and vitamins to 1-2% of the whole diet. Vegetables, leaves and whole grains are good sources of fiber and all are encouraged to use them in plenty. Minerals like Se, Zn and Ca are particularly necessary to protect our body[33,37] from the action of carcinogens. Lee Wattenberg[38] reviewed the role of non-nutrients (food components with no known role in the growth or maintenance of body) as possible sources of anticarcinogenic substances. **When crude diet fed mice and semipurified diet (that is devoid of non-nutrients) fed mice were subjected to a tobacco carcinogen NNK (4-(methylnitrosamino) = 1,3 (pyridyl)1-butanone)by Hecht and his team[39], the number of mice that developed tumour were thrice in the latter group as compared to that in the former. Here the protection offered against tumour by the non-nutrients is self evident.**

The sources of anticarcinogenic substances are many. The protective effects of sulphur containing compounds of onion, and garlic were reported by Belman[40], Wargovich[41] Sumiyoshi[42] and Lau[43] and that of cabboage type vegetables by Wattenberg[44] and that of the terpenes in citrus fruit oil by Elson[45] and that of curcumin in turmeric by Ramadasan Kuttan[46] and that of tannins in green tea by Fujiki and his team[47]. All these non-nutrients significantly inhibited chemically induced tumours in experimental animals. The non nutrients are now called as nutraceuticals.

The importance of garlic as a source of anticarcinogenic compounds was suggested after an epidemiological study reported by Mei and his team in China[48]. According to the study in the province of Shandong the incidence of stomach cancer in Qixia was 3 times in a population that rarely used garlic as compared to a neighbouring population in Cagsham that used about 20 gm garlic/person/day i.e. 40 and 13 per 100,000 people developed stomach cancer respectively.

Further it was found that Cagshan residents had lower concentrations of nitrites in their gastric juice than those in Qixia. Nitrites are precursors of certain carcinogens that induce cancer. Pan[49] in China has shown that a garlic compound diallyl trisulphide can inhibit the growth of stomach cancer in tissue culture as effectively as did some chemotherapeutic drugs. Lau[50] in California has demonstrated that deodourised garlic and its compounds like ajoene and diallyl sulphide can prevent the activities of carcinogens like aflatoxin B1 and Benzo(a) pyrene and increase their detoxification. Lipid lowering effects of garlic products may also contribute to the anticancer effects of garlic[51].

According to many researchers[44] the sulphur compounds in these vegetables not only prevent lipid accumulation in tissues, but they inhibit activation of several carcinogens and enhance their detoxification. Thus their hypolipidemic effects and counteraction with carcinogens may be held responsible for their anticarcinogenic action. Similar or related mechanism of action are ascribed to terpenes of Caraway seed and orange oils and tannins, flavanoids and isoflavanoids of various plant products that act as anticarcinogens[52]. Hence plenty of fruits and vegetables, like pomegranate, papaya, carrots, onions, garlic, cabbage, soyabeans and edible leaves and spices e.g. turmeric, asafoetida, ginger etc. must be included in the diet with plenty of fiber i.e. 20-30 g/day. Scientists in U.K have developed a super broccoli that can help combat colon cancer and a tomato that may help fight heart disease and boost immune system. Addition of citrus fruit terpenoids viz, nomilin and limonin to the diet inhibited Benzopyrene induced lung tumor formation in A/J mice. The inhibition of tumor was correlated with inhibition of the formation of BP-DNA adducts[53(a)] genistin, the major isoflavanoid in soyabean were shown to induce p450 level in streptomyces grisens. Biochanin A an isoflavone in red clouer has been shown to inhibit the metabolism of Benzo(a) pyrene and its binding to DNA[53(b)]. Adulterated food and vegetables polluted with insecticides may be avoided, to keep our body healthy and immunoresistant to cancer. Exercise and occasional fasting may keep your system absolutely clean. At Amala Hospital, Trichur a team is investigating on the anticarcinogenic effects of garlic and certain other plants.

Cancer Prevention and Cure by Vegetables

Beneficial effects of pomegranate juice (PJ), has been reported for men with rising prostate specific antigen following surgery or radiation for prostate cancer[54]. Further the beneficial role of this fruit juice for chemoprevention and chemotherapy of prostate cancer was studied by Malik et. al.[55] also. Fresh juice of pomegranate contains 85% water, 10% total sugars, 1.5% pectin, small amounts of ascorbic acid and polyphenolic flavonoids[56]. The soluble polyphenol content varies within the limits of 0.2-1.0 % depending on the variety and includes mainly anthocyanins, catechins, ellagic tannins and gallic and ellagic acids[57,58]. Claudia Napoli's group, Filomena de Nigris et. al.[59] have earlier shown that intervention with antioxidants contained in pomegranate juice can reduce oxidative stress, atherogenesis, and activation of redox-sensitive genes (ELK-1 and P-JUN) with a concommittant increase in endothelial NO synthase (eNOs) expression in cultured endothelial cells and in atherosclerosis prone areas of hypercholesterolemic mice. These findings suggest that PJ is beneficial to prevent not only various cancers but also atherosclerosis that predisposes any one to CHD. Pomegranate has been shown to reduce systolic blood pressure by inhibiting serum angiotensin-converting enzyme (ACE)[60]. Others research suggests that PJ may be effective against prostate cancer and osteoarthritis. In 2007 six clinical trials in U.S, Israel and Norway have been approved to examine the effects of PJ consumption on parameters of prostate cancer or prostatic hyperplasia, diabetes or lymphoma[61].

Vegetables like broccoli and cabbage known as cruciferous vegetables contain glucosinolate. When this is broken down into active sulforane compounds we get several anticarcinogenic polyphenols that were studied by scientist at John Hopkins University in 1992. Dr. Jed Faheys team demonstrated in mouse model that sulphoraphane could inhibit cancer causing Helicobacter infections and block the formation of gastric tumours[62]. He stated "if future clinical studies show that a food can relieve or prevent diseases associated with this bacterium in people, it could have significant public health implications in the United States and around the world". Research on indole-3-carbinol a component present in broccoli, showed that this compound helps in deactivating a potent oestrogen metabolite (4- hydroxy esterone) that promotes tumor growth, especially in estrogen sensitive breast cells[63], while at the same time increasing the level of 2-hydroxy estrone, a form of estrogen that can be cancer preventive.

The research team led by Yanaka[64] in Japan found that in patients with H.pylori infection, a diet including 100 g broccoli sprouts per day (about 3 ounces) resulted in a significant reduction of H.pylori and pepsinogen (a biomarker in the blood indicating the degree of gastritis). These workers think the beneficial results are due to sulforaphane present in the vegetable and which can protect against oxidative damage in cells that in turn can damage DNA, potentially causing cancer.

Broccoli and tomatoes–two vegetables separately recognized for their cancer-fighting capabilities are even more successful against prostate cancer when working as a team in the daily diet, as per the research of Canene-Adams et. al.[65].

Garlic (Allium sativum)

A host of studies provide compelling evidence that garlic and its organic allyl sulfur components are effective inhibitors of the cancer process. These studies[66-70] reveal that the benefits of garlic are not limited to a specific species, to a particular tissue, or to a specific carcinogen. **Of 37 observational studies in humans using garlic and related allyl sulfur components, 28 studies showed some cancer preventive effect. The evidence is particularly strong for a link between garlic and prevention of prostate and stomach cancers among various populations who**

consumed or did not consume garlic as a component diet. A study conducted at the school of Chinese medicine also shows that a crude extract of garlic induces a caspase-3-gene expression that leads to apoptosis of human colon cancer cells. A large scale epidemiological Iowa women's Health study looked at the garlic consumption in 41,000 middle aged women. Results showed that women who regularly consumed garlic has 35 % lower risk of developing colon cancer. It is thought that the allyl sulphur compounds in garlic prevent cancer by slowing or preventing the growth of the cancer tumor cells. Recently researchers in Pennsylvania have shown that by injecting a compound called diallyl disulphide (DADS) that tumors can be reduced by half and that a further compound (S-allyl cysteine) can stop cancer causing agents from binding to human breast cells. Many physicians think that the inhibitory action of garlic on putrefaction in the intestines together with the secretion stimulating effect, brought about detoxification and an increase in resistance. Stimulation of gastric juice secretion and restoration of the intestinal flora, combined with the resulting prevention of gastro intestinal autointoxication, may help to remove at least one of the possible causes of cancer. Garlic may therefore be useful as a cancer preventative agent, and its application as an anticancer drug is based on this assumption (garlic @mistral.co.uk)

The only known study in which garlic has been used to treat patients with advanced stages of cancer was conducted by Spivak (1962). A garlic juice preparation was administered in doses of 0.2-2.0 ml intravenously or 1-5 ml intramuscularly daily for 3-7 days. Of 35 patients with cancer at various sites (lung, Cervix, stomach, lower lip, mammary gland, larynx, and leukemia), 26 showed positive treatment results of varying degrees, though complete healing was not achieved in any case. There is a single case report, however of a man whose pituitary tumor shrank by 50 % during the 5 months in which he ate 5-7 gs fresh garlic daily. This was the first case ever reported of reduction of this type of tumor without chemotherapy or surgery (Rainov & Burkert 1993). The anticancer effects of garlic are likely due to both allicin or allicin derived compounds as well as to unidentified compounds not related to allicin.

Garlic against Infections

A natural weapon against infection, the research findings reported in Antimicrobial Agents and Chemotherapy revealed allicin disables dysentery causing amoeba's by blocking two groups of enzymes, cysteine proteinases and alcoholdehydrogenases. Cysteine proteinase enzymes are among the main culprits in infection, providing infectious organisms with means to damage and invade tissues. Alcohol dehydrogenase enzymes play a major role in these harmful organisms' metabolism and survival. Because these groups of enzymes are found in a wide variety of infectious organisms such as bacteria, fungi and viruses, this research provides a scientific basis for the notion that allicin is a broad spectrum antibiotic, capable of warding off different types of infections. **"It has long been argued that garlic can fight a wide range of infections and now we have provided biochemical evidence for this claim"** the authors wrote. (compiled by the garlic information centre. Sabardene House, Church Road. Catsfield Battle. East Sussex. TN 339 DP. Phone 01424-892440). Garlic may be provoking the B lymphocytes, T lymphocytes and various killer cells in the body to produce immunoglobulins that destroy various viruses. BHS Lau (Garlic for health 1988 Lotus Publication Japan)

Garlic and Smokers

Yet another study in China reported that smokers with high garlic intake have a relatively lower stomach cancer-risk than smokers with low garlic intake. The beneficial effects of garlic and onion oils and a precursor of the former i.e. S-allyl cysteine sulfoxide have been reported by our team of researchers in nicotine, lead salt or alcohol treated rats[71-73].

Garlic Key Message

In order to get the maximum health benefits of garlic, it is suggested to wait 15 mins, between peeling (better smashing) and cooking garlic to allow the enzymatic reaction to occur so that the active ingredient of garlic i.e. allicin is formed by the action of an enzyme alliinase. If you use garlic supplements, use the enteric coated tablets, so that the healthy ingredients can survive the gastric action and could be absorbed into the blood stream in the small intestines. Avoid the use of garlic along with blood thinners such as aspirin and warfarin as the garlic principles are also blood thinners. Further it may be noted that garlic and garlic products may be discontinued from at least 7 days prior to surgery as they may increase bleeding.

Effects of Vitamin E and some Antioxidants with relation to Cancer

Numerous properties suggest that antioxidants and carotenoids may be valuable chemopreventive agents. A population based case control study of 952 rectal cancer cases and 1,205 controls from Northern California and Utah was conducted between 1997 and 2002 by Murtaugh, Ma et. al.[74]. Detailed diet history, medical history and life style factors were recorded. Dietary antioxidants were not associated with rectal cancer risk in men. For women low intake of dietary lycopene or vitamin E was associated with an increased risk of rectal cancer. No association of lutein, betacarotene, vitamin C or selenium from dietary sources with risk of rectal cancer was found for either men or women. Vitamin supplement use was also not associated significantly with rectal cancer in younger women or men. **The association between Vitamin E and rectal cancer was stronger for women aged 60 years or older than for younger women. Associations with lycopene, beta carotene, vitamin C and Se did not vary by age for men or women.**

Further assessment of types of vitamin E showed that all forms except delta-tocopherol were associated with a decreased risk of rectal cancer in women, but not in man. Assessment of tocopherols by age showed that β-tocopherol was associated with rectal cancer in both younger and older women, while other forms of tocopherols were associated with rectal cancer in older woman only. At the lowest level of intake, α- tocopherol was associated with a 3.6 fold increased risk, γ- tocopherol was associated with a 5.3 fold increased risk and Δ- tocopherol was associated with a 1.9 fold increased risk.

Estrogen Status

It was determined by a combination of menopausal status and use of hormone replacement therapy. Women who were pre or post menopausal and reported hormone replacement therapy use were considered estrogen positive.

Given the gender specific associations observed with some antioxidants and carotenoids, the researchers evaluated the associations for women by estrogen status. They found no differences in the associations of lutein, vitamin C and Se by estrogen status. However estrogen status appeared to modify the associations of β-carotene, lycopene and Vitamin E with rectal cancer in women. The combined effect of being estrogen negative and having low intakes of lycopene, β- carotene and vitamin E was greater than any of these factors independently. For lycopene and vitamin E lower dietary intakes were associated with approximately a third fold increase in risk of rectal cancer in estrogen-negative women to estrogen positive women with high intakes; for β-carotene, there was an approximate two fold increase in risk of rectal cancer in estrogen-negative women. These results suggest that vitamin E and lycopene may modestly reduce the risk of rectal cancer in women.

Both age and estrogen for women appeared to modify the associations of lycopene and vitamin E with risk of rectal cancer. However, age and estrogen status are tightly related, making it difficult to evaluate whether their influences are independent or whether estrogen status influences the relation of age to risk of rectal cancer. Inadequate data hampered the efforts to clearly distinguish this issue, however, the association of lycopene with hormone sensitive cancers[75-76]. Certainly points to the plausibility of an independent influence of estrogens, as do the gender-specific associations.

On a perusal of earlier work by others significant associations have been reported for α-carotene and lycopene with breast cancer[75]. α- carotene, β-Carotene and lycopene with ovarian cancer[76], lycopene with prostate cancer[77,78], lycopene with ovarian and colorectal cancer[79], lutein with proximal colon cancer[80], and vitamin E with colon cancer[81-84]. On the other hand, some observational studies and clinical trials have shown that β-carotene supplementation increases the risk of cancer especially among smokers[85,86]. In general, it can be concluded that the associations of antioxidants with colorectal cancers are inconsistent and studies have primarily focused on colon cancer. However a few studies have reported associations between antioxidants/ carotenoids (mostly β-Carotene) and rectal cancer[87-89]. Bostick et. al.[83] reported significant associations between colon caner and total vitamin E intake (diet and supplements in a cohort of older women) but associations were stronger for women aged 55-59 years versus 60-64 years. A study of incident rectal cancer found no association with dietary vitamin E for men or women[88].

In a review of tocopherols and colon cancer[89], it was suggested that both α and γ tocopherols may be important in the prevention of colon cancer. Further according to these studies antioxidants in fecal material may be effective in preventing DNA damage in epithelial cells lining the colon. It has been suggested that fecal bacteria contribute to colon cancer risk by producing carcinogens or procarcinogens[90]. It is possible that gamma-tocopherol is involved in reducing the risk of rectal cancer via this mechanism. Cramer et. al.[76] reported an inverse association of lycopene with risk of ovarian cancer, predominantly among postmenopausal women. Similarly in Murtaugh's study[74] the present study the highest intakes of lycopene were associated with a decreased risk of rectal cancer in women only and the association was stronger for estrogen negative women. It has been suggested that the actions of higher levels of prooxidant catechol estrogens prior to menopause could be countered by the free radical quenching activity of lycopene[75]. Other possibilities for the detected association include up-regulation of the cytochrome P450 enzyme system[91] and of the proteins that enable cell to cell communication at high levels of lycopene intake[92]. Findings of the recent study[74] conflict with previous reports of an inverse association of β carotene with rectal cancer. With the highest intake of β-carotene a 46% reduction in risk was reported for Chinese[93] and a 68% reduction in risk was reported for Italians[87]. Recent findings of Murtaugh[74] further agree with those of Australian case- control study in which no significant associations were detected[94]. However in the study for estrogen-negative women versus estrogen-positive women[74], the lowest intakes of β-carotene were associated with a two fold greater risk of rectal cancer. β-carotene exposure has been linked to production of reactive oxygen species in the colon that may act in either a pro oxidant or antioxidant capacity depending on the cellular environment[95]. It is possible that the association of β-carotene with rectal cancer is through regulation of cell. Availability of β-carotene as a precursor of vitamin A and the maintenance of cell integrity may be more important for estrogen positive women, since estrogen may increase cell proliferation.

References

1. Seidman H., *Environ. Res.* 3 (1970) 234
2. Haenszel. W. *In. J. Med Sci* 7 (1971) 143
3. Cunningham A.S. Lymphomas and animal protein consumption. *Lancet* 2 (1976) Nov.27; 2 1184-6.
4. Franceschi, S; Serraino D; Carbone. A et. al. Dietary factors and non-Hodgkin's lymphoma: a case control study in the north eastern part of italy. *Nutr. Can.* 12(1989) 333-41.
5. Ursin, G; Bjeike, E Heuchi, I et. al. Milk consumption and cancer incidence: a norwegian prospective study. *Br J. Cancer* 61 (1990) 456
6. Schwartz. R. S; *N. Engl. J. Med.* 293(1975) 181.
7. Drasar. B.S; Irving D; Environmenal factors and cancer of the colon and breast. *Br.J.Cancer.* 27;(1973) 167
8. Miller. A.B; Kelly A. *Am.J Epidemiol.* 107 (1978) 499
9. Goodwin. P.J. and Boyd N.F; *J. Natl Cancer. Inst.* 79 (1987) 474.
10. Prentice, R.L; Kakar, F; Hursting, S. et. al. Aspects of the rationale for the women's health trial. *J. Natl. Cancer Inst.*80(1988)802.
11. Kelsey J and Berkowitz, G. Breast cancer epidemiology. *Canc. Res.* 48(1988) 5615-5623.
12. Howe G.R; Hirohata, T; Hislop T.G. et. al. Dietary factors and risk of breast cancer: combined analysis of 12 case-control studies. *J. Natl. Cancer. Inst.* 82 (1990) 561
13. Schatzkin, A; Jones D.Y and Hoover. R.N et. al. Alcohol concumption and breast cancer in the epidemiologic follow-up study of the first national health and nutrition survey. *N Engl. J. Med.* 316(19)(1987)1169-1173.
14. Alexopoulos, C.G; Blatsios, B and Avgerinos A. Serum lipids and lipoprotein disorders in cancer patients. *Cancer* 60(1987)3065
15. Willett, W. C; Stampfer, M, J; Coldditz, G. A et. al. *N Engl. J. Med* 323(1990)1664
16. Ames B, N; Science 221 (1983) 1256

17. Tornberg, S.A; Holm, L.E; Carstensen, J.M and Eklund, G.A. Risks of cancer of the colon and rectum in relation to serum cholesterol and betalipoprotein. *N Eng. J.Med* 315(1986)1629-33.

18. Scott, D; *Cancer Res*. (Suppl) 52 (1992) 5492s.

19. Hill, M.J, Crowther, J.S; Drasar, B.S et. al. Lancet 95 (1971) 100.

20. Brattsand, R and Lundholm, L. The effect of nicotinic acid and pentaerythritolteranicotinate upon experimental atherosclerosis in the rabbit. *Atherosclerosis*. 14. (1971) 91-105.

21. Erlanader, S.R. Enzymologia 28 (1964)139.

22. March BE and Biely, J. Vitamin A and cholesterol absorption in the chicken. *J.Nutr*.79(4) (1963) 474.

23. Kasatkina, L.V; Lobova, N.M et. al. in A. Myasnikov (ed) Atherosclerosis and Thrombosis Mir, Publishers, Moscow p. 39(1967).

24. Boutwell, R.K.J. Am. Acad. Dermatol. 6(1982) 796.

25. Harisiadis, L;Miller, R.C; Hall, E.J et. al. A vitamin A analogue inhibits radiation-induced oncogenic transformation. Nature 274(1978) 486.

26. Hennekens, C.H; Mayrent, S.L; Willet., W. Vitamin A, Carotenoids and Retinoids. Cancer 58 (1986) 1837.

27. Bullock, C. Biochem. Edn. 18(1960) 62

28. Wattenberg, L.W. Chemoprevention of cancer, Cancer Res.45(1985)1.

29. Chida, K; Hashibam. H;Suda, T and Kurok T. *Cancer Res*. 44 (1984)342.

30. Kryptopolulose. S.A; *Am. J Clin. Nutr*.45(1987) 1374.

31. Carr B.L. Cancer 55 (1985)218.

32. Greenwald P., Lanza E., Eddy G.A."Dietary fiber in the reduction of colon cancer. J.Am. Diet. Assoc. 87(a)(1987) 1178.

33. Wattenberg, L.W; Inhibitors of chemical carcinogenesis. Adv. Cancer Res. 26(1978)197-226.

34. Ip.C.J.Am.Call. Toxicol 5 (1986) 7.

35. Reynoso, G; In Cancer Medicine Holland J.F.Frei. E.111(eds) lea& Febiger Philadelphia P. 373 (1982)

36. Garland, C; Shekelle, R.B; Barrett-Conner E.et. al. Lancet 1 (1985) 307.

37. Gangadharan, B and Rajan, A. Amala Res. Bulletin 12 (1992) 25.

38. Wattenberg, L.W. Inhibitors of carcinogenesis by minor dietary constituents. Cancer Res. 52 (1992) Suppl. 2085S-2691S.

39. Hect. S.S. et. al. Carcinogenesis 10 (1989) 1901.

40. Belman S; Block, E et. al. Proc. Am. *Assoc Cancer Res*. 28 (1987) 166.

41. Wargevich M.J. Carcinogenesis, 8 (1987) 487.

42. Sumiyoshi, H and Wargovich. M.J. Chemoprevention of 1,2-dimethylhydrazine-induced colon cancer in mice by natural occurring organosulfur compounds. *Cancer. Res*, 50. (1990) 5084-5087.

43. Lau, B. in garlic for health P.37.Lotus light publications. Wilmot. Wl. printed in japan (1988)

44. Wattenberg, L. W et. al. Inhibition of carcinogenesis by some minor dietary constitutents in Hayashi, Y. et. al. (eds). Diet, *Nutrition and Cancer* P 193 (1985) Tokyo japan. Soc. Press.

45. Elson, C.F, et. al. Carcinogenesis 9 (1988)331

46. Ramadasan Kuttan, Bhanumathy, P; Nirmala, K. and George M.C. Cancer Letters 29 (1985) 197.

47. Fujiki, H. et. al. New Antitumour Promoters (-)epigallocatechin gallate and Sarcophytols A and B. In Y. Kuroda, M Shankel M.D Waters (eds) Antimutagens and anticarcinogenesis mechanism II.P.205 New York Plenum Publishing Corp. 1990.

48. Mei X, et. al. Acta Nutr. *Sinica* 4. (1982)53

49. Pan. X. Y et. al. Chung-Hua Chung Liu *Tsa-Chih* 7(1985)103.

50. Lau B, Garlic Reserch up date. P. 15. by odyssey phblishes Inc. 2135. West 45h. venue Vancouver, *B.C.Canada.*

51. Augusti K.T. Therapeutic and Medicinal values of onions and garlic. In Onions a Crops. Nol.3 Biochemistry, Food. Science and minor crops. J.L. Brewster, H.D. Rabinowtich [Eds] p.93. C.R.R. press, Inc. *Boca Raton Florida* (1990).

52. Bhattacharryya, S; Don't lose heart, Yet. I.U Lifeline, A weekly feature of medicine and popular health, *Indian express publication* p 9. 24th April Kochi 1993.

53. (a) Luke K.T Hasegawa in Food Phytochemicals for cancer prevention II 209-219 *American Chemical Societ*, Washington D C (1994).

    (b) Zhane Y Cassady Z B M. *Chem. Biol interact* 82(1992) 181-193.

54. Pantuck, A.J; Leppert, J.T. et. al. Phase II study of pomegranate juice for men with rising prostate–specific antigen following surgery or radiation for prostate cancer. Clin. Cacer Res. 12(3) (2006) 4018-26.

55. Malik, A; Afaq F. et. al. Pomegranate fruit juice for chemoprevention and chemotherapy of prostate cancer. PNAS. 102(41) (2005) 14813-18

56. Aviram, M; Dornfeld, L. et. al. Am. J. Clin. Nutr. 71(2000) 1062-76.

57. El-Nemr, S.E; Ismail, I.A and Ragab, M. Nahrung, 34 (1990)601-606.

58. Narr Ben, C; Ayed, N and Metche, M, Quoted in Z. Lebensm Uters, F.A. 203(1996) 374-378.

59. de Nigris, F; Lerman, L.O. et. al. Proc. Natl. Acad. Sci. USA 100(2003) 1420-25.

60. Aviram, M; Dornfeld, L. Pomegranate juice consumption inhibits serum angiotensin converting enzyme activity and reduces systolic blood pressure. Atherosclerosis 158(1)(2001) 195-98

61. [edit] Notes. Can pomegranates prevent prostate cancer? A New study offers promise, 26 Sept. 2005. Also refer "htt://en.wikipedia.org/wiki/pomegranate".

62. Fahey. J.W; Haristoy, X et. al. Sulforaphane inhibits extracellular, intracellular, and antibiotic-resistant strains of Helicobacter pylori and prevents benzopyrene-induced stomach tumors. Proc. Nat. Acad. Sci.USA 99(11) (2002) 7610-15

63. Meng, Q; Goldberg, I.D. et. al. Inhibitory effects of Indole-3-carbinol on invasion and migration in human breast cancer cells. Breast Cancer Res. Treat. 63(2) (2000) 147-52.

64. Yanaka, A; Zhang, S et. al. Role of the nrf-2gene in protection and repair of gastric mucosa against oxidative stress. Inflammopharmacology. 13 (2005) 83-90.

65. Canene- Adams, K; Lindshield, B.L et. al. Combinations of tomato and broccoli enhance antitumor activity in dunning γ 3327-h prostate adenocarcinomas. Cancer Res. 67(2) (2007) 836-43. Epup.2007.Jan.9 PMID.17213256

66. Anagase, H; Petesch, B.L et. al. "Intake of garlic and its bioactive components" J.Nutr.131(2001) 955S.

67. Fleischauer, A.T and Arab, L. Garlic and Cancer: a critical review of the epidemiologic literature. J. Nutrition 131(2001) 1032 S-1040S

68. Milner, J.A. Mechanisms by which garlic and allyl sulfur compounds suppress carcinogen bioactivation. Garlic and carcinogenesis. Adv. Exp. Med. Biol. 492(2001) 69-81

69. "Allium Vegetables and organosulfur compounds: Do they help prevent cancer?" http://ehpnetl.nichs.nih.gov/members/2001/109 p 893-902 bianchini/bianchini-full.html.

70. "Garlic: Effects on cardiovascular Risks and Disease, Proliferative effects against cancer, and clinical Adverse effects". http://www.ahrg. gov/clinic/ epcsums/garlic sum.htm.

71. Helen A; Rajasree, C.R. et. al. Antioxidant role of oils isolated from garlic (Allium Sativum Linn) and onion (Allium cepa Linn) on nicotine induced lipid peroxidation. Vet. Human Toxicol 41(5)1999, 316-319.

72. (a) Helen, A; Krishnakumar, K et. al. A comparative study of antioxidants S-allyl cysteine sulfoxide and vitamin E on the damages induced by nicotine in rats. Pharmacology. 67(2003) 113-117.

(b) Bindu, M.P; Sreekanth K.S. et. al. Effects of S-allyl cysteine sulphoxide on lipid metabolism and free radical scavengers in alcohol fed rats. Current Science 82 (2002) 628-631

73. Augusti. K.T. Beneficial effects of active principles isolated from alliums, F. bengalensis Linn and S. Oblonga Wall. In various experimental conditions in rats. Abstracts of the National Symposium on current trends in the development of Herbal drugs. 27th Annual Conference of IABS .2006 P.76. Thiruvananthapuram.

74. Murthaugh, M.A,; Khe-ni Ma et. al. Antioxidants, Carotenoids and risk of rectal cancer. Am. J. Epidemiol 159(2004)32-41

75. Hulten, K; Van Kappel, A.L et. al. Carotenoids, α-tocopherols and retinol in plasma and breast cancer risk in northern Sweden. Cancer Causes Control.12(2001)529-37.

76. Cramer, D.W, Kuper, H et. al. Carotenoids and ovarian cancer risk in pre and post menopausal women. Int. J. Cancer 94(2001) 128-34

77. Vogt, T.M; Mayne, S.T. and Graubard, B.I et. al. Serum lycopene other serum carotenoids and risk of prostate cancer in US Blacks and Whites. Am. J. Epidemiol.155(2002)1023-32

78. Giovannucci E; Rimm, E.B. Liu Y, et. al. A prospective study of tomato products, lycopene and Prostate cancer risk. J. Natl Cancer Inst 94(2002)391-98.

79. La Vecchia C. Tomatoes, lycopene intake and digestive tract and female hormone-related neoplasms. Exp Biol Med. 227(2202)860-63.

80. Slattery, M.L, Benson J, et. al. Carotenoids and colon cancer. Am. J. Clin. Nutr.71(2000) 575-82.

81. Slattery, M.L., Edwards, S.L., Anderson K, et. al. Vitamin E and colon cancer; is there an association? Nutr Cancer. 30(1998)201-06

82. Wu K, Willet WC, Chan J.M et. al. A prospective study on supplemental vitamin E intake and risk of colon cancer in women and men. Cancer Epidemiol Biomarkers Prev. 11(2002)1298-304.

83. Bostick, RM, Potter, J.D. et. al. Reduced risk of colon cancer with high intake of vitamin E; The Iowa Women's Health Study. Cancer Rs. 53(1993)4230-37.

84. Ghadirian, P; Lacroix, A et. al. Nutritional factors and colon Carcinoma: a case control study involving French Canadians in Montreal, Quebec, Canada. Cancer 8(1997) 858-64.

85. Albanes, D; Heinonen, O.P; et. al. Alpha-tocopherol and beta-carotene supplements and lung cancer incidence in the alpha-tocopherol, beta-carotene cancer prevention study: effects of base-line characteristics and study compliance. J. Natt Cancer Inst. 88(1996)1560-70.

86. Omenn, G.S.; Goodman, G.E. Thornquist,M.D. et. al. Risk factors for lung cancer and for intervention effects in CARET, the beta-carotene and retinol efficacy trial. J. Natl. Cancer Inst. 88(1996)1550-59.

87. Ferraroni M, La Vecchia C.D'Avanzo B, et. al. Selected micronutrient intake and the risk of colorectal cancer. Br. J. Cancer 70(1994)1150-55.

88. Freudenheim, J.L; Graham, S, Marshall J.R. et. al. A case – control study of diet and rectal cancer in Western New York. Am. J. Epidemiol, 131(1990) 612-24.

89. Stone, W.L. and Papas A.M. Tocopherols and the etiology of colon cancer. J. Natl Cancer Inst. 89(1997) 1006-14.

90. Guarner, F; Malagalada. J.R. Gut Flora in health and disease. Lancet 361(2003) 512-19

91. Bendich, A. Recent advances in clinical research involving carotenoids. Pure Appl. Chem. 66(1994)1017-24

92. Zhang, L.X; Cooney, R.V. et. al. Carotenoids up-regulate connexin, 4-3 gene expression independent of their provitamin A or antioxidant properties. Cancer Res.52 (1992) 5707-12

93. Lee, H.P.; Gourley, L; Colorectal cancer and diet in an Asian population – a case control study among Singapore Chinese. Int. J. Cancer 43(1989) 1007-16.

94. Potter, J.D McMichael, A.J. Diet and Cancer of the colon and rectum; a case-control study. J. Natl. Cancer Inst. 76(1986)557-69.

95. Palozza. P, Calviello G, et. al. β-carotene at high concentration induces apoptosis by enhancing oxy-radical production in human adenocarcinoma cells. Free Radic Biol. Med. 31(2001)1000-07.

8.3 Nutrition, Nutraceuticals Vs Health and Aging

Drs. D. S. Sheriff and P.T. Annamala,

Department of Biochemistry, Jubilee Mission Medical College, Thrissur, Kerala.

It is noteworthy to remember the quotation of John Russo Jr. "Let food be thy medicine and medicine be thy food: what every health care professional should know about nutraceuticals and functioned foods".

Food is essential for survival, growth and reproduction. Humans have over the years selected a wide range of nutrients of animal and vegetable origin. Selected nutrients are supposed to provide essential dietary components, requisite calories and other physiologically important compounds required for life and health. Diet therefore plays a vital role in maintaining health or in precipitating disease. A defective diet is considered as one of the major causative factors linked to coronary heart disease (CHD), non-insulin dependent diabetes mellitus (NIDDM), atherosclerosis, certain types of cancer and stroke.

Food technology and nutrition science have evolved over a period of time to identify the active ingredients of nutritive value as well as non-nutritive components that promote physiological functions in health and disease. Leaves, flowers, bark and root, the plant components have been used to treat patients. The development of technology helped to isolate the beneficial components, develop corporate pharmaceutical industries to manufacture and convert them into pharmaceutical agents.

This has resulted in a multi-billion dollar pharmaceutical giants who rule the world of medicine. The expenditure, the long wait for approval of drug design, manufacture and marketing led to the development of food industry that concentrates on designer food that promote health, prevent disease and supplement nutritional requirements.

The market is crowded with food products in the name of antioxidants, phytochemicals, fibers, cholesterol free diet, isolated components like glucosamine, performance enhancing components like creatine and even oxygen as spray in Japan. The combination of food technology with pharmaceuticals led to the development of **nutraceuticals,** a term coined to indicate

"any substance considered as food or part of a food that provides medical or health benefits, including the prevention and treatment of disease".

These may include isolated nutrients, dietary supplements, genetically engineered designer foods, herbal products, processed products such as cereals, soups and beverages.

Medical foods are complex formulated products specially designed to support the medical condition as a complete or dietary supplement or as a product to suit the physiological need of the patient who should consume it only under the supervision of a physician.

What is a dietary supplement?

A product intended for ingestion as a tablet, capsule, liquid, powder, soft gel or labeled as a dietary supplement

A drug or antibiotic or a biologic marketed as a dietary supplement

A food that is not considered as food additive

A preparation that help to increase total intake of components to provide energy, mineral, a herb, or botanical, an aminoacid, a dietary substance for use by man like.

Antihypertensives, Antioxidants, Antimutagens, Antimicrobial or antiviral agents, Enhancers of GI function including dietary fiber, Probiotics, Prebiotics, Colonic microflora, Immunomodulators, Phytoestrogens, Hypocholeserolemic agents, Neuroregulatory substances, Food components with diminished allergenicity.

The Little Helpers

Vitamins and minerals are just as important as the carbohydrates, proteins and fats for good nutrition. However you only need them in small amounts. Vitamins and minerals usually function as coenzymes and cofactors which means they help the chemical reactions in the body go a lot faster. For example, many of the B complex vitamins help your body burn carbohydrates for energy. *Vitamin A is needed for vision, zinc is involved in many metabolic processes and vitamin C helps keep connective tissue strong and your immune system functioning.*

Your diet needs to provide adequate amounts of all of these little helpers. A healthy, balanced diet will provide you with lots of vitamin and minerals. An unhealthy diet may make your body deficient in one or more of these helpers.

Above and Beyond the Basics

Good nutrition provides more than energy, structural components, vitamins and minerals. There are other substances in the foods that you eat that have become better known over the last few years. Phytochemicals are found in the colorful parts of fruits and vegetables. Although they aren't required for the functions in your body, they may have a very powerful impact on your health. For example, quercetin found in apples functions like an antihistamine and as an antiinflammatory. Resveratrol, found in grape skins and seeds, is a powerful antioxidant.

Antioxidants help protect your body from damage that comes from the sun, pollution, smoke, and poor dietary choices. They are found in the phytochemicals of fruits and vegetables, plus some of the vitamins and some amino acids.

Complex carbohydrates (fiber rich) are good for health, but plenty of sugars are not good for health. *An example of a good source of carbohydrates would be almost any fruit or vegetable. You still get the carbohydrates you need for energy, plus fiber for a healthy digestive system, vitamins, minerals and anti-oxidants.* About half of your daily calories should come from carbohydrates. Those carbohydrates should come from fruits, vegetables and 100 percent whole grain breads and cereals, not from candy, sodas and pastries.

This concept works with proteins and fats too. A healthy protein source is one that does not add extra unhealthy fats and hopefully offers some fats that are good for you. For an example of a healthy protein, think of navy beans. These beans will provide protein, fiber, vitamins, minerals and carbohydrates. **An unhealthy protein source would be something like bacon. Lots of saturated fats which are bad for your heart, lots of calories that aren't good for your waistline and processed meats like this have been linked to an increased risk of cancer.**

Healthy fats come from foods that contain polyunsaturated fats, as well as monounsaturated fats like olive oil, fish, walnuts, soy, flax seeds and canola oil. While fats contain a lot of calories, you do need the fatty acids that fats and oils provide. Unfortunately there are a lot of unhealthy fats to be aware of. Saturated fats in red meats (if consumed more than 8% of the required calories) and trans fats found in some stick margarines, baked goods and processed foods are very bad for your health.

Good Nutrition Means Good Health

A healthy diet will give your body right amount of energy, enough raw materials and all of the little helpers you need to stay healthy. Good nutrition will also provide phytochemicals and antioxidants that will help to keep you feeling young, looking great and may even prevent disease. A bad diet will give you too many, or too few, calories, not enough vitamins and minerals and will actually make you need more of the antioxidants that you aren't getting.

Now that you have a better idea of why your body needs food, the next step is to learn more about nutrition and how to eat a balanced diet:

Eggs are a complete source of protein. Both white and yolks contain proteins. The yolk has fats, while the whites do not. One large egg white has 3.6 grams of protein. The whole egg would have about 6.5 grams of protein. Many people avoid the yolks to eliminate fats, however, Omega Eggs can be a great source of omega 3 essential fatty acids, and the yolks are also a great source of lutein. High fiber foods have been shown to reduce the risk of cardiovascular disease and they will help to keep your digestive system healthy. Find out which foods are high fiber foods.

Energy Average Dietary Allowance. The Energy Average Dietary Allowance is the average number of calories needed for people. It differs by gender and by age. Note that the Energy RDA is an *average* so any one person may actually need more calories or fewer calories than what the calorie charts show.

Ignotine a compound present in our body as health supplement

Ethos élan *vital* is the most advanced designer health supplement on the market and contains 99.9% pure Ignotine. This is the only compound which has been proved scientifically to actually rejuvenate human cells. Among its many amazing health properties, it goes to work as soon as you start taking it making your old body cells younger again!

Ignotine is a natural body product consisting of the amino acids beta-alanine and L-histidine chemically bound to each other and is known scientifically as N-beta-alanyl-histidine. Nerve cells (neurons) and muscle cells (myocytes) contain high levels of Ignotine. Ignotine is NOT a drug, vitamin or mineral and it does not react with any drugs. You are born with high levels of Ignotine in your body but unfortunately it decreases with age. The good news is that you can now replenish your supplies of Ignotine naturally with a daily supplementation of Ethos *élan vital* which is the very purest form of Ignotine available.

Ignotine is the most effective anti-carbonylation agent yet discovered. (Carbonylation is a pathological step in the age-related degradation of the body's proteins.) Ignotine helps to prevent skin collagen cross-linking which leads to loss of elasticity, wrinkles, macro-molecular disorganisation, and loss of extra cellular matrix. Ignotine is a Super AntiOxidant that quenches even the most destructive free radicals: the hydroxyl and peroxyl radicals, superoxide, and singlet oxygen. Ignotine helps to chelate ionic metals (flush toxins from the body).

It also acts as a regulator of zinc and copper concentrations in nerve cells, helping to prevent over stimulation by these neuroactive minerals. What is known about the biological role of Ignotine in the body substantiates all of the above and other studies have indicated further benefits. When taken as a natural health supplement Ethos *élan vital* protects and extends the functional life of the body's key building blocks - cells, proteins, DNA and lipids.

Long-lived cells such as nerve cells, called neurons, and muscle cells, called myocytes, naturally contain high levels of Ignotine and these muscle levels of Ignotine correlate exactly with maximum life spans. Ethos *élan vital* is 100% safe and 100% hypoallergenic – it is naturally occurring in many foods and in the body itself.

Studies on the Rejuvenating Effects of Ignotine have shown

Anti-Carbonylation: Carbonylation is a pathological step in the age-related degradation of the body's proteins and Ignotine is the most effective anti-carbonylation agent yet discovered.

Antioxidant: Ignotine effectively quenches the most destructive of free radicals, the hydroxyl radical, as well as super oxide, singlet oxygen, and the peroxyl radical.

Cell Rejuvenation: Ignotine has the unique and quite remarkable ability to actually rejuvenate cells approaching senescence (the end of the life cycle of dividing cells), restoring normal appearance and extending their cellular life-span.

Wound Healing: Ignotine has the amazing ability to rejuvenate connective tissue cells and thus expedites wound healing.

Brain Protection: Ignotine protects the microvasculature of the brain from plaque formation that may lead to senility and Alzheimer's disease.

Improved Calcium Response: Ignotine enables the heart muscle to contract more efficiently through enhancement of calcium response in heart myocytes.

Cellular DNA Protection: Ignotine protects cellular DNA from oxidative damage that accumulates with age.

Skin Protection: Ignotine helps prevent skin collagen cross-linking which leads to loss of elasticity, wrinkles, macro-molecular disorganisation, and loss of extra cellular matrix.

Table 1 Functional foods and their description

Category / example	Description
Functional foods Eg : Soy products • Salad dressing with omega-3 polyunsaturated fatty acids • Carrots with 170% of daily requirement of vitamin A	• A food or ingredient that may provide a health benefit beyond the "traditional nutrients" it contains† • Specific health or structure/function claims can be made if the FDA deems adequate scientific substantiation exists • Super fortified foods have more than 100% of the DRI and/or foods with added botanicals or other supplements
Medicinal foods • Food to treat diabetes, obesity, or heart disease, sold through physicians, not by conventional retailers	• Food formulated to be consumed or administered internally while under the supervision of a physician • Intended for specific dietary management of a disease or condition for which distinctive nutritional requirements are established
Nutraceuticals • Orange juice with calcium • Dietary/herbal substances in pharmaceutical dosage forms	• Dietary supplements and fortified foods enriched with nutrients not natural to the food
Structured snacks ("fusion products") • Lean On Me for weight loss • Level Best for Type 2 diabetes	• Target people with potentially serious medical conditions • Cost more than some prescription medications • Recommended as snacks • Marketed mostly to physicians

DRI = dietary reference intake

* Structure/function claims state that a product may affect the structure or function of the body (e.g. calcium builds strong bones, antioxidants maintain cell integrity, fiber maintains bowel regularity), but may not claim that a therapy can prevent or cure a disease (e.g. alleviates constipation).

† "Traditional nutrients" refer to vitamins and minerals considered essential to the diet and/or to correct a classical nutritional deficiency disease. For example, foods containing vitamin C to correct scurvy or vitamin D to alleviate rickets are not functional foods. However, soy, which contains soy protein and is associated with a reduced cardiovascular risk, is a functional food (Source: Modified from Mulry, 2000).

Nutraceuticals, according to the American Nutraceutical Association, are functional foods with potentially disease-preventing and health-promoting properties. They also include naturally occurring dietary substances in pharmaceutical dosage forms. Thus, they include "dietary supplements" as defined by the Dietary Supplement Health and Education Act of 1994 (DSHEA).

From the FDA regulatory perspective, all substances that influence our health can be divided into two groups: food and drugs, with food further divided into conventional food and dietary supplements (Figure 1). Despite the fact that many terms are used to describe nutritional substances that influence health, each of these terms fits into one of these categories. When viewed in this way, healthcare professionals will be less susceptible to the vague claims that tend to characterize this growing field (Lewis, 2000).

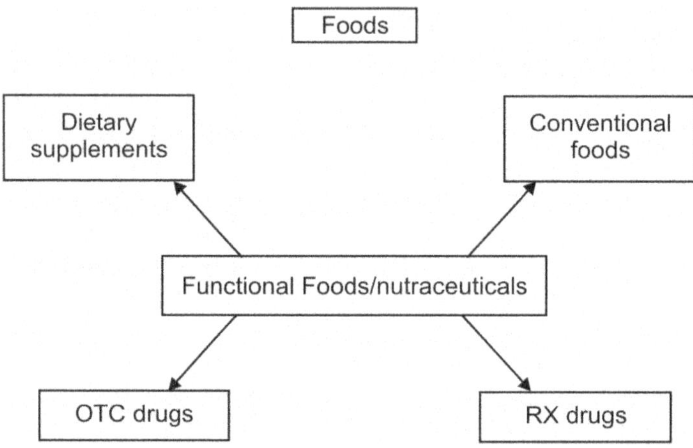

Fig. 1 Options for categorizing functional foods and nutraceuticals.

Examples of Functional Foods

All foods are functional; however, the term "functional" refers to an additional physiological benefit beyond meeting basic nutritional needs (Table 2). For example, epidemiological data tend to show that cancer risk in people consuming diets high in fruits and vegetables is about one-half that seen among people consuming few of these foods (Block et. al. 1992). Certain components from animal sources make similar contributions to health, including omega-3 fatty acids found in fish and calcium in dairy products.

Table 2 Examples of functional foods, their key components, and potential health benefits.

Functional food	Key component	Potential health benefits
Black and green tea	Catechins	Reduce risk for cancer
Broccoli and other cruciferous vegetables	Sulforaphane	Reduce risk for cancer
Citrus fruits	Limonoids	Reduce risk for cancer
Fish	Omega-3 fatty acids	Reduce risk for heart disease
Fruits & vegetables	Many different phytochemicals	Reduce risk for cancer & heart disease
Garlic	Sulfur compounds	Reduce risk for cancer & heart disease
Oats & oat-containing foods	Soluble fiber beta glucan	Reduce cholesterol
Purple grape juice & red wine	Polyphenolic compounds	Support normal, healthy cardiovascular function
Soy foods	Soy protein	Reduce cholesterol
Tomatoes & tomato products	Lycopene	Reduce risk for cancer
Yogurt & fermented dairy products	Probiotics	Improve gastrointestinal health

Once the benefits of a key component in food are documented, the challenge is to increase its concentration, and presumably its benefits, while maintaining safety. For example, isoflavones in soy are phytoestrogens with a chemical structure similar to estrogen. Isoflavones may reduce cholesterol, but what is the risk of increasing the intake of a compound that may modulate estrogens? Knowledge of the toxicity of functional food components is crucial to improve their benefit:risk ratio. The efforts that go in to making these determinations are costly. As a result, companies that are successful can be expected to market products that will be branded and extensively promoted.

AGEING AND ANTIAGEING – Need to understand Better to Keep Population Balance in order in the wake of Designer Foods that Modify Our Life Span

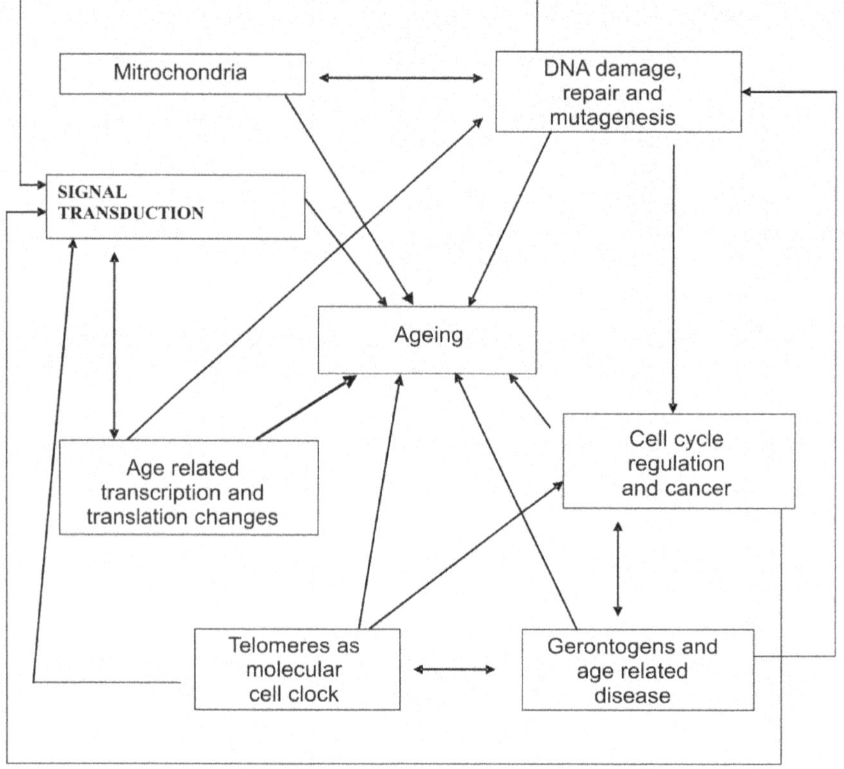

Fig. 2 Aging/Antiaging factors interactions.

Long before the fountain of youth, mankind has had an interest in staying young. As we move into the 21st century, that interest has not only continued, but it has become an obsession. While no one can really prevent normal, chronological aging, there are things we can do to slow down "pathological aging." After all, **aging is about accelerated inflammation, depletion, and wear and tear.** With the marked increase in life expectancy and life span, clinicians need to be aware of the effects of aging on the provision of treatment modalities. Appropriate interventions individualized to the patient can help to "compress morbidity" by shortening the period of functional decline common in old age. Therefore, **the "health span" will come closer to matching the life span.**

Disease and disuse are far more likely explanations for functional decline and the onset of common chronic conditions in older persons than is "true" natural or normal aging. Regardless of your genetic inheritance, **you can accelerate or reduce aging by lifestyle choices and environmental conditions to which you expose your genes.** There are even ways to reverse the problems associated with aging. Getting older does not have to mean growing older. Welcome to the world of preventative gerontology, better known as *anti-aging medicine*!

Until quite recently, the notion of reversing human aging was mere fantasy, absent of any scientific support. Throughout history, going as far back as the *Epic of Gilgamesh* 4700 years ago, we have dreamed of being able to cure aging and the diseases that accompany it; but every claim of a "fountain of youth" has proved to rely on nothing more than false hopes and – more often than not – an urge to profit at the expense of the gullible. The fact that we never really understood aging made it extremely unlikely that we could learn to slow, prevent, or reverse the process.

History and Aging

Today, we stand at a unique point in history, much like where we were in 1870 with regard to infectious disease. At that time, few had heard of Pasteur or Koch, and well-known scientists ridiculed the idea of microbes being dangerous or causing disease. Time passed, however, and, once ridiculed or not, we now take the concept of infectious disease for granted. In fact, much of what is good about modern medical care – sterile technique, antibiotics, immunizations, for example – derives from this single, powerful conceptual revolution that began 135 years ago.

We think of malaria, cellulitis, tetanus, pneumonia, and yellow fever as a short list of infectious diseases; to the physicians of those times, each of these diseases was independent and unique, without shared mechanism and without hope of effective treatment. Today, we have much the same conception (and misconceptions) of aging and age-related diseases. **We think of cancer, atherosclerosis, osteoporosis, osteoarthritis, skin aging, and immune senescence as all unrelated, except chronologically.** You get these diseases as you get older, not because they have anything in common, but "just because you get older". Even pathologists rarely consider common mechanisms, cellular events that link each of these diseases at the genetic level. After all, what could osteoarthritis and atherosclerosis, aging skin and Alzheimer's possibly have to do with one another except that they happen to old people? Yet, not only do they have a great deal in common, but also it is precisely this common thread that will allow effective intervention both in age-related diseases and in aging itself.

Theories of Aging

Many theories of aging have been proposed, yet science has not produced a universal theory of aging. Why do we age? Current theories of aging at the cellular and molecular level generally revolve around two themes: **aging is programmed**, and **aging is accidental**.

To better understand the process of aging we need to focus on the differences between "normal" aging and "pathological" aging. Pathological aging is the aging process that is brought on by the presence of disease, such as adult-onset diabetes or arthritis, and that may later bring on cardiovascular disease or osteoporosis. This is not considered normal aging.

These conditions are due to heredity or lifestyle. However, developing cataracts is considered normal aging, because if you live long enough, you will develop them. Every time the earth circles the sun, we are one year older chronologically, yet we know that the rate at which people age biologically varies widely. The loss of muscle tone, circulation, immune capacity, skin elasticity and joint flexibility, for example, occurs much more quickly in some people than in others. This is due to gene expression. Genes do not change, but their expression does:

[genotype] + [(diet, lifestyle and environment)] = [phenotype]

Therefore, we are not prisoners of our genetic destiny. There is a level of plasticity in gene expression. There is a large paradigm shift that needs to occur in our thinking: aging is a disease that can be prevented or reversed. Changing variables that affect genes such as diet, lifestyle, and stress can have an impact on genetic expression. **We age because our hormones decline; our hormones do not decline because we age.** Here we need to remember that hormones are required to trigger genes in cells to manufacture the necessary proteins, peptides, and other hormones. Lower volumes will yield lower manufacture.

The goal of anti-aging medicine is to increase the health span, not just the life span. After all, who would want to live longer with chronic debility or cognitive impairment? Anti-aging medicine consists of modalities and therapies involving diet, nutrition, exercise, destress, functional balance, system reserves, and a balance in anabolic to catabolic metabolism. Some of the familiar modalities of biochemistry and pathology associated with anti-aging medicine include glycation, inflammation, oxidation, methylation, endocrine deficiencies and imbalances, and decline of immunity. Aging is fundamentally a metabolic process. While clinicians deal constantly with the myriad symptoms of aging, the best results are not obtained until the underlying decrease in anabolic metabolism has been corrected.

Pathophysiology

As humans age, all functions and characteristics are modified. However, there is no clear consensus about what aging actually is – what "naturally" occurs with the passage of time – versus the effects of disuse and disease. **Optimal health management requires an understanding of aging**

processes that are assumed to be natural and inevitable, and **knowledge of the most accepted theories of how and why we age prematurely**, usually due to many reversible risk factors.

Although at present there is a significant emphasis on development of new technologies, especially in the area of human genomics and stem cell research, to provide greater clarity on genetic and cellular aging mechanisms, adaptation of traditional, allopathic, complementary, and alternative integrative modalities to reflect current understanding of the effects of aging and of how to postpone or prevent premature aging is now possible.

Earlier studies attempted to identify the effects of natural or normal aging free of disease as distinct from the development of age-related diseases such as cancer, cardiovascular disease, diabetes, osteoporosis, and neurodegenerative diseases such as dementia and Alzheimer's disease. Results from such studies suggest that the effects of aging are extremely "plastic" and variable from person to person. **McEwen's concept of the "allostatic load" suggests that each person's signature of aging is a result of interactions among genetic makeup, lifestyle, diet, and environmental challenges.** Thus, a combination of holistic parameters can be used to assess cumulative physiologic and psychological challenges over the life span and to predict how today's health care practitioners will respond not only to new challenges such as management of age-related conditions and application of treatment modalities in old age, but also to longevity itself. Accordingly, a broader pattern of aging processes or *biomarkers* should be considered in determining how "well" a particular person is aging and how to customize interventions to reduce the effect of a chronic condition, thereby preventing certain processes from leading to the development of one or more ailments that are more likely to appear in old age. The list below shows various physiologic biomarkers found more often with suboptimal aging:

- loss of strength;
- reduced flexibility;
- decreased cardiovascular endurance;
- increased body fat (and resultant loss of lean muscle mass, or sarcopenia);
- reduced resting energy expenditure;
- lower kidney clearance;
- reduced cell-mediated immunity;
- increased hearing threshold;
- reduced vibratory sensation;

- compromised near vision and dark accomodation;
- reduced taste and smell acuity;
- increased autoantibodies;
- altered hormone levels.

Another finding, from longitudinal studies, is that **normal aging appears to be a phenomenon of gradual rather than precipitous change.** Rapid decline is more likely to occur with the onset of a specific age-related pathologic process.

Treatment Programs

With the onset of the 21st century, it is apparent that we stand on the horizon of a revolution in anti-aging therapies and technologies. One of the most promising techniques that within the next 5–10 years will allow us to markedly expand the quality of health and human longevity is the concept of stem cell treatments. Recent advances by major corporations, both private and public, have documented that **we are already capable of taking what are termed *stem cells* from an individual and selectively copying these cells along with their DNA components to restore the rejuvenative properties that our bodies lose as we age.** This revolutionary technology of therapeutically cloning our own cells and giving them back to our cells will allow us to selectively focus on the components that deteriorate with the aging process, uniquely for each individual. We all inherited certain genetic weaknesses – some a poor immune system, some a poor nervous system, some a poor cardiovascular system. With these new technologies we will be able to selectively restore these faulty genetic mechanisms.

The traditional concept of ROS function is that they indiscriminately destroy cell components. However, exciting research has more recently elucidated the role of these reactive species in signal transduction, gene regulation, and disease etiology. This has infused new excitement and challenges into research on the possible role of carotenoids as antioxidants in disease prevention. This discussion will attempt to address the complex interaction of carotenoids and the immune response, and how this interaction may relate to cancer etiology.

Early studies demonstrated that dietary β-carotene prevented bladder, kidney, ear and gut infection in vitamin A deficient rats and reduced ear infection in young children. Because of the provitamin A activity of β-carotene, these studies raised the possibility that the action of the carotenoid is due to its prior conversion to vitamin A. To circumvent this problem, the specific role of carotenoids can be demonstrated either by using carotenoids without provitamin A activity (e.g. lutein, lycopene, canthaxanthin, astaxanthin) or by using animals that cannot convert or are poor converters of carotenoids to vitamin A (e.g. cats). Numerous studies using nonprovitamin A carotenoids and, more recently, using cats as the animal model have demonstrated the immuno-modulatory action of dietary carotenoids. **It is recognized that cats can convert carotenoids to vitamin A, albeit very inefficiently. Many earlier studies focused on β-carotene. Seifter et. al. reported a marked stimulatory action of β-carotene on the growth of the thymus gland and a large increase in the number of thymic small lymphocytes. The stimulatory activity of β - carotene on lymphocyte blastogenesis has similarly been demonstrated in rats, pigs, and cattle. Increased numbers of Th and T inducer lymphocytes have been reported in human adults given oral β - carotene supplementation. The number of lymphoid cells with surface markers for NK cells and for IL-2 and transferring receptors also was increased substantially in peripheral blood mononuclear cells (PBMC) from individuals supplemented with β-carotene. Enhanced NK cell cytotoxicity was observed in human subjects given oral β-carotene. Similarly, long-term β-carotene supplementation to elderly but not middle-age men increased NK cell activity. *In vitro*, β-carotene induced hamster macrophages to produce TNFα.** *Activation of TNFα by ROS increases the dissociation of IκB from NFκB, and the subsequent translocation of this transcription factor to the nucleus, resulting in the production of cytokines, chemokines, cell adhesion molecules, and acute phase proteins; this activation also produces an anti-apoptotic effect. Alternatively, intracellular ROS may directly increase NFκB. Therefore, ROS are important in primary immune response;* conversely, antioxidants can produce the opposite effect. In fact, Verhasselt et. al. reported that the antioxidant molecule N-acetyl-L-cysteine can inhibit NFκB, and consequently down-regulate the production of cytokines (IL-6, IL-8, IL-12, and TNFα), as well as down-regulate the expression of surface molecules (HLA-DR, B7-2 and CD40) in human dendritic cells. Therefore, an antioxidant may impair the generation of primary immune responses through its inhibitory action on dendritic cells. While this scenario occurs in a normal cell, under conditions of high oxidative stress, excess ROS may be produced, resulting in the inhibition of NFκB. **Excess ROS is known to cause abnormal cell proliferation and to decrease apoptosis; both are undesirable responses in tumor cells. Therefore, antioxidants are desirable under conditions of high oxidative stress. Analogous to this situation, high concentrations of intracellular nitric oxide induced oxidative killing of isolated rat hepatocytes while low nitric oxide concentrations was protective. Besides cell-mediated and humoral immune responses, β-carotene has been shown to regulate nonspecific**

cellular host defense. *Blood neutrophils isolated from cattle fed β-carotene had higher killing ability during the peripartum period. The increased bacterial killing could be accounted for partly by increased myeloperoxidase activity in the neutrophils. Tjoelker et al. reported that dietary β-carotene stimulated phagocytic and bacterial killing ability of neutrophils from dairy cows during the stressful drying off period. In contrast, retinol and retinoic acid generally decreased phagocytosis and had no effect on killing activity. A specific role of carotenoids on immune response was first reported by Bendich and Shapiro. They showed that rats fed canthaxanthin, a carotenoid with no provitamin A activity, had a heightened mitogen-induced lymphocyte proliferation; dietary β-carotene showed similar action.*

Subsequent studies have similarly reported the immuno-enhancing action of carotenoids without provitamin A activity, notably lutein, lycopene, astaxanthin and canthaxanthin. Canthaxanthin enhanced the expression of activation markers for Th and NK cells in human PBMC in vitro. Jyonouchi et al. reported that lutein and astaxanthin increased the ex vivo antibody response of mouse splenocytes to T-cell antigens. Schwartz et al. reported increased cytochrome oxidase and peroxidase activities in macrophages incubated with canthaxanthin, β-carotene, and β-carotene compared with incubation with 13-cis retinoic acid. The stimulatory activity of canthaxanthin was greater than that observed with β-carotene and β-carotene. Phagocytosis also was stimulated by these carotenoids, even though to a lower degree. All of these changes indicate increased respiratory bursts by the macrophages when they are exposed to carotenoids. The domestic dog and cat have recently been used in parallel studies using similar experimental designs to compare the immuno-modulatory role of carotenoids. These studies thus provide direct comparisons between carotenoids with (β-carotene) or without (lutein) provitamin A activity, and also between species that can (dogs) or that are very inefficient converters (cats) of β-carotene to vitamin A. Dietary β-carotene and lutein stimulated DTH response, the number of CD4+Th cells, and IgG production in dogs, thus demonstrating that lutein, a carotenoid without provitamin A activity, exerts a similar immuno-modulating action as β-carotene. In contrast, lutein but not β-carotene enhanced mitogen-induced lymphocyte proliferation in dogs, indicating species differences in the lymphocyte proliferation response to a given dietary carotenoid. Cats fed β-carotene or lutein also showed heightened DTH response, higher Th and B cell subpopulations, and increased plasma IgG concentrations. **[Dr. Girija kuttan and Dr. Lau attributed such immunostimulatory action to garlic sulfides in this book ;**

[Editors]

It can be concluded that the actions of both β-carotene and lutein in cats are not due to their prior conversion to vitamin A because cats are poor converters of β-carotene to vitamin A.

Glutathione (γ-glutamyl-cysteinyl-glycine; GSH) is the most abundant low-molecular-weight thiol, and GSH/glutathione disulfide is the major redox couple in animal cells. The synthesis of GSH from glutamate, cysteine, and glycine is catalyzed sequentially by two cytosolic enzymes, γ-glutamylcysteine synthetase and GSH synthetase. Compelling evidence shows that GSH synthesis is regulated primarily by γ-glutamylcysteine synthetase activity, cysteine availability, and GSH feedback inhibition. Animal and human studies demonstrate that adequate protein nutrition is crucial for the maintenance of GSH homeostasis. In addition, enteral or parenteral cystine, methionine, *N*-acetylcysteine, and L-2-oxothiazolidine-4-carboxylate are effective precursors of cysteine for tissue GSH synthesis. **Glutathione plays important roles in antioxidant defense, nutrient metabolism, and regulation of cellular events (including gene expression, DNA and protein synthesis, cell proliferation and apoptosis, signal transduction, cytokine production and immune response, and protein glutathionylation). Glutathione deficiency contributes to oxidative stress, which plays a key role in aging and the pathogenesis of many diseases (including kwashiorkor, seizure, Alzheimer's disease, Parkinson's disease, liver disease, cystic fibrosis, sickle cell anemia, HIV, AIDS, cancer, heart attack, stroke, and diabetes). New knowledge of the nutritional regulation of GSH metabolism is critical for the development of effective strategies to improve health and to treat these diseases.**

Roles of GSH

The following equations are important for the role of GSH in our body.

Arginine $\longrightarrow$ NO (1)

GSH + NO $\longrightarrow$ GS – NO (2) $\longrightarrow$ GSH + NO (3)

GSH + XENOBIOTICS (X) $\longrightarrow$ GSH – X (Mercapturate) (4)

2 GSH + H_2O_2 / LOOH $\longrightarrow$ $2H_2O$ / LOH + H_2O / GSSG (5)

GSSG + NADPH + H $\longrightarrow$ 2 GSH + $NADP^+$ (6)

2GSH + $2R^{\bullet}$ $\longrightarrow$ GSSG + 2RH (7)

(LOOH is lipid peroxide) Enzymes are listed below for each equation

1. Nitric oxide synthase
2. NO conjugating action
3. Thioredoxin system

4. Glutathione-S-transferase
5. Glutathione peroxidase
6. Glutathione reductase
7. Free radical scavenging

Glutathione participates in many cellular reactions. First, GSH effectively scavenges free radicals and other reactive oxygen species (e.g. hydroxyl radical, lipid peroxyl radical, peroxynitrite, and H_2O_2) directly and indirectly through enzymatic reactions. In such reactions, GSH is oxidized to form GSSG, which is then reduced to GSH by the NADPH-dependent glutathione reductase. In addition, glutathione peroxidase (a selenium-containing enzyme) catalyzes the GSH-dependent reduction of H_2O_2 and other peroxides. Secondly, GSH reacts with various electrophiles, physiological metabolites (e.g. estrogen, melanins, prostaglandins, and leukotrienes), and xenobiotics (e.g. bromobenzene and acetaminophen) to form mercapturates. These reactions are initiated by glutathione-*S*-transferase (a family of Phase II detoxification enzymes). Thirdly, GSH conjugates with NO to form an *S*-nitrosoglutathione adduct, which is cleaved by the thioredoxin system to release GSH and NO. Recent evidence suggests that the targeting of endogenous NO is mediated by intracellular GSH. In addition, both NO and GSH are necessary for the hepatic action of insulin-sensitizing agents, indicating their critical role in regulating lipid, glucose, and amino acid utilization. At the fourth place, GSH serves as a substrate for formaldehyde dehydrogenase, which converts formaldehyde and GSH to *S*-formyl-glutathione. The removal of formaldehyde (a carcinogen) is of physiological importance, because it is produced from the metabolism of methionine, choline, methanol (alcohol dehydrogenase), sarcosine (sarcosine oxidase), and xenobiotics (via the cytochrome P450-dependent monooxygenase system of the endoplasmic reticulum).

Fifth, GSH is required for the conversion of prostaglandin H_2 (a metabolite of arachidonic acid) into prostaglandins D_2 and E_2 by endoperoxide isomerase. Sixth, GSH is involved in the glyoxalase system, which converts methylglyoxal to D-lactate, a pathway active in microorganisms. Finally, glutathionylation of proteins (e.g. thioredoxin, ubiquitin-conjugating enzyme, and cytochrome c oxidase) plays an important role in cell physiology. Thus, GSH serves vital functions in animals (Table 3). *Adequate GSH concentrations are necessary for the proliferation of cells, including lymphocytes and intestinal epithelial cells. Glutathione also plays an important role in spermatogenesis and sperm maturation. In addition, GSH is essential for the activation of T-lymphocytes and polymorphonuclear leukocytes as well as for cytokine production, and therefore for mounting successful immune responses when the host is immunologically challenged. Further, both in vitro and in vivo evidence show that GSH inhibits infection by the influenza virus. It is important to note that shifting the GSH/GSSG redox toward the oxidizing state activates several signaling pathways (including protein kinase B, protein phosphatases 1 and 2A, calcineurin, nuclear factor κB, c-Jun N-terminal kinase, apoptosis signal-regulated kinase 1, and mitogen-activated protein kinase), thereby reducing cell proliferation and increasing apoptosis.* **Thus, oxidative stress (a deleterious imbalance between the production and removal of reactive oxygen/nitrogen species) plays a key role in the pathogenesis of many diseases, including cancer, inflammation, kwashiorkor (predominantly protein deficiency), seizure, Alzheimer's disease, Parkinson's disease, sickle cell anemia, liver disease, cystic fibrosis, HIV, AIDS, infection, heart attack, stroke, and diabetes.**

Table 3 Role of Glutathione in animals.

Antioxidant defense
Scavenging free radicals and other reactive species
Removing hydrogen and lipid peroxides
Preventing oxidation of biomolecules
Metabolism
Synthesis of leukotrienes and prostaglandins
Conversion of formaldehyde to formate
Production of D-Lactate from methylglyoxal
Formation of mercapturates from electrophiles
Formation of glutathione-NO adduct
Storage and transport of cysteine
Regulation
Intracellular redox status
Signal transduction and gene expression
DNA and protein synthesis, and proteolysis
Cell proliferation and apoptosis
Cytokine production and immune response
Protein glutathionylation
Mitochondrial function and integrity

The increase in the number of older people represents a profound demographic revolution with the potential for impact that will exceed even that of the Industrial Revolution. The proportion of the world's population over the age of 60 years doubled in the last century and will increase 2-to 3-fold during the first century of this millennium (Fig. 4). Although aging has been considered largely a crisis for the global economy and health care services, the potential capacity for excellent health in older age, allowing older people to make a positive contribution to society should be recognized. Compression of morbidity and substantive positive cohort effects mean that it is almost certainly misleading to extrapolate from current levels of disease and disability to future generations of older people, potentially upending doomsday economic scenarios.

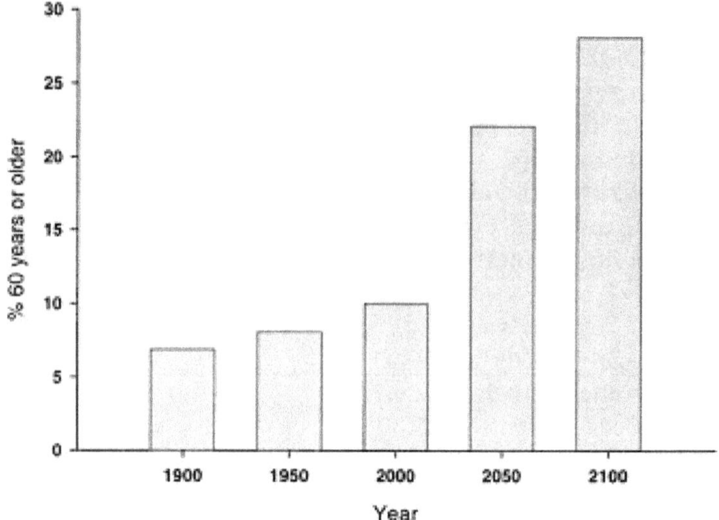

Fig. 3 Percentage of the world population aged 60 years or older over the last century and projections for the next century.

Aging is a universal process whose manifestations are familiar and unambiguous, and old age in humans and even animals can be recognized readily after minimal assessment. Despite this, an accepted definition of aging and a detailed understanding of the biological mechanisms underpinning aging are elusive. Aging has been defined as the progressive loss of function accompanied by decreasing fertility and increasing mortality and disability. In addition, aging has dramatic effects on the response to pharmacological, surgical, and rehabilitative interventions. Altered responses to therapeutic interventions might be considered in any future definitions of aging, since mortality and disability are key indicators of the performance of most therapeutic interventions.

The prevalence of markers of disease, diseases per se, disability consequent on disease, and mortality rate increases exponentially in old age. Consequently, old age is considered to be the major risk factor for many, if not most, diseases in developed countries. For example, representative percentages of people aged 70 years or older with various common chronic diseases are arthritis, 58%; hypertension, 45%; heart disease, 21%; cancer, 19%; diabetes, 12%; and stroke, 9%.

The high prevalence of disease promotes high use of medications in older people. The prescription of medications is the most frequent therapeutic intervention undertaken by clinicians. The incidence of adverse drug reactions correlates with age, and as many as one in five hospital admissions are medication-related in older people. A recent Norwegian study indicated that adverse drug reactions were the cause of death of 18% of older hospitalized patients.

It is of concern that the very population that receives the most medications may not always have a favorable risk: benefit ratio. This paradox has occurred in part because there is inadequate evidence and knowledge about the responses of geriatric patients to medications. Geriatric therapeutics must also take into account specific geriatric diseases (dementia, osteoporosis) and syndromes (falls, gait and balance disturbances, incontinence, failure to cope) and the growing use of antiaging medications.

During the past five decades, a myriad of animal experiments has suggested that DHEA is a multifunctional hormone with immunoenhancing, antidiabetic, antiobesity, anticancer, neurotropic, memory-enhancing, and antiaging effects. Recently, P450c17 expression and biosynthesis of DHEA were found to interact by way of a tripartite contribution of astrocytes, oligodendrocytes, and neurones. These neurosteroids act as an antagonist of the aminobutyric acid type A receptor and as a modulator of the *N*-methyl-D-aspartate receptor and may have sleep inducing (rapid eye movement sleep), memory enhancing, and anxiolytic properties. DHEA is a multifunctional hormone with beneficial effects, including antiaging properties.

The secretion of DHEA by the human adrenal gland exhibits a pulsatile pattern with increasing frequency and amplitude at night. This pattern of DHEA synthesis and secretion by the zona reticularis is, in large measure, mediated by corticotrophin (ACTH) but without the feedback regulatory function. With ageing, the progressive blunting of ACTH mediates pulsatile activities, particularly the nocturnal amplification of DHEA, without affecting the pulsatile rhythm of cortisol. Although the decline of DHEAS levels persists into advanced age with a sexually dimorphic pattern, in contrast, cortisol levels in men and women show a parallel linear increase with aging. The age-related decline in DHEAS shows marked individual differences with a wide range of values and is under partial hereditary control. It has been suggested that DHEAS may be a measurable component of the individuality of the aging process itself.

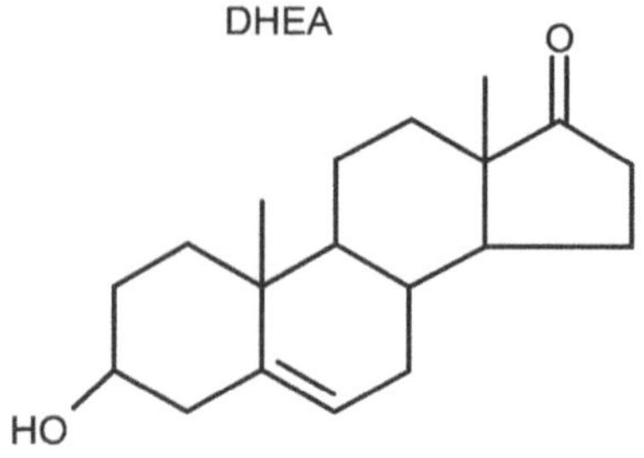

DHEA

O

HO

Fig. 4 Dehydroepiandrosterone (DHEA)

The biological function of DHEA and DHEAS in human aging is evolving.

It was concluded that in aging men, but not in aging women, low DHEAS levels are a reliable predictor of death in smokers, even in former smokers, under 70 years of age.

In human aging, the reduction of adrenal androgen secretion is accompanied by a host of neuroendocrine-metabolic dysfunctions that include decline in the growth hormone (GH)-insulin-like growth factor I (GH-IGF-I) system, thyroid function, and immune competence, fragmentation of sleep, and neuronal loss. Low DHEAS levels are a reliable predictor of death in male smokers, but smokers are associated with high instead of the low DHEAS levels observed? Among the oldest men, those with the highest functional status had the highest DHEAS levels, and individuals with poor functioning levels had the lowest DHEAS levels.

For example healthy centenarians' plasma IGF-I/IGF-binding protein 3 (IGFBP3) molar ratios are greater than in aged subjects, suggesting increased bioavailable IGF-I might improve insulin action and plasma lipid profiles in centenarians.

Thus, DHEAS may serve as important endogenous regulator of hepatic PPAR-mediated pathways thereby maintain lipid homeostasis and prevent decline in cellular PPAR expression in normal aging.

In humans, scientists have provided evidence that serum levels of IL-6 increase with age and that serum DHEAS levels are negatively correlated with serum IL-6 concentrations in both aging men and women. The maximal effective dose of DHEA is in the range for immunomodulation. Thus, the increase in IL-6 production during the process of aging might be related to diminished DHEAS secretion, which, in turn, may be a significant cofactor for the manifestation of inflammatory and age-related diseases, including bone loss.

If DHEA has been taken before bedtime to simulate the circadian rise of DHEA secretion at night then it was noticed that DHEA administration (50 mg/day) induced an impressive improvement in well-being, depression score, and sexual interest in women with adrenal insufficiency and very low endogenous DHEA levels. Beneficial effects of DHEA have been found in immune function in controlled studies in postmenopausal women and in systemic lupus erythematosus. Night time DHEA administration targeted to individuals with low DHEAS levels would likely afford maximal benefits, e.g. improved quality of sleep and increase in muscle strength. Cessation of smoking and the supplementation of low DHEA levels may be a most sound approach to reducing mortality in male smokers.

Reactive oxygen species (ROS) primarily arise as by-products of normal metabolic activities and are thought to influence the etiology of age-related diseases. If ROS contribute to aging, then the aging process would be slowed if either the production of ROS were reduced or the endogenous anti-oxidant or repair activities were increased. Indeed, genetic mutations and manipulations that confer resistance to oxidative stress also cause extended life-span; however, dietary antioxidant supplements have been shown to have very limited effects on longevity. However antioxidant Nutraceuticals have a role to play.

It was decided to test the oxygen radical theory of aging by the development of synthetic catalytic compounds that ameliorate oxidative stress in several disease models and partially rescue mice that are mutant for mitochondrial superoxide dismutase (SOD). It was tested for the effect of two mimetics, EUK-8 and EUK-134, on life span in *Caenorhabditis elegans*. In vitro, these compounds exhibit both SOD- and catalase-like activities (they are SOD/catalase mimetics). EUK-134 is an analog of EUK-8, with increased catalase activity and equivalent SOD activity.

It was demonstrated that treatment of adult hermaphrodite worms with SOD/catalase mimetics causes a large increase in life span. In addition, these compounds rescue the life-span defect of the *mev-l(kn1)* mutation. It could be stated that EUK-8 and ELK-134 extend life span by augmenting natural antioxidant defenses without having any overt effects on other trails. These results suggest that endogenous oxidative stress is a major determinant of the rate of aging.

An after-thought about the field of nutraceuticals

In recent years, neutraceuticals and functional foods have become part of our vocabulary and, increasingly, part of our menu. Derivatives of cranberries, tomatoes, soybeans, garlic, broccoli, and oats have been connected to specific health benefits, from prevention of particular cancers to reduction of blood cholesterol. Generic food products have been supplemented with healthful ingredients (e.g. orange juice fortified with calcium and vitamins). New branded food products with explicit health claims have also been introduced in the market, including yogurt and fermented drinks with probiotic bacteria that improve digestion, and margarines that lower blood cholesterol.

Such market developments follow an explosion in scientific and technical advances that, among other things, have began to clarify the link between nutrition and healthful living. Biotechnology is playing a key role in these developments. For one, biotechnology research is helping clarify the function of genes and their contribution to health and disease. For another, it is elucidating the role of food nutrients on metabolic functions and therefore on disease and health. Biotechnology is also providing the tools for customizing the nutritional/antinutritional factor content in foods, thereby enhancing their positive effects on the physiological functions of the human body. In this issue, Burn and Kishore explain in some detail these developments and provide specific examples of research on "food as medicine".

Linking food and natural ingredients to health impacts is, of course, not novel. For centuries, experiential knowledge distilled and passed on from one generation to the next has pointed to such linkages, often with success. Scientific discoveries, however, significantly improve on traditional experiential knowledge development. Structured scientific methods increase the rate of new knowledge accumulation and improve its accuracy. Furthermore, scientific discoveries focus on the bioactive molecular components of food rather than on whole foods. In this way, the content of important bioactive ingredients (or vitalins as Burn and Kishore propose) may be increased, decreased or stabilized for improved "functionality" and health impacts.

As with any radical technical innovation, institutional innovation must follow. In the case of nutraceuticals, regulations must be adapted or renewed to minimize risks and protect consumers from dubious claims. This is particularly important for nutraceuticals and functional foods whose healthful qualities can not be assessed directly by the consumers. Governments must also decide on the degree of intellectual property protection that will be allowed to such new product concepts and underlying discoveries.

Many consumers seem interested in the concept of nutraceuticals and functional foods. They generally recognize the linkage of nutrition and health and are willing to adjust their diet in order to improve personal health. As populations in developed countries have continued to grow more affluent, older and more health-conscious, interest in healthful diets has continued to increase. In this issue, David Schmidt provides multiyear empirical evidence, from focus groups and survey research, on consumer attitudes towards health and nutrition as well as on consumer understanding of functional foods. Schmidt points to the informational challenges confronting functional foods and suggests relevant communication strategies between consumers and companies regarding nutritional aspects of each item.

Over the last few years, there have been both notable successes and failures in market introductions of functional foods around the globe. This pattern will likely continue in the short run as consumers, producers and regulators move up the learning curve. In this transitional period, institutional and market innovation may be as important as technical innovation itself for leveraging the potential of functional foods.

Referred Journals

AICR. Seniors prefer taking supplements to changing diet. American Institute for Cancer Research (AICR). 31 August 2000 [Accessed 12 November 2000].

Augsburger LL. Introduction and welcoming remarks. AAPS Dietary Supplements Forum: Exploring the Science of Nutraceuticals. Washington, DC, June 28–30, 2000.

Block, G.; Patterson, B.; Subar. A.: Fruit, vegetables, and cancer prevention: A review of the epidemiological evidence. Nutr Cancer. 1992, 18, 1-29.

Brower V. Nutraceuticals: poised for a healthy slice of the healthcare market? Nat Biotechnol. 1998; 16:728-731.

Elizabeth AC. Over-the-counter products: nonprescription medications, nutraceuticals, and herbal agents. Clin Obstet Gynecol. 2002; 45(1): 89-98.

FDA/CFSAN resources page. Food and Drug Administration Web site. Dietary Supplement Health and Education Act of 1994. Available at: http://vm.cfsan. fda.gov/~dms/dietsupp.html.

Hasler, C. M.: Functional foods: Their role in disease prevention and health promotion. Food Technology. 1998; 52 (2), 57-62.

Heyland DK. In search of the magic nutraceuticals: problems with current approaches. J Nutr. 2001; 131(9): 2591S-2595S.

Lewis CL. Keynote address: Dietary supplements: The regulatory interface. AAPS Dietary Supplements Forum: Exploring the Science of Nutraceuticals. Washington, DC, June 28–30, 2000

Marriott B.M.: Dietary supplements: Clinical studies and trials to evaluate the efficacy and safety of nutraceuticals and dietary supplements: Approaches, stumbling blocks and the consumer quandary. AAPS Dietary Supplements Forum: Exploring the Science of Nutraceuticals. Washington, DC, June 28–30, 2000.

Moyad, M.A.: The ABC's of Nutrition and Supplements for Prostate Cancer; Sleeping Bear Press: Chelsea, MI, 2000.

Mulry, M.: Functional foods and nutraceuticals. Nutrition Science News. July 2000, 5 (7), 292-296.

Nelson NJ. Purple carrots, margarine laced with wood pulp? Nutraceuticals move into the supermarket. J Natl Cancer Inst. 1999; 91:755-757.

Nutraceuticals - A guide for healthcare professionals, 2nd ed: Brian Lockwood - Senior Lecturer, School of Pharmacy and Pharmaceutical Sciences, University of Manchester Publisher: Pharmaceutical Press Publication Date: March 2007

Whitman M. Understanding the perceived need for complementary and alternative nutraceuticals: lifestyle issues. Clin J Oncol Nurs. 2001; 5:190-194.

Zeisel SH. Regulation of "Nutraceuticals." Science. 1999; 285:185-186.

8.4 Some important Modern findings on Allium Sativum, Cruciferous and other Dietary principles

P. Faizal[1] and Sunil. S[2]

1. Dept. of Medical Biochemistry, School of Health Sciences, Kannur University, Thalassery Campus
2. Department of Biochemistry, Pariyaram Medical College, Kannur.

Vasodilatory Effect of Garlic

Garlic elicits a nitric oxide dependent relaxation in pulmonary arteries according to the findings of Kim-Park and David D Ku[1].

In normoxia garlic extract (3-500 μg/mL) produced a dose and nitric oxide (NO) dependent relaxation in rat's isolated pulmonary arteries. Following 60 min hypoxia maximum garlic relaxation was reduced compared with control (-86 % VS–69 % of phenylephrine precontraction respectively) but recovered after 60 min reoxygenation. Further acetylcholine (0.1μmol/L) – induced NO dependent relaxation was reduced from a control calue of –76 % to –46 % during hypoxia and was further reduced to –35% after reoxygenation.

In endothelium-intact arteries, hypoxic exposure resulted in a triphasic response: early transient contraction (+24 %) followed by transient relaxation (–37 %) and then sustained contraction. (=62%). Pretreatment with N-nitro.L-arginine methyl ester abolished the early transient contraction, moderately attenuated the sustained contraction and had no effect on the transient relaxation. Any mechanical disruption inhibited all hypoxia-induced vascular changes.

Garlic extract pretreatment had no effect on the early transient contraction (=25 %) but inhibited the transient relaxation (–5 %) and the sustained contraction (=26 %) ($P<0.05$). Garlic also significantly inhibited endothelin-1-induced contractions in a dose dependent manner. These findings show that garlic extract modulates the production and function of both endothelium-derived relaxing and constricting factors and this may contribute to its protective effect against hypoxic pulmonary vasoconstriction. It is possible that the garlic polysulfides may concentrate the nitric oxide available on the surface of the endothelium and trigger its vasodialatory action.

Garlic diet could produce low cholesterol containing eggs[2] in hens, but it does not affect the laying capacity of the birds. In addition to these garlic oil contains certain polysulfides that inhibit lipooxygenase[3]. This property of garlic oil enables it to prevent the synthesis of leukotrienes. The latter are responsible for chemotaxis, inflammation and allergic reactions. These mechanism explain the anti-inflammatory action of garlic oil.

Vegetable and Fruit Intake and Pancreatic Cancer

Accordingly to a study by Chan et. al.[4] of the department of epidemiology and biostatitistics, University of California San Francisco in 2005 they observed inverse associations between consumption of dark leafy vegetables, cruciferous vegetables, yellow vegetables, Carrots, beans, onions, garlic, citrus fruits and juice etc., and incidence of pancreatic cancer. Out of these beans, onions, and garlic were found to be better than others in preventing pancreatic cancers and that too with more than nine servings per day in various dishes.

Dietary Agents in the Chemoprevention of Prostate Cancer

Shukla and Gupta[5] report that according to epidemiological evidences use of plant based dietary agents decrease the risk. Intake of 400-600 g/day of fruits and vegetables is found to be associated with reduced risk of several cancers. Cosiderable attention has been devoted to identify plant-based dietary agents that may serve as natural inhibitors of prostate tumorigenesis. Pant derived dietary agents such as flavonoids, indoles, isothiocyanates, phenolics, monoterpenes etc., are recommended for prevention and management of prostate cancer.

Beneficial Effects of Virgin Coconut Oil on Lipid Parameters and *in vitro* LDL Oxidation

Nevin and Rajmon[6] conducted a study on the effects of consumption of Virgin Coconut Oil (VCO) on various lipid parameters in comparison with mature coconut oil (C.O). In addition to that, the preventive effect of polyphenol fraction (PF) from test sample of VCO on copper induced oxidation of LDL and Carbonyl formation was also studied.

A 45 day feeding of 8% each of groundnut oil (GNO), CO or VCO mixed with a semisynthetic diet to make albino rats gave the following results.

No significant change in body weights was observed for any of the groups. The concentrations of cholesterol, TAG and PL in serum, Liver and Heart of VCO treated group were significantly lower compared to the other two groups. In VCO fed group HDL cholesterol was increased and L.D.L cholesterol was reduced significantly as compared to the other two groups.

PF of the oils was isolated as follows by the method of Vasquez Ronecro et. al[7]. 10 g oil was dissolved in 50 ml hexane and extracted thrice with 20 ml portion methanol (60%) successively. The combined extracts were vacuum dried. This was used. PF content was estimated by Folin Ciocalteau reagent[8]. In *in vitro* oxidation studies the PF of VCO was found to be more beneficial than the PF of CO and GNO in preventing the copper-induced oxidation of LDL as indicated by the low TBARS formation and reduced carbonyl formation. The differences in the biological effects of the three oils may be due to the differences in the concentrations of certain antioxidants in each of them. VCO contains a higher polyphenol content (80 mg/100g) than CO (64.4 mg/100g). PF contains some α-tocopherol as part of the oils. Other studies have shown that α-tocopherol (Vitamin E) has a synergic effect in association with some phenolic compounds having significant antioxidant activity[9,10]. The biological effects of the minor components in CO was not studied elsewhere[11]. GNO and CNO at 20% level in diet was found to be atherogenic by Augusti et. al.[12] and the former was also found to be harmful by others[13].

Determination of Carbonyl content in the copper oxidized samples of PF from the three oils[6,14] was carried out. The order of inhibition on the carbonyl formation in the *in vitro* study with PF samples was VCO>CO>GNO. This result agrees with the antioxidant status of each oil. The source of carbonyl groups[15] are from the proteins of LDL undergone oxidation. These polyphenols might trap ROS in aqueous components such as plasma and interstitial fluid of the arterial wall thereby inhibiting LDL oxidation and showing anti-atherogenic activity[16]. In addition these compounds are capable of reversing cholesterol transport and reducing its intestinal absorption[17]. The decreased oxidation of LDL is due to the presence of antioxidants in PFs[6]. These results highlifht the antiatherogeni effects of VCO as well as the Kernel of tender coconuts.

Role of Glucosinolates and Indoles in Chemoprevention of Cancer

In cancer prevention studies it was discoversd that adding cruciferous vegetables to the diet produced a marked decrease in the incidence of breast tumor in animals. This was shown for Dimethyl (a) Benzanthracene induced tumors[18] as well as MCF-7 breast tumor metastasis in athymic mice[19]. Glucosinolates are found in cruciferous vegetables. The hydrolysis of the glucosinolate glucobrassiein by the plants own enzymes leads to the formation of various indoles including Indol-3-Carbinol and Indol-3-acetonitrile. It has been suggested that indoles may protect against breast cancer by way of their effect on oestrogen metabolism.

In one human clinical trial women were given a massive daily dose of 500 mg (approximately 50 times the estimated average daily intake in the USA) indole derivative resulted in a shift in oestrogen metabolism towards the production of relativey more of a less potent form of oestrogen as stated by Rajesh kumar[20]. Thejas and Kuttan[21] studied the inhibitory effects of two naturally occurring isothiocyanates allyl and phenyl isothiocyanates that occur in cruciferous vegetables e.g; Brassica nigra, Lepidum sativum, Wasabia japonica etc on the production of nitric oxide (NO) and tumor necrosis factor-α (TNF- α) in vivo as well *in vitro* systems. Kim Park attributes a role of vasodilatory effect of NO[1]. Nitric oxide is a multifunctional species that is implicated in a wide variety of physiological and pathological processes[22,23]. It is an essential physiological signaling molecule mediating various cell functions but also induces cytotoxic and mutagenic effects, when present in excess, thus pointing its dual role in biological system[23].

NO reacts rapidly with superoxide anion to form peroxy nitrite which may be cytotoxic by itself or easily decompose to the highly reactive and toxic hydroxyl radical and nitrogen dioxide[24]. A family of three isoenzymes called nitric oxide sunthase produces NO from L-Arginine[23,25]. NO released by constitutive nitric oxide synthase acts as an important signaling molecule in the cardiovascular and nervous systems[23] and that produced by the immune system has been shown to be Cytostatic/Cytotoxic for tumor cells[26]. Two of the isomeric enzymes are responsible for NO production that causes vasodilation.

TNF-α a mediator of induction of NO synthesis, possesses multifunctional activities and is one of the most important pro-inflammatory and proimmuno cytokines[27,28]. Lipopolysaccharide (LPS) obtained from gram negative bacteria has been shown to be a potent inducer of TNF-α[29]. Concavalin A which is a lectin activates T lymphocytes and induces the release of IFN- α and other cytokines.

Isothyocyanates (ITCS) occur in cruciferous vegetables like cabbage as thioglucoside conjugates called glucosinolated. Many of these principles protect against chemically induced tumours in a variety of animals. Phenethyl and Benzyl isothiocyanates ($C_6H_5CH_2CSN$ and C_6H_5CSN) inhibited carcinogenesis induced by carcinogens such as diethyl nitrosamine (DEN), dimethyl benzo (a) anthracene (DMBA) or benzopyrene (BP)[30] The mechanism involved in the inhibition of carcinogenesis by ITCs is most likely due to the blocking of the activation of carcinogens through the inactivation of P450 enzymes and activation of Phase II enzymes. Allyl isothiocyanate (C_3H_5CSN) and phenyl isothiocyanate (C_6H_5CSN) have showed immunomodulatory and antimetastatic activity according to the earlier work of Manesh and Kuttan[31]. Allyl isothyocyanate has been shown to strongly induce glutathione-S-transferase activity by Boggards et. al.[32]

According to Thejus and Kuttan's work elevated level of nitrite (Precursor of NO) produced by macrophages stimulated with a lipopolysaccharide (LPs) of gram negative bacteria in *in vitro* was significantly reduced from 119.39 ± 0.63 μm to 42.27 ± 1.45 μm and 48.46 ± 1.51 μm when treated with allyl isothiocyaanate (AITC) and phenyl isothiocyanate 9PITC) (*in vitro* dose of 5 μg/ml) respectively. Similarly drastically elevated level of nitrite in the serum of LPS stimulated BALB1c mice was significantly reduced from 83.25 ± 0.8 μm to 23.25 ± 0.62 μm and 25.27 ± 0.88 μm by the treatment of AITC and PITC respectively at a dosage of 25 μg/animal. Both the isocyanates also significantly reduced the drastically enhanced level of nitrite stimulated with concavalin A. A similar reduction in the level of TNF-ά in LPS and Con. A stimulated animals was observed on treatment with either of the isothiocyanates. The results *in vitro* condition of macrophages with LPS or Con A also showed a similar pattern of reduction in TNF-ά with the addition of nutraceuticals.

Thus the above studies clearly demonstrated the inhibitory effects of AITC and PITC on the production of NO and TNF-ά which were induced by LPS and Con A both *in vitro* as well as *in vivo* systems. Bioassay of TNF-ά and NO production with isocyanates confirmed their down regulating activity on TNF-ά and NO levels. In such a system TNF-ά sensitive L 929 cells exihibited only normal growth pattern and NO dependent angiogenesis slowly retarded. These cascade process of isocyanates in series with down regulated TNF-ά and NO explains how mechanistically the cruciferous vegetable products can interfere with tumorigenesis if we use any of them regularly.

Tumor Reducing and Anticarcinogenic Activity of Selected Spices

Tumour reducing activity of methanol or aqueous extracts of eight commonly used spices in India viz: black pepper, asafoetida, pippali, garlic, mustard, horse gram, Sesame and ginger, were studied in mice transplanted intraperitoneally with Ehrich ascites tumour or Dalton's lymphoma ascites tumour[33]. Intraperitoneal administration of the extracts did not significantly change the life span of the animal with the former type of tumour although sesame could raise the life span by 19%. However this spice significantly raised the lifespan of mice with the latter type tumour by 39%. Whereas oral administration of the extracts from six of them viz: black pepper, asafoetida, pippali, garlic, mustard and horse gram significantly raised the life span of the animals with Ehrlich tumour by 65%, 53%, 47%, 41% 29% & 24% respectively.

In a second type of experiment topical application of aqueons extracts of asafoetida and methanol extract of garlic for sixteen weeks reduced significantly (P<0.001) the number of animals developed DMBA induced papilloma by 20% and 30% respectively as well as their onset. (DMBA= 7, 12 dimethyl benzanthraccne. Application of this carcinogen along with croton oil on mice skin induce papilloma formation).

These results indicate the potential use of the above six spices. Along with them sesame and ginger could also be considered as useful spices as they produced considerable effects next to the six others i.e. 18% and 12% in life span of animals with Ehrlich ascites tumour.

The antioxidant property of many spices make them not only useful preservatives but also possible antitumour promoters although some of them in excess may produce mucosal irritation and promote mutagenicity. The active ingredient of turmeric viz; curcumin has been shown to inhibit the tumour promotion brought about by TPA (12-0 – Tetradecanoyl Phorbol – 13-acetate) and croton oil[34]

Various nutraceuticals or alkaloids present in the spices may be responsible for their anticarcinogenic effects. Terpenoids and polysulphides and their related principles may be present in most of them and alkaloids may be the active principles in pippali and black pepper. The last two spices were proved to be highly cytotoxic by Amla Cancer Research Team. These studies explain the role of spices as beneficial ingredients in our food. Of course they should be just optimum in concentrations.

Refences

1. Sang Ae Kim-Park and David D Ku. Garlic elieits A Nitric oxide-dependent relaxation and inhibits hypoxic Pulmonary vasoconstriction in rats Clinical and Experimental Pharmac. And Physiol 27(2000)780.
2. Chowdhury, S.R; Chowdhury, S.D; Smith, T.K.; Effects of dietary garlic on cholesterol metabolism in laying hens. Poult. Sci. 81(2002)1856-1862.
3. Block; E, Iyer, R; Grisoni, S; Saha, C; Belman, S- Lipoxygenase inhibitors from the essential oil of garlic. Markowinikoff addition of the allyldithio radical to olefins. J. Am. Chem. Soc. 110(1988)7813-27.
4. Chan J M, Wang F et. al. Vetgetable and fruit intake and Pancreatic Cancer in a population-based case-control study in the Sanfrancisco bay area. Cancer Epidemicology … Prov. 14(9)2005.2093-97.
5. Shikla, S and Gupta, S. Dietary agents in the chemo prevention of prostate Cancer. Nutr Cancer 53(1)(2005) 18-32.
6. Nevin, K.G. and Rajmohan, T. Beneficial effects of Virgin Coconut Oil on lipid parameters and invitro LDL Oxidation. Clinical Biochem. 37(2004) 830-835.
7. Vazquez ronecro, A; Janer Del Valle, L and Janer del Valle, C. Determination of Olive oil total polyphenols. Grassa Acetes 24(1973)350-55.
8. Gut finger, T. Polyphenols in Olive oil. J. Am oil chem.. Soc. 1(1981) 966-68.

9. Servili.M; Baldioli. M; Miniati, E; Montedoro, GF. Antioxidant activity of new phenolic Compounds extracted from virgin olive oil stability measured by rancimat. J. Agri. Food Chem. 47(1999) 4150-55.

10. Galli, C; Pettroni, A; Visioli, F. Natural antioxidants, with special reference to those in olive oil and cell protection. Eur. J.Pharm Sci.2(1994) 67-68.

11. Pehwich, D.J; Gones, A, V; Barnes, J.A. Fatty acid composition and possible health effects of coconut constituents. West India. J. Med. 49(2000) 128-29.

12. Augusti, K.T; Aswathy,N et. al. Beneficial effects of garlic (Allium sativum Linn) on rats fed with diets containing chiolesterol and either of oil seeds, cocnuts or gound nuts. Indian J Exp. Biol 39(2001) 661-67.

13. Elaine, B; Feldman, M.D. Those scientific evidence for a beneficial health relation ship between walnuts and coronary heart disease. J. Nutr. 132(2002) 1062, S-101.S.

14. Levine, R.L; Garland, D, Oliver C.N et. al. Determination of carbonyl content in oxidatively modified proteins. Methods. Enzymol 186(1990) 464-80.

15. Teresa, C.P.D; conceicao, L.S; Leonor, M.A. The apo Protein is the preferential target for peroxy nitrite-induced LDL damage protein by dietary pehnolic acids. Free radical Research 36 (2002) 531-43.

16. Tebib, K; Bitri, L. et. al. Pohymeric garape seed tannins prevent plasma cholesterol changes in high cholesterol fed rats. Food Chem. 49(1994)403-06.

17. Tebib, K; Besancon, P and Rouanet, J.M. Dietary grape seed tannins effect lipoproteins, lipoprotein lipase and tissue lipids in rats fed by perecholesterolemic diets.

18. Stockwrand, G; Anderson, J.L; Musion, L. Cancer letters 30 (1988) 199-207.

19. Scholar, E.M, Wolterman, K; Birt, D.F; E. Nutr. Cancer 12(1989)121-126.

20. Rajesh Kumar, N.V. Cancer Chemoprevention by phytochemicals in Fruits and Vegetables. Amala Research Bulletin 18 (1998) 141-149.

21. Thejass. P. and Kuttan G. Effect of allyl isothiocynate (AITS) and phenyl isothiocyanate (PITC) on the inhibition of nitric oxide (No) and tumour factor-α (TNF-α) Production. Amala Res. Bulletin 25(2005)213-221.

22. Carla B, Patrizia F, Sergio A.T et. al. Vitamin E Serum levels and gastric cancer: results from a cohort of patients in Tuscany, Italy. Cancer Lett. 151 (2000) 15-18.

23. Jenkins D.C, Charles I.G, Thomsen, L.L. Moss D.W. et. al. Role of NO. in tumour grough. Proc. Natl Acad Sci.USA. 92(1995) 4393-4396.

24. Feinstair, D.L. Galece, E et. al. Induction of nitric oxide Synthase in rat C_6 glioma cells. J. Neurochem. 62 (1994)315-321.

25. Ignarro, L.J; Buga, G.M. et. al. Role of arginine-No Pathway in the regulation ofvascular smooth muscle cell proliferation. Proc. Natl Acad Sci. USA 98 (2001)4202-4208.

26. Vakkala, M; Kahlos, K, Lakari, E et. al. Inducible nitric oxide synthase expression, apoptosis and angiogenesis in insitu and invasive breast carcinoonas. Clini. Cancer Res.6 (2000) 2408-2416.

27. Fimiani, C; Mattocks d, et. al. The role of endogenous IFN-C and TNF-a in LPS INDUCED No. release in a mouse model. Cytokine 10( )115-123.

28. Mc Dermott, M.F. TNF and TNFR biology in health and disease Cell Mole Biol. 47(2001)619-635.

29. Beutler, B. Han, J, and Krays. V. Coordinate regulation of TNF biosynthesis at the levels of transcription and translation. Patterns of TNF experession invivo in tumour necrosis factor; The molecules and their engineering, role in medicine. Ed: Raven press, Newyork 1992. PP.2542-47.

30. Wattenberg, L.W., Inhibitory effects of benzyl isothiocynate administered shortly before diethyl nitrosamine or benzo(a) pyrene on pulmonary and forestomach neoplasia in A/J mice Carcinogenesis, 8 (1987) 1971-1983.

31. Manesh, C and Kuttan, G. Effect of naturally occurring allyl and phenyl isothiocyanates in the inhibition of experimental pulmonary metastasis induced by $B_{16}F_{10}$ melanoma cells. Fitoterapia. 74(2003)355-363.

32. Boggards, JJP, Verhagen, H, Willems, M.I. et. al. Consumption of Brussels sprouts results in elevated a- class glutathione S-transferase levels in human blood plasma. Carcinogenesis. 15(1994)1073-1075.

33. Unnikrishnan, M.C. and Kuttan, R. Tumor reducing and anticarcinogenesis activity of selected spices. Cancer Letters. 51(1990)85-89.

34. Huang, M.T; Smart, R>C et. al. Inhibitory effect of curcumin, chlorogenic acid, caffeic acid and Ferulic acid on tumour promotion, in mouse skin by 12-O-tetra decanoyal phorbol – 13- acetate. Cancer Research 48(1988) 5941-46.

Chapter – 9

Laboratory Experiment

9.1 Antidiabetic and related Effects of Solvent Extracted Oils of Alliums and a Synthetic Disulfide in Experimental Diabetes Mellitus

S. Paramesha
* Dept. of Biochemistry, Hassan Institute of Medical Sciences, Hassan - 573201, Karnataka;

R.T. Kasinath,
Dept. of Biochemistry, Basaveshwara Medical College, Chitradurga, Karnataka 577502.

*This work was done at the Dept. of Biochemistry, Dr. B.R. Ambedkar, Medical College, Bangalore-45 under the guidance of Dr. Kasinath in 2003.

Garlic and onion principles are hypoglycemic and insulinogenic agents and they control diabetes mellitus by preventing loss of weight, glycosuria, derangement of enzymes and disorders of carbohydrate, lipid and protein metabolism[1-4]. In the present experiment we have tested the biochemical effects of aqueous and hexan soluble fractions of onion and garlic and also that of a synthetic disulfide called diaceto dibutyl disulfide (DADBDS) originally synthesized by Joseph and Kasinath in 1989 at St.John's Medical College, Bangalore for a previous study and also at present in alloxan diabetic rats.

Material and Methods

Normal and alloxan diabetic rats were used in the study. Male albino rats from the stock colony of animals at Dr. B.R. Ambedkar Medical College, Bangalore were selected and a large number of them were made diabetic with alloxan injection as depicted below. 24 hr fasted rats were given 80 mg/kg alloxan in distilled water through tail vein. These rats were kept fasting for a further period of 8 hrs. Later they were maintained on stock rat feed and water *ad libitum*. Next day their urine sugar was tested. Rats with glycosuria were separated and their blood sugar was estimated using orthotoluedene reagent with a modified method.[5] Rats with blood glucose in the range of 200-460 mg/dl were used in the experiments. Various doses of aqueous extracts viz; 1-3 g/kg and that of hexane extracts of onions and garlic and DADBDS in the range of 100-400 mg/kg were used in order to find an effective dose of each that controls diabetes to a reasonable level.

Preparation of Onion and Garlic Extracts/oils Aqueous extracts:

Fresh onion or garlic homogenates were extracted with water and the filtered fractions were used for the present study.

Hexan Extracted Onion and Garlic Oils

Fresh onion or garlic homogenates were kept over might in methanol at room temperature and the filtered fractions were evaporated to dryness and these residues were **extracted** thrice with diethyl ether. The ethereal oil was prepared from these extracts on evaporation in each case and the same was dissolved in methanol and kept for 4 days at 25°C. It was then extracted with hexane and the solvent was distilled off. Hexane soluble fractions of onion and garlic contains Allicin type compounds (R-S-S(O)-R) and their polymers DADS, DATS, DATTS with a difference in the location of double bonds between carbon linkages viz; allyl in garlic oil (CH_2=CH-CH_2^-) and propenyl in onion oil (CH_3CH=CH-) as the case may be. For this study six rats in each group were taken for the following experiment. One normal and one diabetic groups of control rats were fed daily with 30 ml normal saline per kg body weight intragastrically using a stomach tube daily for 10 days. Some groups of alloxan diabetic rats were given daily different doses of aqueous extracts of onion and garlic in the range of 1g to 3g/kg respectively for 10 days using the stomach tube as above. Similarly some other groups of alloxan diabetic rats were fed with hexane extracts of onion (HEO) or garlic (HEG) at a dose of 0.2 g/kg body weight for 10 days. In the same way, a group of alloxan diabetic rats was also fed within DADBDS at a dose of 0.1 g/kg body. Hexan extracts shall be called as oils.

After 10 days feeding of normal saline or test doses of extracts/DADBDS to various groups they were kept for fasting over night and their blood glucose was determined[5]. On the 12th day all the groups were sacrificed by decapitation and their blood and liver tissue were collected. Certain blood and tissue parameters including marker enzymes were estimated by standard procedures[6]. Only the values of selected groups fed with effective doses are given below.

Results

Table1 gives the plasma levels of blood glucose, aminoacid nitrogen (AAN), free fatty acids (FFA), total cholesterol (TC), triacylglycerol (TAG), phospholipids (PL) and insulin values of normal and diabetic control groups and also those of various treated groups. All values except that of PL and insulin were significantly increased by diabetes and insulin level was significantly decreased. On treatment with onion and garlic oils or aqueous extracts of garlic (AEG) these deranged values were ameliorated significantly and DADBDS showed beneficial effects only selectively.

Fig.1 Cross section of pancreas in normal group. Normal pancreas showing islet cells and acinar cells.

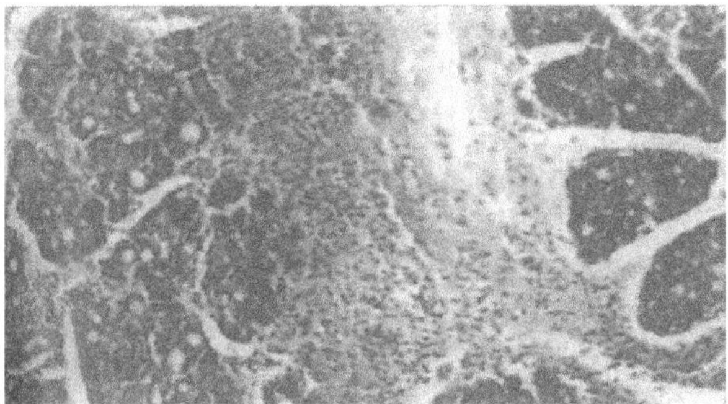

Fig.2 Cross section of pancreas of alloxan diabetic rat. (Control). Severe insulitis showing dense lymphocytic infiltration.

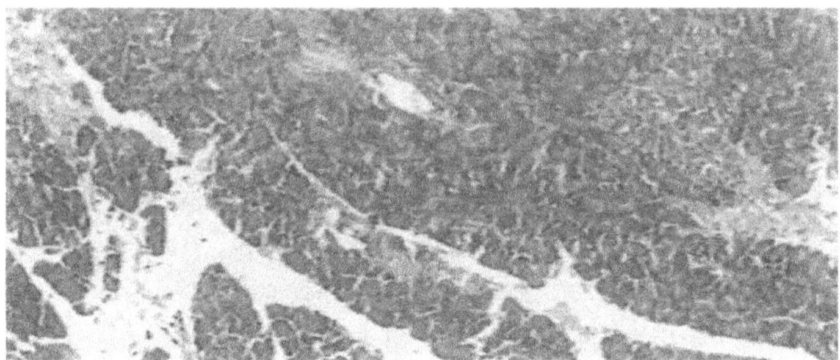

Fig. 3 Cross section of pancreas of alloxan diabetic rat treated with Garlic oil (HEG), Pancreas showing mild inflammation and insulities.

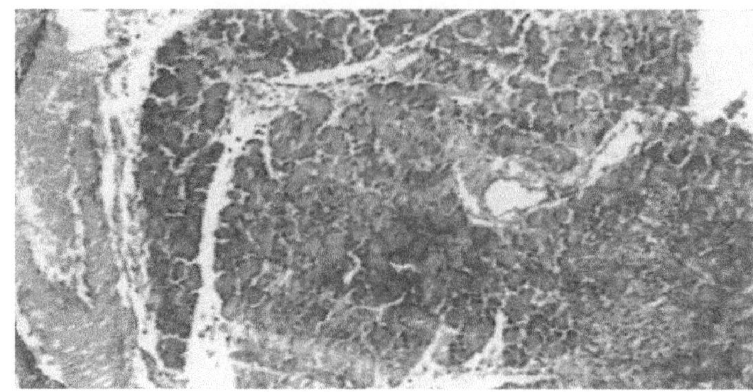

Fig. 4 Cross section of pancreas of alloxan diabetic rat treated with onion oil (HEO) pancreas showing mild inflammation and insulitis.

Plasma levels of Alanine transaminase (ALT), Aspartate transaminase (AST) and Alkaline phosphatase (ALP) and liver tissue lipid peroxidation values as thio- barbituric acid reacting substances (TBARS) and total thiol groups (-SH) of various groups of rats are given in Table 2. Significant increases of ALT, AST, ALP and TBARS values were observed in alloxan diabetic rats and their tissue –SH values also increased similarly. On treatment with AEG and garlic or onion oils or with DADBDS all the altered values were significantly ameliorated. These values were statistically analysed by student's t-test and the level of significance was determined in each case.

Discussion

The beneficial effects of garlic and onion principles for the control of diabetes were reported by various workers[7,8]. In their exhaustive work Augusti and Mathew[9], Itokawa et. al.[10] and Sumiyoshi[11] also accounted on the hypolipidemic effects of garlic. Augusti[3] and Block[12] suggested that allicine type compounds in garlic and onion viz; C_3H_5 S-S(O)C_3H_5 and CH_3-S-S(O)CH_3 and their polymers like ajoene are responsible for their antidiabetic, hypolipidemic, antiatherogenic and hypotensive actions. Many others showed the insulinogenic[13] and hypolipidemic[14] actions of allium principles in experimental animals.

As per a request of Augusti, Omkar et. al.[15] studied and reported the inhibitory effects of a garlic oil component, diallyl disulfide (DADS) on HMGCoA reductase which is the rate limiting enzyme for cholesterol synthesis. This enzyme's active site contains a thiol group and thiol disulfide interaction is known.

Probably Two or More Types of Interactions are Possible

2RSH + R1-S(O)S-R1 → R-S-S-R+R1-S-S-R1+H2O

RSH+R1-S-S-R1 → R1-SH+R1S-S-R

RSH stands for any thiol group of the body.

A third possibility for the interaction of RSH with the allyl group should be looked into

2RSH+CH_2=CH-CH_2-S-S-CH_2-CH=CH_2 →

R-S-CH_2-CH_2-S-S-CH_2-CH_2-CH_2-S-R and so on.

Gebhardt[16] also demonstrated the inhibitory effects of various garlic polysulfides including vinyl dithiins on HMGCoA reductase.

A better action with garlic oil rather than with onion oil in the control of diabetes may be due to the presence of two allyl groups in the former rather than the propenyl groups as observed in onion oil. Probably –SH group enzymes can interact with allyl group compounds more quickly than with propenyl group as the double bond is in the exterior part of the former as against that is present in the interior part of the latter. This type of double bonds are absent in DADBDS and that may be one of the reasons that the synthetic disulfide is a poor blood sugar and cholesterol lowering agent.

In a separate study the authors also showed the prophylactic effects of treatment of rats with garlic and onion oils and DABDS, prior to alloxan injection. In both cases the oils protected the rats from the induction of diabetes by alloxan. It is known that sulfur compounds especially cysteine and such other organic sulfur compounds could give protection to animals from chemically induced diabetes mellitus. The results of the present study uphold the medicinal effects of onion and garlic with a far better action of the latter on diabetes.

Treated group values were compared with those of diabetic control. All values except that of insulin and PL decreased significantly. On treatment with various fractions of Alliums and DADBDS the affected values were significantly decreased or increased as the case may be.

Table 1 Plasma levels of B.S., AAN, FFA,TC,TAG, PL and insulin are given in normal, diabetic control and treated groups. Values are mean ± S.D. of six rats in each group

	Groups	BS (mg/dl	AAN (mg/dl)	FFA (mEq/L)	TC (mg/dl)	TAG(mg/dl)	PL (mg/dl)	Insulin (mIU/ml)
1	Normal	95±6	4.3±0.4	0.168±0.02	127±7	108±15	42±16	4.5±0.8
2	Diabetic control	451±16	9.8±0.7	0.38±0.05 *	299±9 *	177±9*	73.5±27	0.8±0.2 *
3	Aqueous extract of garlic (AEG) group (Dose 3g/kg)	105±9*	5.3±0.4*	0.181±0.02*	85±12 *	107±7 *	45±17	5.1±0.62*
4	Onion oil (HEO) group (Dose 0.2g/kg)	128±6*	3.5±0.3*	0.136±0.01*	127±7.5*	125±9*	42±15	6.1±0.4*
5	Garlic oil (HEG) group (Dose 0.2g/kg)	91±4*	4±0.25*	0.157±0.01*	87±8*	103±8*	41±15	6.6±1.1*
6	DADBDS Group (dose 0.1g/kg)	201±4*	5±0.4*	0.28±0.04*	245±8*	159±9N.S	50±18N.S	3.8±0.07*

Statistical analysis by student's t-test.: Alloxan diabetic group values were compared with the normal values.
*P<0.001 as compared to each of their control. N.S. = Nonsignificant

Table 2 Plasma levels of ALT, AST, ALP and liver tissue values of TBARS and total-SH groups in various groups of rats as shown below. Values are mean ± S.D. of six rats in each group.

	Groups	ALT (IU/ml)	AST (IU/ml)	ALP (KAU)	Liver TBARS (μ mol/g)	Liver total-SH (μmol/g)
1	Normal	18.2±2.5	15. 6±3.4	11.5±1.4	3.7±0.3	35.6±2.1
2	Diabetic Control	95.2±9.3*	81.3±3.7*	54.6±2.9*	14.8±0.3*	11.5±1.4*
3	AEG Group	71.7±6.4*	70.8±8.1^{s}	45±2.7*	8.2±0.7*	21.8±1.9*
4	HEO Group	28.6±4.1*	26.5±4.5*	35.6±3*	8.2±0.5*	21.6±2.8*
5	HEG Group	44.2±4.5*	65.2±3.9*	37.8±2.8*	8.3±0.7*	21.4±2.1*
6	DADBDS Group	19.8±2.3*	18.8±4.7*	15±2.7*	4.4±0.6*	31.9±2.3*

Statistical analysis is by student's t- test and comparison of groups are as in table 1.
*P < 0.001 as compared to each of their control.

References

1. (a) Brahmachari H.D. and Augusti K.T. Orally effective hypoglycemic agent from onions. J.Pharm.Pharmacol 13(1961) 128

   (b) Brahamchari. H.D. and Augusti. K.T. Orally effective hypoglycemic agents from plants J.Pharm.Pharmacol.14(1962)254-255.

2. Augusti. K.T. and Benaim M.E. Effect of Essential oil of onion on blood glucose, free fatty acids and insulin levels of normal subjects. Clinica Chemia Acta 60 (1975) 121-123

3. Augusti. K.T. Therapeutic values of onion (Allium Cepa L) and garlic (Allium Sativam L) 1996. Indian Jour. Expt-Biol 3(1966) 634-640.

4. Kumud Kumari, Biju C Mathew, Indian Jour. Biochem & Biophys. Antidiabetic and Hypolipedemic effects of S-methyl cysteine sulfoxide isolated from Allium cepa Linn. 32(1995) 49-54

5. Rechard. J.Henry, Donald, C.Connan and James. W.Winkelman (1974). Chapter 28. Lipids pp 1436-1441 and Chapter 25 Carbohydrates pp 1285-1289 in Clinical Chemistry. Principles and practice. 2nd 1974. Harper-Row Publishers, New York.

6. S. Paramesha. Hypoglycemic effect of Disulfides in Experimental diabetes mellitus. Ph.D Thesis submitted to the Rajiv Gandhi University of Health Sciences, Bangalore in Aug. 2003 PP 54-82

7. Sheela, C.G; Kumud Kumari and Augusti.K.T., Antidiabetic effects of onion and garlic sulfoxide amino acids in rats. Planta Med 61(1995) 356-357

8. Kumud Kumari and Augusti. K.T., Antidiabetic effects of S-methyl cysteine sulfoxide on alloxan diabetes. Planta Med.61(1995) 72-74.

9. Augusti. K.T. and Mathew.P.T. Effect of long term feeding of the aqueous extracts of onion and garlic on normal rats. Indian Jour. Expt Biol.11(1973)239-241.

10. Itokawa.Y; Inoue. K.; Sasagawa. S and Fujiwara. M. Effect of S-methyl cysteine sulfoxide, S-allyl cystein sulfoxide and related sulfur containing aminoacids on lipid metabolism of experimental hypercholesterolemic rats. J.Nutr 103 (1973)88-92

11. Sumiyoshi. H. New Pharmacological activities of garlic and its constituents. Nippen Yakurigaku Zaashi 110 (1997)Suppl (1)93

12. Erick Block. Organosulfur chemistry of the genus Allium-Implications for the organic chemistry of sulfur. Angew Chem. Int. Ed.Engl. 31 (1992) 1135-1178.

13. Chang. M.L.W and Johnson. M.A.; Effect of garlic on Carbohydrate metabolism and lipid synthesis in rats. J. Nutr.110 (1980) 931-936.

14. Lau.B.H.S.et al. Allium Sativum (garlic) and atherosclerosis; A Review Nutrition Res.13 (1983) 119-128.

15. Kumar. R.V.O; Banerji.A, Kurup.C.K.R and Ramasarma.T. The nature of inhibition of 3-hydroxymethyl glutaryl CoA reductase by garlic derived diallyl disulfide. Biochim Biophys Acta 1078 (1991) 209.

16. (a) Gebhardt. R; Beek.H, Wagner. K.G. Inhibition of Cholesterol biosynthesis by allicin and ajoene in rat hepatocytes and $HepG_2$ cells. Biochem Biophys Acta 1213 (1994) 57-62.

(b) Gebhardt R and Beek.H. Differential inhibitory effects of garlic derived organosulfides on cholesterol biosynthesis in primary rat hepatocyte culture. Lipid, 31 (1996) 1269.

9.2 Nutraceutical Effects of Garlic Oil, its Nonpolar Fraction and a Ficus Flavonid as compared to Vitamin E in CCl_4 induced Liver damage in Rats

Anuradha, KT Augusti[1], SP Prabha, KB Smitha, M Sudheesh, Anu George and MC Joseph[2]

Departments of Medical Biochemistry and Medical Laboratory Technology, School of Med. Edn.(M.G. University Centre) Kottayam-686 008,Kerala.

1. Corresponding author E-mail – ktaugustei@yahoo.co.hk
2. Rtd. Prof. of Patholoyg, Medical College Kottagam and Honarary Professor to SME

Abstract

Carbon tetrachloride feeding (3.2 g/kg/72hr) for one month increased significantly the serum and tissue lipid profile and deranged the enzyme levels Viz; (ALP), (ALT), (AST), (GSSG reductase), (HMGCoA reductase), Catalase, Gluc.6.PDH and Malic enzyme in rats. Simultaneously the lipid peroxidation level in liver was also raised.

On administration of garlic oil, and also its major non polar fraction (NPFGO), a flavonoid isolated from the bark of Ficus bengalensis Linn, Viz; leucopelargonin derivative and Vitamin E respectively to different groups (100 mg / kg / day of the former three and 50 mg/kg of the vitamin)) along with Carbon tetrachloride (3.2 g/kg/72 hr.) for a month, the deleterious effects of CCl_4 were significantly ameliorated. The liver damage by CCl_4 was satisfactorily prevented by the nutraceutical samples as effectively as Vitamin E (50 mg/kg/day). The results prove that important nutraceuticals (Phyto nutrients) like bioflavonoids and theols i.e. allylic sulfide rich fractions give protection from toxins like CCl_4.

The order of beneficial effects of the drugs are:

Leucopelargonin > NPFGO > Garlic oil and their effects are comparable to that of vitamin E used at a minimal dose. (Published in Indian. Jour. Exp. Biol. 43 (2005) 437-444. Reproduced here with the permission from NISCAIR, New Delhi.)

Introduction

The role of free radical has been implicated in several diseases. The damages produced by certain toxic chemicals or hepatotoxic agent like carbon tetrachloride (CCl_4) were found to be due to its metabolism in the liver. CCl_4 binds to cytochrome P_{450} reductase. The enzyme substrate complex then loses a chloride ion and a free radical ($CCl^{\cdot}_3$) intermediate is generated.

$$CCl_4 \xrightarrow[\text{Cytochrome } P_{450} \text{ reductase}]{\text{NAPDH}} CCl_3^{\cdot} + Cl^-$$

The above free radical then reacts with oxygen or takes a hydrogen from a suitable donor to yield a secondary radical or reacts with lipids or proteins.

$$CCl_3^{\cdot} + O_2 \longrightarrow CCl_3 - O\text{-} O^{\cdot} \text{ (methyl peroxy radical)}$$

The methyl peroxy radical is much more reactive than $CCl_3^{\cdot}$ and is the main initiating species for lipid peroxidation that causes tissue injury in the hepatotoxicity of CCl_4.

$$RH + CCl_3 - O\text{-} O^{\cdot} \longrightarrow R^{\cdot} + CCl_3 - O\text{-}OH$$

$$R^{\cdot} + O_2 \longrightarrow ROO^{\cdot} \text{ (lipid peroxide)}$$

Kupffer cells play a role in the mechanism of action of CCl_4, e.g. CCl_4 elevates Ca^{2+} and the release of toxic eicosanoids and cytokines by Kupffer cells is calcium dependent[1].

There are certain naturally occuring antioxidants that can give protection to liver from hepatotoxins. Schisandrin B an active ingredient of the fruit of Schisandra chinesis can enhance the hepatic glutathione antioxidant system in mice against CCl_4 toxicity[2]. Similarly, oral administration of ellagic acid (a polyphenolic acid anhydride) to rats was found to reduce significantly the elevated levels of lipid peroxides and liver hydroxy proline after CCl_4 induced liver damage. Treatment with ellagic acid rectified the liver pathophysiology and significantly reduced CCl_4 toxicity and subsequent fibrosis. Adequate liver protection by several defined constituents of garlic was shown with freshly prepared rat hepatocytes that had been treated with CCl_4, a strong toxicant. S- allyl cysteine sulfoxide (alliin) and related sulfur compounds in garlic were found to be effective in the neutralization of cytotoxicity. Further, S-allyl mercaptocysteine and S- methyl mercapto cysteine ($R\text{-}S\text{-}S\text{-}CH_2.CH(NH_2)$ $COOH$ or RS-Cysteine, where $R = CH_3$ or C_3H_5) showed remarkable protection *in vitro* to heaptocytes against the toxic effects of CCl_4 and galatosamine[3]. Garlic oil (mixtures of RSS(O)R and RS_nR) and possibly ajoene (a polymer of allicin i.e. $C_3H_5\text{-}S(O)\ CH_2.CH{=}CH\text{-}S\text{-}S\text{-}C_3H_5$) are also involved in the protective action of garlic principles. Another group of compounds viz; polyphenols and bioflavonoids have been found to exert their chemopreventive role through multiple pathways including free radical scavenging. Bhardwaj et. al.[4] found that fistein and resveratrol (a flavonoid and a polyphenol respectively) were as effective as vitamin E in their inhibitory action on lipid peroxidation. A Ficus flavonoid leucopelargonin was proved as a good hypoglycemic agent and an antioxidant[5]. As many flavonoids were shown to inhibit CCl_4 induced microsomal lipid peroxidation, leucopelargonin was also selected for the present study. The flavonoids have a keto (=CO) function in the 4th place of the oxide ring and flavanoids have a methylene ($-CH_2$) group in that place and both are polyphenols. In the present study garlic oil, its nonpolar fraction and leucopelargonin, a ficus flavanol derivative have been used. Flavanol derivatives are also termed flavonoids as a class. As the yield of the polar fraction of garlic oil was very poor (10% of the oil) its effects were not studied. **These compounds with biological action in our food are newly termed as nutraceuticals. They are functional foods.**

Materials and Methods

Preparation of garlic oil and its nonpolar fraction (NFGO): One kg of locally purchased fresh garlic (*Allium sativum* Linn) was cleaned and homogenized. Enough methanol was added to keep it fully immersed and left in a conical flask overnight. Mixture was filtered and the extract collected. The residue left behind was further extracted with methanol twice as before. Methanol was distilled off and the oil left behind was collected. This oil was extracted thrice with diethyl ether to get the soluble fraction and the ether was evaporated off on a water bath and the left over oil was collected and a part of this garlic oil (yield 4 g/kg) was used for one experiment and the remaining was used for the preparation of the non polar fraction for another experiment.

Nonpolar fraction of garlic oil (NPFGO) was prepared from the above oil by extracting it with hexane thrice and the hexane soluble fraction was collected by filtration. Hexane was evaporated off on a water bath and the oil left behind was collected as nonpolar fraction (yield 3.5 g/kg fresh garlic). Vitamin E (Sigma Chemicals Co St. Louis Mo) was used as a standard at a minimum dose.

Preparation of leucopelargonin derivative: A glycoside of pelargonidin (leucopelargonin derivative) was isolated from the bark of banyan tree (*F.bengalensis* Linn) according to the method of Prema and Misra[6]. This compound was found to be a secretagogue of insulin and hence hypoglycemic in action. It is a flavanol derivative (yield 5g/kg) under the general group flavonoids.

Experimental animals: Adult male albino rats (Sprague Dawley strain) weighing around 100 g were divided into 6 groups of 6 in each. They were maintained on Gold Mohur rat feed. The oral dose of CCl_4 (Sisco Laboratories Bombay containg 1.6 g/ml) was 3.2 g/kg/72 hr according to the method of Recknagel and Glende[7] for developing cirrhosis in the test groups. Other treatment details are listed below for each group.

Group I : Normal rat feed was supplied with water *ad libitum*

Group II : Normal rat feed + CCl_4 i.e. 0.2 ml of CCl_4 was dissolved in 0.2 ml ground nut oil/100g body weight and administered po, every 72 hr for one month.

Group III : Normal rat feed + CCl_4 as above + garlic oil 100 mg/kg body weight and dissolved in 0.2 ml ground nut oil was administered ip,. daily.

Group IV : Normal rat feed + CCl_4 as above + NPFGO, 100 mg/kg body weight and dissolved in 0.2 ml ground nut oil was administered ip, daily

Group V : Normal rat feed + CCl_4 as above + leucopelargonin derivative, 100 mg/kg body weight and suspended in 0.2 ml ground nut oil was administered ip, daily.

Group VI : Normal rat feed + CCl_4 as above + Vitamin E, 50 mg/kg body weight, dissolved in 0.2 ml ground nut oil was administered ip, daily.

Chronic administration of CCl_4 for developing cirrhosis was carried out for groups II to VI along with treatment for one month as described. The rats were sacrificed by decapitation after over night fasting. Blood was collected in centrifuge tubes and was allowed to clot. Clear serum was separated by centrifugation and various estimations were carried out. Liver and heart were also collected in ice cold containers for various estimations. Lipids from tissues were extracted by Folch's procedure.

Total cholesterol, LDL cholesterol, HDL cholesterol, TAG (Triacylglycerol) and FFA in serum and tissue lipid extracts as the case may be and protein and A/G ratio in serum, TBARS (thiobarbituric acid reacting substances), conjugated dienesand activities of ALP (alkaline phosphatase), glutathione redcutase, glucose –6-phosphate dehydrogenase, malic enzyme and HMGCoA reductase in liver homogenates and activities of ALT and AST (alanine and aspartate transamianses) and catalase in heart and liver homogenates were estimated by standard methods. In TAG determination florisil column was used to remove phospholipids. All the data were statistically analysed according to student's t-test.

Liver tissues fixed in 10% formalin were processed for routine histopathological examination. Sections (5 μm thickness) were cut and stained with routine haematoxyline and eosin.

Results are given in Tables 1-3 and in Figures 1 and 2.

The order of their effects on deranged lipid profile as shown in table 1 is – Leucopelargonin > NPFGO > Garlic oil > Vitamin E, as compared to the minimum standard dose of vitamin E. Serum protein level was significantly reduced in the CCl_4 fed group and both vitamin E and the drugs raised the A/G ratio significantly; the former by 1.5 fold and the latter by two fold.

Enzyme activities in serum and liver (ALP, ALT and AST) which were raised significantly by CCl_4 and ameliorated by drugs are presented in Table 2. Treatment with vitamin E and the above drugs significantly decreased the activities of the above enzymes. Here again the order of effects of each drug is more or less the same as mentioned above.

CCl_4 feeding very significantly reduced the activities of the antioxidant enzymes viz; catalase and glutathione reductase and very significantly increased the activities of HMGCoA reductase and the lipogenic enzymes viz; glucose 6- phosphate dehydrogenase and malic enzyme as depicted in Table 3.

Treatment with each drug very significantly improved the activities of both the antioxidant enzymes. However vitamin E did the same to a highly significant level only in the case of catalase. Treatment with each drug and vitamin E very significantly lowered the activities of the remaining enzymes viz; HMGCoA reductase and the two lipogenic enzymes. In this experiment near normal activities for most of the enzymes were obtained in the groups treated with the leucopelargonin derivative. The effects of each drug were comparable to that of vitamin E and the order of their effects were more or less the same as stated above.

CCl_4 feeding increased, to a significant degree both TBARS and conjugated dienes in the liver tissue (Fig 1). On treatment with each drug or vitamin E, lipid peroxidation was significantly decreased to various levels. Leucopelargonin derivative produced the maximum effect by bringing down the levels of TBARS and CD significantly in liver. This was followed by NPFGO and garlic oil. The corresponding effects of vitamin E were also significant with the least effect on TBARS in liver. Histopathological changes of the liver in control and test groups revealed that the treatment prevented the damages by CCl_4 (See Fig 2).

Table 1 Effects of G.O., NFGO and leucopelargonin on lipids and proteins as compared to Vitamin E in CCl_4 induced liver damage in rats. [Values are Mean ± S.D of rats].

Groups of rats	Serum* lipids and proteins							Liver** lipids		Heart** Cholesterol
	TAG	Total chol.	HDL chol.	LDL chol.	FFA	Protein	A/G ratio	Total chol.	TAG	Total chol.
I. Normal Group	52.76±1.2	70.64±2.14	36.58±1.12	23.52±1.58	72.32± 1.51	10.16± 1.1	2.0±0.03	351.8±4.11	440.7±3.58	232.7± 2.87
II.Carbontetrachloride group	88.25±1.78^a	117.68±2.14^a	43.9±1.97^a	56.13±2.45^a	95.43±1.62^a	7.34±0.89^a	0.84±0.07^a	643.72±4.01^a	602.2±3.99^a	496.25±2.83^a
III. CCl_4 + garlic oil	58.76±1.21^a	95.6±2.99^a	56.25±1.25^a	27.59±2.92^a	78.42±1.75^a	9.88±1.2^b	1.61±0.16^a	407.09±3.62^a	462.65±3.24^a	288.98±2.35^a
IV. CCl_4 + NPFGO	58.43±1.22^a	94.28±3.11^a	58.54±1.58^a	24.05±1.82^a	81.86±1.68^a	9.88±1.15^b	1.61±0.19^a	408.40±3.76^a	460.35±3.25^a	290.4±4.36^a
V. CCl_4 + Leucopelargonin	54.36±1.25^a	85.38±3.2^a	60.0±1.36^a	14.51±2.02^a	76.32±1.54^a	10.02±1.35^c	1.62±0.18^a	379.78±2.47^a	458.45±3.12^a	263.7±3.4^a
VI. CCl_4 + Vitamin E	62.32±1.56^a	102.83±3.7^a	51.22±1.27^a	39.14±1.76^a	85.45±1.72^a	9.6±0.95^b	1.29±0.10^a	438.46±4.81^a	467.32±4.01^a	319.0±3.18^a

Student's t – test

IInd group Vs Ist group and IIIrd to VIth groups Vs IInd group are compared.

^{a}P<0.001 and ^{b}P<0.01 and ^{c}P<0.05 as compared to each control.

(Units* mg/100ml serum and ** mg/100g liver /heart tissue)

Table 2 Effects of nutraceuticals on certain enzymes as compared to vitamin E in CCl_4 induced liver damage in rats [Values are Mean ± S.D. of 6 rats] . Enzyme activities are expressed as IU/L serum and for the liver ALP as μmol/min/mg protein. ALT & AST as IU/100g wet tissue.

Groups	Alkaline phosphatase (ALP)		Alanine transaminase (ALT)		Aspartate transaminase (AST)	
	Serum	Liver	Serum	Liver	Serum	Liver
I. Normal Group	23.03±3.38	1.49±0.59	22.68± 1.2	73.12± 1.99	29.32 ±1.99	43.81± 2.25
II. CCl_4 group	45.87±1.99 ^{a}	4.25±1.12 ^{b}	46.5± 1.7 ^{a}	145.42± 2.25 ^{a}	50.05± 2.5 ^{a}	65.7± 2.61 ^{a}
III. CCl_4 + garlic oil	25.70±3.42 ^{b}	1.67± 1.26 ^{b}	33.0 ±1.31 ^{a}	76.78 ±2.10 ^{a}	35.57± 1.99 ^{a}	51.21± 1.5 ^{b}
IV. CCl_4 + NPFGO	25.73±3.65 ^{a}	1.82± 0.28 ^{b}	34.10± 1.32 ^{a}	74.60± 2.15 ^{a}	35.97± 2.0 ^{a}	51.61± 1.58 ^{b}
V. CCl_4 + Leucopelargonin	24.99±3.87 ^{a}	1.52± 1.64 ^{c}	31.96± 1.12 ^{a}	74.64± 2.12 ^{a}	33.47± 1.8 ^{a}	49.65± 1.98 ^{b}
VI. CCl_4 + Vitamin E	28.54±2.67 ^{a}	1.96± 0.87 ^{b}	39.37± 1.5 ^{a}	78.75 ±2.46 ^{a}	40.61± 2.12 ^{a}	55.21± 1.99 ^{b}

Student's t – test

IInd group Vs I^{st} group and IIIrd to VIth groups Vs IInd group are compared.

$^{a}P<0.001$ and $^{b}P<0.01$ and $^{c}P<0.05$ as compared to each control

Enzyme activities are expressed as I/L serum and for the liver ALP as μmol/min/mg protein, ALT of AST as Iu/100 g wet tissue.

Table 3 Effects of nutraceuticals on antioxidant and lipogenic enzymes activities in liver as compared to vitamin E in CCl_4 induced liver damage in rats [Values are Mean ± S.D. of 6 rats] .

Units of enzyme activities are expressed as noted below.

Groups	Glutathione reductase	Catalase	HMGCoA reductase	Glucose 6 phosphate dehydrogenase	Malic enzymes
I. Normal Group	5.51± 0.22	65.25 ±0.78	0.30 ±0.06	65.53 ±1.79	8.39± 0.51
II.Carbontetrachloride group	3.58 ±0.20^a	32.37 ±1.2^a	0.99 ±0.03^a	92.88 ±3.94^a	14.97± 0.70^a
III. CCl_4 + garlic oil	4.27 ±0.16^a	91.14 ±1.12^a	0.35 ±0.03^a	47.7 ±2.48^a	10.76 ±0.36^a
IV. CCl_4 + NPFGO	4.45 ±0.13^a	95.34 ±1.05^a	0.35 ±0.05^a	74.67 ±2.67^a	10.78 ±0.24^a
V. CCl_4 +Leucopelargonin	4.57 ±0.13^a	75.76 ±0.99^a	0.33 ±0.03^a	70.94 ±2.18^a	10.75 ±0.28^a
VI. CCl_4 + Vitamin E	4.05 ±0.09^b	69.16± 1.51^a	0.44 ±0.02^a	82.89± 1.79^a	12.22± 0.45^a

Student's t-test

IInd group Vs Ist group and IIIrd to VIth groups Vs IInd group are compared. Level of significance $^aP<0.001$ and $^bP<0.01$ as compared to each control.

Units of enzymes in liver. Glutathione reductase as values x 10^{-2} μmol of NADPH oxidized/min.

Catalase as values x 10^{-3} velocity constant /second. HMGCoA reductase as the ratio of Mevalonate / HMGCoA

Glucose 6 – phosphatase DH & malic enzyme as change in O.D of 0.01/unit/min mg protein

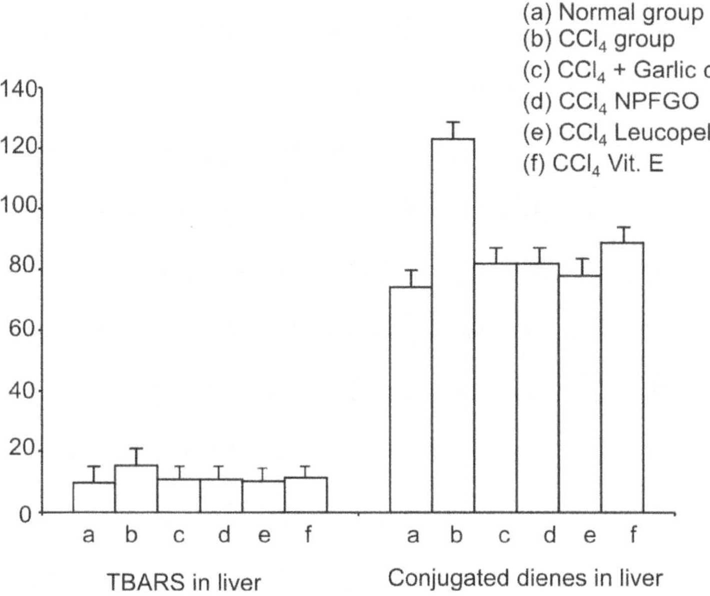

Fig. 1 Lipid peroxidation values in liver.

Values of TBARS (mg/100g wet tissue) and conjugated dienes (mM/100g wet tissue) levels in the liver of rats. (Values are Mean ± S.D. of 6 rats). Comparison is made between groups I and II and between group II Vs groups III to VI for each parameter.

[Level of significance for TBARS $P<0.05–0.02$; Conjugated dienes $P<0.01–0.001$]

Discussion

The thiyl radical (RS$^{\cdot}$) helps in the repair of free radicals and it does not react with critical molecules, hence it serves as a very good scavenger of free radicals. Flavonoids act as metal chelators and also as stimulators of microsomal activating enzymes. Pancreatic β cell stimulation by flavonoids and insulin sparing action by garlic sulphur compounds were known.

Organic disulphides oxidize NADPH which is necessary for cholesterol and fatty acid synthesis[8].

$$RSSR + NADPH + H^{+} \longrightarrow 2RSH + NADP^{+}$$

This reaction of disulphides explains the hypolipidemic effects of garlic allyl disulphides ($C_3H_5 – S\text{-}S\text{-}C_3H_5$) and its polymers in NPFGO.

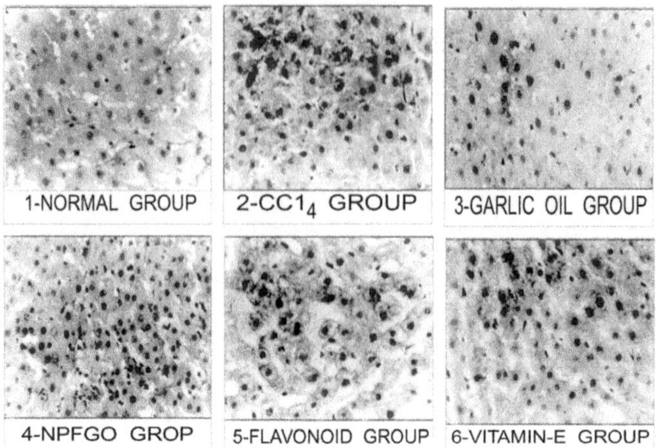

Fig. 2 Diagram of liver sections.

1. Normal - No pathologicalo changes were observed
2. Carbon tetrachloride group. A striking alteration of the normal lobular architecture could be seen in liver sections from CCL_4 fed rats. Liver sections showed mild grades of fatty degeneration (fd), focal cellular necrosis (cn) and periportal fibrosis (pf).

   3-6 Liver sections of garlic oil, NPFGO, flavonoid(leucopelargonin) and vitamin E treated groups respectively showed very mild grades of fd (white patches), pf (diffused shades), cn (fused dark spots) or any related pathological changes. Here garlic oil showed the best results in preventing liver followed by NPFGO, flavonoid and vitamin E.

In a classical work by Hikino et. al.[3] they demonstrated that the volatile oil of garlic inhibited galactosamine induced liver injury and CCl_4 induced free radical formation and lipid peroxidation in rats, more efficiently than that with vitamin E and it also indicated that the factor responsible for the inhibition of liver damage is the volatile oil of garlic which contains a mixture of both polar and nonpolar sulphur compounds. Cardioprotective action of garlic has also been reported by many workers, viz; garlic dialysate has a significant antiarrhythmic effect in both ventricular and supraventricular arrhythmias[9] The electron capture and related antioxidant actions of organic poly sulfides as found in garlic and onions are depicted by equations by Klanns-Dieter[10]. Hence the use of these vegetables may protect all types of tissues from oxidative stress.

The variation in the protective capacities of these nutraceuticals and vitamin E on liver/heart may be explained based on their various biological effects. Even though leucopelargonin is not lipid soluble, it is freely water soluble and endowed with antioxidant actions of flavonoids and such compounds were once termed by Szent Gyorgi as vitamin P. Since the association of reduced risk for diseases like cancer, CHD, ageing etc with a diet high in fruits and vegetables is strong, dietary constituents other than vitamin C and E or β carotene e.g. the above theols and flavonoid type compounds or polyphenols and terpenes may be making a greater contribution to this effect. Hence we suggest that if garlic and ficus compounds are used as dietary components or herbal preparations they may give hepato and cardioprotective actions. Further study is warranted on all nutraceuticals including the above.

Acknowledgement

The authors acknowledge with thanks the founder Director of the School of Medical Education, Dr.P.G.R. Pilla for his encouragement and also NISCAIR New Delhi for the permission granted to include the relevant parts of the published paper (Indian Jour. Exp. Biol. 43/2005/437-444) in this book.

(This paper was presented at the international seminar on alliums at Beijing by Dr. K.T.Augusti in 2004)

References

1. Edwards MJ, Keller BJ, Kauffman FC & Thurman RG. The involvement of Kupffer cells in carbon tetrachloride toxicity. Toxicol App- Pharmacol 119(2) (1993) 275.
2. Nakagawa S, Kasuaga S & Matsuur W.H. Prevention of liver damage by aged garlic extract and its components in mice. Phytother.Res. 3(1989)50.
3. Hikino H, Tohkin M, Kiso Y, Namiki T, Nishimura S & Takeyama K. Antihepatotoxic actions of *Allium sativum* bulbs. Planta Med. 53 (1986) 163.
4. Bhardwaj A, Hundal MK, Pathania V, Syal N, Sohi KK & Khanduja KL. Evaluation of antioxidant and antiradical activity of resveratrol. Paper presented at the 19th annual convention of Indian Assoc. for Cancer Res & Symposium on Cancer Biology 21-23 Jan 2000. Abstracts Session 8 P49. Amala Cancer Hospital & Res Center, Amalanagar, Thrissur, Kerala.
5. Reji Susan Daniel, Biju C Mathew, Devi KS & Augusti KT. Antioxidant effect of two flavonoids from the bark of *Ficus bengalensis* Linn in hyperlipidemic rats. Indian J. Exp. Biol. 36(1998)902.

6. Prema MS & Misra GS. Chemical constituents of *Ficus bengalensis*. Indian. J. Chem. 15B. (1977) 762.
7. Recknagel RO & Glende EA (Jr). Carbon tetrachloride induced hepatotoxicity. In: Hand book of physiology, (ed, DK. Lee.) American Physiological Society, Bethesda (1977). p.591.
8. Black S. Reduction of sulfoxide and disulfides. Methods. Enzymol 5. (1962) 992.
9. Martin N, Bardisa L, Pantoja C, Vargas M, Quezada P & Valenzuela J, Anti-arrhythmic profile of a garlic dialysate assayed in dogs and isolated arterial preparations. J.Ethnopharmacol 43, (1994) 1.
10. Klanns-Dieter A; Sulfur content free radicals In: Radio protectors and anticarcinogens. Nygaard OF and Simic MG (Eds) (1983) pp.23-42 Acad. Press New York.

9.3 Beneficial Effects of Onion and Garlic Oils against damages induced by Nicotine in Rats

Krishnakumar K, Vijayammal PL, Helen A and Augusti KT;
Dept. of Biochemistry, University of Kerala, Thiruvananthapuram

Abstract

Onion oil is mainly composed of dipropyl and dipropenyl disulfides, their polysulfides and oxides of the nature of ajoene. Similarly garlic oil contains mainly diallyl disulfide, their polysulfides and oxides of the nature of ajoene. All of them are strong antioxidants and their oxides are strong antibiotic, antiatherogenic, hypolipidemic and hypoglycemic agents. Garlic oil at a dose of 100 mg/kg/day is more potent in action than onion oil of the same dose as the former contains more reactive allyl groups and the latter contains only less reactive propenyl groups.

In nicotine injected (S.C) rats, free fatty acid release from liver is significantly raised and on treatment with the above oils, FFA level decreased in serum significantly towards normal. Similarly lipid peroxidation in terms of TBARS, conjugated dienes and hydroperoxides in liver increased significantly on nicotine injection and these parameters decreased significantly by treatment with the above oils. On the contrary the level of antioxidant enzymes viz, superoxide dismutase (SOD), catalase, glutathione peroxidase and glutathione reductase decreased significantly in the liver of the nicotine treated rats. On administration of garlic or onion oil to other nicotine treated groups, the decreases in the levels of antioxidant enzymes were prevented and their activities viz, SOD, Catalase, GSH Pxase, GSSG reductase were raised significantly. Side by side the GSH content of liver also increased significantly. Garlic oil showed slightly better effects than onion oil and the antioxidant effects of the sulfur rich oils of garlic and onion are reflected in this study.

Table 1 Concentration of lipid peroxide products (mM/100g wet tissue)

Group	TBARS	Conjugated dienes	Hydroperoxides
I Normal	0.72 ± 0.06	75.0±9.0	40.17±3.12
II Nicotine	1.06±0.10	123.0±14.8[a]	54.50±4.24
III Nicotine + O.O	0.73±0.10[b]	111.6±13.4	29.74±2.31[b]
IV Nicotine + G.O	0.86±0.11[b]	50.7±6.1[b]	38.78±3.01[b]

Values are mean±S.D of 6 rats. $P<0.01$,
a = vs normal and b=vs nicotine
O.O = onion oil G.O = garlic oil

Table 2 Activity of superoxide dismutase (units/mg protein), catalase (values × 10^{-3} units/mg protein), glutathione peroxidase (units/mg protein) and glutathione reductase (values × 10^{-2} units/mg protein) and the level of glutathione (mM/100g wet tissue).

Group	SOD	Catalase	GSH Pxase	GSSG Rase	GSH
I	7.51±0.37	65.28±7.02	0.147±0.01	5.13±0.52	477.9±39.0
II	4.63±0.13[a]	38.56±4.20[a]	0.098±0.01[a]	3.14±0.30[a]	492.6±39.0
III	10.4±0.72[b]	95.74±10.2[b]	0.129±0.01[b]	3.64±0.50	563.1±32.9[b]
IV	9.08±0.45[b]	92.8±9.97[b]	0.165±0.01[b]	3.97±0.47	602.0±29.2[b]

a = vs Normal & b = vs nicotine;

This is taken from the Post Doctoral work of Drs. K. Krishna Kumar and A. Helen. It was supported by ICMR.

Garlic is Effective against Tuberculosis also!!!

Dr. Ritu Singh, Professor of Lady Hardinge Medical College, Delhi personally told the senior author (KTA) at a conference at Tirupathi (Dec. 2007) that regular consumption of 25-30 g raw garlic syrup daily for three years in early 1940s completely cured the tuberculosis of her maternal grand father in his old age. According to her the x-ray film of his lungs was clear of T.B and he continued the use of garlic for many more years till his death. She said it was a wonderful effect of garlic as a medicine.

9.4 Ampicillin resistant Staphylococcus Aureus and the synergistic effects with extracts of garlic and other plants

Vinod. N.V, and Sadasivan. C.
School of Life sciences, Kannur University

Introduction

The antibiotic resistance is the naturally acquired ability of a microorganism to overcome the inhibitory effects of an antibiotic. Most of the resilient microbes are likely to develop resistance to the antibiotic in our communities. Ampicillin is a penicillin group of antibiotics containing a beta lactam ring. They inhibit the transpeptidoglycan synthesis and prevent the growth of bacteria. The ampicillin resistant *Staphylococcus aureus* is used in this experiment. Types of resistance seen in the organisms are Natural Resistance and Acquired Resistance. In the natural resistance the microorganism lacks the structures that the antibiotic inhibits or the cell wall structure or cytoplasmic membrane of an organism may be impermeable to an antibiotic. In acquired resistance a resistant organism may produce a substance that inactivates the antibiotic, as occurs in strains of *Staphylococcus aureus* in producing the enzyme penicillinase, which disrupts the penicillin molecule or a gradual accumulation of mutations in chromosomal DNA may result in cellular structures that will not bind the antibiotic. Strains resistant against beta lactam antibiotics appear to contain enzymes, betalactamase capable of hydrolyzing beta lactam antibiotics. Most strains produce both extracellular and cell membrane-bound form of beta lactamase. Around 90% of *Staphylococcus aureus* isolates currently recovered from clinical specimens produce beta lactamase. Beta lactamase vary in their activity against different beta lactams

When the antimicrobial activity of a combinations of antibiotics is studied, several results are possible, the combined effect may be greater than that of either agent alone could achieve is synergistic, if the combined effect may be reduced it is called antagonistic and the combined effect is equal to that of more active compound it is indifference.

The synergistic effects implying the beneficial interaction between two drugs exceeding simple additive effects, may take several forms. One compound may potentiate the activity of the other at a biochemical level. One may assist the other to penetrate into the bacterial cell. One may protect the other from destruction. Each compounds may act on separate sections of bacterial population.

Materials and Methods

Plants chosen for the study

Mimosa pudica, Adathoda vasica, Azadirachta indica, osimum sanctum, Allium sativam, Alliumcepa and Eupatoriu *odoratum*

Preparation of Plant Extract

About 20 gram of plant materials were crushed and extracted with solvents such as hexane, ether, acetone and water. Paper discs of 4 mm diameter soaked in the extract and dried at room temperature to remove the solvent. The discs were applied in the lawn culture of the organism to determine the antibiotic activity. The experiments were repeated in presence of ampicillin, to get the synergistic effect we incorporated different plant extracts (*Piper longum*, *Ocimum sanctum, Mimosa pudica, Eupatorium odoratum, Allium cepa*, and *Allium sativam*) in the growth media. The experiment has been repeated by adding ampicillin in the growth media. Acetone extract of *Allium sativum* (garlic) showed the best inhibitory effect among the plant extracts tried. It showed an inhibitory zone of 1.4 mm without the antibiotic, which increased to 2.1 mm in the presence of the antibiotic. Among the aqueous extracts only that of garlic has showed an inhibitory zone of 1.2 mm diameter in the absence of antibiotics while it has increased to 1.5 mm in the presence of ampicillin (0.25 mcg/ml of growth media). The study indicates that some of the compound present in garlic show synergistic effect with the ampicillin against *Staphylococcus aureus*. *Allium sativum* gave inhibitory zone in the absence of ampicillin showing its strong antibiotic activity against *Staphylococcus aureus*. *Azadirachta indica* and *Allium cepa* gave inhibitory zone only in the presence of ampicillin – showing their synergistic effects. Increased inhibitory zone was observed in presence of *Allium sativum* – showing a better synergistic effect. It indicates that the *Azadirachta indica*, *Allium sativum, Allium cepa* contains some compounds which promotes the antibacterial activity of ampicillin against *Staphylococcus aureus*. This is a clear indication of synergistic effect of the plant products with ampicillin. If the compound is isolated it can be used with ampicillin against the resistant *Staphylococcus aureus.*

Results

Antibacterial activity and synergistic effects of some plant extracts

S.I No	Organic solvent used	Diammeter of inhibitory zone (without antibiotic)	Diammeter of inhibitory zone (with antibiotic)
Neem (*Azhadiracta indica*)			
1	Hexane extract	none	8 mm
2	Ether extract		9 mm
3	Acetone extract		4 mm
4	Water extract		8 mm
Garlic (*Allium sativum*)			
1	1 Hexane extract	1.3 mm	1.8 mm
2	Ether extract	1.2 mm	1.4 mm
3	Acetone extract	1.4 mm	2.1 mm
4	Water extract	1.2 mm	1.5 mm
Onion (*Allium cepa*)			
1	Hexane extract	None	8 mm
2	Ether extract		8.5 mm
3	Acetone extract		9 mm
4	Water extract		8 mm

*Acetone extract of garlic showed the maximum synergistic effect.

References

Aburjai T and Natsheh F.2003 Plants used in cosmetics Phytotherapy Research. 17,987-1000.

Adebolu. T.T and Salau Abiola Oladimeji. 2005 Antimicrobial Activity of Leaf Extracts of Ocimum Gratissium on selected Diarrhoea Causing Bacteria in South Western Nigeria. African journal of Biotechnology. 4, 682-684.

Ahmad I., Mehmood Z and Mohammad F.1998 Screening of some Indian medicinal plants for their antimicribial properties. J. Ethnopharmacol. 62,183-93

Bedi K.L., Zutshi U., Chopra C.L and Amla V.1989 Picrorhiza kurroa, an Ayurvedic herb, may potentiate photochemotherapy in vitigo. Jethnopharmacol. 27,347-352

Chapter – 10

Certain Functional Foods in the Prevention of Diseases

10.1 Edible Mushrooms and Nutraceutical properties

Drs. Pushpalatha, P.B. and Indira, V.
College of Horticulture, Kerala Agricultural University, Vellanikkara Thrissur, 680656.

Mushrooms are primitive organisms known as fungi. They are fruit bodies or reproductive structures emanating from the mycelium, which under natural conditions, lie buried in the soil or in the substrate where conditions are favorable for their growth. This mycelium forms the fleshy structures, the fruit bodies, which are generally called as mushrooms. There are about 20 genera of mushrooms being cultivated, the world over, either commercially or in laboratories.

In India, mainly three types are cultivated on commercial scale, giving thrust to food value. They are (1) Button mushroom (*Agaricus bisporus*), (2) Oyster mushroom (*Pleurotus spp.*), (3) Paddy straw mushroom (*Volvariella volvacea*).

Apart from this many different types of mushrooms gained importance due to their nutraceutical properties.

Nutraceutical Properties of Mushrooms

The high protein content, associated with low starch and sugar make it a delight of the diabetic. In addition to proteins (3.7%) they also contain carbohydrate (2.4%), fat (0.4%), minerals (0.6%) and water (91%). They also contain Vit. B and C which include thiamine, riboflavin, niacin, biotin and pantothenic acid. Folic acid and Vitamin B_{12} which are normally absent in vegetable foods are present in mushrooms. They also contain minerals like potassium, sodium and phosphorus in high quantities.

The Table 1 shows the nutritive value of mushrooms. The fat content is low, but they are rich in linoleic acid and deficient in cholesterol, which makes mushrooms as the dieticians choice for heart patients.

Due to the high alkaline and high potassium sodium ratio and high fiber content, they are suitable for the people with hypertension, hyperacidity and constipation. They are reported to have anticancer and blood cholesterol reducing properties. The tables given below show the chemical contents of mushrooms as compared to vegetables.

Table 1 Shows the content of different nutrients present in mushrooms.

Nutrient	Content
Moisture (%)	88.5
Protein (%)	3.1
Fat (%)	0.8
Minerals (g)	1.4
Fibre (g)	1.3
Carbohydrates(g)	4.3g
Energy (kcal)	43
Calcium (mg)	6
Phosphorus (mg)	110
Iron (mg)	1.5
Riboflavin (mg)	0.31

Table 2 Nutrient contents of mushrooms in comparison with vegetables, fruits and milk.

Nutrients	Mushroom	Cabbage	Cauliflower	Potato	Apple	Milk
Moisture (g)	89.9	91.9	90.8	74.7	84.6	87.5
Protein (g)	2.9	1.8	2.6	1.6	0.2	3.2
Fat (g)	0.36	0.1	0.4	0.1	0.5	4.1
Carbohydrate(g)	5.30	4.6	4.0	22.6	13.4	4.4
Fibre (g)	1.10	1.0	1.2	0.4	1.0	-
Energy(cal.)	33.90	27.0	30.0	97.0	59.0	67.0
Calcium(mg)	33.0	39.0	33.0	10.0	10.0	120.0
Phosphorus(mg)	134.8	44.0	57.0	40.0	14.0	90.0
Sodium(mg)	83.7	-	53.0	11.0	28.0	73.0
Potassium(mg)	379.3	-	138.0	247.0	75.0	140.0
Iron(mg)	1.5	0.8	1.23	0.48	0.660	0.2
Thiamine(mg)	0.5	0.06	0.04	0.10	-	0.05
Riboflavin(mg)	0.5	0.09	0.10	0.01	-	0.19
Niacin (mg)	10.9	0.4	1.0	1.2	-	0.1

Mushroom is richer in protein, many minerals, antioxidants and vitamins as compared to vegetables. Preparations of G. lucidum are available as a food supplement with strong medicinal effects.

Ganoderma Lucidum

The Latin word lucidum means 'shiny' or 'brilliant' and refers to the varnished surface of reishi (fruiting bodies of *Ganoderma lucidum*) cap which is reddish orange to black. The stalk is usually attached to the cap at the side. In Japan 99 percent of reishi growing in the wild are found on old plum trees, although wild types are there.

***Ganoderma lucidum* has been reported to infect a large number of trees in Kerala. Fruiting bodies of this fungus commonly known as "Reishi" have been regarded as a panacea for all types of diseases (Jong and Birminghan, 1992). This is perhaps due to the abundance of different triterprines in them. Certain polysaccharides present in them also contribute to their physiological activity and capability to fight against diseases (Miyazaki and Nishijiama, 1981).**

This mushroom has attracted great attention recently due to its antitumor and hypoglycemic actions. Lin and Lin (1995) investigated the free radical scavenging and antihepatotoxic activities of *Ganoderma* spp. occurring in Taiwan. The physiological effects and distinctions of the mushroom are dependent on the environment in which it grows and also its strain (Nishitoba *et. al.* 1986).

Antioxidant and Cytotoxic activities of *G. lucidum* grown in Kerala

Three strains of this mushroom designated G-101, G-106 and G-108 collected from Kerala were analysed for their antioxidant and cytotoxic activities at Amala Cancer Research Centre at Trichur by Jones and Janardhanan (1999). Fruit bodies were dried and defatted with petroleum ether extraction. Fat free sample was further extracted with methanol and water in succession. These extracts were collected and concentrated on a water bath and finally lyophilized. Short term cytotoxicity of the extracts were assayed using Daltons Lymphoma Ascites Cells (DLA) by incubating the cells in PBS at 37°C for 3 hrs by a standard procedure. The viability of the cells afterwards was assayed by trypan blue exclusion using a haemocytometer (Talwar, 1974)

Antioxidant activity based on the inhibition of superoxide was assayed by the Nitro blue tetrazolium (NBT) reduction method of McCord and Fridovich (1969). Hydroxyl radical scavenging activity of the extracts was studied by a standard method and lipid peroxidative index (TBARS) was also measured.

The extracts of the mushrooms of all the three strains did not show any cytotoxic effects against DLA cells. However, methanol and water extracts of *G. lucidum* strains exhibited marked superoxide radical scavenging action. Aqueous extracts of the three strains had uniformly greater superoxide scavenging activity than methanol extracts. G-108 strain showed the maximum activity. Aqueous extracts of the mushrooms also showed a better hydroxyl radical scavenging action. Aqueous extracts of G-101 showed the maximum activity. Lin and Lin (1995) reported on the free radical scavenging activity of *G. lucidum*, *G. formasanum* and *G. neo-japonicum* occurring in Taiwan. However, Kerala variety showed a greater antioxidant activity over the Taiwan variety.

Several polysaccharides isolated from *G. lucidum* were reported to show anti tumor properties. Oxygenated triterpenes isolated from cultured mycelium of this fungus showed cytotoxic effect when tested against hepatoma cells grown *in vitro*. Ganoderma species are also found to possess antihepatotoxic activity. These findings support the claims by others that *G. lucidum* grown in Kerala possesses potential therapeutic uses.

Basidiomycetes Mushrooms

Basidiomycetes mushrooms contain biologically active polysaccharides in fruit bodies, cultured mycelium and culture broth. These polysaccharides belong to the group of glucans. These have β (1,3) linkage in the main chain and additional β (1,6) branch points that are needed for their anti tumor action. High MW glucans appear to be more effective than those of low MW. Chemical modification is often carried out to improve the antitumor activity of polysaccharides and their physical qualities such as water solubility. The main procedures used are oxydoreductohydrolysis (Smith degradation), formolysis and carboxymethylation. **Mushroom polysaccharides prevent oncogenesis, show antitumor activity against various allogenic and syngeneic tumors and prevent tumor metastasis.**

Peptide bound polysaccharides (PSP) extracted from Basidiomycetous fungi are widely used in cancer therapy and has been demonstrated to induce apoptosis in cancer cells *in vitro*. As reported by Sreelekha and Balaram (2006) certain experiments showed that PSP induced apoptosis in human promyelotic leukemia HL-60 cells might be mediated by up regulation of early transcription factors and down regulation of the NF-Kappa B transcription pathways. Other gene expression changes include the increase of several apoptotic or antiproliferation genes (Zeng and Hon, 2005).

Armillariella tabescens

The antitumor polysaccharides containing peptide moieties and an antitumor polysaccharide without peptide link were isolated from hot water extract and alkaline extract of the fruiting bodies of *Armillariella tabescens* (Kiho e.t al. 1992). The major constituent of the former (MW 105,000 Da) a heteroglycan is composed primarily of β (1,6) linked D glucopyranosyl and galactopyranosyl residues and contains their branched residues and terminal sugar (gluco, manno and fucopyranose) residues in addition to β (1,3) linked D-glucopyranosyl residues, while the latter polysaccharide with MW 93,000 Da is chiefly composed of α (1,3) linked D-glucopyranosyl residues.

The influence of a fungal polysaccharide compound (FPC) in inducing human liver cell Bel-7402 apoptosis was observed by another group of workers (Liu and Gao, 2001). The tumor inhibitive gene P_{53} expression in Bel-7402 apoptosis was analysed. With the enhancement of FPC concentration chromatin condensation in some phases accompanying characteristic apoptosis was observed.

Polysaccharide extracts prepared from the fruit bodies of three edible fungal *Flammulina velutipes* (Curt. exfr) Sing (FV), *Lentinus codes* (LE) and *Agaricus bisporus*. Sing (AB) by hot water extractions were purified by removal of protein by ethanol precipitation, trypsin digestion *etc.* by Shi-Ming *et. al.* (1999) for certain experiments. Human hepatoma SMMC-7721 cells were treated with 50 mg/l polysaccharide extracts and mitosis index, mitochondria activity and cell proliferation were detected at different times in both control and experimental groups. The mice with S-180 implanted tumors were injected with polysaccharide extracts at 24 mg/kg wt. for nine days and the tumor weight was measured on the 15th day. The results suggest that the polysaccharide extracts from LE, FV and AB could not only inhibit the growth of inplanted S-180 tumor *in vivo* but also interfere with proliferation of human hepatoma SMMC-7721 cells *in vitro*.

Shiitake (*Lentinula Edodes*)

In the wild, this amber fungus is found on fallen hardwood trees. The caps have nearly ragged gills and an inrolled margin when young and they are covered with a delicate white flocking. The stem may be central or off center. Indigenous to temperate Asia, they are not found in the wild in the United States but are widely cultivated. A similar species occurs wild in Costa Rica.

Medicinal uses: A vast amount of research into shiitake's medicinal properties has been completed and shows that it has the ability to fight tumors and viruses and enhance the immune system.

Shiitake is nonpoisonous, but researchers have observed cases of shiitake induced skin rashes, and some people who work indoors cultivating shiitake experience "mushroom worker's lung", an immune reaction to shiitake spores. A watery extract of the whole mushroom is reported to hinder blood coagulation, so people who bleed easily or who are taking blood thinners should check with their health-care provider before using shiitake or its derivatives for a long period.

The lentinula edodes extract of this mushroom (LEM) has shown no evidence of acute toxicity in more than seventeen years of use in Japan, even in massive doses (more than 50 mg a day for one week), though mild side effects such as diarrhea and skin rashes have been reported. Likewise, lentinan has no known serious side effects. People with allergies may experience adverse reactions due to its histamine-sensitizing properties.

Japanese products containing LEM, a polysaccharide extract from shiitake mushroom are currently undergoing trials in Japan and United states to see whether they are effective treatments for various cancers and AIDS.

Commercial preparations (extracts in capsule form) of shiitake are available in the United States in health-food stores but may be expensive. Dried shiitake mushrooms are available in Asian food stores in the United States, usually at more affordable prices. To avert possible digestive upset from eating large quantities of fresh shiitake, LEM, which is concentrated and easily absorbed, is preferred as medicine.

Maitake (*Grifola Frondosa*)

Maitake means 'Dancing mushrooms" in Japanese. Laboratory studies have shown that Maitake extract can inhibit the growth of tumours and stimulate the immune system of cancerous mice. Human clinical studies of patients with breast and colorectal cancers are underway in the United States. In China, many people who took Maitake extracts in capsule form for three months are reported to show anticancer effect. Further studies are to be taken up to confirm the medicinal properties of Maitake (Smith *et. al.* 2007).

Immunomodulatory Activity of Polysaccharides

PS from certain mushroom do not attack cancer cells directly, but produce their antitumor effects by activating different immune responses in the host. The anti tumor action of PS requires an intact T-cell component, their activity is mediated through a thymus dependent immune mechanism (Wasser, 2002). Polysaccharide and polysaccharide-protein complexes with the linkages of (1,3) (1,6), betaglucans and (1,3) - alpha glucans and as true heteroglucans or as protein bound forms and present in mushrooms/plants are capable of enhancing cell mediated immune response *in vivo* and *in vitro* and they act as biological response modifiers. They are multicytokine inducers that are able to induce gene expression of various immuno-modulatory cytokines and cytokine receptors.

Lentinan is a polysaccharide extracted from a kind of black mushroom shiitake, clinically applied as an anti tumor and anti-metastatic drug and has been reported to prevent both chemical and viral carcinogenesis. Lentinan is known to affect tumorous vascular system resulting in the induction of hemorrhagic necrosis, which is dependent on T-cells in the tumor (Mitamura and Sakamoto, 2000), and the anti tumor action of lentinan is reported to be host mediated. Lentinan is a (1,3)- β-D-glucan with (1,6)- β-D-glucopyranoside branches and its related polysaccharides also found to have marked anti tumor activity. Lentinan is a (1,3)-β-D-glucan with (1,6)-β-D-glucopyranoside branches and its related polysaccharides also found to have marked anti tumor activity.

Lentinan triggers the increased production of various kinds of bio active serum factors associated with immunity and inflammation such as IL-1, CSF, IL-3, Vascular dilation inducer and acute phase protein inducers, by direct impact of macrophages or indirectly via Lentinan - stimulated T-cells. These mediators result in induction of many immuno-biological changes in the host. Augmented IL-1 production amplifies the maturation of immature effecter cells to mature cells capable of responding to lymphokines such as IL-2 and T-cell replacing factors. Because of this mode of action, intact T-cell compartments for antitumor activity of lentinan are required (Chihara and Hamuro, 1987). This PS is also able to increase host resistance to various kinds of bacterial, viral and parasitic infections including AIDs. PS such as lentinan is the most appropriate drug to prevent cancer recurrences (Chihara, 1992).

A polysaccharide peptide complex (PSPC) obtained from submerged mycelia culture of Trichoderma species a local mushroom with a MW of 17 KD in gel filtration and a single band after SDS-PAGE was able to activate the macrophages, stimulate the proliferation of T-cells and inhibit the growth of Sarcoma-180 in mice (Wang and Liu, 1995). It possessed more potent immuno modulatory and anti tumor activities than *Coriolus versicolor* polysaccharopeptide (PSP). The effects of *Ganoderma lucidum* extract using SW 480 human colorectal cancer cellline was evaluated (Xei and Wang, 2006). The anti proliferate activity of GLE-1 and a triterpenoid fraction GLE-2 (without polysaccharide) was evaluated by cell proliferation assay and ^{3}H-thymidine incorporation assay. Both GLE-1 and GLE-2 significantly inhibited the proliferation of SW 480 cells (GLE-2 > GLE-1). GLE-1 inhibited DNA synthesis in the cells and reduced the formation of DPPH radicals. The results showed that that *G. lucidum* extract inhibits proliferation of human colorectal cancer cells and possess antioxidant properties.

The major immunomodulating effects of the active substances derived from mushrooms include mitogenicity and activation of immune effecter cells, such as lymphocytes, macrophages and natural killer cells, resulting in the production of cytokines including ILs, TNF- α and INF-γ. The ability of selective mushroom extracts to modulate differentiation capacity of CD4 + T cells to mature into TH-1 and/or TH-2 subsets was also studied (Lul *et. al.* 2005).

Anti tumor activity of mushroom fruit bodies and mycelial extracts were evaluated using different cancer cell lines. These polysaccharide extracts showed potent anti tumor activity against sarcoma 180, mammary adeno carcinoma 755, leukemia L-1210 and a host of other tumors. The anti tumor activity was mainly due to indirect host mediated immunotherapeutic effect. (Daba and Ezeronye, 2003).

Advantages of Polysaccharides as Anticancer Drugs

One of the greatest limitations of cancer therapy is the development of Multi Drug Resistance (MDR) in patients. Multi drug resistance is caused by an increase in cells production of proteins that transport drugs out of the cell, preventing the drugs from combating cancer. Treatment with anticancer drugs will be also influenced by a variety of factors, including individual variations in patients and somatic cell genetic differences in tumours.

The advantage with polysaccharides is that they bind to a receptor for hyaluronan called CD_{44} and preventing it from a signalling cascade, that would result in drug resistance. Hence polysaccharides can turn into a potential drug in chemotherapy, not only as an adjuvant, but also as monotherapeutic agent.

The antitumour effects of the polysaccharides has been studied at Regional Cancer Centre, Thiruvananthapuram (Sreelekha and Balaram 2006). They reported two classes of polysaccharides viz., β-glucan PSS and Oligosaccharan. β-glucon polysaccharides are biological response modifiers for the adjuvant treatment of cancer and oligosaccharan related oligosaccharides are for the prevention of sun induced skin cancer. Mushroom nutraceuticals may prevent several other diseases also apart from cancer, e.g. inflammation, hepatitis, ulcer, heart diseases etc., as cited by the above workers. Therefore mushroom is a good functional food enriched with nutraceuticals.

References

1. Chihara, G. 1992. Recent progress in immunopharmacology and therapeutic effects of polysaccharides. *Dev. Biol. Stand.* 77: 191-197.

2. Chihara, G.and Hamuro, J. 1987. Antitumor and metasis- inhibitory activities of Lentinan as an immuno modulator: an overview. *Cancer Detec. Prev. Suppl.* 1: 423-443.

3. Daba, A.S. and Ezeronye, O.U. 2003. Anti-cancer effect of polysaccharides isolated from higher basidiomycetes mushrooms. *African Jour. Biotechnol.* 2(12): 672-678.

4. Jones, S. and Janardhanan, K.K. 1999. Antioxidant activity of Ganoderma mushrooms. *Amala Res. Bulletin.* 19: 90-93.

5. Jong, S.C. and Birmingham, J.M. 1992. Medicinal benefits of the mushroom Ganoderma. Adv. Appl. Microbial. 37: 101-134.

6. Kiho, T., Shiose, Y., Nagai, K. et. al. 1992. Polysaccharides in fungi XXIX. Structural features of two antitumor polysaccharides from the fruiting bodies of *Amillariella tabescens. Chem. Phar. Bull.* (Tokyo) 40 (8): 2212-14.

7. Lin, J.M., Lin, C.C. et. al. 1995. Radical scavenger and antihepatotoxic activity of *G. formosanum, G. lucidum* and *G. neojaponicam. J. Ethnopharmacology.* 47: 33-41.

8. Liu, C. and Gao, P. et al 2001. Study of fungus polysaccharides compounds (FPC) in inducing the apoptosis of liver cancer cell Bel-7402. *Sowei Sheng Yan Jin* 30(1): 40-43.

9. Lull, C., Wiehers, H.J. and Savelkoul, H.F.G. 2005. Anti inflammatory and immunomodulating properties of fungal metabolites. *Mediators Inflamm.* (2): 63-80.

10. McCord, J.M. and Fridorich, I. 1969. Superoxide dismutase. An enzymatic function for erythrocuperin. *J. Biol. Chem.* 244: 6049-55.

11. Mitamura, T. and Sakamoto, S. 2000. Effects of Lentinan on colorectal carcinogenesis in mice with ulcerative colitis. *Oncol Rep.* 7(3): 599-601.

12. Miyazaki, T. and Nishijiama. 1981. Studies on fungal polysaccharide XXVII. Structural examination of a water soluble antitumor polysaccharide of *Ganoderma lucidum. Chem. Pharm. Bull.* 29: 3611-16.

13. Nishitoba, T., Salo, H., Shirasu, S. and Sakamura, S. 1986. Evidence on the strain specific terpenoid pattern of Ganoderma lucidum. *Agri. Biol. Chem.* 50: 2151-2154.

14. Shi-Ming, J., Zheng-Ming, X., Zhao-Hui, X. 1999. Inhibitory activity of polysaccharide extracts from three kinds of edible fungi on proliferation of human hepatoma SMMC-7721 cell and mouse implanted S-180 tumor. *World J. of Gastroenterology*. 5(5): 404-407.

15. Smith, E.J., Rowan, N.J. and Sullivan, R. 2007. www.icnet.uk/labs/med_mush/med_mush.html.

16. Sreelekha, T.T. and Balaram, P., 2006. Antitumor and chemopreventive effects of plant polysaccharides - an appraisal. *Amala Res. Bull.* 26: 47-61.

17. Talwar, G.P. 1974. *Hand book of Practical Immunology*, National Book Trust, New Delhi. pp.329-336.

18. Wang, H.X; Liu, W.K. et. al. 1995. Immunomodulatory and antitumor activities of polysaccharides - peptide complex from a local edible mushroom. *Life Sciences.* 57(3): 269-281.

19. Wasser, S.P. 2002. Medicinal mushrooms as a source of antitumor and immuno modulating polysaccharides. *Appl. Microbiol. Biotechnol.* 60: 258-274.

20. Xei,J.T; Wang,C.Z et. al. 2006 Ganoderma lucidum extract inhibits proliferation of SW-480 human colorectal cancer cells. Exp.Oncol. 28(1) 25-29.;

21. Zeng, F., Hon, C.C. et. al. 2005. Molecular characterization of *Coriolus versicolo*r PSP - induced apoptosis in human promyelotic leukemia HL-60 cells using CDNA micro array. *Int. J. Oncology* 27(2): 513-23.

10.2 The fascination of Kombucha

© **Günther W. Frank**
Günther W. Frank, Genossensch.-Str. 10, 75217 Birkenfeld/Germany
Fax (+49) 89-14 88 27 09 87
e-mail frank@kombu.de

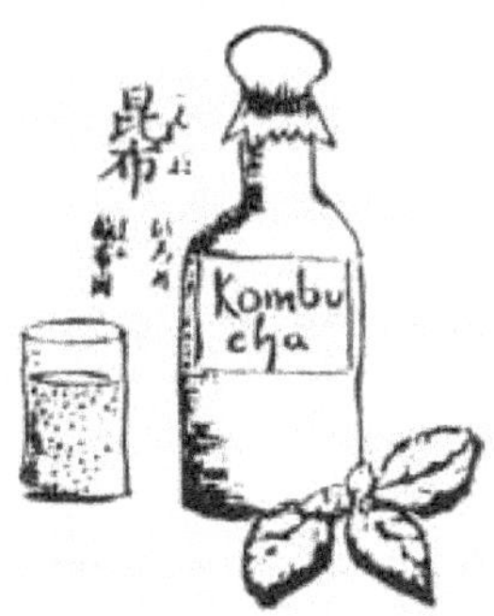

Nowadays we experience a return to healing measures that are close to nature; also remedies and foods of a natural origin – away from industrial packaged products. This may be one of the reasons for the great attractiveness and fascination of the healthful beverage called Kombucha. Communalities of yeasts and bacteria have been used by people, and applied for their well-being, since ancient times in all the world for the creation of health-promoting fermented drinks and foodstuffs

We read already in the Bible (Ruth 2:14) that the land-owner **Boas** invited the Moabite **Ruth**, who later became his wife, during her gleaning of grains: *"Come over here and eat some bread and dip your morsel into the vinegar-drink! And she sat down beside the reapers; and he reached her parched corn and she ate and was sufficed and left"*. This biblical report from around 1000 B.C. not only gives us a hint of their exemplary nutritional habits, although they were modest by our perspective, we see from it also that, even at that time, people prepared beverages with microorganisms of lactic acid and how they served the people for strength and refreshment during the hard work of harvesting.

An ancient, pure relative of these related symbioses of bacteria and yeasts is the tea-fungus called Kombucha. It comes from the area of East Asia and came into Germany via Russia, around the turn of the century. This ancient house-remedy is used more and more also in other countries against all possible defects. The mushroom consists of a gelatinoid and tough mushroom-web membrane in the form of a flat disk. It lives in a nutrient solution of tea and sugar, in which it constantly multiplies through germinating. The fungal disc at first spreads over the entire surface of the tea and then thickens. When one treats the mushroom correctly, it thrives, germinates, and will accompany its owner for life.

During the fermentation and oxidation processes, the mushroom effects diverse complicated reactions in the tea-setting, either one after the other or side by side (these are assimilation- and dissimilation-processes). The tea-mushroom feeds on the sugar and, in exchange, produces other valuable substances which change into the drink: glucuron-acid, acetic acid, lactic acid, vitamins, amino acids, antibiotic substances, and other products. The tea-mushroom is, therefore, a real, tiny biochemical factory.

Kombucha - Remedy for Everything?

There is a treasure of extensive experience regarding the Kombucha mushroom. Besides its use as a refreshing drink, one can read in nearly all reports also of its usage as a remedy. In the reports of oldest and modern times, a large number of diseases are quoted, for which Kombucha-tea is used and praised. The palette reaches from the most harmless indisposition up to the most serious diseases.

These Persons are Kombucha Fans

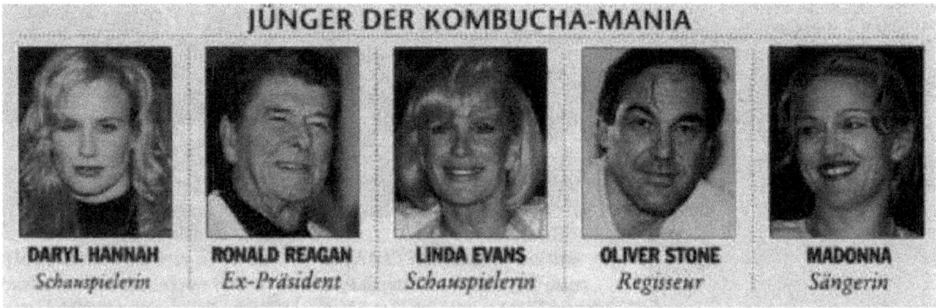

Numerous doctors and scientists have concerned themselves with the effects of the Kombucha-beverage as a home remedy. Many scientific works are at hand concerning Kombucha. They speak of its therapeutic effectiveness as based on glucon-acid, glucuron-acid, acetic acid, lactic acid, acetic acid, as well as the life-supporting vitamins C and the B-group. As has been proven especially by Russian researchers, many of its components have antibiotic and detoxifying characteristics, and they play a decisive role for the biochemical processes in the body.

In contrast to the many pharmaca with unpleasant side effects, the active substances of the Kombucha address themselves to the whole body system; through its friendly metabolistic properties, it can reestablish a normal condition in the cellular membranes without any side-effects and thus promote one's well-being. Let us use these natural powers for maintaining our vitality, activity, as well as our mental and physical capacities!

An Extensive World-Literature

Already **Bacinskaja** (1914) noted that the drink is effective for the stomach-intestinal activity. The authoress recommended that one drink a small glass of it before every meal and to increase the portions gradually.

Professor S. Bazarewski brought forth a report in the "Correspondence for the Association of Nature Researchers in Riga, 1915, that among the Latvian population of the Baltic Russian Provinces of Livland and Kurland, they had a folk-remedy by name of "Brinum-Ssene" Verbally translated, it means "Wonder-mushroom". The Latvian population ascribed to this mushroom "a wonderful healing power for many diseases", according to Bazarewski. Some people asked by Bazarewski insisted that it helps for headaches, but others assured him that "this mushroom is useful for all diseases.

Good for Constipation

Prof. B. Lindner(1917-1918) reported that the remedy is mostly used as regulator of the intestinal activities. Also Hemorrhoids were cured.

Privy Councilor **Prof. Dr. Rudolf Kobert** (1917-18) recollects that an "unfailing remedy against joint rheumatism" was made with this mushroom.

Also **Prof. Dr. Wilhelm Henneberg** (1926) reports that a drink made with tea-mushroom was prepared, called "Teakwass" in Russia, being used in all those areas as a "remedy against all sorts of diseases, especially against constipation".

According to **Dr. Madaus** in the "Biologic Healing Arts" (1927), the mushroom, and its metabolic products, has excellent influence on the regeneration of the cellular walls and is, therefore, an excellent remedy for arteriosclerosis.

General improvement of one's overall condition

H. Waldeck (1927) tells of a chemist he met during W.W.I in Russia-Poland, 1915, with whom he had his quarters, and who cooked for him a "Wonderdrink" against his severe constipation. The chemist entrusted to Waldeck that he always keeps this "Russian secret home remedy" at hand, it being "said that it is good for all kinds of ailments" and "because of its naturally formed acid, it successfully counters aging problems, thus, contributing to life extension".

Prof. Br. Lakowitz (1928) confirms Waldeck's statement that digestive disturbances are quickly removed by the mushroom-tea. Strong headaches and nervous disturbances also are removed experientially. Lakowitz comes to the conclusion: "An extensive spreading of the mushroom-tea for the production of such Tee-Kwasses, as a remedy against digestive disturbances is desirable for all types of people".

In the **"White Flag"** (1928) is reported: 'The refreshing taste of this tea-beverage is generally pleasing, and its effect is ... a very good one. The taste of the fermented tea is very pleasant, being reminiscent of light, sparkling wine or sweet Most (pear juice). The effect of the tea usually shows up very fast. Most of all, it works blood-cleansing and detoxifying and is said ... to give excellent services for facial skin rashes. Further, according to doctor's orders and evaluations, it is very effective for constant headaches, pain in the limbs, gout, rheumatism, and other aging problems. The general effect of the mushroom-tea shows already in a few weeks through an improved general condition and in one's raised performance capacity, which may be connected with the mushroom's high vitamin and hormone effect, which are also emphasized by doctors.

Further, the mushroom stimulates the metabolism ... excellently and, thereby, helps in clearing out the body, i.e. the elimination of all types of disease toxins.

Favorable effect in Arterioclerosis

Dr. Maxim Bing (1928) recommends the Kombucha mushroom as a "very effective remedy for Arteriosclerosis, gout, and intestinal deficiency." "A favorable effect in the sense of lowering blood pressure, cessation of anxiety, of irritability and pains, headaches, dizziness, etc., in arteriosclerosis" occurs from the use of fresh, good cultures. "Intestinal sluggishness and its accompanying effects also can be quickly removed. It gives especially favorable results in calcification of the kidneys and the capillaries of the brain."

Dr. Siegwart Hermann (1929) describes experiments with cats who had been poisoned with Vigantol (an anti-rickets Vitamin B-preparation). He noted a positive influence in their cholesterol level when the animals received Kombucha extracts. This is interesting because in cases of human arteriosclerosis there is also a raised cholesterol level. Hermann's resume based on these experiments is: "The observations by doctors at the sickbed, as also the animal experiments, showed that folk-wisdom quoted effects have been observed in general."

The Glucuronic Acid and its detoxifying action

In my opinion, there are factors speaking for the good effects of the mushroom for gout, rheum, arthritis, etc., as being explainable by the accumulated toxins of the body being made water-soluble and kidney-manageable through their conjugation with the Glucuronic acid in the beverage, and thus being eliminated through the urine. This conjugation is a form of bio-transformation; by it, both endogenic and body-foreign substances become bound with Glucuronic acid into Glucuronoids, also named "paired Glucuronic acid.'

In 1961, **Dr. med. Valentin Köhler** stimulated a discussion on the therapeutic usage of Glucuronic acid through his article titled, "Glucuronic Acid Gives Courage to Cancer-Patients" in the periodical "Medical Practice". Glucuronic acid is one of the products that are produced during the fermentation process in the Kombucha-tea. Dr. Köhler reported at that time about encouraging results in treating cancer patients with Glucuronic acid. **The maximally long effect of Glucuronic acid is able to bring about an increase in the body's own defenses and, possibly, also of the Interferon-production. The detoxifying function of Glucuronic acid goes hand-in-hand with an improvement in the general condition and in the oxidative metabolism.**

Dr. Köhler also noted surprising successes in the treatment of sick trees. Various Institutions were doing scientific tests for resolving the problem of dying trees. By combining nutritious substances, trace-elements, and heavy metals ions a building process was activated or accelerated. The capacity of the Glucuronic acid to enter into combination with both foreign and endogenic toxic substances, effects protection for the plant cell. Over 200 substances can be made harmless by this way, including those which are contained in acidic and radioactive rain, as well as sulfur dioxide, nitrites, ozone. According to Br. Köhler's research, the protective activity connected with Glucuronic acid preserves also the genetics of the plant from growth disturbances or promotes their restoration in the further course of its growth. The insights arising from Dr. Köhler's examinations can be transferred onto all human cells. When the processes of growth and decomposition in the human metabolism are maintained on an optimal level through adding small dosages of Glucuronic acid, as contained in the Kombucha beverage, it presents a combination of scientific data and a product of nature which is currently still much preferred by the laity. Here is a possible aid for a humanity that is more and more threatened through toxic environmental substances. By Glucronic acid, the disturbance products in the human body are disintegrated into end-products, eliminated and, thereby, made harmless. This detoxifying function of Glucuronic acid benefits the variety of cellular functions.

This shows up as increased endogenic capacity towards the toxic and environmental stresses batting us from many sides, as a revival of damaged body cells, and a restoration and firming up of our well-being. When many people say that they use Kombucha not to necessarily heal a particular disease, but they drink it as a beverage for supporting their well-being, we have in this a contact point where scientific insights and folk-wisdom can go hand in hand.

The Normalization of Intestinal Functions

Dr. L. Mollenda (1928) reports that the Kombucha beverage is especially effective for disturbances of the digestive organs, by practically normalizing their functions. Moreover, the drink has proven itself as helpful for gout, rheumatism, and diverse stages of arteriosclerosis. About additional areas of application he writes: "In the case of angina, especially when there is a coating of the tonsils, the drink should not merely be used for gargling but for drinking, and that, for the destruction of bacteria which reach the stomach through food and drink. Such gargling in angina brings fast recovery, and in pains of gout and arteriosclerosis, surprising successes are reached even in serious cases. ... Even though the beverage is acidic, it does not cause any acidic condition in the stomach; it facilitates and noticeably promotes the digestion even of difficult to digest foods. Equally favorable successes after taking Kombucha beverage have also been reached for gouty eczema and for stones in kidneys, urine, and gall".

Dr. E. Arauner (1929) reports of diverse medical reports and evaluations and reaches the following conclusion: "In summary, one can say that the Kombucha mushroom or its extract, has proven itself as excellently prophylactic against diabetes, but especially against aging problems, such as arteriosclerosis, high blood pressure with its consequences such as dizziness, gout, hemorrhoids; for the very least it is a pleasant laxative". Dr. Arauner reports that in his home-country the tea-mushroom has been in usage for centuries by Asian people because of its surprising healing successes, being a most effective, natural home-remedy for tiredness, fatigue, nervousness, beginning aging problems, arteriosclerosis, intestinal lassitude, gout and rheumatism, hemorrhoids, and diabetes.

Arauner adds to this, that not only professors, doctors and biologists have confirmed the surprising healing successes but also those who have imbibed the mushroom-tea report about "entirely excellent effects on the general body functions".

Recommendable for Mental Stress

Hans Irion, who was then the Director of the State-recognized Academy for Chemists in Braunschweig says in his "Course for Druggist Specialty Schools" (1944, Vol. 2, pg. 405): "By the intake of the drink described as

Teakwass, there happens a remarkable invigoration of the body's entire glandular system and a promotion of the metabolisms. Teakwass is recommended as an excellent prophylactic for gout and rheumatism, furunkulosis, arteriosclerosis, high blood pressure, nervousness, intestinal lassitude, and aging problems. It is also very highly recommended for sports-people and those who do strenuous mental work. Through the promotion of the metabolism, undue fat deposits in the body are avoided or removed. With the drink, also microorganisms reach the body which transform damaging deposits, such as uric acid, cholesterol, etc., into easily soluble forms, thus removing them. Foul intestinal bacteria are suppressed."

"Detoxifying in Every Regard...."

The first description having mushroom-tea as it's theme in bookform appeared in 1954. This booklet of 54 pages is written in the Russian language and carries the title "The Tea-Mushroom and its Therapeutic Properties". The author, **G.F.Barbancik** refers in his introduction to the first application of the mushroom-tea decoction (in 1949) as a healing remedy at the therapeutic clinic of the Omsker Hospital for water laborers. He reports of successful therapy for tonsillitis, diverse internal diseases, especially those of inflammatory nature, stomach catarrh due to deficient acid production, intestinal inflammations, dysentery, arteriosclerosis, high blood-pressure, scleroses, etc.

The med. doctor, **Dr. Rudolf Sklenar** of Lich, Oberhessen, reported in 1964 in the periodical "Experiential Healing Science" about his methods of diagnosis and therapy successes: "An outstanding natural remedy is the mushroom beverage named Combucha, which acts detoxifying in every regard and which dissolves microorganisms as well as cholesterol." Dr. Sklenar had developed a biologic cancer therapy in which Combucha, as well as other biologic remedies such as Coli-preparations, held an important place for the sanitization of the intestinal flora.

In a small publication of 8 pages, titled "Cancer Diagnosis Based on Blood and the Treatment of Cancer, Pre-cancerous Conditions, and other Metabolic Diseases with Kombucha and Coli-Preparations", Dr. Sklenar reports that vitamins, lactic acids and glucuronic acid are effective. "They destroy harmful microorganisms (viruses, bacteria, fungi) and dissolve waste matter and toxic deposits (uric acid, cholesterol, etc.)". Kombucha effects "an outstanding detoxification of the organism". Through enjoying this beverage there is, additionally, a "noticeable invigoration of the entire glandular system and enhancement of the metabolism".

Dr. Sklenar reports that he was able to treat successfully with the mushroom-tea: gout, rheum, arteriosclerosis, arthritis, dysbacteria, constipation, impotence, nonspecific draining, obesity, furunculosis, kidney stones, cholesterol, cancer and especially its early stages, etc.

Cancer Killer?

Dr. Veronika Carstens (1987), wife of the former German President, recommends Kombucha in a series titled, "Help from Nature–My Remedies Against Cancer", with the words: "Kombucha detoxifies the organism and enhances the metabolism; this improves the defense capacity".

The Natural Healing specialist **A.J.Lodewijkx** (Homepage: http://www.ngab.nl) of Ermelo, Netherlands, writes about Kombucha in his very recommendable book "Life Without Cancer" (obtainable in the Dutch and German languages): "The Kombucha mushroom has strongly antiseptic properties. The tea purifies the glandular system and promotes elimination; uric acid is neutralized and eliminated through Kombucha tea. Therefore, this tea is an excellent remedy against gout, rheum, arthritis, kidney stones, intestinal dysbacteria, but especially cancer and its early stages because the Kombucha mushroom exerts a mighty influence on the disease-causing endobionts. As we have seen, it is these endobionts which eliminate the red corpuscles when the pH changes unfavorably. In all metabolic diseases and cancer, Kombucha is a unique beverage for the detoxification of the body. Kombucha removes the metabolic dross and normalizes thereby the blood pH".

Gottfried Mueller, founder of the world-wide "Salem Children's and Youth Villages" praises the Kombucha tea-mushroom this way: "A gift from heaven, especially for health emergencies" (in "Salem-Help" 15, Nr. 3, August 1987, page 2).

Judging for One self

In both the literary reports and also in the many personal experiences reported during my focusing on Kombucha, the broad palette of complaints relieved by it is conspicuous. This is explainable on the basis that Kombucha does not target a specific body organ but, rather, it influences the entire organism positively by effecting a stabilization of the metabolic situation and through its detoxifying effect of its glucuronic acid. This leads in many people to a heightened endogenic defense capacity against those toxic influences and environmental stresses which inundate us from many sides, resulting in the invigoration of a damaged cellular metabolism, and the restoration and firming tip of one's well-being.

Some of the health-promoting properties ascribed to Kombucha-tea require further research. However, other active mechanisms are entirely proven both by scientific testings and experientially, such as: regulation of the intestinal flora, cellular strengthening, detoxification and dross elimination, metabolic harmonization, antibiotic effect, facilitating pH-balance.

Make it Yourself! No Problem if You Know How!

The Kombucha beverage can be made in one's home for just pennies. Because the mushroom constantly grows, one can begin with a piece of a mushroom-tea membrane and allow a health-promoting source of drink to bubble tip. The preparation is no problem if one knows how. From ancient days, one prepares the Kombucha beverage right at home and passes the tea-mushroom from family to family as a sign of friendship and mutual helpfulness. Tea-mushroom has high vitality and a great capacity for regeneration. If it did not have this high biologic energy, it would not have survived the long timespan from its reported discovery in the Chinese Empire more than 2000 years ago until now.

Nowadays, there are occasional warnings - mostly coming from ignorance or economic interests - not to make the Kombucha beverage by oneself. Such a warning is justified in so far as the know-how about the precise method, wherewith, and why, etc. had often been lost and people wrongly experimented instead of abiding with proven recipes.

However, when one works clean and abides by proven directions, then there is no hesitation in making the Kombucha drink, as in many generations past. Whoever has the necessary knowledge can deal successfully with the tea-mushroom – just as one deals with other "open" foodstuffs in one's household. When abiding by proven instructions, one can produce an impeccable, tasty, wholesome and effective Kombucha beverage. The mushroom will increase and accompany its owner lifelong and serve him or her well.

The Kombucha Mushroom Protects itself

Whoever treats his mushroom culture according to proven rules with thought and carefulness, need not expect disturbances. In the Russian reports it is even mentioned that no special precautionary measures are needed because the mushroom protects itself against impurities. It has a number of protective features: the organic acids, the low alcoholic content, carbonic acid, the antibiotic products all these jointly block the development of all foreign microorganisms not belonging to the tea-mushroom organism.

The Russian researcher **I.N. Konovalow** mentions in his report of 1959, that the intensive growth of the tea-mushroom leven and bacteria distinctly suppresses the spreading of other yeast and bacterial varities. Also the Russian **Professor G.F.Barbancik** (1958) reports in his book about the tea-mushroom based on laboratory tests which showed that the tea-mushroom bacteria drive out all other microbes energetically (antagonism).

In contrast to other reports this mushroom is easy to multiply and part. Because it grows cheerfully and is parted willingly, all friends and acquaintances can soon benefit. It is a good custom to pass on the Kombucha mushroom to other people as a sign of friendship and mutual helpfulness.

Do you want how to make your own Kombucha tea?

e-mail: buero@ennsthaler.at

WebPage: http://www.ennsthaler.at Author's permission

(by email) to publish the above article

Editor's Comments

The detoxifying effects of glucuronic acid in this beverage may help many who use various drugs for diseases. A quick disposal of the metabolites of the drugs by conjugation with glucuronic acid may have a protective effect on heart, liver, kidney etc. Dr. K.T.Augusti makes this tea wine for personal use.

10.3 Functional Foods as ingredients of Drug preparations

Mohind C Mohan ; Ramalath T; Jamshira M ; Jyolsna R;and Sajna, K.P.

MSc Students, School of Health Sciences Kannur University,Thalassery campus. Kerala 670661.

1. A Decoction to Cure Viral fevers:

(Practised by Late Ayurvedic Physician Dr. Joseph John Kurakkat of Therthally, Kannur District, Kerala, with the permission of his daughter, Mrs. Cillamma Augustine. Cherupuzha, Kannur Dist.).

Garlic Gingeradi Decoction. Weights or numbers of ten items are given in parenthesis Garlic (200 g); Ginger (150 g); Krishna thulasi. (500 g); Palm sugar (100 g); Malabar tamarind (Garcinia cambogia 20 g); Cardamam (20 Nos); Black pepper, (50 g), Turmeric (20 g), Five tea spoon full common salt, and Small variety onions (100 g); All items are cleaned and homogenized separately and mixed with 3.5 liters of water and boiled in an earthern or steel pot for 20 minutes. Filter the same and drink every time half a cup of it, four times a day till the cough and fever are cured. Usualy on the 3 rd day the patient shall be O.K. A three in one preparation as a preventive medicine for CHD, Cancer, jaundice, viral fevers, dementia, tooth ache and other age old problems is described below.

2. A three in one food supplement, similar to a Chinese model

Dr. K.T. Augusti after participation in a seminar on alliums at Beijing (2004) developed a food supplement following a Chinese model of Garlic Ginger syrup in vinegar to prevent cancer, CVD, Viral fevers, Dementia and other old age diseases. The Garlic, Ginger; and Black pepper syrup is made as follows by taking each item respectively in the ratio (4:1:0.25) of cleaned and sliced forms of 40 g. garlic, 10 g. ginger and 2.5 g. black pepper. Homogenize each of them separately with out water and mix them intimately. Keep it in the fridge and consume half a tea spoon of it along with honey, milk or rice porridge every day in the morning for two weeks or more to boost up our immune system, regularly in each month. The above diseases shall be prevented and edema, joint pains etc., after a viral fever attack shall also be cured after regular use of the syrup for 10 or 15 days.

This was experienced by several people in Kerala during the two episodes of the diseases, viz; jaundice in 2005 and viral fever in 2006-2007. Dry Ginger can also be tried in place of raw ginger for achieving a better effect.

Functional Foods Used as Ingredients of Various Drug preparations in Folk Lore and Ayurvedic Systems. Each item is short listed as follows: Garlic(G), Onions (O), Ginger(GR), Turmeric (T), Sesame (S M), Lime Juice(LJ), Honey(H), Palm sugar(PS), Black pepper(BP), Amla (A)or its juice (AJ), Pomegranate juice (PJ), Bitter gourd (BG), Moringa leaves (ML), Krishna thulasi and Thulasi leaves (KTL; TL), Curry leaves (CRL), Coriander leaves or Coriander (CR), Asafoetida (AS), Fenugreek (F), Cardamom (CM) and Cumin(CM). Momordica charantia (MC)

List of functional foods used in the preparation of various Ayurvedic Drugs to cure diseases

Diseases	Functional Foods Used as Ingredients in Different Systems of Medicine.
1. Allergy	T/LJ/A/TL/CN/
2. Anaemia	GR/ H/BP/A/ML/CRL/CM/
3. Angina	GR/CR/CN/
4. Anorexia	GR/LJ/PJ/TL/AS/
5. Asthma	GR/T/SM oil/H/PS/BP/TL/CL/ML/CN/
6. Bleeding nose	G/
7. Blood cholesterol.	G/O/GR/PJ/
8. Boils	BP/
9. Breast milk	H/ML/F/
10. Bronchitis	AS/PJ/
11. Cancer prevention.	LJ/H/SM/A/TL/Thriphala /Black cumin .
12. Centipede poison	Raw turmeric is applied to the wound..
13. Cholera	GR/BP
14. Cold .	GR/T/H/LJ/BP/A/KTL/CN/CM/
15. Coronary artery disease	GR/H/G/O/AS/
16. Cough	O/GR/H/BP/TL/CR/F/CN/Onion juice is inhaled.
17. Diabetes Mellitus	G/T/A/BG/F/MC
18. Diarrhoea	PJ/GR/F/CN/BP/Tender coconut water/
19. Dyspepsia	CN/BP/O/
20. Dysentery	F/PJ/
21. Early greying	A/CL/CL in butter milk/Tea/Apply almonds flour in coconut oil.
22. Edema	GR/G/
23. Epilepsy	G/GR/H/CL/Inhaling onion juice.
24. Gas trouble	G/GR/PS/BP/PJ/CN/

Contd....

Diseases	Functional Foods Used as Ingredients in Different Systems of Medicine.
25. Giddiness	A/CM/
26. Gonorrhea	CN/CM/BP/
27. Head ache	BP/TL/CRL/KTL/CL/ garlic or Pudina leaves as paste on forehead.
28. Haematuria	PJ/
29. Horse ness	GR/H/ML/CN/
30. Hemorrhoids	PJ/
31. Hypertension	G/GR/ML/KTL/AS/F/
32. Hysteria	AS
33. Indigestion	G/GR/H/BP/CN/CR/
34. Intestinal disorders	CR/GR/
35. Jaundice	T/CL/CN/Onion as a sedative.
36. Loose motion	G/LJ/PJ/F/
37. Malarial fever	BP/ .
38. Menopause	G/GR/H/SM/PS/CN/
39. Phlegm	G/O/GR/H/LJ/BP/TL/F/
40. Pneumonia	AS/
41. Pregnancy	SM/
42. Obesity	GR/SM oil/H/A/CL/
43. Ordinary fever	O/GR/H/BP/TL/AS/CN/
44. Osteoporosis	O/CN/
45. Piles	G/Onion fried in oil/GR/T/SM/PS/F/BP/
46. Rheumatism	G/BP/TL/F/
47. Running nose	GR/H/BP/
48. Scorpion poison	PJ/CM/
49. Sinusitis	PS/BP/AS/Inhaling Alma & KTL juices
50. Snake bite	CM as an antidote.
51. Spider poison	T/SM/LJ/TL/
52. Sore throat	H/Garlic paste is applied in front of the throat.
53. Spleen enlargement	F/O/
54. Sprue	O/GR/BP/ Papaya and butter milk/
55. Stomach ache	G/GR/LJ/CL/F/AS/CN/
56. Tooth ache	G/BP/
57. Ulcers	G/GR/H/LJ/A/BP/PJ/ML/
58. Urinary stone.	PJ/Juice of plantain inflorescence
59. Urinary system disorder	BP
60. Viral fevers	G/O/GR/T/PS/BP/TL/CN/
61. Vomiting	G/H/TL/ML/CM/CR/
62. Whooping cough	O/GR/LJ/H/AS/
63. Wounds	T/PS/ML/O/GT/

Mangiferin an Antioxidant Present in Mango Tree and Fruits

Roopesh N.P. (Lecturer) and Aparna G.S SHS Kanuur University.

Mangiferin is a naturally occurring nutraceutical made of C- glycosyl xanthone which was first extracted from the leaves of Mangifera indica Linn (Mango; Anacardiaceae) by Ansari, Reddy et al[1]. This polyphenolic antioxidant is present not only in leaves[2] but also in fruits, stems, and roots of M.indica[3]. (P. 49). Plant parts rich in mangiferin are widely used in India for the treatment of immuno-deficiency diseases such as arthritis, diabetes, hepatitis, cardiac and mental disorders[4]. Being a strong antioxidant it has antilipid peroxidative, immunomodulatory, cardioprotective, diuretic, hypotensive, wound healing, antidegenerative and antidabetic activities[5,6].

Prabhu, Mallika, Jainu et. al.[7] recently reported on the cardio protective effect of mangiferin on myocardial infarction induced by isoproterenol (ISP). ISP is a synthetic catecholamine and beta adrenergic agonist that causes severe stress in the myocardium, which leads to infarction with necrosis of the heart muscle. MI causes generation of free radicals that stimulate lipid per oxidation, which in turn irreversibly damages the myocardial membrane[8]. Recently attention has been focused on nutraceuticals such as flavonoids, alkaloids and xanthones derived from different parts of plants as potential antioxidants for the prevention and management of cardiovascular diseases (CVD)[9].

Prabhu's team took four groups of rats with six in each group. Group 1 was kept as control, and received DMSO (0.2 ml/100g) as a vehicle, i.p, for 28 days. Group 2 was administered ISP (20 mg/100g) suspended in 0.1 ml of normal saline subcutaneously twice daily with an interval of 24 hrs. Group 3 (Drug control) was treated with mangiferin alone (10 mg/100g) i.p, suspended in 0.2 ml DMSO for 28 days. Group 4 was pretreated with mangiferin (10 mg/100 g) i.p, as above for 28 days and ISP was administered as in group 2. After 28 days no DMSO or mangiferin was administered to groups 1 and 3 respectively. Group 2 was not administered with any compound after ISP injection. All groups were maintained on rat feed and water ad libitum for a total of 30 days. On the 31st day all groups were anaesthetized with pentobarbitol sodium (35 mg/kg, i.p) and their blood was collected from the external jugular vein and their heart tissues were dissected out immediately for various estimations and histological studies.

A significant elevation of lipid peroxides both in serum and heart tissue was observed with a concomitant increase in serum AST and ALT activities in ISP injected second group as compared to control group 1. Mangiferin pretreatment in group 4, significantly reduced the level of serum and heart tissue lipid peroxides and the serum marker enzymes AST and ALT as compared to group 2. Treatment with mangiferin alone did not show any significant change in-group 3 as compared to the control group 1.

A significant rise in various marker enzymes such as AST, ALT, CK and LDH and lipid per oxidation was observed in the heart tissue of group 2 rats as compared to the control. Pretreatment with mangiferin retained the activities of these enzymes and LPO level to near normal levels in group 4.

Microscopic examination of heart tissues of groups 1 and 3 showed normal myocardial fibers and muscle bundles, with normal architecture. However heart tissue of ISP injected group 2 rats showed separation of myocardial fibers, with inflammatory mononuclear collections, edema, and myocardial necrosis. Heart tissue of mangiferin pretreated group 4 showed slightly separated myocardial fibers with small focus of inflammatory mononuclear collections with out necrosis. These results clearly establish the cardio protective effects of mangiferin against ISP induced myocardial infarction in rats.

The therapeutic efficacy of mangiferin against ISP induced MI may be due to its antioxidant, antilipid peroxidative, free radical scavenging, immunomodulatory and cardioprotective property. These results further highlight the role of nutraceuticals such as mangiferin in our diet either in pure form or as part of the functional food such as mangoes, mangosteen fruits or as mango leaves which are used for cleaning the teeth that could counteract the bad effects of oxidative stress on our heart. Work by others on the antidiabetic action of mangiferin[10] and cardio protective actions of xanthones[11] further illustrate the benefits of these groups of nutraceuticals in our diet.

References

1. Ansari, M.A; Reddy, K.K; Sastry, K.N.S and Nayudamma, Y. Dicotyledonae anacardiacea. Poly phenols of Mangifera indica, Phytochemistry. 10(1971)2239.
2. Dar, A; Fazi, S; Naqvi, S. et. al. Analgesic and antioxidant activity of mangiferin and its derivatives. The structure activity relationship. Biol. Pharm. Bull. 28(2005) 596.
3. Nunez Selles, A.J; Velez Castro, H.T. et. al. Isolation and quantitative analysis of phenolic antioxidants, free sugars, and polyols from mango (Mangifera indica L), stem bark aqueous decoction used in Cuba as a nutritional supplement. J. Agr. Food Chem 50(2002)762.
4. Ichiki, H; Miura, T; Kubo, M. et. al. New antidiabetic compounds, mangiferin and its glycoside. Biol. Pharm. Bull 12(1998)1389.
5. Ghosal, S; Rao, G; Saravanan, V. et. al. A plausible chemical mechanism of the bioactivities of mangiferin. Indian J.Chem.35 B(1996) 561.

6. Andreu, G.P; Delgado, R et. al. Iron complexing activity of mangiferinh, a naturally occurring glucosyl xannthone,inhibits mitochondrial lipid per oxidation induced by Fe(2+)-citrate. Eur. J. Pharmacol, 513(2005)47.
7. Prabhu, S; Jainu, M; Sabitha, K.E and Shyamala Devi, C.S. Cardioprotective effect of mangiferin on isoproterenol induced myocardial infarction in rats. Indian Jour. Exp. Biol. 44(2006) 209.
8. Senthil Kumar, H; Anandan, R. et. al. Cardioprotective effects of Picrorrhizia kurrora against isoproterenol induced myocardial stress in rats. Fitotherapia . 72(2001) 402.
9. Pauletti, P.M; Castro-Gamboa, I. et. al. New antioxidant C-glucosyl xanthones from the stems of Arrabidaea samydoides. J. Nat.Prod. 10(2003)1284.
10. Muruganandan, S; Gupta, S. et. al. Mangiferin protects the streptozotocin –induced oxidative damage to cardiac and renal tissues in rats. Toxicology. 176(2002)165.
11. He, Q; Xu, S and Peng, B. Mechanism of Cascora lucidissama xanthones against arrhythmia induced by myocardial ischemia – reperfusion in rata. China J. Chin Mater Med. 23(1998)556.

Asafoetida Has Similar Effects to that of Alliums as It Contains many Polysulfides.

Health Benefits of Asafoetida

Jeena Antony, SHS. Kannur university.

Asafoetida, one of the most pungent of all spices, is obtained from the rhizomes and roots of the shrub Ferula assa-foetida (Apiaceae) native to the South West Asian region. It is rich in Oleo-gum-resin made up of 6-17 % volatile oils, 40-64 % resin and 7-25 % gum. The volatile oil contains disulfide compounds similar to those in garlic. The resin consists of farnesiferols-sesquiterpenoid coumarins-along with ferulic acid and asaresin –atannols[1]. Asafoetida is an essential component of a vegetable curry preparation called Samber daily used by South Indians. It mainly contains drum sticks, potato, urad dhal,tomatoe, ladies finger and asafetida. Bordia and Arora[2] studied the ameliorating effects of the volatile oil of asafeotida on alimentary lipemia. These results warrant further research on this spice for evaluating its therapeutic effects for preventing diseases like CVD.

References

1. Bradley, P.R(ed)1992. British Herbal Compendium, Vol, British Herbal Medicine Association Bournemouth.
2. Effect of essential oil (active principle of asafetida) on alimentary lipemia. Bordia, A and Arora, SK. Ind J Med Res. 63(1975) 707-711.

10.4 Medicinal values of Moringa Oleifera

K Sumesh and K V Sreejith,
Dept of Medical Microbiology, SHS, Kannur University, Thalassery Campus

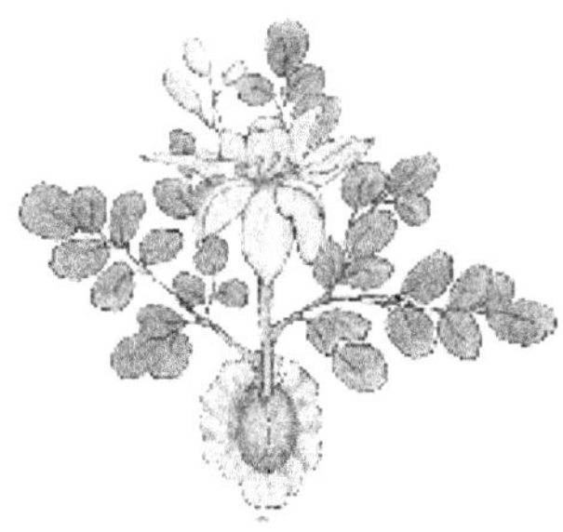

Moringa is a food, with amazing healing properties. Moringa is one of the most powerful health-enhancing plants. India's ancient tradition of ayurveda medicine sites 300 diseases that are treated with the leaves of the Moringa tree. Recent scientific research has proven that these humble leaves are in fact a powerhouse of nutritional value

The Miracle of Moringa Tree Leaves (Moringa Oleifera), commonly called the 'drumstick tree", and 'horseradish tree' is native to India but has been planted around the world and is naturalized in many locales[1].

Moringa nutritional uses

Almost every part of the plant is of value for food. Seed is said to be eaten like a peanut in Malaya. Thickened root used as substitute for horseradish. Foliage eaten as greens, in salads, in vegetable curries, as pickles and for seasoning.

Folk Medicine

According to Hartwell (1967–1971), the flowers, leaves, and roots are used in folk remedies for tumors[2], the seed for abdominal tumors. The root decoction is used in Nicaragua for dropsy. Root juice is applied externally as rubefacient or counter-irritant. Leaves applied as poultice to sores, rubbed on the temples for headaches, and said to have purgative properties.

Bark, leaves and roots are acrid and pungent, and are taken to promote digestion.

Chemistry

Per 100 g, the pod is reported to contain 86.9 g H_2O, 2.5 g protein, 0.1 g fat, 8.5 g total carbohydrate, 4.8 g fiber, 2.0 g ash, 30 mg Ca, 110 mg P, 5.3 mg Fe, 184 IU vit. A, 0.2 mg niacin, and 120 mg ascorbic acid, 310 μg Cu, 1.8 μg I. Leaves contain 7.5 g H_2O, 6.7 g protein, 1.7 g fat, 14.3 g total carbohydrate, 0.9 g fiber, 2.3 g ash, 440 mg Ca, 70 mg P, 7 mg Fe, 110 μg Cu, 5.1 μg I, 11,300 IU vit. A, 120 μg vit. B, 0.8 mg nicotinic acid, 220 mg ascorbic acid, and 7.4 mg tocopherol per 100 g. Estrogenic substances, including the anti-tumor compound, β-sitosterol, and a pectinesterase are also reported. Leaf amino acids include 6.0 g arginine, 2.1 histidine, 4.3 lysine, 1.9 tryptophane, 6.4 phenylalanine, 2.0 methionine, 4.9 threonine, 9.3 lucine, 6.3 isoleucine, and 7.1 valine/16 gN. Pod amino acids include 3.6 g arginine, 1.1 g histidine, 1.5 g lysine, 0.8 g tryptophane, 4.3 g phenylalanine, 1.4 g methionine, 3.9 g threonine, 6.5 g leucine, 4.4 g isoleucine, and 5.4g valine/16 gN. Therefore the protein is biologically rich. Seed kernel (70–74% of seed) contains 4.08 H_2O, 38.4 g crude protein, 34.7% fatty oil, 16.4 g N free extract, 3.5 g fiber, and 3.2 g ash. The seed oil contains 9.3% palmitic, 7.4% stearic, 8.6% behenic, and 65.7% oleic acids among the fatty acids. Myristic and lignoceric acids have also been reported[3]. The cake left after oil extraction contains 58.9% crude protein, 0.4% Cao, 1.1% P_2O_5 and 0.8% K_2O. Pterygospermin, a bactericidal and fungicidal compound, isolated from Moringa has an LD_{50} subcutaneously injected in mice and rats of 350 to 400 mg/kg body weight. Root-bark yields two alkaloids: moringine and moringinine. Moringinine acts as cardiac stimulant, produces rise of blood-pressure, acts on sympathetic nerve-endings as well as smooth muscles all over the body, and depresses the sympathetic motor fibers of vessels in large doses only.

Other uses : The roots are acrid, digestive, anthelmentic, constipating, anodyne, bitter alexipharmic stimulant and vesicant. They are useful in paralysis, inflammations, fever, cough, cold, bronchitis, pectoral diseases, epilepsy, hysteria. Its leaves are useful in scurvy, vitiated conditions of kapha and vata. The seeds are acrid, bitter, anti inflammatory, purgative, and are useful in neuralgia, inflammations and intermittent fevers.

The immature green pods, called "drumsticks" are probably the most valued and widely used part of the tree. They are commonly consumed in India, and are generally prepared in a similar fashion to green beans and have a slight asparagus taste. The seeds are sometimes removed from more mature pods and eaten like peas or roasted like nuts. The flowers are edible when cooked, and are said to taste like mushrooms. The roots are shredded and used as a condiment in the same way as horseradish, however it contains the alkaloid spirochin, a potentially fatal nerve paralyzing agent, so such practices should be strongly discouraged.

The leaves are highly nutritious, being a significant source of beta-carotene, Vitamin C, protein, iron and potassium. The leaves are cooked and used like spinach. In addition to being used fresh as a substitute for spinach, its leaves are commonly dried and crushed into a powder, and used in soups and sauces. Murungakai Tamil as its locally known in Tamil Nadu is used in Siddha medicine. Its leaves are full of medicinal properties. The tree is a good source for calcium and phosphorus. In Siddha medicine, the drumstick seeds are used as a sexual virility drug for treating erectile dysfunction in men and also in women for prolonging sexual activity.

The Moringa seeds yield 38–40% edible oil (called ben oil, from the high concentration of behenic acid contained in the oil) that can be used in cooking, cosmetics, and lubrication. The refined oil is clear, odorless, and resists rancidity at least as well as any other botanical oil. The seed cake remaining after oil extraction may be used as a fertilizer or as a flocculant to purify water.

The bark, sap, roots, leaves, seeds, oil and flowers are used in traditional medicine in several countries. In Jamaica, the sap is used for a blue dye.

The flowers are also cooked and relished as a delicacy in West Bengal and Bangladesh, especially during early spring. There it is called sojne ful and is usually cooked with green peas and potato[3].

Useful against Malnutrition

Interest is growing in the use of moringa in addressing malnutrition in developing areas of the world. Also because of its high vitamin and mineral content, in Africa it has become popular as a locally produced nutritional supplement for individuals infected with the HIV/AIDS virus. It can be grown cheaply and easily, so several governments in Africa have promoted Moringa oleifera as locally produced food beneficial to HIV-positive individuals.

In Kerala, tribals use Moringa leaves to increase breast milk. In addition it has been used successfully to combat malnutrition among infants and women of childbearing age. In Africa, also nursing mothers have been shown to produce far more milk when Moringa leaves have been added to their diet, while severely malnourished children have made significant weight gains when the leaves have been added to their diets. It is commonly added to porridge increase its nutritional content.

One doctor in Senegal (West Africa) explained: "We have always had problems with the classical approach to treating malnourished children. This was based on industrial products: whole milk powder, vegetable oil and sugar. All these things are expensive. When you tell a parent to go out and buy these things—this can be truly costly for him. On the other hand, with Moringa the resource is locally available. The people themselves can produce it. We have done experiments in treating malnourished children with this plant and the results have been really spectacular".

Rajangam et. al.[4] Report that India is the largest producer of Moringa trees

The moringa pod is known as drumstick or saragwa or saragwe in India. In South India[5], it is used to prepare a variety of sambar and is also fried. It is also preserved by canning and exported worldwide. In other parts of India, especially West Bengal and also in a neighboring country like Bangladesh it is enjoyed very much. It can be made into varieties of curry by mixing with coconut, poppy seeds and mustard. It can just be boiled, until the drumsticks are semi-soft and consumed directly without any extra processing or cooking. It is used in curries, sambars, kormas, and dals, although it is also used to add flavor to cutlets, etc.

Tender drumstick leaves, finely chopped, make an excellent garnish for any vegetable dishes, dals, sambars, salads, etc. One can use the same in place of or with coriander, as these leaves have high medicinal value..

Philippines

In the Philippines, the leaves are widely eaten[6]. Bunches of leaves are available in many markets, priced below many other leaf vegetables. The leaves are most often added to a broth to make a simple, and highly nutritious soup.

On September 14, 2007, Loren Legarda campaigned for the popularization of moringa, after a recent scientific report that it boosts male potency. She asked the government to make moringa among its priority crops for propagation. Research at the Bureau of Plant Industry (BPI) found that a steady consumption of its fruit increases sperm count: "helps to raise sperm count and mobility, which both translate to increased opportunity for the sperm to fertilize an egg". It is also rich in vitamins C and A, iron, and high density lipoprotein (HDL) or good cholesterol. The BPI report stated that, weight per weight, moringa leaves have the calcium equivalent of 4 glasses of milk, the vitamin C content of 7 oranges, potassium of 3 bananas, 3 times the iron of spinach, 4 times the amount of vitamin A in carrots, and 2 times the protein in milk. Moringa also helps to purify water, a cheaper alternative to mechanical filtration[7,8].

References

1. Duke, J.A. 1978. The quest for tolerant germplasm. p. 1–61. In: ASA Special Symposium 32, Crop tolerance to suboptimal land conditions. Am. Soc. Agron. Madison, WI.
2. Hartwell, J.L. 1967–1971. Plants used against cancer. A survey. Lloydia 30–34.
3. Verma, S.C., Banerji, R., Misra, G., Nigam, S.K. 1976. Nutritional value of moringa. Current Sci. 45(21):769–770.
4. Rajangam J., et. al. Status of Production and Utilisation of Moringa in Southern India. In "Development potential for Moringa products", October 29th - November 2nd, 2001, Dar es Salaam, Tanzania
5. Food and Agriculture Organization of the United Nations, The Vegetable Sector in Thailand, 1999
6. Food and Agriculture Organization of the United Nations, Country Pasture/Forage Resource Profiles: Philippines
7. Inquirer.net, Legarda pushes for malunggay, her beauty soup
8. AHN, Philippine Lawmaker Urges Agriculture Department To Propagate Highly Potent Malunggay Vegetable

For more details refer Wikipedia, the free Encyclopedia.

Phytochemicals Additional Informations

Ajoene

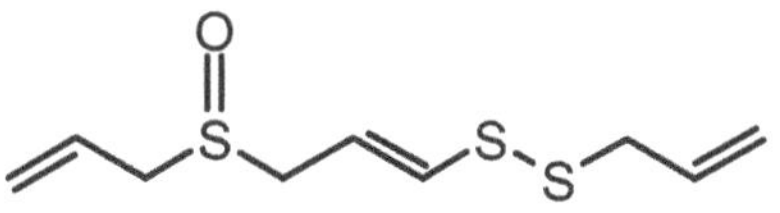

Mohind. C. Mohan, Nufaila, K.M, Sangeetha, R and Shimya vasu. SHS. Kannur University.

Source; Garlic (*Allium sativum*)

Uses ; It functions as an antioxidant, by inhibiting the release of superoxide. Ajoene also has antithrombotic (anti-clotting) properties, which helps prevent platelets in the blood from forming blood clots, potentially reducing the risk of heart disease and stroke in humans. Ajoene is also known to have effective broad-spectrum antimicrobial (antibacterial and antifungal) properties, helpful in preventing yeast infection (*Candida albicans*) and treating athlete's foot (*tinea pedis*), for example. Ajoene has even been shown effective in inhibiting tumor cell growth by targeting the microtubule cytoskeleton of such cells.

Allicin

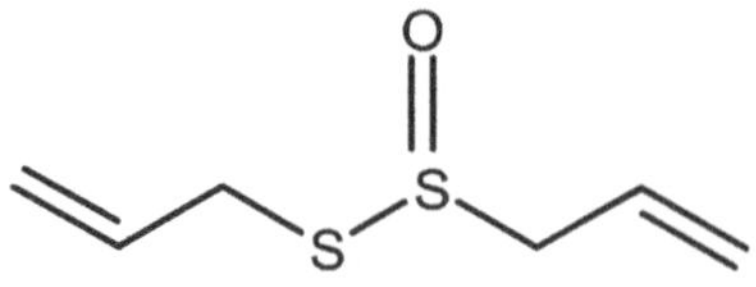

Source; Garlic (*Allium sativum*)

Uses: it helps fighting arteriosclerosis, it has the ability to dissolve fats and it can also be used as an antioxidant to some extent

Quercetin

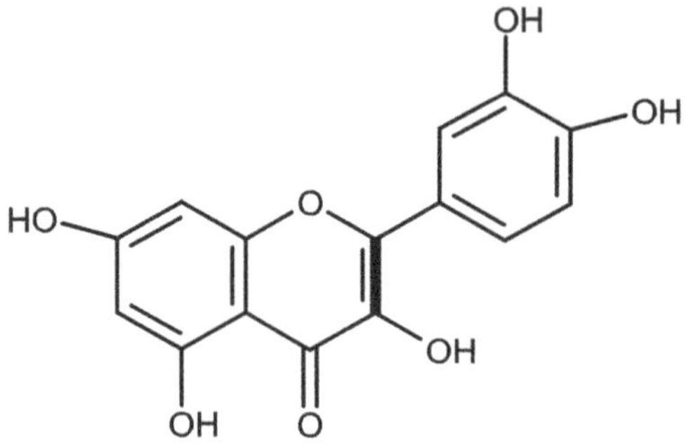

Sources; apples, black & green tea, onions, red wine, red grapes, citrus fruits, broccoli & other leafy green vegetables, cherries, and a number of berries including raspberry, bog whortleberry, lingonberry, cranberry, chokeberry (sweet rowan (85 mg/kg), rowanberry (63 mg/kg), sea buckthorn berry (62 mg/kg), crowberry (53 and 56 mg/kg)[1], and the fruit of the prickly pear cactus. A study by the University of Queensland, Australia, has also indicated the presence of quercetin in varieties of honey, including honey derived from eucalyptus and tea tree flowers.

Quercetin may have positive effects in combating or helping to prevent cancer, prostatitis, heart disease, cataracts, allergies/inflammations, and respiratory diseases such as bronchitis and asthma.

Phytosterols

1. **Beta-sitosterol**

   Sources : Serenoarepens (saw palmetto), Pygeum africanum, rice bran, wheat germ, corn oils, Pumpkin seed and soybeans.

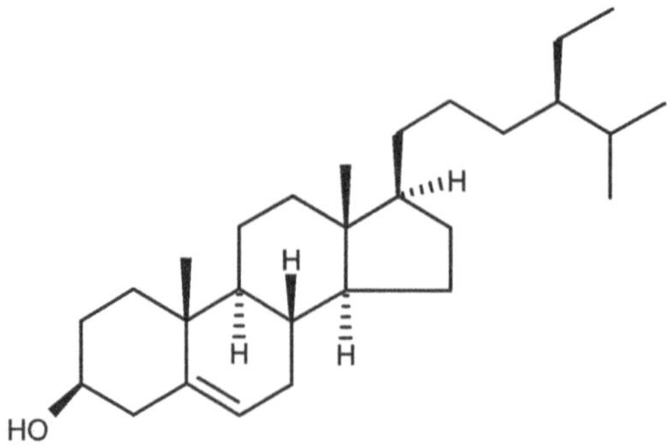

uses: β-sitosterol reduces blood levels of cholesterol. There is some belief that it plays some role in the possible benefits of herbal therapy of benign prostatic hypertrophy (BPH). β-sitosterol itself is used as a medicine in Europe for BPH.

β-sitosterol

2. Ergosterol

Sources ; Shiitake mushrooms. Biological precursor to Vitamin D_2.

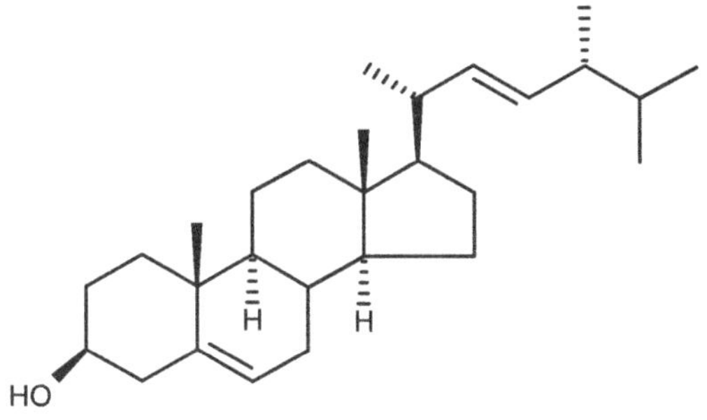

Uses : antifungal drugs. Ergosterol is also used as fluidiers in the cell membranes of some protists, such as trypanosomes. This explains the use of some antifungals against West African sleeping sickness.

Ergosterol

3. Brassicasterol

Sources; unicellular algae (phytoplankton) and some terrestrial plants *e.g.* oil seed rape. Use. Hypocholesteralemic agent.

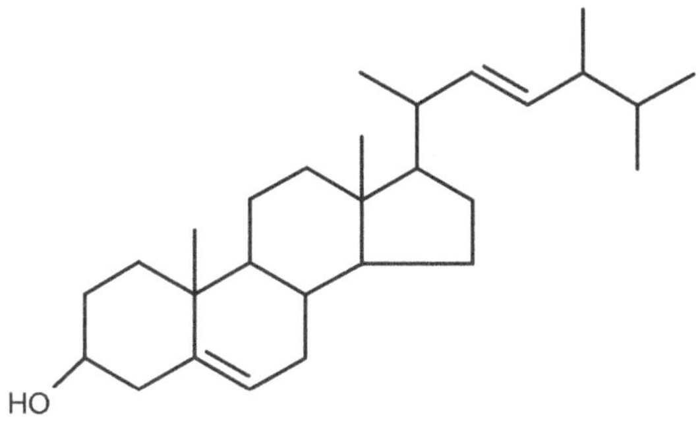

Carotenoids

β-Carotene

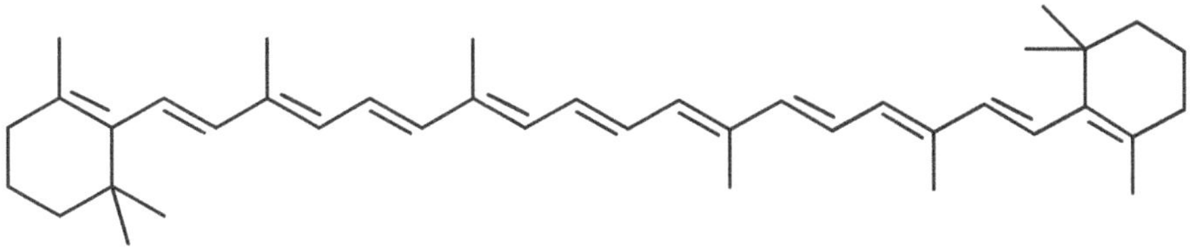

Sources : β-Carotene is the more common form and can be found in yellow, orange, and green leafy fruits and vegetables. These can be carrots, spinach, lettuce, tomatoes, sweet potatoes, broccoli, cantaloupe, oranges, and winter squash. As a rule of thumb, the greater the intensity of the color of the fruit or vegetable, the more β-carotene it contains.

Uses : β-Carotene is an anti-oxidant and as such can be useful for curbing the excess of damaging free radicals in the body. However, the usefulness of β-carotene as a dietary supplement (i.e. taken as a pill) is still subject to debate. β-Carotene is fat-soluble and a precursor of vitamin A

THIOLS

Dithiothreitol(DTT) is a reducing agent and it is frequently used to reduce the disulfide bonds of .proteins and more frequently to prevent intramolecular and intermolecular disulfide bonds from forming between cysteine residues of proteins.

Grapefruit mercaptan

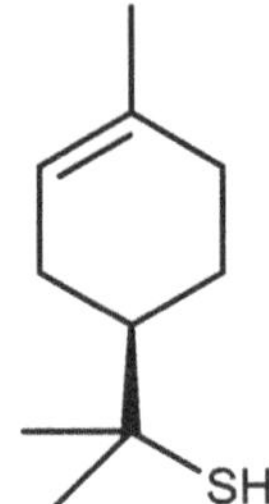

Uses : Pure grapefruit mercaptan, or citrus-derived oils rich in grapefruit mercaptan,are some times used in perfumary and the flavour industry to impart citrus aromas and flavors.

Terpenes

Limonene

Sources: Citrus fruits, black pepper.

Uses: It is present in citrus fruits and black pepper as a useful antioxidant. Therefore limes, limons, oranges and grape fruit work as functional foods. Limonene is increasingly being used as an environmentally friendly alternative to mineral oils as a solvent for cleaning purposes, such as the removal of oil from machine parts, being more easily biodegradable than mineral oils, and produced from a renewable source (citrus oil, as a byproduct of orange juice manufacture). Limonene works as paint stripper when applied to painted wood. The (*R*)-enantiomer is also used as botanical insecticide.

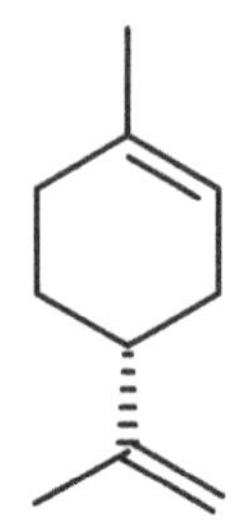

Limnoids induce activity of the detoxifying enzyme ghtathione. S traferase. Hence they are good nutraceuticals.

Cembrene,

Uses : **Cembrene**, or sometimes neocembrene, is a natural monocyclic diterpene. It is a colorless oil with a faint wax-like odor.

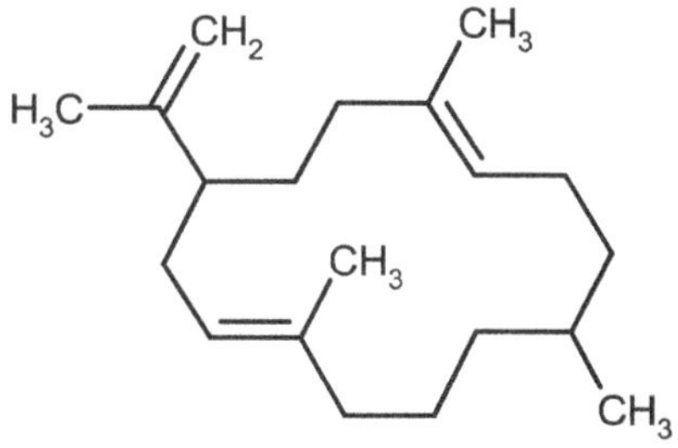

Cembrene itself has little importance as chemical entity, being a trail pheromone for termites; however, the chemical structure of cembrene is central to a very wide variety of other natural products found both in plants and in animals.

Phytosterols (See the structures given in 48-49

These are plant derived sterols and stanols which are mainly divided into three classes. They are (1) Isoflavonoids. (2) Coumestans (Saturated steroids with a methyl group on carbon 24) and (3) Lignans (Phenyl polymers) with variuos nutraceutical effects.

1. Isoflavonoids

The main isoflavones are genistein, diadzein & glycitein present in soybeans and its products.

2. Coumestans

The most common coumestans is coumesterol. Sprouts including mung bean, soybean & alfalfa sprouts are richest sources of coumesterol.

3. Lignan Precursors (They are bound forms of phytosterols)

Lignan precursors, secoisolariciresinol and matairesinol are ubiquetous in plant food. The sources are grains, cerials, oilseeds, nuts, berries, fruits, vegetables, tea, coffee & wine.

Functions:

- Phytosterols inhibit intestinal absorption of cholesterol.
- It lowers serum LDL cholesterol.
- Phytosterols are associated with decreased cancer risk.
- Low doses can improve urinary tract symptoms related to benign prostatic hyperpalsia.

10.5 An Apple A Day prevents Brain-Cell damage

Lalbin. S,
Dept. Medical Biochemitry, Kannur University Campus at Thalassery.

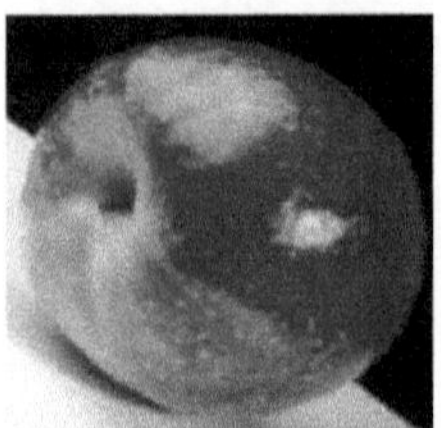

An apple may supply major bioactive compounds, which reduce the risk of neuro-degenerative disorders. Various studies show that the chemical quercetin, a so called phytonutrient (Nutraceutical) appears to be largely responsible for protecting rat brain cells when assaulted by oxidative stress in laboratory tests.

Phytonutrients

These compounds such as phenolic acids, and flavanoids, protect the apple against bacteria, viruses and fungi and provide the fruit's anti-oxidant and anti-cancer benefits. This group of chemicals found in apples, onions, berries etc., could protect the brain from the type of damage that triggers such neurodegenerative diseases as Alzheimer's and Parkinsonism, according to two new studies from Cornell University food chemists.

Quercetin is a major flavanoid found in apples. Antioxidants help prevent cancer cell-damaging free radicals and inhibiting the production of reactive substances such as hydroxy radicals that could damage normal cells. The studies show that additional apple consumption not only may help reduce the risk of cancer, as previous studies have shown, but also that an apple a day may supply major bioactive compounds, which may play an important role in reducing the risk of neurodegenerative disorders says, Chang, Y. Cy Lee, Professor of food science at Cornell University's New York State Agricultural Experiment station in Geneva, N.Y. In a study published in the Journal of Food Science (2004) Lee et. al. compared how two groups of rat neuronal cells fared against hydrogen peroxide, a common oxidative stressor. Only one of the group was pretreated with different concentrations of apple phenolic extracts. The researchers found that the higher the concentration of apple extract, the greater the protection was for the nerve cells against oxidative stress. What they found was that the apple phenolics found in fresh apples can protect nerve cells from neurotoxicity induced by oxidative stress.

Main Agent

When Lee et. al. looked at quercetin they found that it appeared to be the main agent responsible for the beneficial effect. In fact quercetin worked better in protecting nerve cells against oxidative stress than vitamin C a naturally occurring antioxidant known to help prevent cell and tissue damage from oxidation. Hence not only apple, even our cashew fruit (Indian apple), all colored fruits, e.g. berries and even onions can protect our body from all types of oxidative damages, as they contain flavonoids related to quercetin.

10.6 A Good News about Vanilla as an agent for Relaxation and Weight Reduction

Deepa. P. Mohan & Fathimath Safoora,
SHS, Thalassery campus of Kannur University.

Vanilla, a flavoring substance derived from orchids is considered a strong aphrodisiac and has been used medicinally time and again, to calm an uneasy stomach or treat respiratory disorders. Vanilla has also wide spread use in aroma therapy, for being soothing to the nervous system and mind. More recently, however research has shown that some vanilla compounds have strong properties that can prevent cancer and work at a deep level to reverse early cancer through a mechanism of DNA strand repair as reported in the New Sunday Express on 20th May 2007.

Though the predominant compound responsible for the flavor and smell of vanilla is vanillin, a minor component of the essential oil is piperanol (Heliotropin) which also affects the odor of vanilla. In 1991, the Sloan-Kettering cancer center in New York announced that heliotropin present in vanilla was the most relaxing and pleasant of the five fragrances tested for reduction of anxiety during a difficult medical procedure.

In a study, 85 patients who went through Magnetic Resonance Imaging (MRI) scan were exposed to heliotropin fragrance. Patients were asked to sit in motionless for up to an hour for the MRI and anxiety is the most common reason for them to terminate the scan midway. In the study, patients experienced 63 % less anxiety than those who were not given the fragrance during the scan. Dr. Sakshi Chawla, senior dietician, Fortis, Noida ascribes the medicinal properties of vanilla e.g. prevention of cancer to its antioxidants. According to her if vanilla essence is mixed in a cold drink, it helps in neutralizing the acidity in the stomach. A recent study at the St. George Hospital in London indicates that vanilla may help people lose weight.

Another study at Tubingen Univerity in Germany showed that vanilla frgrance reduced the startle reflux in humans and animals. Various studies have confirmed that vanillin can restore appetite in dogs after surgery and encourage calmness and raise the appetite of pigs.

10.7 Garlic Protein is as good as Soy Protein to prevent Diseases

Dr. C.R. Rajasree

Research Fellow Dept. of Biochemistry, University of Kerala. Kariavattom, TVM.

Nitha Pavithran,

Former student of Medical Biochemistry, SHS, Thalassery Campus of Kannur University.

Biju, Daniel and Augusti[1] reported that the composition of garlic protein (GP) is almost similar to that of soy protein (SP) and that on incorporation of 16 % of the former in the diet of rats lowered the lipid profile in hypercholesterolemic rats to a significant level. Sakono, Yoshida et. al.[2] reported on the hypolipidemic effects of soy protein in rats maintained on high fat diet. Senior author under the supervision of Augusti[3] showed the atherogenic activity of coconut oil, sun flower oil and dalda in the order **CNO > Dalda > SFO**.

Amino acid contents in garlic and soy proteins are closely related as given below. Sulfur aminoacids viz; Cysteine, cystine and methionine are three fold in GP over SP. Histidine, Phe. alanine, isoleucine, threonine etc., are also more in GP than in SP. These proteins have a comparable composition with that of casein. Simultaneous feeding of 500 mg / kg/day of GP for three months to rats fed a diet containing 15% edible fats i.e. CNO, Dalda or SFO for the same period, decreased significantly cholesterol, TAG and PL in serum and tissues. Dalda is a hydrogenated oil. GP also decreased the activity of liver HMGCo A reductase (regulatory enzyme for cholesterol synthesis) and increased the level of HDL chol. with a concomitant decrease in LDL and VLDL chol. levels. This is an antiatherogenic effect of GP.

According to previous reports most of the unsaturated fats as compared to saturated fats on feeding to rats showed higher fecal sterols and bile acid excretions. Srikantiah and Gopalan[4] and Nath and Brahmachari[5], reported on an increased excretion of bile salts in human subjects receiving unsaturated fats. Unsaturated fats promote intestinal growth of microorganism which increases conversion of cholesterol to beta cholestanol and coprostanol and that is very pertinent in the light of the results. A study on the effects of GP in a diet containing saturated oils showed similar effects as that of soy protein especially in lowering hepatic level of TAG. Therefore GP and SP with similar medicinal effects are good as functional foods to prevent heart diseases [3,4].

An American Heart Assoc. Review (2006) states that soy products may be beneficial to heart only because of their high content of PUFA, fiber and vitamins and not due to isoflavones and such other compounds (The last mentioned items are good to prevent breast cancer). This means that less content of SAFs and high fiber in soy products may add to the merits of tofu, soy butter, soy nuts and burgers. Hirao's team[6] reported on the immunoboosting effect of a small MW protein of garlic. Therefore garlic and soy products rank among first class functional foods.

References

1. Biju. C. Mathew; Daniel. R.S. and Augusti, K.T. Hypolipidemic effect of garlic protein substituted for casein in diet of rats compared to those of garlic oil. Ind. Jour. Exp. Biol. 34(1996)337-340.
2. Sakono, M Yoshida, K; Yahiro, M. J. Nutr. Sci & Vit. 39(1993)335.
3. Rajasree, C.R. Biochemical Effects of garlic protein on alcohol fed and oil fed rats. Ph.D. Thesis submitted to University of Kerala, 1998 and Degree was awarded. Pp, 91-112.
4. Srikantiah, S.C and Gopalan, C. Indian J. Med. Res. 48 91960)503.
5. Nath, C and Brahmachari, D.M. Proc. Exptl. Biol. Med. 108(1961) 337.
6. Hirao, Y. Sumioka, I, et. al. Activation of Immunoresponder cells by the protein fraction from aged garlic extract. Phytotherapy Research, 1(1987)161-164.

Index

A

B

C

D

E

F

G

H

I

K

L

M

N

O

S

T

V

W

X

Y

Z

www.ingramcontent.com/pod-product-compliance
Ingram Content Group UK Ltd.
Pitfield, Milton Keynes, MK11 3LW, UK
UKHW021326190726
13845UKWH00003B/50

9 789352 300617